Katzenstein and Askin's Surgical Pathology of
Non-Neoplastic Lung Disease

Fourth edition

Dedication

To my family
Michael, Tom and Kristen Mazur,

and to the memory of my parents,

Hildegarde Arnold MD (1906–1994)
and
Rolf Ewald Katzenstein MD (1909-1975)

Commissioning Editor: Michael J. Houston
Development Editor: Sheila Black
Editorial Assistant: Liz Brown
Project Manager: Glenys Norquay
Design Manager: Erik Bigland
Illustration Manager: Bruce Hogarth
Illustrator: Hardlines Studios
Marketing Managers: Leontine Treur (UK/NL), Lisa Damico (USA)

MPP

13

Anna-Luise A. Katzenstein MD

Professor and Vice Chairman of Pathology
Director, Anatomic Pathology
SUNY Upstate Medical University
Syracuse, New York
USA

Katzenstein and Askin's Surgical Pathology of
Non-Neoplastic Lung Disease

MAJOR PROBLEMS IN PATHOLOGY

FOURTH EDITION

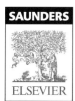

SAUNDERS

ELSEVIER

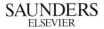

SAUNDERS
ELSEVIER

Saunders is an affiliate of Elsevier Inc.

First edition 1982
Second edition 1990
Third edition 1997

© 2006, Elsevier Inc. All rights reserved.

ISBN-13: 978-0-7216-0041-3
ISBN-10: 0-7216-0041-7

British Library Cataloguing in Publication Data
A catalogue record for this book is available from the British Library

Library of Congress Cataloging in Publication Data
A catalog record for this book is available from the Library of
Congress

Notice
Medical knowledge is constantly changing. Standard safety
precautions must be followed, but as new research and clinical
experience broaden our knowledge, changes in treatment and drug
therapy may become necessary or appropriate. Readers are advised
to check the most current product information provided by the
manufacturer of each drug to be administered to verify the
recommended dose, the method and duration of administration, and
contraindications. It is the responsibility of the practitioner, relying
on experience and knowledge of the patient, to determine dosages
and the best treatment for each individual patient. Neither the
Publisher nor the author assumes any liability for any injury and/or
damage to persons or property arising from this publication.
The Publisher

Printed in China

Last digit is the print number: 9 8 7 6 5 4 3 2 1

Contents

Preface

It does not seem possible that over two decades have passed since the first edition of *Surgical Pathology of Non-Neoplastic Lung Disease* was published in 1982. There have been many changes over these years not only in pulmonary pathology, but also in supporting ancillary services. For example, computers were not widely used for word processing until the mid 1980's, and therefore the first edition was entirely produced with a typewriter. Revisions for the second edition were hand-written on actual book pages that were pasted onto larger blank paper leaving room for changes, and some parts were completely retyped. "Cut" and "paste" were literally done with scissors and tape. Currently, all aspects are computerized, including both text and figures, and the final copy is submitted on discs. Photomicrographs and other pictures in earlier editions, of course, were all in black and white. When I first discussed a 4th edition with the editor in 2000 I was told that color was not possible except for a few color plates, but by mid 2002 the publisher asked that all photographs be submitted in color.

Many concepts in pulmonary pathology have changed over the years and others continue to evolve, especially in the areas of interstitial pneumonia and lymphoproliferative disease. As in other disciplines, immunohistochemistry has largely replaced electron microscopy in evaluating most diseases. Nomenclature has also changed, but rather than becoming simpler, it is often more complicated with complex and intricate classification schemes that are difficult even for the experts to follow. There has also been an explosion of new articles in the literature, and they are so numerous that it is difficult just to read them all, and nearly impossible to critically evaluate them. Despite these issues, and also because of them, I have attempted to maintain the aim of the first edition which was to provide a practical guide for the general surgical pathologist in interpreting non-neoplastic lung biopsy specimens. A generous bibliography is also provided so that the reader can obtain more in depth details if desired. Hopefully, the information furnished will be sufficient to enable general surgical pathologists to diagnose the majority of non-neoplastic lung diseases without the need for an "expert" opinion.

Anna-Luise A. Katzenstein
2006

Acknowledgements

Dr Ola El-Zammar, previously a Pulmonary Pathology fellow with me and currently an Assistant Professor at SUNY Upstate Medical University, extensively researched recent articles on drug toxicity and updated the chapter on drug induced lung disease, which is co-authored with Dr Jeffrey Myers, the A. James French Endowed Professor of Diagnostic Pathology, and Director of Anatomic Pathology at the University of Michigan Medical School, Ann Arbor, Michigan. Dr Myers additionally contributed several color photographs of rare diseases. Dr Frederic Askin, Professor of Pathology at Johns Hopkins School of Medicine in Baltimore was supportive, as always, and he provided a number of photographs of pediatric lung diseases.

As in the previous edition, I am indebted to Cheryl Dickinson who single-handedly typed (and retyped) the many changes and corrections, and completed all this work in her home after normal working hours. As I review some of my scribbles, circles, arrows, and notes, I still cannot help but wonder how she managed to interpret them and flawlessly arrange them in the text. Deborah Rexine in the Medical Photography Department tirelessly scanned in hundreds of projection slides for the new color photographs, and she spent countless hours arranging them, cataloging them, and making necessary changes. My children, Tom and Kristen Mazur, enthusiastically contributed (for a small fee, of course) by renumbering all the many references both in the bibliography and in the text. I would also like to thank the Elsevier staff, especially Michael Houston, Sheila Black and Glenys Norquay, who were extremely helpful and supportive.

HANDLING AND INTERPRETATION OF LUNG BIOPSIES

A variety of methods have been described to obtain lung tissue for diagnostic purposes.[41] They range from formal thoracotomy and open lung biopsy[8,18,36,42,44] to less invasive endoscopic[2,3,6,17,34,38] or percutaneous[5,12,46] techniques. Although mortality is low with all methods, complications and morbidity differ for each, and their usefulness will vary depending on the clinical situation.

OPEN LUNG BIOPSY AND THORACOSCOPIC LUNG BIOPSY

Open lung biopsy traditionally has been the standard technique for obtaining lung tissue when other less invasive techniques have failed to produce a diagnosis.[7,8,13,18,28,36,44,48] Video-assisted thoracoscopic surgery (VATS) is a less invasive technique that currently is used more often.[1,4,13,14,25,29,30,48] It supplies equivalent tissue to formal thoracotomy specimens, and the diagnostic yield is similar.[4,25] The advantages include less patient morbidity and shorter hospital stays.[4,16] Both procedures also usually provide sufficient tissue for a variety of studies in addition to routine hematoxylin and eosin (H and E)-stained sections.

Site for Biopsy

The site for taking a lung biopsy will vary depending on the nature and distribution of the underlying lung disease. For patients with diffuse lung disease, especially diffuse interstitial lung disease, the best approach is to sample *moderately abnormal* parenchyma while avoiding areas of end-stage scarring or honeycomb change.[8] The chest radiograph and computed tomography (CT) examination can be useful guides for identifying an appropriate site.[35] The presence of ground glass attenuation in CT studies appears to indicate foci of active inflammation. Although the lingula has traditionally been considered inappropriate for biopsy, evidence suggests that it is the tip of any lobe rather than the lingula specifically that should be avoided.[22,31,33,47] The surgeon, therefore, should be advised to avoid the scarred tips of any lobe and to attempt to biopsy deeper portions of lung. Taking biopsies from multiple lobes is important to adequately sample cases of diffuse interstitial lung disease.

The approach is slightly different in patients with localized or patchy lung disease, since the most abnormal zones of the lung (rather than intermediate or moderately involved areas) should be sampled in these cases. Although it may be helpful to biopsy the interface with normal lung, it is more important that representative areas of active disease be adequately sampled. When patients have nodular densities, the surgeon should be encouraged to remove an entire nodule, if possible, rather than attempting to biopsy a small piece from the edge.

Handling of Open Lung Biopsy or Thoracoscopic Biopsy Specimens

All biopsy specimens should be routinely cultured for bacteria, fungi, and acid-fast bacilli, and this function can be accomplished by the surgeon in the operating room. Viral cultures can also be taken in selected cases. Once cultures have been performed, the specimen can either be placed in formalin or sent unfixed to the pathology laboratory for frozen section. In either case, care should be taken to handle the tissue gently to avoid artifactual collapse. Before sectioning, the staple line should be removed by cutting along the lung surface adjacent to the staples with small scissors. A new sharp scalpel or razor blade should be used to serially section the specimen perpendicular to the long axis using a gentle sawing motion. The sectioning should always begin at the lung margin and proceed toward the pleural surface. Since the pleura is firmer than the underlying lung, beginning the sectioning at the lung rather than the pleural surface will produce less atelectasis. A technique for inflating the specimens with formalin or other fixative by means of a small syringe has been described.[9,21] In our experience, this procedure is not necessary if specimens are carefully handled. Also, it is associated with its own artifacts, including overexpansion of airspaces and dilatation of lymphatic spaces.

Frozen Sections

Although not mandatory, frozen section can provide useful information (Table 1–1). First, and most important

Table 1–1   Role of Frozen Section in Lung Biopsy
I. Diagnosis (especially in acutely ill patients)
II. Determining the need and saving tissue for additional studies such as: Immunofluorescence in alveolar hemorrhage syndromes (snap-frozen aliquot) Flow cytometry (fresh tissue), and B-5 fixation in lymphoid lesions Analytic techniques in suspected pneumoconiosis (either snap-frozen aliquot or in formalin)
III. Assessing adequacy of the biopsy specimen

for acutely ill patients, a specific diagnosis may be determined within minutes of biopsy. Immunocompromised patients are especially prone to develop acute pneumonic processes that rapidly progress to involve both lungs. These patients are usually desperately ill, and lung biopsy is undertaken in hopes of finding a treatable disease, particularly an infection. Routine stains for infectious organisms can be done on frozen sections, and rapid-acting stains for *Pneumocystis carinii* and fungi are also available (see Chapter 10). The diagnosis of infection can thus be made quickly for prompt institution of therapy. Similarly, if recurrent malignancy or evidence of drug toxicity is seen on frozen section, other more appropriate therapy can be initiated. Frozen sections are equally important for quickly providing a diagnosis in immunologically intact patients who are acutely ill. Goodpasture's syndrome, eosinophilic pneumonia, Wegener's granulomatosis, and infections such as Legionnaire's disease and miliary tuberculosis are but a few examples of diseases that may require immediate therapy. Frozen sections can also be used to assess the need for special stains, which can be cut and stained along with the routine sections the next day. Thus, organism stains can be ordered if infection is suspected, immunohistochemical stains for a possible carcinoma or lymphoma, and so forth.

Another use for frozen section is to assess the need for other more sophisticated diagnostic techniques. For example, if intraalveolar hemorrhage suggestive of Goodpasture's syndrome or another alveolar hemorrhage syndrome is found, a piece of lung can be snap-frozen in liquid nitrogen for immunofluorescence studies. If a lymphoid infiltrate is found, an additional fixative such as B-5 may be chosen, and fresh tissue can be sent for flow cytometry. If the biopsy suggests an occupational lung disease, part of the specimen may be stored for tissue analysis.

A final important role for frozen section is to assess the adequacy of the tissue obtained and to determine whether or not it is representative of the disease process. This function is especially important when the process in the lung is patchy or focal, but it can be difficult and requires prior communication with the surgeon and knowledge of the clinical and radiographic findings. In such cases, the pathologist should assess whether the frozen section findings correlate with the clinical and radiographic manifestations, and, if not, additional tissue can be requested. It is also important in diffuse interstitial lung diseases where areas of nondiagnostic, end-stage, honeycomb lung are sometimes biopsied. If honeycomb lung is the only finding on a frozen section, the surgeon should be advised to obtain additional (preferably deeper) tissue for diagnosis.

Other Studies

An important role for the surgical pathologist at the time of biopsy is to make certain that sufficient tissue is maintained for routine light microscopic examination. Although in the past aliquots were routinely taken for electron microscopy, the advent of immunohisto-chemistry has largely replaced the need for this procedure. Therefore, aliquots need not be saved for electron microscopy unless there is some specific indication (such as a storage disease or unusual infection, for example). Likewise, as mentioned earlier, snap-frozen tissue for immunofluorescence is indicated only if there is clinical (hemoptysis) or morphologic (at frozen section) evidence of an alveolar hemorrhage syndrome. Even when tissue aliquots are indicated for these and other studies as outlined earlier, it should be remembered that the diagnosis will rest in most cases on routine light microscopy, and care should be taken to *keep the majority of the tissue for light microscopy.*

LOBECTOMY/PNEUMONECTOMY SPECIMENS

Occasionally, lobes or even whole lungs may be excised for non-neoplastic diseases. For routine study, the tissue should be inflated through the bronchi with formalin and allowed to fix for 1 to 2 hours. The authors use gravity drainage to fill the lungs. In this technique, a plastic tube is extended from a tank of formalin located 2 to 3 feet above the specimen. The tube is wedged into each major bronchus, and the formalin is allowed to flow until the lung is maximally expanded. The bronchi should not be clamped after inflation. A more precise method of inflation has been described for studying lung volumes and requires the use of a pump that maintains constant infusion pressure at 25 to 30 cm H_2O.[23] This procedure is not necessary, however, for routine cases. Tissue for microbial culture should be taken from these large specimens before fixation. Excision of small peripheral pieces of lung will not significantly interfere with inflation.

In exploring the relationship of lesions to the bronchial tree in lobectomy or pneumonectomy specimens, a dissection technique using intrabronchial probes is helpful. The lobe or lung is first inflated with formalin, as described previously. After fixation for 1 to 2 hours, metal probes are placed in two bronchi that are located in approximately the same plane. The lung is then sectioned by cutting with a long, sharp knife placed at a 45° angle against the probes (Fig. 1–1). In this way, the bronchi are bisected along their length, and the intervening parenchyma is exposed in a flat plane (Fig. 1–2). The process can be repeated by placing the probes in consecutively deeper bronchi until a lesion is identified or all bronchi are opened.

A variety of special techniques are available for demonstrating vascular or bronchial anomalies in unfixed lobectomy or pneumonectomy specimens. Most require specialized equipment and supplies, and are not practical for routine cases.[23,43] Radiopaque material such as micropulverized barium (Micropaque), with or without gelatin filler, can be used to fill vessels. Other injection media such as multicolored silicone rubber (Microfil) or Dow-Corning Silastic rubber may also be useful. Most of these compounds will not interfere with routine sectioning and processing, and the specimen can still be inflated with formalin through the bronchi. Bronchography can also be performed using radiopaque contrast media. For specimens in which the parenchyma can be sacrificed, the vinylite plastic cast technique is an excellent method. For teaching and radiologic correlation, whole-mount giant paper sections, so-called Gough-Wentworth sections, can be useful.

TRANSBRONCHIAL AND PERCUTANEOUS LUNG BIOPSY SPECIMENS

Tissue fragments taken by a less invasive technique, such as bronchoscopy or percutaneous biopsy, are small. Transbronchial biopsy specimens measure 1 to 2 mm in greatest dimension, while percutaneous needle

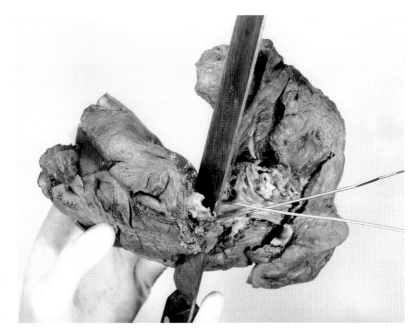

Figure 1–1 Technique for sectioning the lung along the bronchi. Metal probes are placed in two bronchi of a formalin-fixed lung or lobe. The bronchi chosen are those that course in approximately the same plane. The lung is sectioned with a knife angled against the probes.

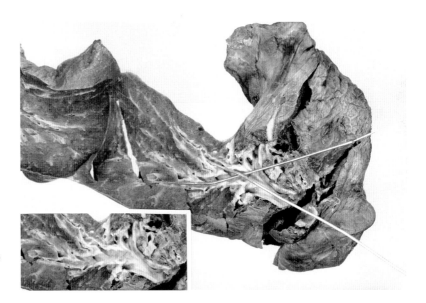

Figure 1–2 Appearance of the lung shown in Figure 1–1 after the bronchi have been bivalved. A portion of the bisected lung has been reflected to the left. *Inset*: Appearance of the bronchi with the probes removed.

biopsies measure 1 to 2 cm in length but less than 1 mm in diameter.[2,3,6,17] The handling of transbronchial lung biopsies is discussed in detail in Chapter 17. In general, such specimens must be placed immediately in formalin by the clinician performing the procedure. The pathologist should retrieve them from the formalin and wrap them in moist lens paper before placing them in a cassette. They should not be placed between sponges since this causes both atelectasis and so-called sponge artifact (irregular geometrically shaped spaces related

to indentation from the sponge). Serial H and E-stained sections should be obtained initially,[32] and special stains can be ordered subsequently if indicated by the clinical history or histologic findings. Although special techniques such as immunofluorescence can be performed in selected cases, we discourage saving fresh tissue for this function in these small biopsy specimens. At the discretion of the bronchoscopist, either bronchial washings or brushings can be sent to the microbiology laboratory for culture or, if indicated, a tissue piece can be sent. Similarly, a fragment of needle biopsy can be sent for culture. The clinician, however, should be advised to save as much of the specimen as possible for light microscopy.

INTERPRETATION OF LUNG BIOPSIES

Clinicopathologic Correlation

Knowledge of the pertinent clinical history and chest radiographic findings is important for interpreting non-neoplastic lung biopsy specimens. Table 1–2 lists some clinical findings that are especially useful. Knowing whether or not the patient is immunocompromised is essential since the microscopic approach to specimens differs depending on the immune status (see Chapter 10). The nature of the onset and the presence or absence of systemic symptoms are factors that may help narrow the histologic differential diagnosis in difficult cases and confirm the histologic impression in others.

While the pathologist should be aware of the radiographic findings, it is not necessary to personally review each film. A brief description from the clinician should be adequate in most cases, especially whether there are diffuse or localized infiltrates and whether they are airspace or interstitial. The findings on high-resolution CT (HRCT) scans are especially important. Ground glass opacities usually connote active inflammation with minimal fibrosis, while honeycomb change is indicative of irreversible fibrosis. A superficial knowledge of pulmonary function test results may also be helpful.[45] Restrictive defects are found in the diffuse interstitial lung diseases and include a decrease in lung volumes [vital capacity (VC), total lung capacity (TLC), functional residual capacity (FRC), and residual volume (RV)] as well as decreased diffusion capacity (DLCO). Knowledge of these values can help in difficult cases, especially when there is a question about specimen adequacy. For example, if histologic changes are minimal on a small biopsy yet the patient has severe restrictive defects, the biopsy may not be representative. Conversely, if the biopsy contains extensive scarring but the patient has minimal functional abnormalities, the changes likely represent focal, nonspecific, subpleural scarring rather than a form of diffuse interstitial lung disease.

In busy practices, obtaining a clinical history from the clinician can be difficult. In many cases, however, a brief sentence on the pathology requisition form may suffice. For example, the clinical impression of 'probable IPF' would indicate a patient with chronically progressive diffuse interstitial lung disease (see Chapter 3). Alternatively, 'lung mass' or 'rule out tumor' may be enough information in other circumstances.

Careful correlation of clinical and pathologic findings in all cases can save the pathologist from making an erroneous (and sometimes foolish) diagnosis. It should be remembered, however, that microscopic examination remains the gold standard for diagnosis, and the pathologist must be prepared to stand by the histologic diagnosis when it is straightforward, regardless of the clinical findings.

Normal Morphology

A general knowledge of normal lung structure and, in some cases, of lung growth and development is necessary for interpreting lung biopsies, and detailed reviews of lung morphology are available elsewhere.[11,20,43] Knowledge of the following few basic facts, however, is essential for the surgical pathologist and can be very helpful in interpreting lung biopsy specimens:

1. *Pulmonary arteries and bronchioles course together.* Using this information, the pathologist can infer that a particular blood vessel is a pulmonary artery (rather than a vein), for example. Conversely, if an area of scarring or inflammation is present next to an artery, it can be inferred to represent the remnant of a damaged bronchiole.
2. *Pulmonary veins are located within interlobular septa.*
3. *Pulmonary arteries contain two distinct elastic tissue layers, while pulmonary veins have only one.* This fact can help when topography cannot be appreciated in routine H and E-stained slides.

Table 1–2 Helpful Clinical Infozrmation for Diagnosing Non-Neoplastic Lung Disease
• **Patient's immune status** – immunocompetent/ immunocompromised
• **Onset of disease** – acute, subacute, insidious
• **Presence/absence of systemic symptoms** – fever, weight loss
• **Radiographic findings** – localized, diffuse If localized – nodules (mass-like) or infiltrates (pneumonia-like), solitary or multiple If diffuse – interstitial, airspace, ground glass, honeycomb areas
• **Pulmonary function tests** – restrictive, obstructive, normal

4. *Pulmonary lymphatics are found within the bronchovascular bundles, interlobular septa and pleura;* hence, a 'lymphangitic distribution' connotes distribution along these pathways.

5. *Alveolar epithelium is not normally detectable by light microscopy, and the finding of easily visible alveolar lining cells suggests interstitial lung disease.* The main cells covering alveolar septa under normal circumstances are the type 1 pneumocytes that contain small flattened nuclei and long cytoplasmic processes and cannot be seen by light microscopy. In many interstitial lung diseases the type 1 cells are replaced by hyperplastic type 2 pneumocytes. These cells have large round nuclei and a hobnail shape that are easily visualized by light microscopy.

Microscopic Approach to Lung Biopsy Specimens

The interpretation of lung biopsy slides can be facilitated by an organized, systematic approach to their examination. As outlined in Table 1–3, the slides first should be scanned at low magnification to determine the predominant site of involvement as well as the extent and distribution of changes. The lung can be simplistically viewed as containing two main compartments – interstitium and airspace – and it helps to determine initially whether one or both are primarily affected.

Table 1–3 Microscopic Approach to Lung Biopsy Interpretation

I. Examination at low magnification

    A. Determine predominant site of involvement
        Airspace
        Interstitial
        Mixed airspace–interstitial

    B. Assess extent – patchy or diffuse?
        If patchy, determine distribution pattern:
            Random
            Specific (bronchiolar, lymphangitic, arterial)

II. Examination at high magnification
    Evaluate nature of process
        Cellular
            Reactive (inflammatory/infectious)
            Neoplastic
        Necrotizing/non-necrotizing
        Metabolic

Some processes involve the lung diffusely, whereas others are focal or patchy, and the extent of the changes is another important feature to evaluate. If the lesion is patchy, the next step is to attempt to identify a characteristic pattern of distribution. A patchy process, for example, may be randomly distributed, or it may follow the distribution of certain landmarks such as bronchioles, pulmonary arteries, or lymphatics. Lymphoid interstitial pneumonia is an example of a predominantly interstitial process that is diffuse, whereas hypersensitivity pneumonia is a patchy interstitial process that tends to be accentuated around bronchioles. Sarcoidosis is another patchy interstitial lesion, but it follows lymphatic pathways. Pulmonary alveolar proteinosis, *Pneumocystis carinii* pneumonia, eosinophilic pneumonia, and pulmonary hemorrhage are examples of airspace-filling lesions that tend to involve the lung diffusely. Bronchiolitis obliterans–organizing pneumonia is another airspace-filling lesion, but it is patchy, involving predominantly peribronchiolar airspaces. Diffuse alveolar damage is an example of a mixed interstitial–airspace lesion that is usually diffuse. Certain viral pneumonias (herpesvirus and adenovirus, for example) also involve both airspace and interstitium but tend to be distributed in a peribronchiolar location.

Once the location, extent, and distribution of the lesion have been determined at low magnification, the nature of the process can be more carefully examined at higher magnification. Whether a cellular infiltrate is inflammatory, reactive, or neoplastic, and whether the process is necrotizing or non-necrotizing, should be assessed. For example, eosinophilic granuloma is a patchy, usually peribronchiolar, predominantly interstitial process, and the diagnosis is established by finding the morphologically distinct Langerhans cells. Low-grade lymphoma of mucosa-associated lymphoid tissue (MALT) is a patchy interstitial lesion that follows a lymphatic distribution and is composed mainly of mature lymphocytes. The pulmonary vasculitides are mixed airspace–interstitial lesions that may be distributed around arteries or randomly, and they are usually necrotizing. Determining the type of the cellular infiltrate present and whether or not well-formed granulomas are seen helps distinguish them from the superficially (at low magnification) similar process, lymphomatoid granulomatosis. Occasionally, infiltrative lung lesions may be caused by processes other than cellular infiltrates. For example, alveolar septal amyloidosis is a diffuse interstitial process involving alveolar septa in which amorphous eosinophilic amyloid is deposited and cells are sparse. Diffuse calcification is another similar example of a relatively acellular interstitial lesion.

Common Artifacts or Incidental Findings of Little Significance

The pathologist frequently encounters changes on lung biopsy specimens that, while not 'normal', have little or no clinical relevance (see Table 1–4).[11] They are important to recognize, however, because they may confound pathologic interpretation.

Areas of *artifactually collapsed lung* are common and can be minimized by careful handling of the specimen, as emphasized earlier in this chapter.[25] Although collapsed lung may sometimes mimic interstitial lung disease, careful attention to the adjacent parenchyma should sort out the problem; that is, finding normal lung

Table 1–4 Commonly Encountered Microscopic Findings of Little Significance

Architectural changes	Atelectasis, fresh hemorrhage, intraalveolar macrophage accumulation
Structural variations	So-called chemodectomas, carcinoid tumorlets, intraparenchymal lymph nodes
Curious, but irrelevant, findings	Corpora amylacea, megakaryocytes, bone marrow emboli, focal ossification, various cytoplasmic inclusions (blue bodies, smokers' pigment, crystals), Hamazaki-Wesenberg bodies

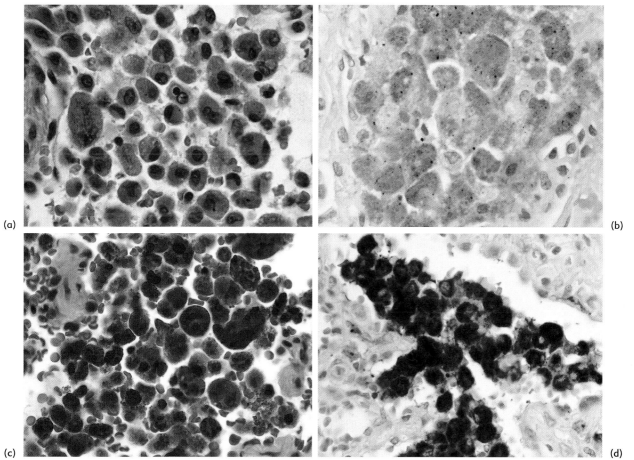

(a) (b) (c) (d)

Figure 1–3 Intraalveolar macrophage accumulation – smokers' pigment versus hemosiderin. Smokers' pigment appears finely granular, light golden brown (a), and stains unevenly light blue–green with Prussian blue (b). Hemosiderin is coarsely granular and dark brown (c). Individual granules are well defined and often surrounded by a distinct darkly staining rim. They stain uniformly deep blue in Prussian blue (d).

on the edge of a questionably abnormal focus with no intervening transition zone would indicate collapse. The absence of type 2 alveolar pneumocyte hyperplasia (a phenomenon characteristic of interstitial lung disease) also favors collapse. Immunohistochemical staining for cytokeratin can help in difficult cases since it outlines type 1 pneumocytes along apposed but otherwise normal alveolar septa.

Fresh *intraalveolar hemorrhage* is extremely common in all types of lung biopsy specimens.[25] In the absence of a history of hemoptysis clinically or hemosiderin deposition microscopically, it should be ignored.

Intraalveolar macrophage accumulation is common, especially in distal subpleural areas and around scars. This phenomenon is accentuated in cigarette smokers, in whom peribronchiolar airspaces are preferentially involved (*respiratory bronchiolitis*, see Chapter 3). The macrophage cytoplasm in cigarette smokers contains golden brown, coarsely granular pigment that should not be confused with hemosiderin (Fig. 1–3). It differs

from hemosiderin in that it is lighter brown with a yellow tint, and the granules are smaller and lack the distinct, often geometric shapes that are characteristic of hemosiderin. Both granule types stain with the Prussian blue iron stain, but hemosiderin has a more uniform dark blue appearance compared with a lighter blue–green appearance and more variable staining of smokers' pigment.

So-called chemodectomas are common stellate-shaped proliferations of bland, oval cells within the interstitium (Fig. 1–4).[10,19,24,27,40] Most are microscopic findings, although they can reach several millimeters in diameter and may be visible grossly. Despite their light microscopic appearance suggestive of 'cell ball' formation, ultrastructural and immunohistochemical studies have failed to demonstrate neuroendocrine differentiation (Fig. 1–5).[19,24,40] Most stain for vimentin and about one-third also stain for epithelial membrane antigen (EMA), while they are uniformly negative for cytokeratin and neuroendocrine markers. These findings have suggested

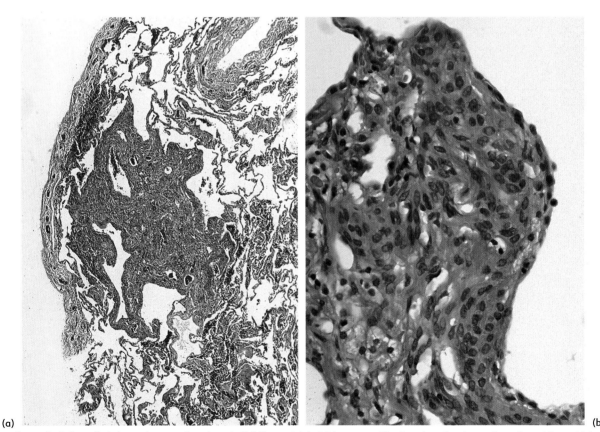

(a)   (b)

Figure 1–4 So-called chemodectoma (meningothelial-like nodule). (a) Low magnification view showing stellate-shaped interstitial nodule with surrounding traction emphysema. **(b)** Higher magnification showing the characteristic nests of epithelioid cells beneath the alveolar lining cells (right).

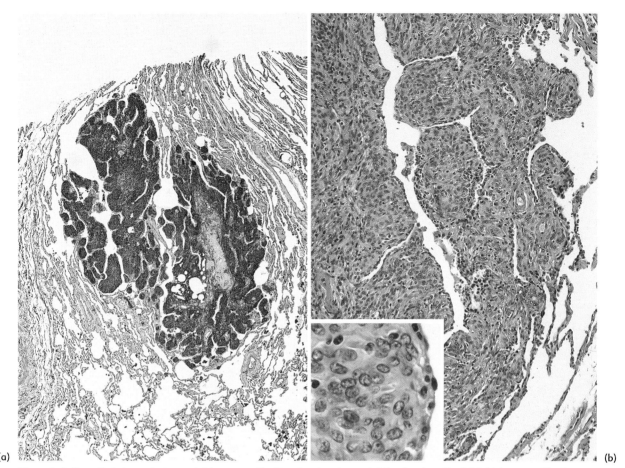

Figure 1–5 So-called chemodectoma. (a) Low magnification showing strong staining for vimentin. **(b)** A higher magnification shows the typical nests of uniform, oval-shaped cells in the interstitium. The location of the cell nests beneath the alveolar lining cells is better illustrated in the inset.

similarity to meningiomas, hence the synonym *'pulmonary meningiothelial-like nodules'*,[19] although one study utilizing mutational analysis failed to show common major genetic events with meningioma.[24] Their origin, therefore, remains uncertain.

Carcinoid tumorlets are microscopic proliferations of Kulchitsky-like cells, usually occurring around damaged or destroyed bronchioles or in areas of scarring (Fig. 1–6). They are composed of small nests of oval- to spindle-shaped cells with characteristic coarsely granular ('salt-and-pepper') nuclear chromatin (Fig. 1–7). Evidence of neuroendocrine origin can be demonstrated by both immunohistochemistry and electron microscopy.

Intraparenchymal *lymph nodes* are discussed in Chapter 9. They show changes similar to extrapulmonary lymph nodes (hyperplasia, granulomas, metastatic carcinoma, and so forth) and have no other inherent significance. They may be solitary or multiple and are

sometimes biopsied since they may be visualized on CT scans and may raise the clinical suspicion of a tumor.

Corpora amylacea are large, round eosinophilic structures that may fill an entire alveolus. They can be numerous, and are sometimes surrounded by histiocytes. They should not be confused with inhaled exogenous material (Fig. 1–8).[15] Careful examination in well-processed cases reveals both concentric circumferential lines and radiating lines extending from the center to the periphery (Fig. 1–9). Often, a darkly staining polarizable structure is seen in the center. Their origin is unknown, but they occur mainly in older adults and may represent a degenerative phenomenon.

Cytoplasmic inclusions are sometimes encountered in alveolar macrophages. The golden brown granules in cigarette smokers have already been described. *Blue bodies* are round, often laminated, blue–grey structures found within macrophages (Fig. 1–10).[26] They stain

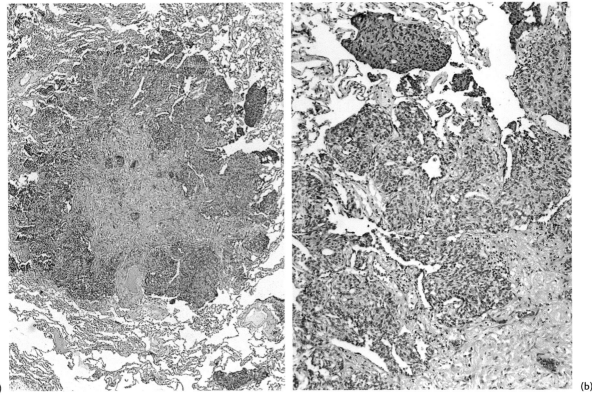

(a) (b)

Figure 1–6 Carcinoid tumorlet. (a) A proliferation of Kulchitsky-like cells emanates from a central scar that has replaced a bronchiole. A small pulmonary artery is seen at the bottom. **(b)** Higher magnification showing the typical nests of neuroendocrine cells extending along alveolar septa at the periphery of the scar. In contrast to the cells in so-called chemodectomas, the cells of carcinoid tumorlets are not covered by alveolar epithelium.

weakly for iron and are positive with von Kossa stain for calcium. They are thought to represent breakdown products of cell metabolism, and they occur in any chronic process containing abundant macrophages. Large, *polarizable crystals* can sometimes be found within histiocytes, usually within granulomatous foci, and are described in Chapter 7.

Megakaryocyte nuclei are often found within alveolar septal capillaries (Fig. 1–11). They are usually irregularly shaped and darkly staining, and they can be numerous. They tend to be most prominent in febrile illnesses, sepsis, and cardiovascular diseases and are also associated with metastatic malignancies.[37,39]

Although *bone marrow emboli* are most commonly found at autopsy, where they are related to chest trauma (broken ribs) during resuscitation attempts, they are also occasionally found in open lung biopsy specimens (Fig. 1–12). Presumably their pathogenesis in this situation is also related to rib trauma. No adverse clinical effects have been reported despite the fact that they sometimes involve numerous arteries.

Small foci of *osseous metaplasia* can be encountered in biopsies from a variety of conditions. This phenomenon is discussed in Chapter 16.

Small, oval-shaped structures known as *Hamazaki-Wesenberg bodies* are frequently encountered in peribronchial and mediastinal lymph nodes, especially when histiocytes are prominent or when granulomas are present (Fig. 1–13). They usually are found within sinusoids, and they stain strongly with Gomori's methenamine silver (GMS) and appear golden brown in H and E. Their only known significance is that they can be confused with histoplasma organisms. They differ in that they are more irregular in shape and they vary in size. The H and E appearance helps in difficult cases since histoplasma does not appear brown.

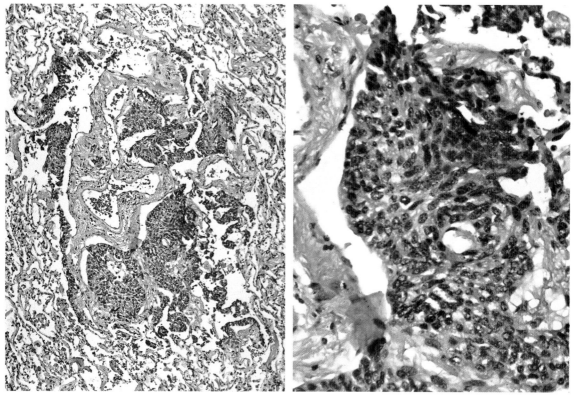

(a)   (b)

Figure 1–7 Carcinoid tumorlet. (a) In this example, nests of Kulchitsky-like cells replace a small bronchiole in the absence of scarring. The pulmonary artery is at the center. **(b)** Higher magnification shows the characteristic finely granular, 'salt-and-pepper' chromatin pattern of the component cells.

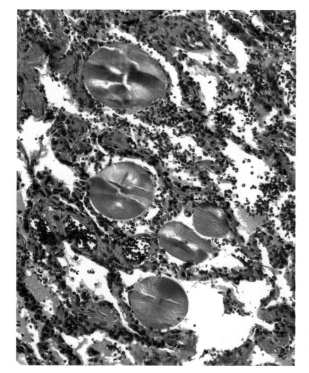

Figure 1–8 Corpora amylacea are seen within several alveolar spaces in this case.

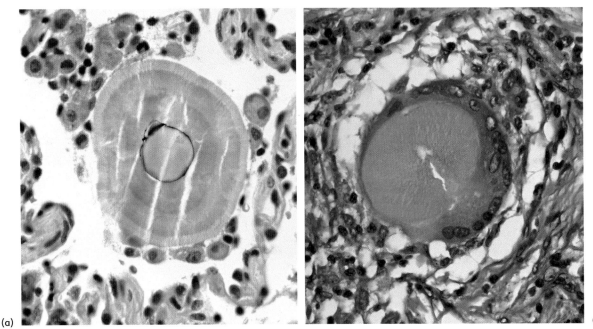

(a)　　　　　　　　　　　　　　　　　　　　　　　　　　　(b)

Figure 1–9 Higher magnification of corpora amylacea. The typical concentric rings are illustrated in **(a)**, while a foreign body giant cell reaction to the structure is seen in **(b)**.

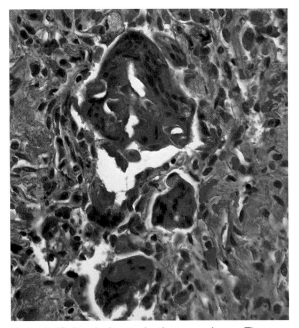

Figure 1–10 Blue bodies in alveolar macrophages. These blue–grey, sometimes laminated structures are common in any situation where alveolar macrophages are numerous.

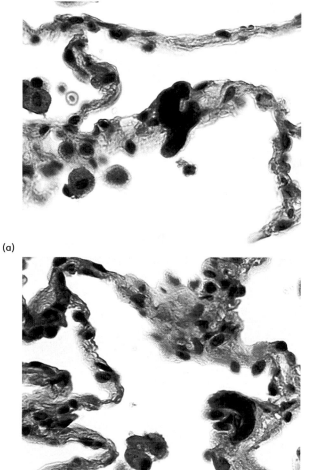

(a)

(b)

Figure 1–11 Megakaryocytes within the interstitium. (a), (b).
The nuclei are large, darkly staining, and irregular shaped,
and they bulge from alveolar capillaries.

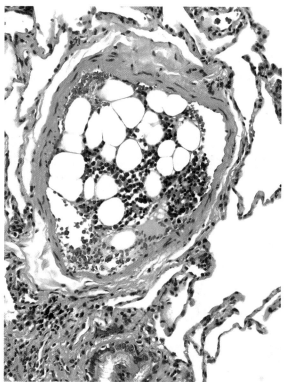

Figure 1–12 Bone marrow emboli are common incidental
findings in surgical lung biopsy specimens.

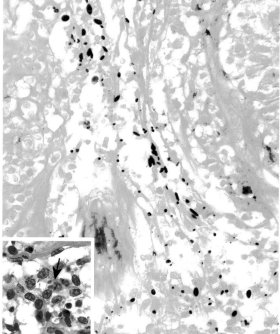

Figure 1–13 Hamazaki-Wesenberg bodies. GMS stain shows
the variable-sized oval-shaped structures within a lymph node
sinus. The inset (arrow) shows the golden brown appearance
in H and E.

REFERENCES

1. Allen MS, Deschamps C, Jones DM, et al: Video-assisted thoracic surgical procedures: The Mayo experience. Mayo Clinic Proc 71:351, 1996.

2. Anders GT, Johnson JE, Bush BA, Matthews JI: Transbronchial biopsy without fluoroscopy. A seven year perspective. Chest 94:557, 1988.

3. Anderson H: Transbronchial lung biopsy for diffuse pulmonary diseases. Results in 939 patients. Chest 73:734, 1978.

4. Bensard DB, McIntyre RC Jr, Waring BJ, Simon JS: Comparison of video thoracoscopic lung biopsy to open lung biopsy in the diagnosis of interstitial lung disease. Chest 103:765, 1993.

5. Berquist T, Bailey P, Cortese D, Miller W: Transthoracic needle biopsy. Accuracy and complications in relation to location and type of lesion. Mayo Clinic Proc 55:475, 1980.

6. Blasco LH, Hernández IMS, Garrido VV, De Miguel Poch E, Delgado MN, Abreu JA: Safety of the transbronchial biopsy in outpatients. Chest 99:562, 1991.

7. Blewett CJ, Bennett WF, Miller JD, Urschel JD: Open lung biopsy as an outpatient procedure. Ann Thorac Surg 71:1113, 2001.

8. Chechani V, Landreneau RJ, Shaikh SS: Open lung biopsy for diffuse infiltrative lung disease. Ann Thorac Surg 54:296, 1992.

9. Churg A: An inflation technique for open lung biopsies. Am J Surg Pathol 7:69, 1983.

10. Churg A, Warnock ML: So-called "minute pulmonary chemodectoma": a tumor not related to paragangliomas. Cancer 37:1759, 1976.

11. Colby T, Yousem S: Pulmonary histology for the surgical pathologist. Am J Surg Pathol 12:223, 1988.

12. Conces DJ Jr, Schwenk GR Jr, Doering PR, Glant MD: Thoracic needle biopsy. Improved results utilizing a team approach. Chest 91:813, 1987.

13. Deshmukh SP, Krasna MJ, McLaughlin JS: Video assisted thorascopic biopsy for interstitial lung disease. Internat Surg 81:330, 1996.

14. Dijkman JH, Van der Meer, JWM, Bakker W, et al: Transpleural lung biopsy by the thoracoscopic route in patients with diffuse interstitial pulmonary disease. Chest 82:76, 1982.

15. Dobashi M, Yuda F, Narabayashi M, et al: Histopathological study of corpora amylacea pulmonum. Histol Histopathol 4:153, 1989.

16. Ferson PF, Landreneau RJ, Dowling RD, et al: Comparison of open versus thoracoscopic lung biopsy for diffuse infiltrative pulmonary disease. J Thorac Cardiovasc Surg 106:194, 1993.

17. Fraire AE, Cooper SP, Greenberg SD, et al: Transbronchial lung biopsy. Histopathologic and morphometric assessment of diagnostic utility. Chest 102:748, 1993.

18. Gaensler E, Carrington C: Open biopsy for chronic diffuse infiltrative lung disease: Clinical, roentgenographic, and physiological correlation in 502 patients. Ann Thorac Surg 30:411, 1980.

19. Gaffey MJ, Mills SE, Askin FB: Minute pulmonary meningothelial-like nodules: A clinicopathologic study of so-called minute pulmonary chemodectoma. Am J Surg Pathol 12:167, 1988.

20. Gail DB, L'Enfant CJM: Cells of the lung: Biology and clinical implications. State of the art. Am Rev Respir Dis 127:366, 1983.

21. Gianoulis M, Chan N, Wright JL: Inflation of lung biopsies for frozen section. Mod Pathol 1:357, 1988.

22. Gianoulis M, Wright JL: An autopsy study of the structure of the small vessels in biopsies from the lingula and upper and lower lobes: Implications for vascular assessment. Mod Pathol 3:567, 1990.

23. Hasleton PS, ed: *Spencer's Pathology of the Lung*, 5th ed, New York, McGraw-Hill, 1996, pp 1211–1219.

24. Ionescu DN, Sasatomi E, Aldeeb D, et al: Pulmonary meningothelial-like nodules: A genotypic comparison with meningiomas. Am J Surg Pathol 28:207, 2004.

25. Kadokura M, Colby TV, Myers JL, et al: Pathologic comparison of video-assisted thoracic surgical lung biopsy with traditional open lung biopsy. J Thorac Cardiovasc Surg 109:494, 1995.

26. Koss MN, Johnson FB, Hochholzer L: Pulmonary blue bodies. Hum Pathol 12:258, 1981.

27. Kuhn C 3rd, Askin FB: The fine structure of so-called minute pulmonary chemodectomas. Hum Pathol 6:681, 1975.

28. Lettieri CJ, Veerappan GR, Helman DL, et al: Outcomes and safety of surgical lung biopsy for interstitial lung disease. Chest 127:1600, 2005.

29. McKeown PP, Conant P, Hubbell DS: Thoracoscopic lung biopsy. Ann Thorac Surg 54:490, 1992.

30. Miller DL, Allen MS, Trastek VF, et al. Video thoracoscopic wedge excision of the lung. Ann Thorac Surg 54: 410, 1992.

31. Miller RR, Nelems B, Muller NL, et al: Lingular and right middle lobe biopsy in the assessment of diffuse lung disease. Ann Thorac Surg 44:269, 1987.

32. Nagata N, Hirano H, Takayama K, Miyagawa Y, Shigematsu N: Step section preparation of transbronchial lung biopsy; Significance in the diagnosis of diffuse lung disease. Chest 100:959, 1991.

33. Newman SL, Michel RP, Wang NS: Lingular lung biopsy: Is it representative? Am Rev Respir Dis 132:1084, 1985.

34. Poletti V, Patelli M, Poggi S, et al: Transbronchial lung biopsy and bronchoalveolar lavage in diagnosis of diffuse infiltrative lung diseases. Respiration 54(Suppl 1):66, 1988.

35. Remy-Jardin M, Giraud F, Remy J, et al: Importance of ground glass attenuation in chronic diffuse infiltrative lung disease: Pathologic CT correlation. Radiology 189:693, 1993.

36. Shah SS, Tsang V, Goldstraw P: Open lung biopsy: A safe, reliable and accurate method for diagnosis in diffuse lung disease. Respiration 59:243, 1992.

37. Sharma GK, Talbot IC: Pulmonary megakaryocytes: "Missing link" between cardiovascular and respiratory disease. J Clin Pathol 39:969, 1986.

38. Shure D: Transbronchial biopsy and needle aspiration. Chest 95:1130, 1989.

39. Soares FA: Increased numbers of pulmonary megakaryocytes in patients with arterial pulmonary tumour embolism and with lung metastases seen at necropsy. J Clin Pathol 45:140, 1992.

40. Torikata C, Mukai M: So-called minute chemodectoma of the lung: An electron microscopic and immunohistochemical study. Virchows Archiv A Pathol Anat 417:113, 1990.

41. Utz JP, Perrella MA, Rosenow EC III: Lung biopsy. Adv Intern Med 37:337, 1991.

42. Walker WA, Cole FH Jr, Khandekar A, et al: Does open lung biopsy affect treatment in patients with diffuse pulmonary infiltrates? J Thorac Cardiovasc Surg 97:534, 1989.

43. Wang N-S: Anatomy. In: Dail DH, Hammar SP, eds: *Pulmonary Pathology*, 2nd ed, New York, Springer-Verlag, 1994, pp 21–44.

44. Warner D, Warner M, Divertie M: Open lung biopsy in patients with diffuse pulmonary infiltrates and acute respiratory failure. Am Rev Respir Dis 137:90, 1988.

45. West JB: *Pulmonary Pathophysiology: The Essentials*, 6th ed, Baltimore, Lippincott, Williams & Wilkins, 2003.

46. Westcott JL: Percutaneous transthoracic needle biopsy. Radiology 169:593, 1988.

47. Wetstein L: Sensitivity and specificity of lingular segmental biopsies of the lung. Chest 90:383, 1986.

48. White DA, Wong PW, Downey R: The utility of open lung biopsy in patients with hematologic malignancies. Am J Respir Crit Care Med 161:723, 2000.

ACUTE LUNG INJURY PATTERNS: DIFFUSE ALVEOLAR DAMAGE AND BRONCHIOLITIS OBLITERANS–ORGANIZING PNEUMONIA

The lung reacts in a similar fashion to various types of acute injury, regardless of etiology. The changes produced are related to initial epithelial and endothelial necrosis followed by alveolar collapse and eventually fibrosis. The light microscopic appearance varies depending both on the time interval between injury and biopsy and on the extent and localization of the injury. For example, hyaline membranes or proteinaceous exudates are prominent soon after injury, whereas fibroblasts predominate after a few weeks. Widespread injury to distal alveoli produces diffuse alveolar damage (DAD), while more localized injury to peribronchiolar parenchyma produces bronchiolitis obliterans–organizing pneumonia (BOOP). We use the term *acute lung injury pattern* in a general sense to encompass these two histologic manifestations.

Terminology

Acute lung injury (ALI) is defined clinically as the rapid alteration of alveolar walls with resultant impaired gas exchange that follows a toxic insult to the lung. The extent of injury varies, and the resultant functional impairment ranges from mild to severe. The most severe cases are classified as the acute respiratory distress syndrome (ARDS) based on the degree of hypoxemia.[27,34] The ratio of the partial pressure of arterial oxygen to the fraction of inspired oxygen (PaO_2/FIO_2) is used as an objective measurement to separate cases of ARDS from ALI, with values of less than 200 for ARDS and less than 300 for ALI. By definition, both ALI and ARDS patients have bilateral lung infiltrates on chest radiographs in the absence of cardiac failure.

Diffuse alveolar damage (DAD) is the underlying pathologic finding in most cases of ALI and ARDS.[1] Conversely, most patients with DAD on biopsy specimens have ARDS clinically, and therefore the terms are often used interchangeably. It should be remembered, however, that ALI and ARDS are defined clinically, while DAD describes the pathologic changes. Findings other than DAD, such as BOOP, acute eosinophilic pneumonia, malignancies, and infections, for example, can cause the clinical picture of ARDS.[8,33,39] Therefore, the terms DAD and ALI/ARDS should not be used synonymously.

We include BOOP along with DAD under the category of *acute lung injury pattern* because both can be caused by a large variety of toxic insults while some are idiopathic, their pathogenesis is similar, and fibroblast proliferation is often present histologically in both. The conditions are quite distinct, however, clinically, and are usually easily distinguished pathologically. Sometimes, especially at autopsy, but also occasionally in open lung biopsy specimens, overlapping features of DAD and BOOP occur and the changes can only be descriptively diagnosed as acute lung injury pattern. This difficulty in classification should not be surprising, since some toxic agents would be anticipated to affect both the peribronchiolar and the more distal lung parenchyma. In fact, it almost seems more surprising that this overlapping pattern of lung injury is not more common.

Another use for the term 'acute lung injury pattern' is in the interpretation of small biopsies, especially transbronchial biopsies, when, because of sampling problems, the changes may not be unequivocally classifiable as DAD or BOOP. This term is helpful in such cases since it communicates to the clinician the need to search for a source of injury, and it also suggests a possible role for corticosteroid therapy. Because it encompasses only two entities – and their therapy is similar – obtaining a larger tissue specimen for a more specific diagnosis may not be necessary.

DIFFUSE ALVEOLAR DAMAGE

Diffuse alveolar damage is a descriptive term for the pathologic sequence of events that follows severe ALI caused by any one of a variety of toxic insults.[17] The name is confusing, because the adjective 'diffuse' is usually interpreted as synonymous to 'widespread', and 'diffuse alveolar' is thus inferred to mean all the alveoli in the lung. Used in this manner, therefore, the changes of DAD, by definition, would involve the entire lung.

However, as envisioned by Liebow, the word 'diffuse' refers to changes in a single alveolus and indicates that all parts of the alveolus (epithelium, endothelium, and interstitial space) are affected by the process (i.e. the alveolus is *diffusely* involved). Used in this way, the process of DAD may involve the lung either diffusely or focally. The term *regional DAD* has been used for cases of localized DAD,[48] but this descriptor is not necessary when one understands the intended meaning of DAD. The clinically important forms of DAD involve the lung diffusely, however, and the following discussion applies to them.

Pathologic Findings in DAD

The exact histologic appearance of DAD varies, depending on the time interval between the onset of symptoms and lung biopsy. As first defined by Nash et al[79] in patients exhibiting oxygen toxicity, and subsequently confirmed by other studies, DAD may be divided into two fairly discrete, but overlapping, stages.[9,19,35,62,72,75,76,104,105,107,121] An *early, acute,* or *exudative stage* is most prominent in the first week after injury and is characterized by edema and hyaline membranes. A *later, proliferative,* or *organizing stage* in which fibrosis predominates occurs after 1 to 2 weeks. Figure 2–1 illustrates schematically the temporal relationship of the two stages in the evolution of DAD. It should be noted that the changes of DAD are not necessarily progressive from the acute to the organizing stage, since the process may cease and

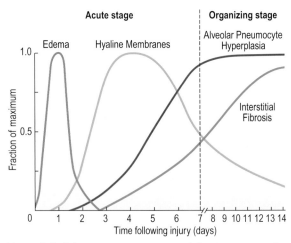

Figure 2–1 Schematic representation of the time course of the evolution of DAD. This graph is meant to illustrate the relative, rather than absolute, time of appearance of various features of DAD and also to emphasize the overlap between *acute* and *organizing* DAD. The numbers on the abscissa are only crude approximations and should not be considered accurate.

recovery occur at any stage. There is some evidence that local factors such as hydrodynamic and hydrostatic forces and intraalveolar pressure (rather than simply the length of time following injury) may influence the progression of acute to organizing DAD.[2]

Acute Stage of DAD

The earliest light microscopic changes in the acute stage of DAD are visible 12 to 24 hours following injury and consist of interstitial and intraalveolar edema with varying amounts of hemorrhage and fibrin deposition. By electron microscopy, cytoplasmic swelling and other degenerative changes are seen in capillary endothelial cells and alveolar epithelial cells, and interstitial edema is prominent. Hyaline membranes, the histologic hallmark of the acute stage, may be seen as early as 12 hours following injury but are most numerous after 3 to 5 days (Fig. 2–2). They appear as homogeneous, amorphous eosinophilic, structures that are plastered along the alveolar septa (Fig. 2–3). An intraalveolar, proteinaceous exudate containing cellular debris often

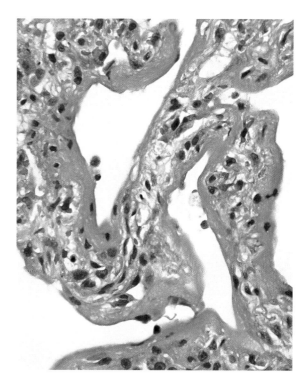

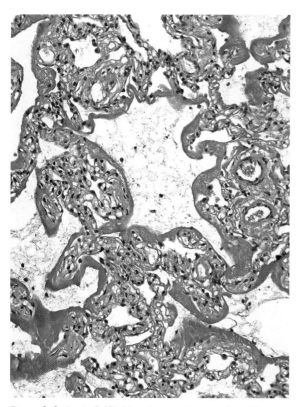

Figure 2–2 Acute DAD. Note the prominent eosinophilic hyaline membranes plastered along edematous alveolar septa. Intraalveolar edema characterized by feathery proteinaceous exudate within alveolar spaces is also present in this example of early DAD.

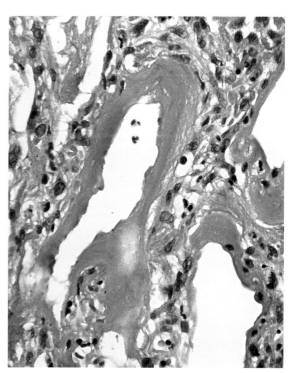

Figure 2–3 Hyaline membranes in two cases of acute DAD. Note the homogeneous eosinophilic appearance of the hyaline membranes. The adjacent alveolar septa are mildly thickened and contain scattered fibroblasts in addition to scant chronic inflammatory cells.

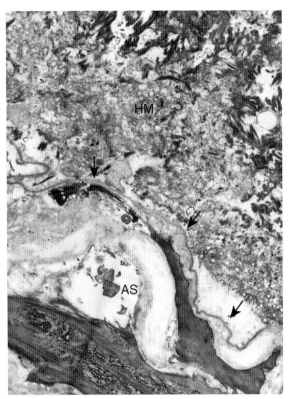

Figure 2–4 Ultrastructure of acute DAD. Note the heterogeneous appearance of the hyaline membrane (HM), which contains a mixture of fibrin and cellular debris. The alveolar basement membrane (arrows) is denuded of the alveolar lining epithelium. A myofibroblast (bottom) is present in the alveolar septum (AS).

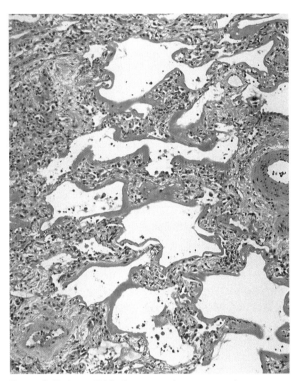

Figure 2–5 Acute DAD. Low magnification view showing extensive hyaline membrane formation. Note also the uniform alveolar septal thickening containing a mild chronic inflammatory cell infiltrate.

accompanies the hyaline membranes. Electron microscopy at this time demonstrates sloughing of alveolar lining cells and denudation of the epithelial basement membrane associated with areas of alveolar collapse (Fig. 2–4).[6,18] The hyaline membranes, although appearing homogeneous by light microscopy, ultrastructurally contain abundant cytoplasmic and nuclear debris from sloughed epithelial cells admixed with small amounts of fibrin. A sparse interstitial inflammatory cell infiltrate consisting predominantly of lymphocytes, plasma cells, and macrophages accompanies the other changes and is most prominent after 1 week (Fig. 2–5). Fibrin thrombi in various stages of organization are often present in small pulmonary arteries and they may be numerous (Fig. 2–6).[40,45] They are thought to occur secondary to endothelial damage.

Alveolar lining cell hyperplasia develops approximately 3 to 7 days following injury (Fig. 2–7). This feature is most prominent toward the end of the acute stage of

DAD and persists throughout the organizing stage. It is characterized by proliferation along the alveolar septa of regularly spaced cuboidal cells that often protrude into the alveolar spaces in a hobnail fashion (Fig. 2–8). Considerable atypia may be encountered and is characterized by nuclear enlargement, clumped nuclear chromatin, large eosinophilic nucleoli, and cellular pleomorphism, and it can lead to concern for malignancy on cytologic specimens.[4,42] Mitotic figures may be numerous, and atypical forms are sometimes present. Other abnormalities have also been described, including intracytoplasmic lipid accumulation and cytoplasmic hyaline change similar to Mallory hyaline in liver cells (see Chapter 3).[41,47] The proliferating alveolar lining cells have been shown by immunohistochemistry and electron microscopy to represent type 2 pneumocytes or their precursors.[44] The presence of p53 and WAF1, nuclear proteins important in cell cycle regulation, and BAX has been demonstrated in the hyperplastic pneumocytes. Tumor necrosis factor alpha (TNFα) has also been found in their cytoplasm.[10,11,28] They frequently exhibit ultrastructural features of ongoing injury such

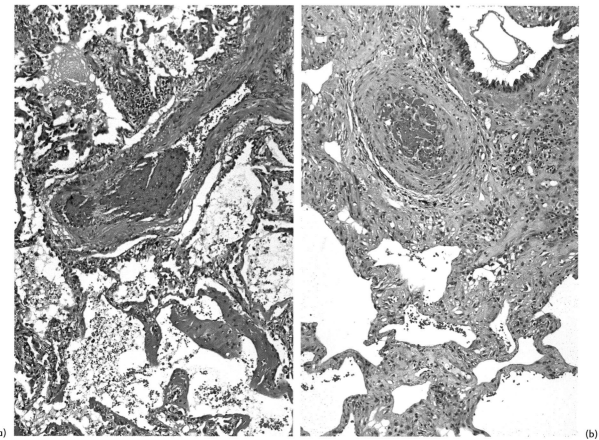

(a)   (b)

Figure 2–6 Arterial thrombi in DAD. (a) A recent thrombus is seen in a pulmonary artery in this example of acute DAD. Note the hyaline membranes at the bottom. **(b)** An organizing thrombus is seen in this example of organizing DAD.

as intracellular edema and dilatation of endoplasmic reticulum. The number of lamellar bodies may be decreased or increased, and they may be abnormally large or small. This proliferation of type 2 pneumocytes is thought to be a reparative phenomenon in that the type 2 cells replace sloughed type 1 cells, and they have the capacity to differentiate into type 1 cells once the initial insult has passed. There is also some evidence that the type 2 pneumocytes may protect the lung from further injury. The pneumocyte proliferation sometimes occurs over the luminal surface of the hyaline membranes, thus incorporating the hyaline membranes into the alveolar septa and contributing to the interstitial thickening (Fig. 2–9).

Organizing Stage of DAD

The organizing stage of DAD is characterized by fibroblast proliferation, mainly within the interstitium but also focally within airspaces (Fig. 2–10). It begins after one or more weeks but is most prominent two or more weeks following injury. Interstitial inflammation and alveolar lining cell hyperplasia are still present, but edema and hyaline membranes are not prominent. Phagocytosis of hyaline membrane remnants and other debris by alveolar macrophages is common. Some of the residual alveolar exudate is incorporated into the alveolar septa,[22,105] and remnants of hyaline membranes can sometimes be identified in the thickened septa. In some cases, the exudate undergoes organization and active fibrosis occurs on the luminal surface of alveolar walls (Fig. 2–11). This fibrosis may show a striking localization around alveolar ducts.[19,35] Eventually, extensive interstitial fibrosis develops that is characterized by loosely aggregated fibroblasts and myofibroblasts admixed with scattered mononuclear inflammatory cells but with minimal associated collagen deposition (Fig. 2–12). Staining of the fibroblasts and myofibroblasts has been demonstrated for alpha-smooth muscle actin, Bcl-2,

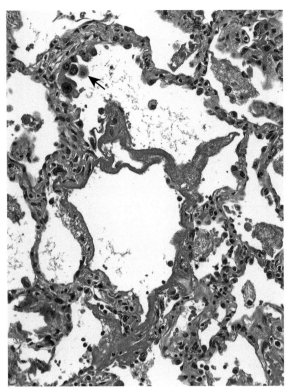

Figure 2–7 Alveolar pneumocyte hyperplasia in DAD. In this example, alveolar pneumocyte hyperplasia (arrow) is becoming confluent along alveolar septa. Hyaline membranes are still prominent.

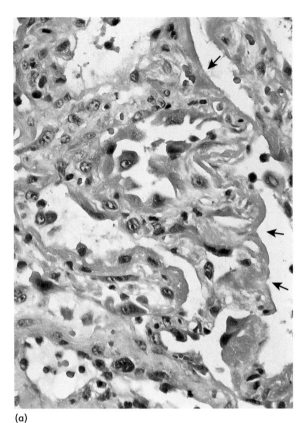

(a)

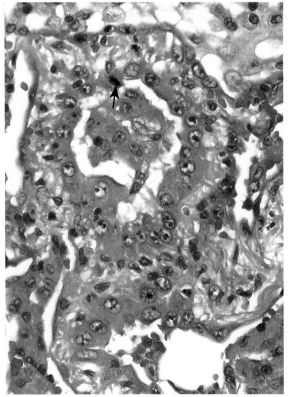

(b)

Figure 2–8 Extensive alveolar pneumocyte hyperplasia in DAD. **(a)** Prominent alveolar pneumocyte hyperplasia covers most of the alveolar septa in this example. Remnants of hyaline membranes are seen on the right and at the top (arrows). **(b)** Significant cytologic atypia is seen in the proliferating alveolar pneumocytes in this case. Note the prominent nucleoli and the mitotic figure (arrow).

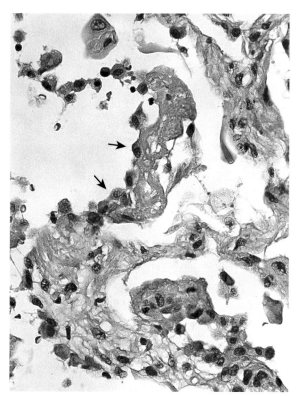

Figure 2–9 Proliferation of alveolar pneumocytes along the luminal surface of hyaline membranes (arrows). This process contributes to alveolar septal thickening by incorporating the hyaline membrane material into underlying alveolar septa.

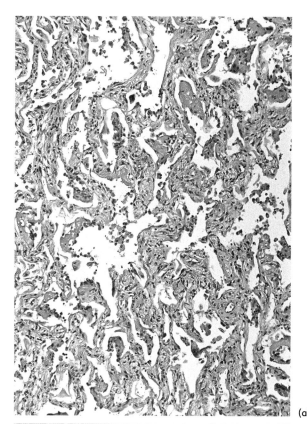

(a)

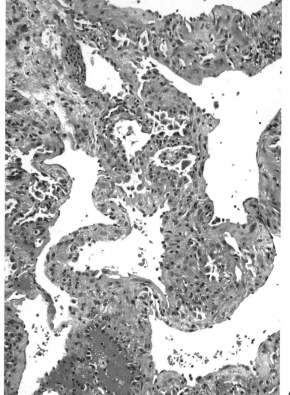

(b)

Figure 2–10 Organizing DAD. (a) Prominent alveolar septal thickening by fibroblasts and scant chronic inflammatory cells is seen in this example. There are also remnants of hyaline membranes present within alveolar lumens. (b) More striking alveolar septal fibroblast proliferation is present in this example. Hyaline membranes are not seen. Note the striking alveolar pneumocyte hyperplasia that lines many of the residual alveolar spaces.

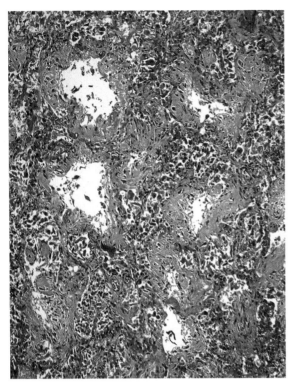

Figure 2–11 Organizing DAD. Prominent fibrosis is seen along alveolar ducts and alveolar spaces in this example. The changes likely represent organization of hyaline membranes. This pattern is usually only seen at autopsy.

versican, decorin, and type I procollagen by immuno-histochemistry.[3,10,12,21,32] Elastic fiber deposition has also been noted in alveolar septa.[29,37] Ultrastructurally, in addition to the prominent fibroblast proliferation, collapse and apposition of alveoli can be appreciated (Fig. 2–13).[18] The collapsed alveoli are permanently apposed when they are reepithelialized by proliferating alveolar pneumocytes, and this process contributes to the interstitial thickening (Figs 2–14 and 2–15). In fatal cases, fibrosis may progress for several weeks with extensive restructuring of lung parenchyma and formation of honeycomb lung (see Chapter 3, Fig. 3–28). As in the acute stage, acute and organizing thrombi continue to be present (see Fig. 2–6). Additional arterial changes are seen late in the course and consist of medial hypertrophy and intimal fibrosis with eventual obliteration of large portions of the vascular bed.[40,45,75,116]

Bronchiolar epithelium commonly shows evidence of injury in DAD. In the early stages, necrosis of the mucosal cells may occur. Later, there is regrowth of the epithelium, and the regenerating cells may extend along adjacent alveolar septa. Squamous metaplasia is a frequent alteration in the new epithelium, and cytologic atypia is common (Fig. 2–16). The regenerative atypia can be so severe in some cases that a malignancy is considered in the differential diagnosis.[30]

The separation of DAD into an acute and an organizing stage is helpful for understanding the pathogenesis and evolution of the various pathologic changes that occur. The two-stage theory is supported by animal models but is somewhat artificial in humans, since the precise time of onset of the lesion is difficult to determine in patients. Also, alveolar injury may continue or recur after the initial injury, so that different areas in the same biopsy may sometimes show different or overlapping stages of DAD. For instance, patients with DAD, regardless of etiology, usually require high concentrations of oxygen for adequate ventilation, and their clinical course may be complicated by hypotension, sepsis, or disseminated intravascular coagulation (DIC) – all factors that by themselves can cause DAD. Some investigators have suggested that local factors such as interstitial hydrostatic and hydrodynamic forces and intraalveolar pressure related to mechanical ventilation may influence the development of organization from acute DAD and thus account for coexisting areas of acute and organizing DAD.[2]

Clinical Features, Treatment, and Prognosis in DAD

Patients with DAD present with the rapid onset of shortness of breath and diffuse lung infiltrates in the absence of heart failure, and ventilator therapy with high concentrations of inspired oxygen is usually required. DAD is rarely encountered in patients who are not on a ventilator, and the diagnosis should be made with caution in such patients. The mortality associated with DAD is high, with mortality rates averaging 35–50% and ranging from 10% to 90% depending on the cause. Follow-up studies in survivors show surprisingly few abnormalities, with mild pulmonary functional abnormalities, especially decreased carbon monoxide diffusing capacity (DLCO).[15] Chest computed tomography (CT) scans may show a residual reticular pattern, however, and health-related quality of life appears to be decreased.[15,16a,31] There is no correlation between the severity of morphologic changes on biopsy specimens and the severity of subsequent functional abnormalities.[43] Recurrent DAD has been reported occasionally,

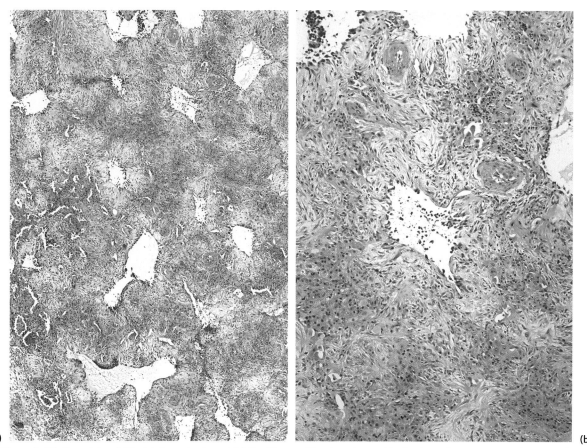

(a)   (b)

Figure 2–12 Organizing DAD. (a) Extensive interstitial fibroblast proliferation along with alveolar collapse is seen in this example. Note the solid appearing areas containing slit-like, collapsed alveolar spaces between residual enlarged airspaces. **(b)** Higher magnification showing the prominent fibroblast proliferation in the interstitium around a residual alveolar duct.

most often in patients receiving narcotic therapy for chronic pain management.[38]

There are no specific pathologic features for predicting prognosis, although the presence of extensive fibrosis on biopsy specimens appears to be associated with the greatest mortality.[23,26] Nonetheless, three of 13 such patients in a study by Lamy et al[23] survived with minimal or no residual functional abnormalities. Therefore, even extensive fibrosis found in a lung biopsy should not be considered irreversible and should not preclude continued treatment with aggressive support measures.

The role of corticosteroids or cytotoxic drugs in the treatment of patients with DAD is controversial. Although some studies have shown a beneficial effect with corticosteroids, others have suggested that this therapy has no effect or may even be harmful.

Pathogenesis of DAD

Numerous experimental studies have shown the importance of epithelial and endothelial cell injury in the pathogenesis of DAD, although the relative susceptibility of each of these cell types to injury varies according to species.[17] Figure 2–17 summarizes the probable sequence of events in the evolution of DAD. Endothelial cell damage results in fluid leakage from the capillaries into the interstitium and eventually into the alveolar spaces. The destruction of alveolar lining cells adds to the intraalveolar exudate and contributes to the subsequent formation of hyaline membranes. The epithelial basal lamina is denuded in this process but remains intact and thus forms a framework for lung repair that is initiated by the proliferation of type 2 pneumocytes. Collapse and coalescence of alveoli occur in the areas

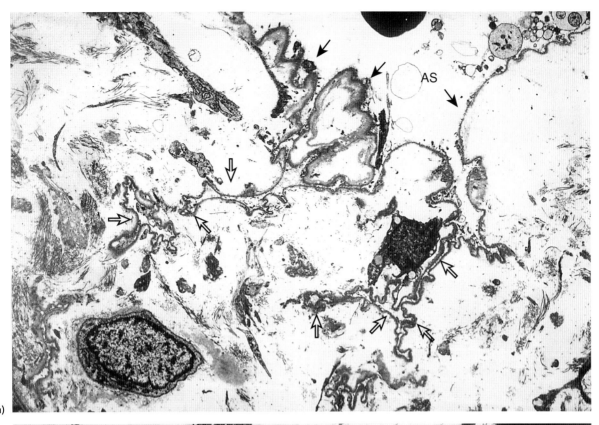

(a)

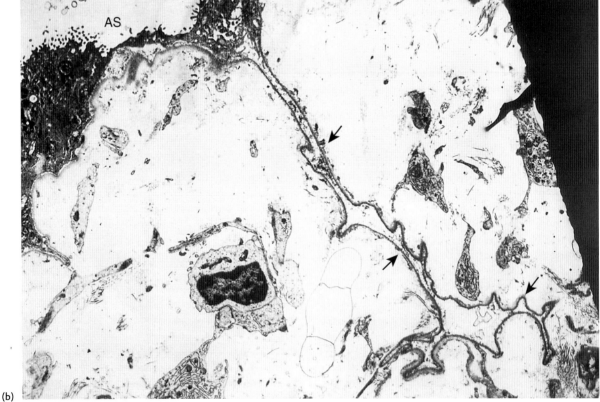

(b)

Figure 2–13 Ultrastructure of organizing DAD. (a) There is complete denudation of the alveolar epithelial basement membrane (black arrows), and long invaginations of the denuded membrane resulting from alveolar collapse extend deeply within the alveolar septa (open arrows). (b) Reepithelialization and permanent apposition of collapsed alveoli. A type 2 alveolar pneumocyte proliferates along the alveolar surface (top) of a collapsed alveolus (arrows indicate invaginated denuded alveolar basement membrane), thus causing permanent apposition of collapsed alveolar walls. (AS – alveolar space)

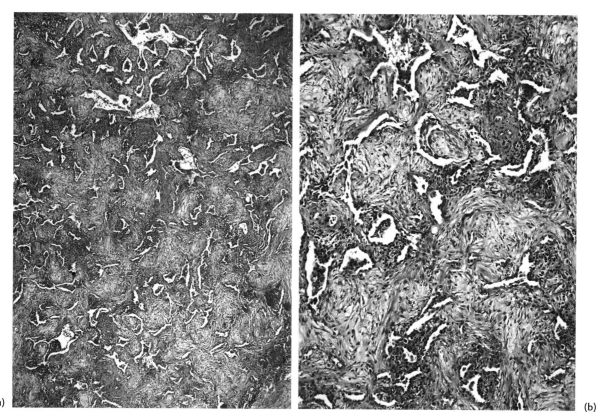

Figure 2–14 Extensive interstitial fibrosis in organizing DAD. (a) Low magnification view showing nearly solid appearance with only slit-like remnants of alveolar spaces. Note the light staining appearance of the stroma in areas. **(b)** Higher magnification showing lightly staining myxoid appearing stroma containing spindle-shaped fibroblasts and myofibroblasts that thicken alveolar septa. The slit-like remnants of alveolar spaces are lined by hyperplastic alveolar pneumocytes.

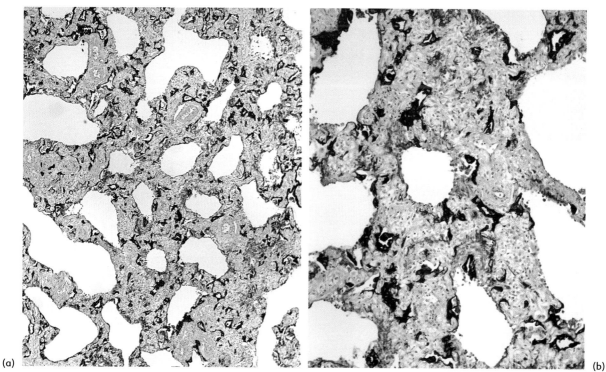

Figure 2–15 Cytokeratin staining in organizing DAD. (a) Low magnification showing remnants of collapsed alveoli that are highlighted by strong staining within alveolar septa. **(b)** Higher magnification showing lighter staining remnants of hyaline membranes within the alveolar septa in addition to the collapsed alveoli.

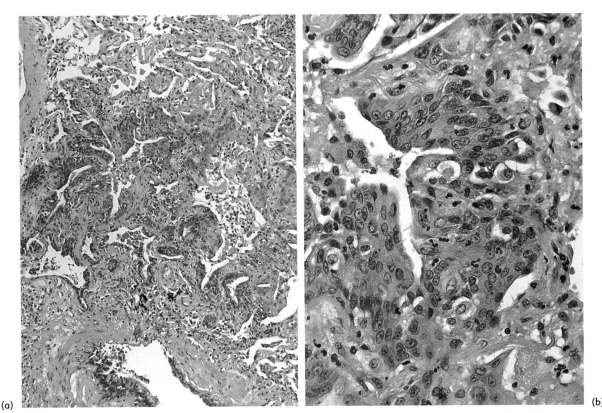

(a)   (b)

Figure 2–16 Squamous metaplasia in DAD. (a) Low magnification showing prominent squamous metaplasia. Note the remnants of hyaline membranes along with the alveolar septal fibroblast proliferation at top. A bronchiole with regenerative epithelial changes is seen at the bottom. **(b)** Higher magnification of the squamous metaplasia, showing mild cytologic atypia.

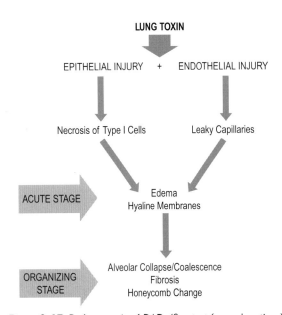

Figure 2–17 Pathogenesis of DAD. (See text for explanation.)

of denuded basal lamina and partly account for the appearance of interstitial thickening.[6,18,22] Interstitial inflammation accompanies these changes and is followed by fibroblast proliferation. The fibrosis occurs predominantly in the interstitium but is present to some extent in the airspaces as well. An additional mechanism of alveolar septal thickening is related to the incorporation of hyaline membranes and other intraalveolar exudates into the interstitium. This occurs when the type 2 pneumocytes proliferate along the alveolar luminal, rather than the septal, side of the hyaline membranes.[9,18,22]

The precise mechanism of cell injury in DAD is uncertain, but neutrophils are thought to have a central role in at least some examples.[13,25,36] One theory suggests that neutrophils stimulated by activation of the complement system or recruited by various chemotactic agents are aggregated in lung capillaries, where noxious substances such as elastase or oxygen radicals are released that directly damage endothelium and also attract additional inflammatory cells. Although this theory is appealing, it is not the entire explanation, since DAD can occur in neutropenic patients.[24] There is evidence that other oxidants, such as peroxynitrite, might also contribute to lung damage.[26] Additional factors, including circulating toxins, platelet aggregates, cytokines such as tumor necrosis factor or interleukins, and various lipid mediators, may also be important in producing or magnifying the injury.[27,28] The eventual fibroblast proliferation that occurs in the later stages of DAD is thought to be related to the release of several substances that stimulate replication of these cells, such as platelet-derived growth factor (PDGF), basic fibroblast growth factor (bFGF), insulin-like growth factor-I, and fibronectin.[14,21] A role for metalloproteinases and their tissue inhibitors has also been postulated.[12]

Etiology of DAD

A large variety of potential toxic insults can cause DAD and are listed in Table 2–1. Unfortunately, a specific cause usually cannot be determined from the histologic findings alone, and its identification requires knowledge of clinical history and laboratory data. Even with this information, however, a specific etiologic agent may not be identifiable, because the cause is often multifactorial.[7] For example, patients with malignancies may receive several chemotherapeutic drugs, their subsequent clinical course may be complicated by sepsis or DIC, and their treatment may require ventilator therapy with high concentrations of oxygen. Similarly, the course of patients following severe trauma may be complicated by a combination of hypotension, fat embolism, DIC, and/or sepsis. In rare cases, DAD occurs in previously healthy individuals with no identifiable inciting cause. Such cases are known as *acute interstitial pneumonia* or *Hamman–Rich disease*. This condition is a fulminant, often fatal disease and it is discussed along with the idiopathic interstitial pneumonias in Chapter 3. The following sections discuss the most common etiologies of DAD.

Infection

Among infectious agents, viruses most consistently produce DAD (see Chapter 10). Influenza is a classically described cause of the lesion, but other viruses, including adenovirus, herpesvirus, cytomegalovirus, hanta virus, severe acute respiratory syndrome (SARS) associated corona virus, and, rarely, respiratory syncytial virus, may produce similar changes.[17,50–52,54–57,60] DAD due to *Mycoplasma pneumoniae*[53] and certain rickettsiae (as in Q fever)[59] has been reported, and biopsies in Legionnaire's

disease (see Chapter 10) may show this lesion. DAD may contribute to the respiratory failure that has been occasionally reported following treatment of advanced pulmonary tuberculosis.[58] In immunocompromised patients, DAD can be caused by virtually *any* infection, although *Pneumocystis carinii* is most commonly implicated (see Chapter 10).[49] This fact emphasizes the necessity of carefully examining special stains for organisms in all immunocompromised patients with DAD.

Oxygen Toxicity and Other Toxic Inhalants

Pulmonary changes attributed to high concentrations of inspired oxygen were first noted in patients by Pratt in 1958.[81] The pathologic changes were subsequently described in more detail and the frequent finding of hyaline membranes emphasized.[65,68,72,76,78,79,84] Nash et al[79] were the first to divide the lesions caused by oxygen toxicity into the characteristic acute, or exudative, and organizing, or proliferative, stages. Similar changes have also been described in neonates and are generally included in the term *bronchopulmonary dysplasia* (see Chapter 14).[61,62,66,80,85] It is likely that this condition represents accentuation of the organizing stage of DAD in infant lungs.

Most of the evidence indicating that oxygen can have a direct toxic effect on the lung comes from animal experiments.[17] Although DAD is a common finding in patients receiving mechanical ventilation and inspiring high concentrations of oxygen, these individuals have usually suffered previous lung injury that necessitated such therapy. Any one of the agents listed in Table 2–1 may have precipitated the pulmonary dysfunction. It is therefore difficult to distinguish changes that are due to oxygen from those that are a result of the initial insult.[74,76] Although mild functional abnormalities and evidence of alveolar-capillary leakage have been demonstrated in patients without prior lung injury who received 95–100% oxygen, typical histologic lesions have not been observed in such cases even after exposures lasting almost 2 weeks.[64,70,83] It may be that human lungs are susceptible to severe injury by oxygen only after they are already damaged by other agents. The exact concentration at which oxygen is toxic is unknown, but inspired oxygen at a concentration of less than 40–60% is generally considered safe.[72]

The mechanism of cellular injury by oxygen is thought to be related to the formation of free radical ions that are produced during its metabolism. The superoxide anion (O_2^-) is a highly cytotoxic free radical that reacts with cell products to form other cytotoxic metabolites, including hydrogen peroxide (H_2O_2), the

---

Table 2–1   Causes of Diffuse Alveolar Damage

Infectious Agents
  Any infection in immunocompromised patients, especially
    Pneumocystis pneumonia
  Legionella
  Mycoplasma
  Rickettsia
  Viruses (influenza, SARS, hanta virus, herpes, adenovirus,
    cytomegalovirus, etc.)

Toxic Inhalants
  Amitrole-containing herbicide
  Ammonia and bleach mixture
  Chlorine gas
  Crack cocaine
  Hydrogen sulfide
  Mercury vapor
  Nitric acid fumes
  Nitrogen dioxide
  Oxygen
  Paint remover
  Smoke
  Smoke bomb ($ZnCl_2$)
  Sulfur dioxide
  War gases (phosgene, nitrogen mustard)

Drug Toxicity (see Chapter 4)
  Chemotherapeutic agents
    Azathioprine
    BCNU
    Bleomycin
    Busulfan
    Cytoxan
    Melphalan
    Methotrexate
    Mitomycin
  Other drugs
    Amiodarone
    Gold
    Hexamethonium
    Nitrofurantoin
    Placidyl
    Interferon-gamma
    Penicillamine
  Heroin and other opiates

Ingestants
  Denatured rapeseed oil (toxic oil syndrome)
  Kerosene
  Paraquat

Shock
  Traumatic
  Hemorrhagic
  Neurogenic
  Cardiogenic

Sepsis

Aspiration

Radiation

Exacerbation of Usual Interstitial Pneumonia

Miscellaneous
  Acute pancreatitis[149,157]
  Burns[147]
  Cardiopulmonary bypass[145,156]
  Heat[143]
  High altitude
  Intravenous administration of contrast material[142]
  Leukemic cell lysis[159]
  Partial liquid ventilation with perfluorocarbon[5]
  Molar pregnancy[148,153,160]
  Near-drowning
  Peritoneovenous shunt[146]
  Post lymphangiography[158]
  Scleroderma[152]
  Systemic lupus erythematosus[151]
  Toxic shock syndrome[154]
  Transfusion therapy[150,155]
  Uremia[141]
  Venous air embolism[144]

Unknown Etiology
  Acute interstitial pneumonia
    (Hamman–Rich disease, see Chapter 3)

---

hydroxyl radical (OH•), and singlet oxygen ($^1O_2$). These substances damage cells by inactivating sulfhydryl enzymes, disrupting DNA, and destroying membrane integrity. Several intrinsic biochemical systems are known to be able to protect the cell from oxidant injury: enzymes such as superoxide dismutase, catalase, and glutathione peroxidase; vitamin E, which is a lipid membrane component; and other intracellular compounds such as ascorbate, glutathione, and cysteine. The amount of these substances present within cells, as well as the ability of the cell to manufacture them, may explain the variations in individual susceptibility to oxygen toxicity.

The discovery of practical methods for increasing the concentration of such substances within cells may lead to therapeutic advances for the prevention, or even reversal, of oxygen toxicity.

Exposure to other noxious gases such as phosgene, chlorine, nitrogen mustard, sulfur dioxide, nitric acid, zinc chloride, and mercury vapor, for example, can also produce this reaction.[17,87,69,73,75,77] Smoke inhalation is an important cause of DAD, and DAD is one manifestation of the acute respiratory syndrome related to crack cocaine use (see Chapter 4).[71] Exposure to various other noxious substances such as cleaning fluids containing ammonia and chlorox, certain waterproofing shoe sprays, amitrole-containing herbicides, and paint remover, for example, have been reported to rarely produce this lesion.[63,67,82,86,147]

Drug Toxicity

A wide variety of drugs can cause pulmonary injury manifested by DAD, and this subject is discussed in more detail in Chapter 4.[7,88,90–92] Chemotherapeutic agents constitute the main drugs causing DAD, and pulmonary toxicity is a significant complication of the chemotherapy used both in treating neoplastic and non-neoplastic diseases and for organ transplantation. The most commonly implicated chemotherapeutic agents include bleomycin, busulfan, and BCNU.

Clinically, pulmonary drug toxicity is usually characterized by dyspnea, cough, and diffuse chest infiltrates. Fever may also occur, and the clinical differential diagnosis in addition to drug toxicity includes infection, recurrence of the underlying disease, and radiation pneumonitis. Unfortunately, there are no specific pathologic changes that unequivocally implicate drugs in the etiology of DAD. Although cytologic atypia in alveolar lining cells has been described in toxicity due to busulfan, bleomycin, and several other drugs, this finding is not specific for drug toxicity. Intranuclear tubular structures have been noted ultrastructurally in type 2 pneumocytes of some patients with bleomycin and busulfan toxicity,[89] but similar structures have also been described in cases of bronchoalveolar carcinoma and may occur in usual interstitial pneumonia (UIP). The diagnosis of drug-induced DAD, therefore, must be based on a clinical history of drug therapy and the careful exclusion of other identifiable etiologies.

In addition to chemotherapeutic agents, a large number of other drugs may cause DAD. Nitrofurantoin is the most notorious, but others have been implicated as well, especially amiodarone, gold, and penicillamine. The acute pulmonary edema that occasionally occurs following intravenous heroin administration is probably also a manifestation of DAD.[93,94] Recurrent episodes of DAD have been reported in patients receiving narcotics for chronic pain management.[38]

Other Ingestants

Ingestion of substances such as kerosene, denatured rapeseed oil, and paraquat has been reported to cause DAD.[17,87] *Paraquat* is a potent herbicide sold in a solid granular form (Weedol, containing 2.5% paraquat), in aqueous solutions containing variable concentrations (Ortho paraquat, 29%; Ortho dual paraquat, 42%; and Gramoxine, 20%), and as an aerosol spray (Ortho spot weed and grass killer, 0.44%). Ingestion of even small amounts of the concentrated solutions is associated with high mortality due to the development of respiratory failure.[95–97,101,104]

The initial symptoms of paraquat ingestion are burning of the mouth and throat followed by nausea, vomiting, and diarrhea. Transient liver and kidney dysfunction is common. The onset of hypoxia and chest infiltrates is usually delayed for several days to a week after ingestion, but rapid, inexorable progression to interstitial and intraalveolar fibrosis occurs in fatal cases. The histopathologic findings in most reported cases resemble those of organizing DAD,[96,97,104–106] although acute DAD has been described in the few cases biopsied early in the clinical course.[104] The diagnosis in suspected cases of paraquat poisoning can be confirmed by tissue analysis for paraquat, even at the time of postmortem examination.[95] The toxicity of paraquat is thought to be mediated through the formation of cytotoxic free radical ions, a mechanism similar to that postulated for oxygen toxicity.[101] Various therapies have been attempted to counteract or inhibit the effects of the toxic free radicals, but they have been unsuccessful.[101]

Denatured rapeseed oil is a type of oil denatured with aniline and intended for industrial use. It was illicitly sold in Spain as olive oil in 1981, causing a large outbreak of pneumonitis.[98,99,102] The illness, referred to as *toxic oil syndrome*, affected more than 19,000 persons and caused over 300 deaths. Affected individuals presented with signs of pneumonia, fever, eosinophilia, rash, and gastrointestinal symptoms, and a delayed progressive neuromuscular illness occurred in some cases. Lung findings on biopsy or autopsy specimens resemble those of acute DAD, with edema, hyaline membranes, and epithelial proliferation.[103] Peculiar vascular findings, characterized by endothelial degeneration and proliferation, foam cells, vasculitis, and intimal fibrosis with luminal narrowing, have also been described, and fatal pulmonary hypertension has developed in some cases.[100]

Shock and Trauma (Shock Lung)

The development of respiratory insufficiency is a well-recognized complication of serious extrapulmonary trauma and shock, and was first described in detail in war casualties.[108,109,113,117,120] This condition has been given various names, including *congestive atelectasis, traumatic wet lung, Da Nang lung, respiratory insufficiency syndrome, posttraumatic pulmonary insufficiency, progressive pulmonary consolidation,* and *shock lung.*[108,114,117] A similar syndrome may also occur in nontraumatic shock, such as that resulting from hypovolemia due to hemorrhage, from sepsis (see text following), or from heart failure.[112,122] The clinical presentation is characterized by shortness of breath and diffuse chest infiltrates that develop several hours to days following an episode of shock, often after circulatory stabilization has been achieved. Such patients follow a course typical of ARDS, and mortality is high. The pathologic findings are identical to those of DAD due to other etiologies.[107,115,116,121,123]

The pathogenesis of DAD in patients with shock is not clearly defined, but it is likely that a number of factors are involved. In some cases, direct lung injury may accompany extrathoracic trauma, as in blast injuries or chest wall contusions.[119] In cases that lack evidence of direct lung trauma, a number of other mechanisms for pulmonary damage have been postulated.[107,111,114,115,118,124] Necrosis of peripheral tissues may cause the release of vasoactive peptides that can alter vascular permeability in the lung.[108] Microemboli consisting of platelet and leukocyte masses may be formed by the action of proteolytic agents and other factors released from damaged tissue.[108,111,118] Fat emboli originating from extensive bone fractures or from the mobilization of free fatty acids from damaged soft tissue may lodge in the lung.[118,119] DIC may result in the production of microthrombi.[108,115] Microemboli and microthrombi may damage the lung by either of two mechanisms: (1) mechanical obstruction in the distal capillary bed of the lung, thus impairing gas exchange, or (2) release of platelet factors and leukocyte enzymes that directly injure the capillary endothelial cells. Metabolic acidosis resulting from prolonged hypotension may be another factor that damages the endothelial cells. Decreased pulmonary blood flow per se probably does not cause significant cell damage, however, since DAD rarely follows prolonged cardiopulmonary bypass procedures.[109]

The development of sepsis can aggravate pulmonary insufficiency following trauma, and it is possible that a direct toxic effect of endotoxin on the pulmonary endothelium is operative in such cases.[118] Resuscitative measures used in treating patients in shock may intensify lung damage;[124] for example, rapid fluid administration using large volumes of noncolloid solutions may cause plasma dilution with reduction of oncotic pressure. Overhydration may be another damaging factor. Also, particulate matter in unfiltered blood or blood products may lodge in lung capillaries. The high concentrations of inspired oxygen often required to support such patients may cause additional pulmonary damage.

DAD manifested initially as acute pulmonary edema may follow isolated head injury without other evidence of trauma.[110] The mechanism in such cases is thought to be related, at least in part, to a massive sympathetic neuronal discharge, occurring at the time of injury, that causes pulmonary vasoconstriction. Respiratory failure has been reported in other types of central nervous system dysfunction as well, including drug overdose and cerebrovascular accidents. Hypoventilation and aspiration may be additional etiologic factors in such cases.

Sepsis

DAD is a frequent complication of sepsis, and the mortality is high, approaching 90% in some series.[122] Patients with hypotension accompanying septicemia are more prone to develop DAD, and thrombocytopenia is a common accompanying feature. The pathologic features of DAD occurring in sepsis are indistinguishable from those associated with other predisposing factors, and the pathogenic mechanisms are thought to be similar.[121,123,124]

Radiation (Radiation Pneumonitis)

Radiation injury to the lungs causes either an acute pneumonitis or a chronic fibrotic process.[125,130,132,133] *Acute radiation pneumonitis* complicates therapeutic radiation to the lungs, mediastinum, esophagus, and breast in approximately 10% of patients. It is characterized clinically by dyspnea, cough, and fever occurring from 1 to 6 months following the radiation therapy. Chest infiltrates usually develop in the area of the radiation portal, although they can spread into nonirradiated lung and may rarely involve both lungs.[7,125,131] The development of this complication is related in part to the amount of radiation, the duration of therapy, and the volume of lung irradiated. There is considerable individual variation in susceptibility. Pneumonitis has been described following even low-dose radiation, although several additional factors may add to the toxic effects of radiation, including concomitant chemotherapy, prior history of irradiation, and infection.[126,127,129,136] It has also been related to steroid withdrawal in patients receiving thoracic radiation and combination chemotherapy containing corticosteroids.[127,134] Fatal radiation pneumonitis has been reported in a patient with breast cancer who received only localized irradiation in addition to medroxyprogesterone acetate therapy.[128]

The histopathologic appearance of acute radiation pneumonitis is that of acute or organizing DAD. Hyaline membranes and hyperplasia of type 2 pneumocytes are prominent early, while interstitial fibroblast proliferation is seen later (Fig. 2–18).[125,130] Cytologic atypia of the alveolar lining cells exemplified by hyperchromatic, enlarged nuclei, multinucleated forms, and prominent nucleoli is common but not specific. Abundant, often vacuolated cytoplasm is usually present in these cells. The presence of foam cells within the intima and media of blood vessels is a more specific change, but it is found in only a minority of cases. The pathogenesis of radiation pneumonitis is thought to be related to direct

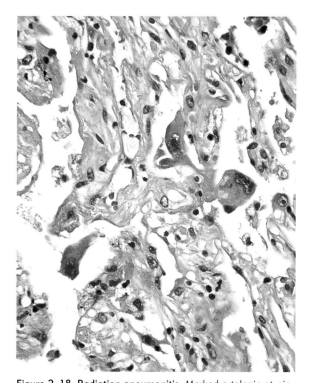

Figure 2–18 Radiation pneumonitis. Marked cytologic atypia is seen in this example. Alveolar pneumocytes are enlarged and contain abundant, often vacuolated cytoplasm. This patient had chemotherapy in addition to radiation, and, as often occurs, it is difficult to pinpoint the specific etiology of the changes.

injury to the capillary endothelium and perhaps also to alveolar lining cells. Corticosteroid therapy appears to ameliorate the syndrome.

Most patients recover from acute radiation pneumonitis and become asymptomatic, although fibrosis is usually found in the affected area after 6 months or longer.[130,135] This *chronic stage* of the disorder causes few symptoms unless a sufficiently large volume of lung is affected. The fibrotic changes may follow clinically apparent acute radiation pneumonitis, or they may develop insidiously without a previous acute illness. The histopathologic appearance is that of nonspecific fibrosis. Hyperplasia and cytologic atypia of type 2 pneumocytes, as described previously, are usually prominent. Vascular changes, including hyalinization and foam cell deposition, are seen more frequently in the chronic than in the acute stage.

Exacerbation of UIP

An acute onset of respiratory failure without an identifiable precipitating factor has been described in patients with UIP, and is referred to as 'accelerated idiopathic pulmonary fibrosis (IPF)', 'acute exacerbation of IPF', or 'acute exacerbation of UIP'.[137,139,139a,139b,140] This occurrence has been reported from 3 months to almost 8 years following diagnosis of UIP. It can also affect patients without a prior diagnosis of UIP, in whom the presence of UIP is first recognized at the time of biopsy for the acute respiratory failure.[139a] The latter cases may explain the reported development of chronic lung disease in patients with acute interstitial pneumonia (see Chapter 3). Some examples of DAD occurring in UIP patients who received interferon therapy (see Chapter 4) may also be due to exacerbation of UIP.[138] Radiographically, ground glass opacities are seen on CT examinations in addition to the typical reticular and honeycomb changes of UIP. Mortality rates are high. There may be a role for cyclosporin in treatment.[139]

The most common pathologic finding is DAD, usually in the acute stage with hyaline membranes, that occurs in a background of UIP (see Chapter 3). The UIP is recognized by the presence of honeycomb areas in addition to the DAD (Fig. 2–19). Sometimes, the typical patchy distribution of interstitial scarring characteristic of UIP can be appreciated as well. If multiple lobes are biopsied, UIP may be present in one while DAD is seen in another. The possibility of underlying UIP should always be considered when end-stage scarring or honeycomb change is present in cases of otherwise typical DAD. Focal bronchiolitis obliterans-organizing pneumonia superimposed on UIP constitutes a less common pathologic finding that is seen in a minority of cases.[139b]

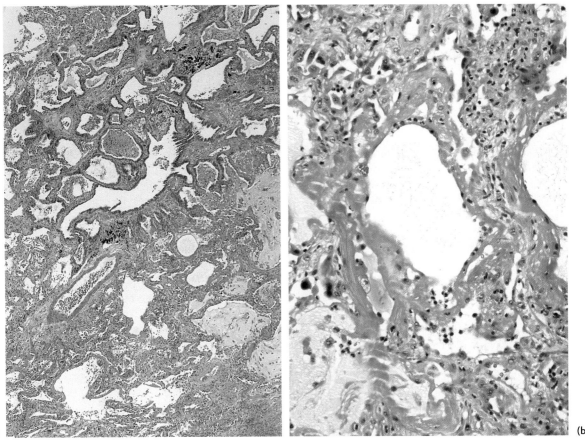

(a)   (b)

Figure 2–19 Acute exacerbation of (UIP). (a) Low magnification view showing an area of end-stage, honeycomb change next to which there is acute DAD (bottom). **(b)** Higher magnification of the DAD in UIP. Note the typical hyaline membrane formation.

BRONCHIOLITIS OBLITERANS–ORGANIZING PNEUMONIA

Bronchiolitis obliterans–organizing pneumonia (BOOP) is a predominantly airspace-filling, active fibrosing process that involves distal bronchioles, alveolar ducts, and peribronchiolar alveoli in varying proportions.[176,180,182] A number of other terms have been used in the past for this lesion, including *bronchiolitis obliterans*,[178,182] *bronchiolitis fibrosa obliterans*, and *organizing pneumonia-like process*,[179] and the different names reflect the bias of pathologists regarding the main site of lung involvement. *Idiopathic BOOP* has become a well-accepted clinicopathologic entity since the report by Epler et al[176] in 1985, and the term *cryptogenic organizing pneumonia (COP)* is used synonymously.[173] The disease, however, is not new and corresponds to cases reported as bronchiolitis obliterans by Gosink et al[178] in 1973 and numerous investigators before that time.

Terminology

Terminology has been confusing for several reasons. First, BOOP is encountered in a number of different settings (Table 2–2), and the same term has been used for all, regardless of etiology. That is, it has been used for both a focal or incidental change of little significance as well as for a more widespread lesion that causes a clinical illness. Some investigators have advocated using the term 'BOOP pattern' to emphasize the nonspecific nature of the pathologic finding and the need for clinicopathologic correlation. This additional term is not necessary, however, if one remembers that 'BOOP' is an entirely generic and descriptive name for a pathologic change. The terms 'idiopathic BOOP' and 'COP' are used for the disease of unknown etiology in which BOOP is the pathologic manifestation.[162,170,173] Some investigators prefer 'COP' over 'idiopathic BOOP' to avoid confusion between the idiopathic disease and the pathologic change.

Table 2–2   Etiologic Considerations in Bronchiolitis Obliterans–Organizing Pneumonia

- **Reaction to a specific injury**
    Prior infection (viral, bacterial, postobstructive)
    Toxic inhalants (nitrogen dioxide in silo-filler's lung, aerosols from spray printing, cocaine, etc.)
    Drug reactions (gold, amiodarone, sufasalazine, minocycline, nitrofurantoin, bleomycin, etc.)
    Radiation of the breast
    Collagen vascular disease (rheumatoid arthritis, lupus, polymyositis, etc.)
    Aspiration

- **Idiopathic disease** (Idiopathic BOOP or COP)

- **Nonspecific reactive change** (edge of granulomas, infarcts, neoplasms, vasculitis, abscesses, etc.)

- **Minor component of other respiratory illness** (hypersensitivity pneumonia, nonspecific interstitial pneumonia, eosinophilic pneumonia, Langerhans cell histiocytosis, etc.)

Another cause of confusion is that different proportions of bronchiolitis obliterans and organizing pneumonia can be found in cases of BOOP. Some investigators have used the term 'bronchiolitis obliterans' synonymously with BOOP, while others restrict it to cases lacking organizing pneumonia.[176,178,182] In fact, examples of 'pure' bronchiolitis obliterans (lacking organizing pneumonia) are uncommon and are of little clinical significance, since most represent inadequately sampled cases of BOOP.[176] Conversely, organizing pneumonia may be the predominant finding, with minimal or even absent bronchiolitis obliterans. The term BOOP encompasses all cases regardless of the proportion of bronchiolar and alveolar involvement.

One other problem is that the term 'bronchiolitis obliterans' has also been used for an unrelated bronchiolar disorder characterized by peribronchiolar fibrosis with luminal narrowing. This entity is now referred to as constrictive bronchiolitis obliterans or bronchiolitis obliterans syndrome and is discussed in Chapters 6 and 16.

Etiology

BOOP is a nonspecific manifestation of ALI that is similar to DAD except that it is localized to the peribronchiolar parenchyma. Like DAD there are a multitude of potential causes (Table 2–2), and the

etiology is seldom identifiable from the pathologic findings. It is important to remember, however, that BOOP is also a common nonspecific reaction occurring on the periphery of a wide variety of unrelated processes ranging from inflammatory reactions to neoplasms. The finding of BOOP, therefore, needs to be interpreted in the overall context of the entire clinical and pathologic picture. This is especially true in transbronchial lung biopsy specimens where it is difficult to be certain whether an actual lesion or only its edge has been sampled.[174,196] BOOP is also frequently encountered as a focal finding in other diseases, such as eosinophilic pneumonia (see Chapter 6), Langerhans cell histiocytosis (see Chapter 15), nonspecific interstitial pneumonia (see Chapter 3), or hypersensitivity pneumonia (see Chapter 6), for example. BOOP in this situation should not cause diagnostic difficulty since it comprises a minor component that is overshadowed by the other characteristic pathologic features of these diseases. The following discussion relates to examples of BOOP that constitute the primary cause of respiratory illness.

A wide variety of infectious, toxic, and inflammatory processes commonly produce BOOP, as outlined in Table 2–2.[162] BOOP has been reported following infectious pneumonias, such as influenza and Legionnaire's disease, for example, and it likely follows other more common pneumonias as well.[168,200] Proximal bronchial obstruction by a tumor or aspirated foreign body may cause changes of BOOP in the distal parenchyma, and the process in this situation represents organization of postobstructive infectious bronchopneumonia.[178] In fact, the main pathologic finding in lobectomy specimens for obstructing intrabronchial tumors is often BOOP, and careful dissection of the bronchial tree may be necessary in such cases to avoid overlooking small tumors. BOOP may result from exposure to toxic fumes, of which silo-filler's disease due to inhalation of nitrogen dioxide is probably the best-known example.[181,197,201] Cases of BOOP were described in the early 1990s in Spanish textile workers who were exposed to aerosols from spray printing techniques.[190,198] The substance Acramin FWR was implicated in the etiology, and this type of spray printing was subsequently banned. BOOP can also be a complication of crack cocaine use.[194] Certain prescribed drugs cause a similar picture, most notably gold and amiodarone (see Chapter 4).[175] BOOP has been reported following radiation of the breast for carcinoma.[163,172,187,203] In this situation it tends to occur outside the radiation field and has been reported from 3 weeks to 18 months after completion of therapy, although most cases occur after several months. Some examples of BOOP are associated with underlying collagen vascular diseases, especially rheumatoid arthritis, systemic lupus erythematosus, and polymyositis (see Chapter 7).[162,176,182,207] Recurrent aspiration of gastric acid related to hiatal hernia, esophageal dysfunction, or gastroesophageal reflux disease may produce BOOP, and there may be associated interstitial pneumonia and fibrosis.[178,188] Rare examples of BOOP occurring at birth or during intrauterine development have been described.[199,204] Possible relation to menstruation was reported in one patient.[205]

Idiopathic BOOP (COP)

Most examples of BOOP that come to biopsy represent examples of idiopathic BOOP. The onset of illness is usually subacute, with symptoms occurring over several weeks to a few months.[162,167,170,171,176–178,180,182,206] Cough, dyspnea, and fever are the most common presenting complaints, and some patients give a history of an antecedent respiratory tract infection. A fulminant course with respiratory failure has been reported in a few cases.[169,192] Patchy airspace opacities that are often multiple and may be bilateral are most

characteristic.[167,171,176,178,193] A peripheral localization has been noted by some investigators.[165] Multiple nodular densities, solitary nodules, and bilateral interstitial infiltrates mimicking the interstitial pneumonias are seen less commonly.[161,177]

The prognosis of idiopathic BOOP is good. Most patients recover within several weeks or months, although death due to progressive disease occurs in about 10–15% of cases.[162,186,206] The presence of interstitial opacities radiographically,[169,171] underlying chronic diseases (connective tissue diseases or malignancies, especially hematologic malignancies) clinically,[176,186,189] or interstitial fibrosis pathologically is associated with a worse prognosis.[208] Corticosteroids are usually used for treatment, although the lesion may regress without therapy. Relapses are common and usually respond to additional corticosteroid therapy.[186] Seasonal recurrences were reported in one series, and those patients also had biochemical evidence of cholestasis.[202]

Pathologic Features

The histologic hallmark of BOOP is a distinct, usually patchy, type of fibrosis that predominantly involves

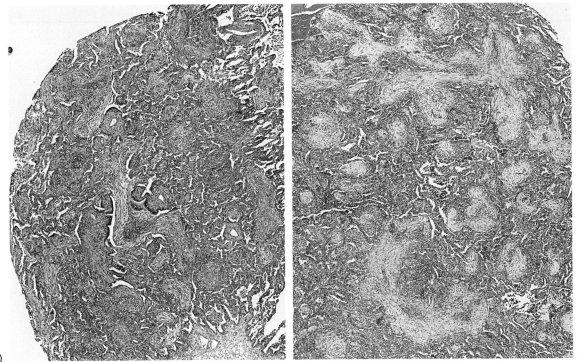

(a) (b)

Figure 2–20 Low magnification view of BOOP. (a) Intraluminal fibrosis involving a respiratory bronchiole (center) and surrounding airspaces is seen in this example. **(b)** This field emphasizes the irregular elongated and serpiginous shapes of some of the fibroblast plugs in BOOP. Note also the lightly stained appearance of the plugs.

bronchiolar lumens and peribronchiolar airspaces (Figs 2–20 and 2–21).[176,178,180,182,195,206] The fibrosis is easily recognized at low magnification because it stains lightly and assumes the round to oval, elongated, branching or serpiginous shapes of the airspaces in which it forms. The process is sharply demarcated from the adjacent areas of normal parenchyma (Fig. 2–21b). The fibrosis is composed of elongated fibroblasts and myofibroblasts arranged in parallel and embedded in a myxoid or pale-staining matrix (Fig. 2–22). The matrix is usually rich in acid mucopolysaccharides and contains variable numbers of lymphocytes, macrophages, plasma cells, and neutrophils in addition to fibroblasts (Fig. 2–23). Increased numbers of capillaries can be demonstrated as well by means of immunohistochemical staining.[183] This mixture of fibrosis and inflammatory cells forms plugs or polyps that occlude distal bronchioles, alveolar ducts, and adjacent alveolar spaces. The polyps may be covered by a lining of bronchiolar or alveolar epithelial cells, and this epithelialization is thought to be a mechanism whereby the polyps are eventually incorporated into the interstitium as the process resolves. Elastic tissue stains can be useful in evaluating

suspected cases of BOOP because they outline the typical discontinuous elastic tissue of bronchioles or alveolar ducts surrounding the fibrous plugs, thus confirming the airspace location of the fibrosis.

Frequently, proteinaceous exudates are seen in some airspaces of otherwise typical BOOP (Fig. 2–24). Yoshinouchi et al[206] noted that prognosis was worse when such proteinaceous areas were prominent. Some investigators use the term 'acute fibrinous and organizing pneumonia (AFOP)' when a proteinaceous or fibrinous exudate predominates (Fig. 2–25).[166] Often, remnants of acute and chronic inflammatory cells are present in such cases and suggest that AFOP may be related to a prior infectious bronchopneumonia. The reaction may also occur in immunocompromised persons. AFOP appears to represent a variant of BOOP in most cases, while some are related to DAD. It may be more meaningful, therefore, to diagnose a variant of BOOP or DAD rather than to suggest a separate entity.

In addition to the fibroblast plugs and proteinaceous exudates, other abnormalities can be found in airspaces in BOOP. Accumulation of foamy, lipid-containing macrophages is common and may be extensive

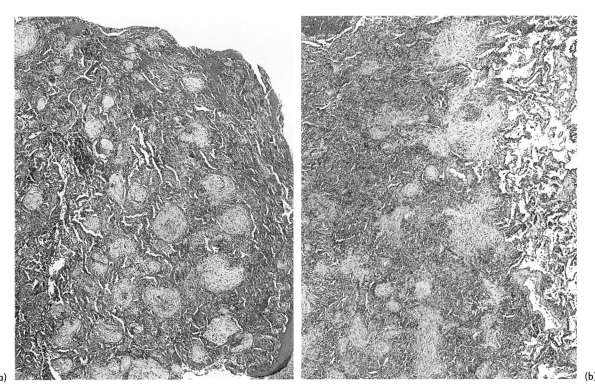

(a)   (b)

Figure 2–21 BOOP. (a) In this focus, most of the fibroblast plugs are round and regular, indicating that they are present within alveolar spaces. This area, therefore, constitutes an area of organizing pneumonia. (b) The process is sharply demarcated from the normal lung on the right.

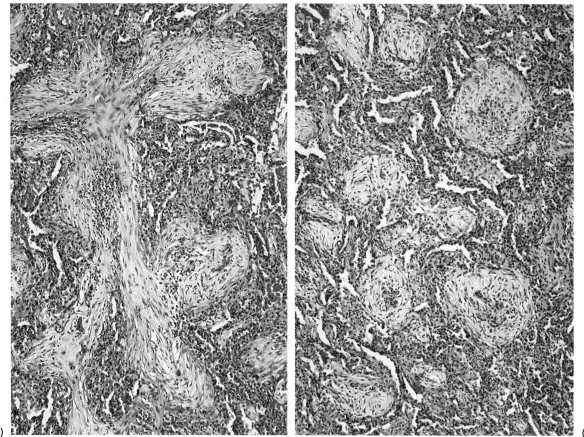

(a)   (b)

Figure 2–22 Fibroblast plugs in BOOP. (a) Higher magnification emphasizing the branching shape of the fibroblast plug that indicates involvement of an alveolar duct. There is a mild chronic inflammatory cell infiltrate admixed with the spindle cells. (b) In this focus, the fibroblast plugs are filling alveoli and appear round and fairly regular.

(Fig. 2–26). It is related to proximal bronchiolar obstruction and represents a form of postobstructive or endogenous lipoid pneumonia (Chapter 16). Focally, neutrophils may be present within alveolar spaces as well, and occasionally eosinophils may be seen, but they are usually not numerous.

While the predominant abnormality in BOOP affects airspaces, the interstitium shows changes as well. The alveolar septa are usually thickened by a chronic inflammatory cell infiltrate of variable intensity along with type 2 pneumocyte hyperplasia (Fig. 2–27). This interstitial pneumonia is usually confined to the area of airspace fibrosis, and, although it may extend slightly more peripherally, it is not a diffuse process.

Although the term BOOP emphasizes the bronchiolar involvement in this disease, sometimes unaffected bronchioles are seen within the areas of airspace fibrosis (Fig. 2–28). This seemingly contradictory finding may cause difficulty in diagnosing BOOP but can be explained by the uneven or interrupted distribution of the fibrosis that occurs within bronchioles. The correct diagnosis can be appreciated in such cases because even if uninvolved bronchioles are present, the process is invariably localized to peribronchiolar parenchyma.

Pathogenesis

Ultrastructural studies in cases of idiopathic BOOP have demonstrated necrosis of alveolar epithelium and evidence of alveolar collapse in peribronchiolar parenchyma.[191] These changes are similar to those described in DAD and support the role of ALI in the pathogenesis. Additionally, proteoglycans such as versican and various growth factors, including vascular endothelial growth factor, bFGF, and PDGF, have been identified in the tissue.[3,164,184] The myofibroblasts stain for smooth muscle actin and often also for type I procollagen.[3]

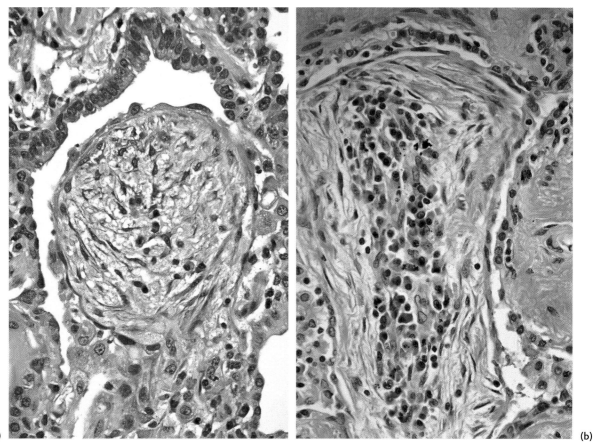

(a)   (b)

Figure 2–23 Variable inflammation in fibroblast plugs of BOOP. (a) Scant chronic inflammatory cells are seen along with the spindle-shaped fibroblasts and myofibroblasts that fill the airway lumen in this example. (b) Numerous plasma cells are seen in this case. Note that the surface of the plugs in both examples is covered by epithelium.

Many of these findings have been demonstrated in organizing DAD and emphasize the similar pathogenesis of these two disorders. Whether the clinical differences between them can be explained by differences in extent of lung injury or in differences in molecular response to injury is uncertain. Some investigators have suggested that differences in vascularization between the intraluminal buds of BOOP and the interstitial organization of DAD may be important.[183]

Differential Diagnosis

Cases of BOOP must be differentiated from other forms of fibrosing lung disease, including, most commonly, organizing DAD and UIP. The latter entities enter the differential diagnosis with BOOP because fibroblast proliferation is seen in both. Helpful features in their differential diagnosis are summarized in Table 2–3.

The most important differential feature of organizing DAD and BOOP is the interstitial location of the fibroblast proliferation in DAD compared with the intraluminal location in BOOP. In difficult cases, histochemical stains for elastic tissue (which outline the walls of bronchioles and alveolar ducts) or immunohistochemical stains for keratin (which outline alveolar epithelium and thus mark the alveolar septa) can help in demonstrating the location of the fibrosis (Fig. 2–29). The fact that changes of BOOP are patchy and peribronchiolar in distribution rather than random or diffuse as in DAD also helps. The presence of other features of ALI, including hyaline membranes, thrombi, and epithelial metaplasia with atypia, is characteristic of DAD but not BOOP. Clinically, the need for ventilator therapy helps, since patients with DAD are usually on a ventilator whereas this therapy is uncommon in BOOP. It should be remembered, however, that in severe ALI, features

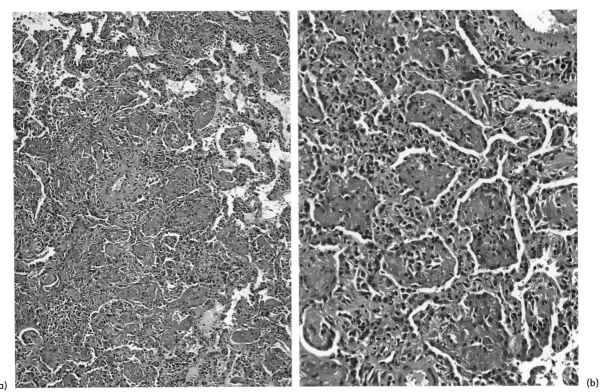

(a)   (b)

Figure 2–24 Proteinaceous exudates in BOOP. (a) At low magnification in this example proteinaceous exudates are present in some alveolar spaces adjacent to more typical BOOP. **(b)** At higher magnification fibroblasts are seen growing into the exudates in addition to chronic inflammatory cells, indicating early organization. Note the associated alveolar septal chronic inflammation (cellular chronic interstitial pneumonia).

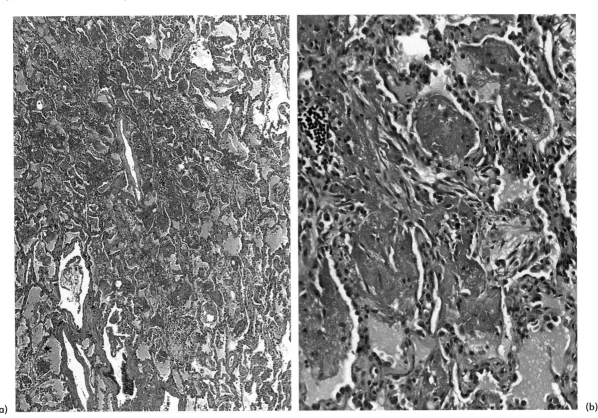

(a)   (b)

Figure 2–25 Acute fibrinous and organizing pneumonia (AFOP). (a) Low magnification showing prominent proteinaceous exudation in peribronchiolar (bottom) parenchyma. **(b)** Higher magnification showing the proteinaceous exudate within alveolar spaces. There is mild thickening of adjacent alveolar septa. The changes most likely represent an early form of BOOP.

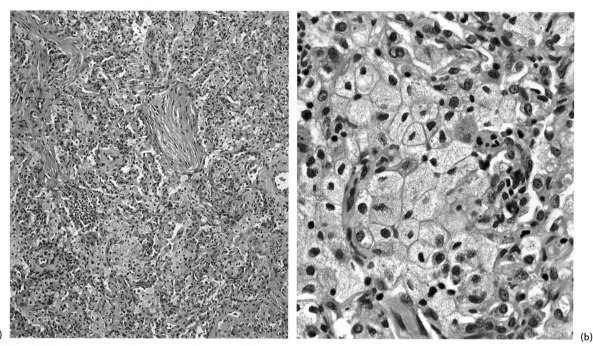

(a)   (b)

Figure 2–26 Foamy macrophage accumulation in BOOP. (a) Large numbers of foamy macrophages fill alveolar spaces in this example. Note the typical intraalveolar fibroblast plug in the center. **(b)** Higher magnification illustrating characteristic foamy cytoplasm of the alveolar macrophages.

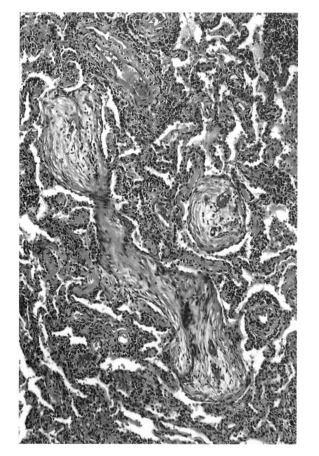

Figure 2–27 Alveolar septal inflammation in BOOP. Note the thickened alveolar septa containing a prominent chronic inflammatory cell infiltrate. This change commonly accompanies BOOP but does not usually extend beyond the areas of intraluminal organization.

of both BOOP and DAD can be found together, and the outcome for such cases will ultimately depend on the extent of the DAD.

Sometimes the fibroblast foci of UIP (see Chapter 3) can be difficult to distinguish from the fibroblast plugs of BOOP. Fibroblast foci are smaller and lack the branching, serpiginous shapes of the fibroblast plugs in BOOP. They are interstitial rather than intraluminal in location and lack a peribronchiolar distribution. In difficult cases, the finding of architectural distortion (interstitial scars and honeycomb change) should suggest UIP. BOOP can occasionally complicate cases of UIP and this occurrence may explain acute exacerbations of some cases of UIP. Such cases are characterized by well-defined areas of intraluminal fibrosis along with the typical temporally and spatially varied fibrosis of UIP (see Chapter 3).

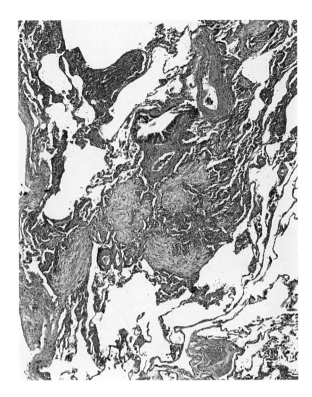

Figure 2–28 Low magnification view of BOOP showing a seemingly unaffected bronchiole adjacent to the BOOP. Unaffected bronchioles are commonly seen in otherwise typical BOOP and should not cast doubt on the diagnosis as long as the intraluminal organization is present within peribronchiolar parenchyma.

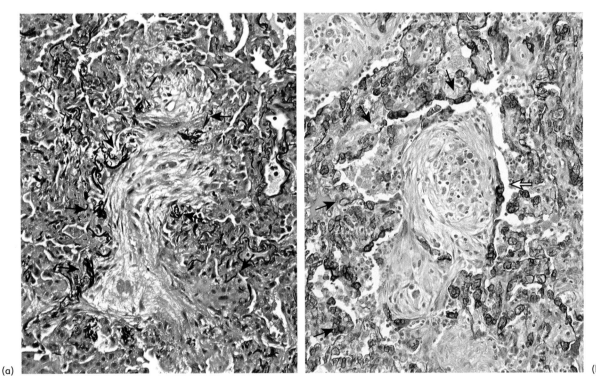

(a)   (b)

Figure 2–29 Special stains in BOOP. (a) An elastic tissue stain outlines the discontinuous elastic layer of a respiratory bronchiole/alveolar duct (arrows). (b) A cytokeratin stain outlines alveolar epithelium (black arrows), indicating that most of the fibrous plug is present within an epithelial-lined space. The plug is focally lined by epithelium (open arrow) that appears to originate from nearby alveolar lining cells.

Table 2–3 Contrasting Features of Acute Lung Injury Patterns and UIP

	Acute DAD	Organizing DAD	BOOP	UIP
Pathologic Findings				
Hyaline membranes	+, extensive	+/–, focal	No	No*
Fibroblast proliferation	No	Yes, extensive interstitial	Yes, patchy intraluminal	Focal, interstitial (fibroblast foci)
Thrombi	Common	Common	No	No
Epithelial metaplasia	Yes	Yes	No	No
Peribronchiolar distribution	No	No	Yes	No
Collagen disposition	No	No	No	Yes
Honeycomb change	No	No**	No	Yes
Clinical Findings				
Onset	Acute	Acute	Subacute	Insidious
Course	Days–weeks	Days–weeks	Weeks–months	Years
Ventilator therapy	Usually	Usually	Not usually	Not usually
Response to steroids	+/–	+/–	Yes	No
Prognosis	Poor	Poor	Good	Poor

*Hyaline membranes can be seen in acute exacerbation of UIP (see text), but are not a feature of uncomplicated UIP.
**Honeycomb change may be encountered in autopsy specimens of DAD (see Chapter 3), but it is usually not a feature in earlier biopsy specimens. It tends to lack the characteristic bronchiolar epithelial lining and collagen deposition seen in the honeycomb change of UIP.

REFERENCES

Diffuse Alveolar Damage

General

1. Ashbaugh D, Bigelow D, Petty T, Levine B: Acute respiratory distress in adults. Lancet 2:319, 1967.
2. Barth PJ, Holtermann W, Muller B: The spatial distribution of pulmonary lesions in severe ARDS. Pathol Res Pract 194:465, 1998.
3. Bensadour ES, Burke AK, Hogg JC, Roberts CR: Proteoglycan deposition in pulmonary fibrosis. Am J Respir Crit Care Med 154:1819, 1996.
4. Beskow CO, Drachenberg CB, Bourquin PM, et al: Diffuse alveolar damage. Morphologic features in bronchoalveolar lavage fluid. Acta Cytol 44:640, 2000.
5. Bruch LA, Flint A, Hirschl RB: Pulmonary pathology of patients treated with partial liquid ventilation. Mod Pathol 10:463, 1997.
6. Burkhardt A: Alveolitis and collapse in the pathogenesis of pulmonary fibrosis. Am Rev Respir Dis 1xck;/40:513, 1989.
7. Doran HM, Sheppard MN, Collins PW, Jones L, Newland AC, Van Der Walt JD: Pathology of the lung in leukemia and lymphoma: A study of 87 autopsies. Histopathology 18:211, 1991.
8. Esteban A, Fernández-Segoviano P, Frutos-Vivar F, et al: Comparison of clinical criteria for the acute respiratory distress syndrome with autopsy findings. Ann Intern Med 141:440, 2004.
9. Fukuda Y, Ishizaki M, Masuda Y, et al: The role of intraalveolar fibrosis in the process of pulmonary structural remodeling in patients with diffuse alveolar damage. Am J Pathol 126:171, 1987.
10. Guinee D, Brambilla, E, Fleming M, et al: The potential role of BAX and BCL-2 expression in diffuse alveolar damage. Am J Pathol 151:999, 1997.
11. Guinee D Jr, Fleming M, Hayashi T, et al: Association of p53 and WAF1 expression with apoptosis in diffuse alveolar damage. Am J Pathol 149:531, 1996.
12. Hayashi T, Setler-Stevenson WG, Fleming MV, et al: Immunohistochemical study of metalloproteinases and their tissue inhibitors in the lungs of patients with diffuse alveolar damage and idiopathic pulmonary fibrosis. Am J Pathol 149:1241, 1996.

13. Heffner JE, Sahn SA, Repine JE: The role of platelets in the adult respiratory distress syndrome. Culprits or bystanders? Am Rev Respir Dis 135:482, 1987.

14. Henke C, Marineili W, Jessurun J, et al: Macrophage production of basic fibroblast growth factor in the fibroproliferative disorder of alveolar fibrosis after lung injury. Am J Pathol 143:1189, 1993.

15. Herridge, MS, Cheung AM, Tansey CM, et al: One-year outcomes in survivors of the acute respiratory distress syndrome. N Engl J Med 348:683, 2003.

16. Honda T, Ota H, Yamazaki Y, et al: Proliferation of type II pneumocytes in the lung biopsy specimens reflecting alveolar damage. Respir Med 97:80, 2003.

16a. Hopkins RO, Weaver LK, Collingridge D, et al: Two-year cognitive, emotional, and quality of life outcomes in acute respiratory distress syndrome. Am J Respir Crit Care Med 171:340, 2005.

17. Katzenstein A, Bloor C, Liebow A: Diffuse alveolar damage. The role of oxygen, shock, and related factors. Am J Pathol 85:210, 1976.

18. Katzenstein A-LA: Pathogenesis of "fibrosis" in interstitial pneumonia. An electron microscopic study. Hum Pathol 16:1015, 1985.

19. Kobashi Y, Manabe T: The fibrosing process in so-called organized diffuse alveolar damage. An immunohistochemical study of the change from hyaline membrane to membranous fibrosis. Virchows Arch A Pathol Anat Histopathol 422:47, 1993.

20. Kooy NW, Royall JA, Ye YZ, et al: Evidence for in vivo peroxynitrite production in human acute lung injury. Am J Respir Crit Care Med 151:1250, 1995.

21. Krein PM, Sabatini PJB, Tinmouth W, Green FHY, Winston BW: Localization of insulin-like growth factor-I in lung tissues of patients with fibroproliferative acute respiratory distress syndrome. Am J Respir Crit Care Med 167:83, 2003.

22. Kuhn C: Patterns of lung repair; a morphologist's view. Chest 99(Suppl):11S, 1991.

23. Lamy M, Fallat R, Koeniger E, et al: Pathologic features and mechanisms of hypoxemia in adult respiratory distress syndrome. Am Rev Respir Dis 114:267, 1976.

24. Laufe M, Simon R, Flint A, Keller J: Adult respiratory distress syndrome in neutropenic patients. Am J Med 80:1022, 1986.

25. Lee WL, Downey GP: Leukocyte elastase. Physiological functions and role in acute lung injury. Am J Respir Crit Care Med 164:896, 2001.

26. Martin C, Papazian L, Payan M-J, et al: Pulmonary fibrosis correlates with outcome in adult respiratory distress syndrome. A study in mechanically ventilated patients. Chest 107:196, 1995.

27. Matthay MA, Zimmerman GA, Esmon C, et al: Future research directions in acute lung injury. Summary of a National Heart, Lung, and Blood Institute working group. Am J Respir Crit Care Med 167:1027, 2003.

28. Nash JRG, McLaughlin PJ, Hoyle C, Roberts D: Immunolocalization of tumour necrosis factor α in lung tissue from patients dying with adult respiratory distress syndrome. Histopathology 19:395, 1991.

29. Negri E, Montes G, Saldiva PH, Capelozzi V: Architectural remodeling in acute and chronic interstitial lung disease: Fibrosis or fibroelastosis? Histopathology 37:393, 2000.

30. Ogino S, Franks TJ, Yong M, et al: Extensive squamous metaplasia with cytologic atypia in diffuse alveolar damage mimicking squamous cell carcinoma: A report of 2 cases. Hum Pathol 33:1052, 2002.

31. Orme J, Romney S, Hopkins RO, Pope D, Chan KJ, Thomsen G: Pulmonary function and health-related quality of life in survivors of acute respiratory distress syndrome. Am J Respir Crit Care Med 167:690, 2003.

32. Pache J-C, Christakos PG, Gannon DE, Mitchell JJ, Low RB, Leslie KO: Myofibroblasts in diffuse alveolar damage of the lung. Mod Pathol 11:1064, 1998.

33. Patel SR, Karmpaliotis D, Ayas NT, et al. The role of open-lung biopsy in ARDS. Chest 125:197, 2004.

34. Piantadosi CA, Schwartz DA: The acute respiratory distress syndrome. Ann Intern Med 141:460, 2004.

35. Pratt P, Vollmer R, Shelburne J, Crapo J: Pulmonary morphology in a multihospital collaborative extracorporeal membrane oxygenation project. Am J Pathol 95:191, 1979.

36. Rinaldo JE: Mediation of ARDS by leukocytes. Clinical evidence and implications for therapy. Chest 89:590, 1986.

37. Rozin GF, Gomes MM, Parra ER, et al: Collagen and elastic system in the remodelling process of major types of idiopathic interstitial pneumonias (IIP). Histopathology 46:413, 2005.

38. Savici D, Katzenstein A-LA: Diffuse alveolar damage and recurrent respiratory failure: Report of 6 cases. Hum Pathol 32:1398, 2001.

39. Schwarz MI, Albert RK: "Imitators" of the ARDS: Implications for diagnosis and treatment. Chest 125:1530, 2004.

40. Snow R, Davies P, Pontoppidan H, et al: Pulmonary vascular remodeling in adult respiratory distress syndrome. Am Rev Respir Dis 126:887, 1982.

41. Sridhar S, Ryan S: Steatosis of granular pneumocytes in alcoholics with acute alveolar injury. Arch Pathol Lab Med 103:522, 1979.

42. Stanley MW, Henry-Stanley MJ, Gajl-Peczalska KJ, Bitterman PB: Hyperplasia of type II pneumonocytes in acute lung injury. Cytologic findings of sequential bronchoalveolar lavage. Am J Clin Pathol 97:669, 1992.

43. Suchyta MR, Elliott CG, Colby T, Rasmusson BY, Morris AH, Jensen RL: Open lung biopsy does not correlate with pulmonary function after the adult respiratory distress syndrome. Chest 99:1232, 1991.

44. Sugiyama K, Kawai T: Diffuse alveolar damage and acute interstitial pneumonitis: Histochemical evaluation with lectins and monoclonal antibodies against surfactant apoprotein and collagen type IV. Mod Pathol 6:242, 1993.

45. Tomashefski JF Jr, Davies P, Boggis C, et al: The pulmonary vascular lesions of the adult respiratory distress syndrome. Am J Pathol 112:112, 1983.

46. Ware LB, Matthay MA: The acute respiratory distress syndrome. N Engl J Med 342:1334, 2000.

47. Warnock M, Press M, Churg A: Further observations on cytoplasmic hyaline in the lung. Hum Pathol 11:59, 1980.

48. Yazdy A, Tomashefski J, Yagan R, Klienerman J: Regional alveolar damage (RAD). A localized counterpart of diffuse alveolar damage. Am J Clin Pathol 92:10, 1989.

DAD Due to Infection

49. Askin F, Katzenstein A: Pneumocystis infection masquerading as diffuse alveolar damage: A potential source of diagnostic error. Chest 79:420, 1981.

50. Ding Y, Want H, Shen H, et al: The clinical pathology of severe acute respiratory syndrome (SARS): A report from China. J Pathol 200:282, 2003.

51. Duchin JS, Koster FT, Peters CJ, et al: Hantavirus pulmonary syndrome: A clinical description of 17 patients with a newly recognized disease. N Engl J Med 330:949, 1994.

52. Franks TJ, Chong PY, Chui P, et al: Lung pathology of severe acute respiratory syndrome (SARS): A study of 8 autopsy cases from Singapore. Hum Pathol 34:743, 2003.

53. Kaufman J, Cuvelier C, van der Straeten M: Mycoplasma pneumonia with fulminant evolution into diffuse interstitial fibrosis. Thorax 35:140, 1980.

54. Lheureux P, Verhest A, Vincent JL: Herpes virus infection, an unusual source of adult respiratory distress syndrome. Eur J Respir Dis 66:72, 1985.

55. Markovic SN, Adlakha A, Smith T, Walker R: Respiratory syncytial virus pneumonitis-induced diffuse alveolar damage in an autologous bone marrow transplant recipient. Mayo Clin Proc 73:153, 1998.

56. Nicholls JM, Poon LM, Kam CL, et al: Lung pathology of fatal severe acute respiratory syndrome. Lancet 361:1773, 2003.

57. Nolte KB, Feddersen RM, Foucar K, et al: Hantavirus pulmonary syndrome in the United States: A pathological description of a disease caused by a new agent. Hum Pathol 26:110, 1995.

58. Onwubalili J, Scott G, Smith H: Acute respiratory distress related to chemotherapy of advanced pulmonary tuberculosis: A study of two cases and review of the literature. Q J Med 59:599, 1986.

59. Torres A, de Celis M, Rodriguez Roisin R, et al: Adult respiratory distress syndrome in Q fever. Eur J Respir Dis 70:322, 1987.

60. Yeldani AV, Colby TV: Pathologic features of lung biopsy specimens from influenza pneumonia cases. Hum Pathol 25:47, 1994.

DAD Due to Oxygen and Other Inhalants

61. Anderson W, Strickland M: Pulmonary complications of oxygen therapy in the neonate. Postmortem study of bronchopulmonary dysplasia with emphasis on fibroproliferative obliterative bronchitis and bronchiolitis. Arch Pathol 91:506, 1971.

62. Anderson W, Strickland M, Tsai S, Haglin J: Light microscopic and ultrastructural study of the adverse effects of oxygen therapy on the neonate lung. Am J Pathol 73:327, 1973.

63. Balkisson R, Murray D, Hoffstein V: Alveolar damage due to inhalation of amitrole-containing herbicide. Chest 101:1174, 1992.

64. Barber R, Lee J, Hamilton W: Oxygen toxicity in man. A prospective study in patients with irreversible brain damage. N Engl J Med 283:1478, 1970.

65. Barter RA, Finlay-Jones LR, Walters MN-I: Pulmonary hyaline membrane: Sites of formation in adult lungs after assisted respiration and inhalation of oxygen. J Pathol Bacteriol 95:481, 1968.

66. Bonikos D, Bensch K, Northway W Jr, Edwards D: Bronchopulmonary dysplasia: The pulmonary pathologic sequel of necrotizing bronchiolitis and pulmonary fibrosis. Hum Pathol 7:643, 1976.

67. Buie SE, Pratt DS, May JJ: Diffuse pulmonary injury following paint remover exposure. Am J Med 81:702, 1986.

68. Cederberg A, Hellsten S, Miorner G: Oxygen treatment and hyaline pulmonary membranes in adults. Acta Pathol Microbiol Scand 64:450, 1975.

69. Charan N, Myers G, Lakshminarayan S, Spencer T: Pulmonary injuries associated with acute sulfur inhalation. Am Rev Respir Dis 119:555, 1979.

70. Davis WB, Rennard SI, Bitterman PB, Crystal RG: Pulmonary oxygen toxicity. Early reversible changes in human alveolar structures induced by hyperoxia. N Engl J Med 309:878, 1983.

71. Forrester J, Steele A, Waldron J, Parsons P: Crack lung: An acute pulmonary syndrome with a spectrum of clinical and histopathologic findings. Am Rev Respir Dis 142:462, 1990.

72. Gould V, Tosco R, Wheelis R, et al: Oxygen pneumonitis in man. Ultrastructural observations on the development of alveolar lesions. Lab Invest 26:499, 1972.

73. Hajela R, Janigan DT, Landrigan PL, Boudreau SF, Sebastian S: Fatal pulmonary edema due to nitric acid fume inhalation in three pulp-mill workers. Chest 97:487, 1990.

74. Hasleton PS, Penna P, Torry J: Effect of oxygen on the lungs after blast injury and burns. J Clin Pathol 34:1147, 1981.

75. Homma S, Jones R, Qvist J, Zapol WM, Reid L: Pulmonary vascular lesions in the adult respiratory distress syndrome caused by inhalation of zinc chloride smoke: A morphometric study. Hum Pathol 23:45, 1992.

76. Kapanci Y, Tosco R, Eggermann J, Gould V: Oxygen pneumonitis in man. Light and electron microscopic morphometric studies. Chest 62:162, 1972.

77. Lilis R, Miller A, Lerman Y: Acute mercury poisoning with severe chronic pulmonary manifestations. Chest 88:306, 1985.

78. Matsubaru O, Takemura T, Nasu M, et al: Pathological changes of the lungs after prolonged inhalation of high concentrations of oxygen. Virchows Arch [A] 408:461, 1986.

79. Nash G, Blennerhassett J, Pontoppidan H: Pulmonary lesions associated with oxygen therapy and artificial ventilation. N Engl J Med 276:368, 1967.

80. Northway W Jr, Rosan R, Porter D: Pulmonary disease following respiratory therapy of hyaline-membrane disease. Bronchopulmonary dysplasia. N Engl J Med 276:357, 1967.

81. Pratt P: Pulmonary capillary proliferation induced by oxygen inhalation. Am J Pathol 34:1033, 1958.

82. Reisz GR, Gammon RS: Toxic pneumonitis from mixing household cleaners. Chest 89:49, 1986.

83. Singer M, Wright F, Stanley L, et al: Oxygen toxicity in man. A prospective study in patients after open-heart surgery. N Engl J Med 283:1473, 1970.

84. Soloway H, Castillo Y, Martin A Jr: Adult hyaline membrane disease: Relationship to oxygen therapy. Ann Surg 168:937, 1968.

85. Stocker JT: Pathologic features of long-standing "healed" bronchopulmonary dysplasia: A study of twenty-eight 3- to 40-month-old infants. Hum Pathol 17:943, 1986.

86. Toor AH, Tomashefski JF, Kleinerman J: Respiratory tract pathology in patients with severe burns. Hum Pathol 21:1212, 1990.

87. Weston J, Liebow A, Dixon M, Rich T: Untoward effects of exogenous inhalants on the lung. J Forensic Sci 17:199, 1972.

DAD Due to Drugs

88. Cooper J Jr, White D, Matthay R: Drug-induced pulmonary disease. Am Rev Respir Dis 133:321, 488, 1986.

89. Gyorkey F, Gyorkey P, Sinkovics J: Origin and significance of intranuclear tubular inclusions in type II pulmonary alveolar epithelial cells of patients with bleomycin and busulfan toxicity. Ultrastruct Pathol 1:211, 1980.

90. Myers JL: Diagnosis of drug reactions in the lung. In: *The Lung: Current Concepts*, USCAP Monograph No. 36, Baltimore, Williams & Wilkins, 1993, pp 32–53.

91. Reed CR, Glauser FL: Drug-induced noncardiogenic pulmonary edema. Chest 100:1120, 1991.

92. Rosenow EC III, Myers JL, Swensen SJ, Pisani RJ: Drug-induced pulmonary disease: An update. Chest 102:239, 1992.

93. Siegel H: Human pulmonary pathology associated with narcotic and other addictive drugs. Hum Pathol 3:55, 1972.

94. Smith W, Glauser F, Dearden L, et al: Deposits of immunoglobulin and complement in the pulmonary tissue of patients with "heroin lung." Chest 73:471, 1978.

DAD Due to Other Ingestants

95. Conradi SE, Olanoff LS, Dawson WT: Fatality due to paraquat intoxication: Confirmation by postmortem tissue analysis. Am J Clin Pathol 80:771, 1983.

96. Copland G, Kolin A, Shulman H: Fatal pulmonary intra-alveolar fibrosis after paraquat ingestion. N Engl J Med 291:290, 1974.

97. Dearden L, Fairshter R, McRae D, et al: Pulmonary ultrastructure of the late aspects of human paraquat poisoning. Am J Pathol 93:667, 1978.

98. Esteban A, Guerra L, Ruiz-Santana S, et al: ARDS due to ingestion of denatured rapeseed oil. Chest 84:166, 1983.

99. Fernandez-Segoviano P, Esteban A, Martinez-Cabruja R: Pulmonary vascular lesions in the toxic oil syndrome in Spain. Thorax 38:724, 1983.

100. Gomez-Sanchez MA, Mestre de Juan MJ, Gomez-Pajuelo C, et al: Pulmonary hypertension due to toxic oil syndrome. A clinicopathologic study. Chest 95:325, 1989.

101. Harley J, Grinspan S, Root R: Paraquat suicide in a young woman: results of therapy directed against the superoxide radical. Yale J Biol Med 50:481, 1977.

102. Kilbourne E, Rigau-Perez J, Heath C Jr, et al: Clinical epidemiology of toxic oil syndrome. Manifestations of a new illness. N Engl J Med 309:1408, 1983.

103. Martinez-Tello FJ, Navas-Palacios JJ, Ricoy JR, et al: Pathology of a new toxic syndrome caused by ingestion of adulterated oil in Spain. Virchows Arch [Pathol Anat] 397:261, 1982.

104. Rebello G, Mason J: Pulmonary histological appearances in fatal paraquat poisoning. Histopathology 2:53, 1978.

105. Takahashi T, Takahashi Y, Nio M: Remodeling of the alveolar structure in the paraquat lung of humans: A morphometric study. Hum Pathol 25:702, 1994.

106. Toner P, Vetters J, Spilg W, Harland W: Fine structure of the lung lesion in a case of paraquat poisoning. J Pathol 102:182, 1970.

DAD Due to Shock and Trauma

107. Bachofen M, Weibel E: Basic pattern of tissue repair in human lungs following unspecific injury. Chest 65(Suppl):14S, 1974.

108. Blaisdell F: Respiratory insufficiency syndrome: Clinical and pathological definition. J Trauma 13:195, 1973.

109. Blennerhassett JB: Shock lung and diffuse alveolar damage: Pathological and pathogenetic considerations. Pathology 17:239, 1985.

110. Fein IA, Rackow EC: Neurogenic pulmonary edema. Chest 81:318, 1982.

111. Jacob HS: Complement-mediated leucoembolization: A mechanism of tissue damage during extracorporeal perfusions, myocardial infarction and in shock – a review. Q J Med 52:289, 1983.

112. Keren A, Klein J, Stern S: Adult respiratory distress syndrome in the course of acute myocardial infarction. Chest 77:161, 1980.

113. Martin A Jr, Simmons R, Heisterkamp C III: Respiratory insufficiency in combat casualties: I. Pathologic changes in the lungs of patients dying of wounds. Ann Surg 170:30, 1969.

114. Martin A Jr, Soloway H, Simmons R: Pathologic anatomy of the lungs following shock and trauma. J Trauma 8:687, 1968.

115. Pietra G: The lung in shock. Hum Pathol 5:121, 1974.

116. Pinet F, Tabib A, Clermont A, et al: Post-traumatic shock lung: Postmortem microangiographic and pathologic correlation. AJR Am J Roentgenol 139:449, 1982.

117. Safar P, Grenvik A, Smith J: Progressive pulmonary consolidation: Review of cases and pathogenesis. J Trauma 12:955, 1972.

118. Schneider R, Zapol W, Carvalho A: Platelet consumption and sequestration in severe acute respiratory failure. Am Rev Respir Dis 122:445, 1980.

119. Tsokos M, Paulsen F, Petri S, et al: Histologic, immunohistochemical, and ultrastructural findings in human blast lung injury. Am J Respir Crit Care Med 168:549, 2003.

120. Wardle EN: Shock lungs: The post-traumatic respiratory distress syndrome. Q J Med 23:317, 1984.

DAD Due to Sepsis

121. Bachofen M, Weibel E: Alterations of the gas exchange apparatus in adult respiratory insufficiency associated with septicemia. Am Rev Respir Dis 116:589, 1977.

122. Clowes G Jr, Hirsch E, Williams L, et al: Septic lung and shock lung in man. Ann Surg 181:681, 1975.

123. Corrin B: Lung pathology in septic shock. J Clin Pathol 33:891, 1980.

124. Tranbaugh R, Lewis F, Christensen J, Elings V: Lung water changes after thermal injury. The effects of crystalloid resuscitation and sepsis. Ann Surg 192:479, 1980.

DAD Due to Radiation

125. Bennett D, Million R, Ackerman L: Bilateral radiation pneumonitis, a complication of the radiotherapy of bronchogenic carcinoma (report and analysis of seven cases with autopsy). Cancer 23:1001, 1969.

126. Braun S, do Pico G, Olson C, Caldwell W: Low-dose radiation pneumonitis. Cancer 35:1322, 1974.

127. Castellino R, Glatstein E, Turbow M, et al: Latent radiation injury of lungs or heart activated by steroid withdrawal. Ann Intern Med 80:593, 1974.

128. DeGreve M, Warson F, Deleu D, Storme G: Fatal pulmonary toxicity by the association of radiotherapy and medroxyprogesterone acetate. Cancer 56:2434, 1985.

129. Einhorn L, Krause M, Hornback N, Furnas B: Enhanced pulmonary toxicity with bleomycin and radiotherapy in oat-cell lung cancer. Cancer 37:2414, 1976.

130. Fajardo L, Berthrong M: Radiation injury in surgical pathology. Am J Surg Pathol 2:159, 1978.

131. Fulkerson WJ, McLendon RE, Prosnitz LR: Adult respiratory distress syndrome after limited thoracic radiotherapy. Cancer 57:1941, 1986.

132. Littman P, Davis L, Nash J, et al: The hazard of acute radiation pneumonitis in children receiving mediastinal radiation. Cancer 33:1520, 1974.

133. Movsas B, Raffin TA, Epstein AH, Link CJ Jr: Pulmonary radiation injury. Chest 111:1061, 1997.

134. Pezner RD, Bertrand M, Cecchi GR, et al: Steroid-withdrawal radiation pneumonitis in cancer patients. Chest 85:816, 1984.

135. Polansky SM, Ravin CE, Prosnitz LR: Pulmonary changes after primary irradiation for early breast carcinoma. AJR Am J Roentgenol 134:101, 1980.

136. Trask CWL, Joannides T, Harper PG, et al: Radiation-induced lung fibrosis after treatment of small cell carcinoma of the lung with very high-dose cyclophosphamide. Cancer 55:57, 1985.

Acute Exacerbation of UIP

137. Ambrosini V, Cancellieri A, Chilosi M, et al: Acute exacerbation of idiopathic pulmonary fibrosis: Report of a series. Eur Respir J 22:821, 2003.

138. Honoré I, Nunes H, Groussard O, et al: Acute respiratory failure after interferon-γ therapy of end-stage pulmonary fibrosis. Am J Respir Crit Care Med 167:953, 2003.

139. Inase N, Sawada M, Ohtani Y, et al: Cyclosporin A followed by the treatment of acute exacerbation of idiopathic pulmonary fibrosis with corticosteroid. Intern Med 42:565, 2003.

139a. Kim DS, Park JH, Park BK, et al: Acute exacerbation of idiopathic pulmonary fibrosis: frequency and clinical features. Eur Resp J 27:143, 2006.

139b. Parambil JG, Myers JL, Ryu JH. Histopathologic features and outcome of patients with acute exacerbation of idiopathic pulmonary fibrosis undergoing surgical lung biopsy. Chest 128:3310, 2005.

140. Rice AJ, Wells AU, Bouros D, duBois RM, Hansell DM: Terminal diffuse alveolar damage in relation to interstitial pneumonias. Am J Clin Pathol 119:709, 2003.

Miscellaneous Causes of DAD

141. Bleyl U, Sander E, Schindler T: The pathology and biology of uremic pneumonitis. Intensive Care Med 7:193, 1981.

142. Bouachour G, Varache N, Szapiro N, L'Hoste P, Harry P, Alquier P: Noncardiogenic pulmonary edema resulting from intravascular administration of contrast material. AJR Am J Roentgenol 157:255, 1991.

143. Brinkmann B, Puschell K: Heat injuries to the respiratory system. Virchows Arch [A Pathol Anat Histol] 379:299, 1978.

144. Clark MC, Flick MR: Permeability pulmonary edema caused by venous air embolism. Am Rev Respir Dis 129:633, 1984.

145. Conti VR: Pulmonary injury after cardiopulmonary bypass. Chest 119:2, 2001.

146. Fenster LF, Wheelis RF, Ryan JA Jr: Acute respiratory distress syndrome after peritoneovenous shunt. Am Rev Respir Dis 125:244, 1982.

147. Hasleton PS, McWilliam L, Haboubi NY: The lung parenchyma in burns. Histopathology 7:333, 1983.

148. Huberman RP, Fon GT, Bein ME: Benign molar pregnancies: Pulmonary complications. AJR Am J Roentgenol 138:71, 1982.

149. Interiano B, Stuard I, Hyde R: Acute respiratory distress syndrome in pancreatitis. Ann Intern Med 77:923, 1972.

150. Lenahan SE, Domen RE, Silliman C, Kingsley CP, Romano PJ: Transfusion-related acute lung injury secondary to biologically active mediators. Arch Pathol Lab Med 125:523, 2001.

151. Matthay R, Schwarz M, Petty T, et al: Pulmonary manifestations of systemic lupus erythematosus: Review of twelve cases of acute lupus pneumonitis. Medicine (Baltimore) 54:397, 1974.

152. Muir TE, Tazelaar HD, Colby TV, Myers JL: Organizing diffuse alveolar damage associated with progressive systemic sclerosis. Mayo Clin Proc 721:639, 1997.

153. Orr J Jr, Austin J, Hatch K, et al: Acute pulmonary edema associated with molar pregnancies: A high-risk factor for development of persistent trophoblastic disease. Am J Obstet Gynecol 136:412, 1980.

154. Paris AL, Herwaldt LA, Blum D, et al: Pathologic findings in twelve fatal cases of toxic shock syndrome. Ann Intern Med. 96:852, 1982.

155. Popovsky MA, Abel MD, Moore SB: Transfusion-related acute lung injury associated with passive transfer of antileukocyte antibodies. Am Rev Respir Dis 128:185, 1983.

156. Ratliff N, Young W Jr, Hackel D, et al: Pulmonary injury secondary to extracorporeal circulation. An ultrastructural study. J Thorac Cardiovasc Surg 65:425, 1973.

157. Rovner A, Westcott J: Pulmonary edema and respiratory insufficiency in acute pancreatitis. Radiology 118:513, 1976.

158. Silvestri R, Huseby J, Rughani I, et al: Respiratory distress syndrome from lymphangiography contrast medium. Am Rev Respir Dis 122:543, 1980.

159. Tryka AF, Godleski JJ, Fanta CH: Leukemic cell lysis pneumonopathy. A complication of treated myeloblastic leukemia. Cancer 50:2763, 1982.

160. Twiggs L, Morrow C, Schlaerth J: Acute pulmonary complications of molar pregnancy. Am J Obstet Gynecol 135:189, 1979.

Bronchiolitis Obliterans–Organizing Pneumonia

161. Akira M, Yamamoto S, Sakatani M: Bronchiolitis obliterans organizing pneumonia manifesting as multiple large nodules or masses. AJR Am J Roentgenol 170:291, 1998.

162. Alasaly K, Müller N, Ostrow DN, et al: Cryptogenic organizing pneumonia. A report of 25 cases and a review of the literature. Medicine (Baltimore) 74:201, 1995.

163. Arbetter KR, Prakash UBS, Tazelaar HD, Douglas WW: Radiation-induced pneumonitis in the "nonirradiated" lung. Mayo Clin Proc 74:27, 1999.

164. Aubert J-D, Paré PD, Hogg JC, Hayashi S: Platelet-derived growth factor in bronchiolitis obliterans-organizing pneumonia. Am J Respir Crit Care Med 155:676, 1997.

165. Bartter T, Irwin RS, Nash G, et al: Idiopathic bronchiolitis obliterans organizing pneumonia with peripheral infiltrates on chest roentgenogram. Arch Intern Med 149:273, 1989.

166. Beasley MB, Franks RJ, Galvin JR, Gochuico B, Travis WD: Acute fibrinous and organizing pneumonia: A histologic pattern of lung injury and possible variant of diffuse alveolar damage. Arch Pathol Lab Med 126:1064, 2002.

167. Bellomo R, Finlay M, McLaughlin P, Tai E: Clinical spectrum of cryptogenic organising pneumonitis. Thorax 46:554, 1991.

168. Chastre J, Raghu G, Soler P, et al: Pulmonary fibrosis following pneumonia due to acute Legionnaire's disease. Clinical, ultrastructural, and immunofluorescent study. Chest 91:57, 1987.

169. Cohen AJ, King TE Jr, Downey GP: Rapidly progressive bronchiolitis obliterans with organizing pneumonia. Am J Respir Crit Care Med 149:1670, 1994.

170. Cordier J-F: Cryptogenic organizing pneumonitis: Bronchiolitis obliterans organizing pneumonia. Clin Chest Med 14:677, 1993.

171. Cordier J-F, Loire R, Brune J: Idiopathic bronchiolitis obliterans organizing pneumonia: Definition of characteristic clinical profiles in a series of 16 patients. Chest 96:999, 1989.

172. Crestani B, Valeyre D, Roden S, et al: Bronchiolitis obliterans organizing pneumonia syndrome primed by radiation therapy to the breast. Am J Respir Crit Care Med 158:1929, 1998.

173. Davison AG, Heard BE, McAllister AC, Turner-Warwick MEH: Cryptogenic organizing pneumonitis. Q J Med 22:382, 1983.

174. Dina R, Sheppard MN: The histological diagnosis of clinically documented cases of cryptogenic organizing pneumonia: Diagnostic features in transbronchial biopsies. Histopathology 23:541, 1993.

175. Epler GR: Drug-induced bronchiolitis obliterans organizing pneumonia. Clin Chest Med 35:89, 2004.

176. Epler GR, Colby TV, McLoud TC, et al: Bronchiolitis obliterans organizing pneumonia. N Engl J Med 312:152, 1985.

177. Flowers JR, Clunie G, Burke M, Constant O: Bronchiolitis obliterans organizing pneumonia: The clinical and radiological features of seven cases and a review of the literature. Clin Radiol 45:371, 1992.

178. Gosink BB, Friedman PJ, Liebow AA: Bronchiolitis obliterans. Roentgenologic-pathologic correlation. Am J Roentgenol Radium Ther Nucl Med 117:816, 1973.

179. Grinblat J, Mechlis S, Lewitus Z: Organizing pneumonia-like process. An unusual observation in steroid responsive cases with features of chronic interstitial pneumonia. Chest 80:259, 1981.

180. Guerry-Force ML, Muller NL, Wright JL, et al: A comparison of bronchiolitis obliterans with organizing pneumonia, usual interstitial pneumonia, and small airways disease. Am Rev Respir Dis 135:705, 1987.

181. Jones GR, Proudfoot AT, Hall JI: Pulmonary effects of acute exposure to nitrous fumes. Thorax 28:61, 1973.

182. Katzenstein A-LA, Myers JL, Prophet WD, et al: Bronchiolitis obliterans and usual interstitial

pneumonia. A comparative clinicopathologic study. Am J Surg Pathol 10:373, 1986.

183. Lappi-Blanco E, Kaarteenaho-Wiik R, Soini Y, Ristelli J, Paakko, P: Intraluminal fibromyxoid lesions in bronchiolitis obliterans organizing pneumonia are highly capillarized. Hum Pathol 30:1192, 1999.

184. Lappi-Blanco E, Soini Y, Kinnula V, Paakko P: VEGF and bFGF are highly expressed in intraluminal fibromyxoid lesions in bronchiolitis obliterans and organizing pneumonia. J Pathol 196:220, 2002.

185. Lazor R, Vandevenne A, Pelletier A, et al: Cryptogenic organizing pneumonia: Characteristics of relapses in a series of 48 patients. Am J Respir Crit Care Med 162:571, 2000.

186. Lohr RH, Boland BJ, Douglas, W, et al: Organizing pneumonia: Features and prognosis of cryptogenic, secondary, and focal variants. Arch Intern Med 157:1323, 1997.

187. Miwa S, Morita S, Suda T, et al: The incidence and clinical characteristics of bronchiolitis obliterans organizing pneumonia syndrome after radiation therapy for breast cancer. Sarcoidosis Vasc Diffuse Lung Dis 21:212, 2004.

188. Miyagawa-Hayashino A, Wain JC, Mark EJ: Lung transplantation biopsy specimens with bronchiolitis obliterans or bronchiolitis obliterans organizing pneumonia due to aspiration. Arch Pathol Lab Med 129:223, 2005.

189. Mokhtari M, Bach PB, Tietjen PA, Stover DE: Bronchiolitis obliterans organizing pneumonia in cancer: A case series. Respir Med 96:280, 2002.

190. Moya C, Antó JM, Newman AJ, et al: Outbreak of organizing pneumonia in textile printing sprayers. Lancet 343:498, 1994.

191. Myers JL, Katzenstein A-LA: Ultrastructural evidence of alveolar epithelial injury in idiopathic bronchiolitis obliterans-organizing pneumonia. Am J Pathol 132:102, 1988.

192. Nizami I, Kissner D, Visscher D, Dubaybo BA: Idiopathic bronchiolitis obliterans with organizing pneumonia. An acute and life-threatening syndrome. Chest 108:271, 1995.

193. Oymak FS, Demirbas HM, Mavili E, et al. Bronchiolitis obliterans organizing pneumonia. Clinical and roentgenological features in 26 cases. Respiration 72:254, 2005.

194. Patel R, Dutta D, Schonfeld S: Free-base cocaine use associated with bronchiolitis obliterans organizing pneumonia. Ann Intern Med 107:186, 1987.

195. Peyrol S, Cordier J-F, Grimaud J-A: Intra-alveolar fibrosis of idiopathic bronchiolitis obliterans-organizing pneumonia: Cell-matrix patterns. Am J Pathol 137:155, 1990.

196. Poletti V, Cazzato S, Minicuci N, Zompatori M, Burzi M, Schiattone ML: The diagnostic value of bronchoalveolar lavage and transbronchial lung biopsy in cryptogenic organizing pneumonia. Eur Respir J 9:2513, 1996.

197. Ramirez RJ, Dowell AR: Silo-filler's disease: Nitrogen dioxide-induced lung injury. Long-term follow-up and review of the literature. Ann Intern Med 74:569, 1971.

198. Romero S, Hernández L, Gil J, Aranda I, Martin C, Sanchez-Payá J: Organizing pneumonia in textile printing workers: A clinical description. Eur Respir J 11:265, 1998.

199. Rosen N, Gaton E: Congenital bronchiolitis obliterans. Beitr Pathol 155:309, 1975.

200. Sato P, Madtes DK, Thorning D, Albert RK: Bronchiolitis obliterans caused by Legionella pneumophila. Chest 87:840, 1985.

201. Sobonya R: Fatal anhydrous ammonia inhalation. Hum Pathol 8:293, 1977.

202. Spiteri MA, Klenerman P, Sheppard MN, Padley S, Clark TJK, Newman-Taylor A: Seasonal cryptogenic organising pneumonia with biochemical cholestasis: A new clinical entity. Lancet 340:281, 1992.

203. Stover DE, Milite F, Zakowski M: A newly recognized syndrome – radiation-related bronchiolitis obliterans and organizing pneumonia. Respiration 68:540, 2001.

204. Sueishi K, Watanabe T, Tanaka K, et al: Intrauterine bronchiolitis obliterans. Report of an autopsy case and review of the literature. Virchows Arch [A Pathol Anat Histol] 362:223, 1974.

205. Yigla M, Ben-Itzhak O, Solomonov A, Guralnik L, Oren I: Recurrent, self-limited menstrual-associated bronchiolitis obliterans organizing pneumonia. Chest 118:253, 2000.

206. Yoshinouchi T, Ohtsuki Y, Kubo K, Shikata Y: Clinicopathological study on two types of cryptogenic organizing pneumonia. Respir Med 89:271, 1995.

207. Yousem S, Colby T, Carrington L: Lung biopsy in rheumatoid arthritis. Am Rev Respir Dis 131:770, 1985.

208. Yousem S, Lohr RH, Colby TV: Idiopathic bronchiolitis obliterans organizing pneumonia/cryptogenic organizing pneumonia with unfavorable outcome: Pathologic predictors. Mod Pathol 10:864, 1997.

IDIOPATHIC INTERSTITIAL PNEUMONIA

The term *interstitial pneumonia* refers to a diffuse, inflammatory, and often fibrosing process in which the histologic abnormality is located predominantly within the alveolar septa rather than in alveolar lumens. The findings are usually not exclusively interstitial, however, since some airspace abnormalities almost always accompany the interstitial changes. Moreover, sophisticated techniques have demonstrated that many processes that appear mainly interstitial by light microscopy may begin within airspaces.

Most interstitial pneumonias are mild, self-limited illnesses that fall into the clinical category of *atypical pneumonia*. The etiology is usually known, including, most commonly, viruses and mycoplasma, and a lung biopsy is not necessary for diagnosis. Occasionally, however, the illness is fulminant or chronic and progressive, and the cause is not apparent. It is these idiopathic forms of interstitial pneumonia in which a lung biopsy may be needed to establish the diagnosis.

Classification of Idiopathic Interstitial Pneumonia

Liebow[6] devised the first detailed pathologic classification of interstitial pneumonia that included five groups as listed in Table 3–1. This classification forms the basis of all current classifications, although it has been modified in recent years as our knowledge of these entities has increased. A multidisciplinary consensus classification sponsored by the American Thoracic Society and the European Respiratory Society (ATS/ERS) expanded Liebow's classification to include seven entities,[1] but we prefer a simplified approach as outlined in Table 3–1.[4,5] Lymphoid interstitial pneumonia (LIP) and giant cell interstitial pneumonia (GIP) are omitted from our classification since the former is a lymphoproliferative rather than inflammatory disorder in most cases and the latter is a form of hard metal pneumoconiosis. These latter entities are reviewed in Chapters 9 and 5,

Table 3–1   Classification of Idiopathic Interstitial Pneumonia

Liebow, 1975[6]	ATS/ERS, 2002[1]	Katzenstein*
UIP	IPF	UIP
DIP	DIP	DIP/RBILD
BIP	RBILD	AIP
LIP	COP	NSIP
GIP	AIP	
	NSIP	
	LIP	

Abbreviations: UIP = usual interstitial pneumonia; IPF = idiopathic pulmonary fibrosis; DIP = desquamative interstitial pneumonia; RBILD = respiratory bronchiolitis interstitial lung disease; BIP = bronchiolitis obliterans interstitial pneumonia; AIP = acute interstitial pneumonia; NSIP = nonspecific interstitial pneumonia; LIP = lymphoid interstitial pneumonia; COP = cryptogenic organizing pneumonia, ATS/ERS = American Thoracic Society/European Respiratory Society.
*Modified from *Katzenstein and Askin's Surgical Pathology of Non-Neoplastic Lung Disease*, 3rd ed, Philadelphia, WB Saunders, 1997.

respectively. Liebow included cases of acute interstitial pneumonia (AIP) under the category of usual interstitial pneumonia (UIP), although there is now good evidence that AIP is a separate entity. Nonspecific interstitial pneumonia (NSIP) likely was lumped with UIP and desquamative interstitial pneumonia (DIP). Bronchiolitis obliterans interstitial pneumonia (BIP) encompassed what is now termed bronchiolitis obliterans–organizing pneumonia (BOOP) or cryptogenic organizing pneumonia (COP), although some cases had associated diffuse alveolar damage (DAD) and thus represented examples of mixed acute lung injury. We do not consider BOOP to be a form of interstitial pneumonia since the main histologic changes occur in the airspaces rather than the interstitium. BOOP is discussed in Chapter 2.

Nomenclature

The classification of the idiopathic interstitial pneumonias was confusing in the past because different terminology was used in the pathologic and clinical literature. For example, the synonymous terms *idiopathic*

pulmonary fibrosis (*IPF*) and *cryptogenic fibrosing alveolitis* (*CFA*) were used by clinicians usually in reference to a slowly progressive, chronic interstitial pneumonia, but they also included more acute processes.[3,4,8,32,92] They thus encompassed several different pathologic entities, including UIP, DIP, and NSIP as well as AIP and BOOP. The lumping together of these different diseases under a single name explains the previously reported vagaries in clinical course, response to treatment, and prognosis of IPF (or CFA).[4] Currently the name IPF (or CFA) is restricted to cases of UIP, and the terms may be used interchangeably.[1,3] All other idiopathic interstitial pneumonias are diagnosed separately.

The following sections describe the clinical characteristics and diagnostic pathologic criteria for each of the idiopathic interstitial pneumonias. Important clinical and pathologic findings are contrasted in Tables 3–2 and 3–3. Honeycomb lung represents the end stage of various interstitial processes and is reviewed in the last section.

Approach to Diagnosis of the Idiopathic Interstitial Pneumonias

The idiopathic interstitial pneumonias differ from most other lung diseases in that they lack a unique and specific single diagnostic finding, such as Langerhans cells in eosinophilic granuloma, smooth muscle bundles in lymphangiomyomatosis, or an identifiable infectious agent, for example. Rather, they are all characterized by varying proportions and arrangements of fibrosis and chronic inflammation. Since fibrosis and chronic inflammation may be nonspecific localized findings in the lung, it is important to correlate the clinical and radiographic findings with the pathologic findings to confirm that the patient has diffuse interstitial lung disease.[36] Specifically, knowledge of the clinical symptoms (dyspnea, cough, etc.), the nature of the onset (acute, subacute, or chronic), the pulmonary function test results (usually restrictive abnormalities with decreased diffusion capacity and exercise-induced desaturation), and the high-resolution computed tomography (HRCT) manifestations is especially useful.

Once the presence of clinical interstitial lung disease is confirmed, evaluation of the pattern, appearance, and distribution of the fibrosis and inflammation should lead to a reproducibly correct diagnosis.[91] Although atypical clinical or radiographic features (in the context of interstitial lung disease) are reason for caution, the pathologist should not be swayed because the pulmonologist or radiologist disagrees with the pathologic

Table 3–2 Contrasting Clinical Features of Idiopathic Interstitial Pneumonias and BOOP

	UIP	NSIP	DIP/RBILD	AIP	BOOP
Onset	Insidious	Insidious to subacute	Insidious	Acute	Subacute
Systemic symptoms	No	Sometimes	No	Usually	Sometimes
Radiographic findings	Interstitial reticular markings, peripheral and basal predominant, with honeycomb change	Diffuse ground glass opacities	Diffuse ground glass opacities	Diffuse consolidation	Patchy airspace opacities
Clinical course	Chronic (years)	Chronic (months–years)	Chronic (years)	Fulminant (days–weeks)	Subacute (weeks–months)
Response to steroids	No	Usually	Usually	Not usually	Usually
Prognosis	Poor	Good	Excellent	Poor	Good

Table 3–3 Contrasting Pathologic Features of Idiopathic Interstitial Pneumonias and BOOP

	UIP	NSIP	DIP/RBILD	AIP	BOOP
Temporal appearance	Variegated	Uniform	Uniform	Uniform	Uniform
Patchwork lung involvement	Characteristic	No	No	No	No
Interstitial inflammation	Scant	Variable	Scant	Scant	Scant
Collagen fibrosis	Prominent	Variable	Mild	No	No
Fibroblast proliferation	Focal, interstitial (fibroblast foci)	Not usually	No	Diffuse, interstitial	Peribronchiolar, intraluminal
Architectural distortion	Yes, prominent	Not usually	Not usually	No	No
Hyaline membranes	No	No	No	Yes	No
Thrombi, epithelial metaplasias	No	No	No	Yes	No

diagnosis. Despite some suggestions to the contrary,[36] pathologic diagnosis remains the 'gold standard' for diagnosing interstitial lung disease. The features of UIP, especially, are so distinct in classical cases that the diagnosis can often be made in the absence of history (a situation encountered sometimes in patients undergoing lobectomy for lung cancer, for example, in whom UIP is unsuspected).

It should be remembered that there are a small number of interstitial pneumonias that show overlapping features or end-stage changes that cannot be pigeonholed into a named idiopathic interstitial pneumonia. These are best diagnosed descriptively ('unclassified interstitial fibrosis', or 'patchy interstitial fibrosis with honeycomb change', for example) and are discussed later on (see Other Idiopathic Interstitial Pneumonias).

USUAL INTERSTITIAL PNEUMONIA

Clinical and Radiographic Features

UIP is the most common idiopathic interstitial pneumonia, comprising over 60% of cases previously included under the category of IPF.[15,39,107] It is characterized clinically by the insidious onset of dyspnea, and it pursues a chronic and progressive downhill course.[6,8,15,32,38,39,42,58,66,92,107] The majority of patients are between 50 and 70 years old, with an average age at onset in the sixth decade. Occasional cases have been reported in younger individuals, with rare patients in their twenties.[88] Familial cases have been described and sometimes occur in younger persons.[11,77,79,95,122] Men are affected about twice as often as women.

Although the disease has been reported in infants and children, we believe that those cases represent other interstitial pneumonias [either NSIP (see text following) or chronic pneumonitis of infancy (see Chapter 14)] that have been misdiagnosed. Collagen vascular diseases, especially rheumatoid arthritis and scleroderma, are frequently present in patients with UIP, and serum auto-antibodies (especially rheumatoid factor and antinuclear antibody) are commonly found whether or not there is an associated collagen vascular disease.[6,119,128,132] Restrictive defects are demonstrated by pulmonary function testing.

HRCT examinations in classic cases show bilateral interstitial reticular markings that are most prominent at the bases and peripherally.[1,8,72,86,94] Traction bronchiectasis and honeycomb change in a similar distribution are usually also present. Evidence has accrued that these radiographic findings in the right clinical setting may be diagnostic of UIP without the need for a surgical lung biopsy.[48,49,78,104] However, they are present in only 50% or less of patients, and other nonspecific changes are common, such as ground glass opacities or a more diffuse or even upper lobe distribution, and honeycomb change may be absent in some cases.[99]

Treatment and Prognosis

The prognosis of UIP is not good. The disease is usually progressive and ultimately fatal in most patients. Acute clinical deterioration may precede death in some patients (see Exacerbation of UIP, Chapter 2).[80] Median survival rates vary, averaging 2 to 3 years in most large series but approaching 4 to 6 years in a few.[7,18,39,42,58,66,92,107,119,128] The presence of an underlying collagen vascular disease is associated with longer survival. While disease progression may be halted in a minority of patients, reversal of pathologic changes and complete recovery do not occur.[18] Increasing age (especially over 60), extensive honeycomb change on HRCT, desaturation during exercise, and worsening pulmonary function tests, especially diffusion capacity and forced vital capacity, are associated with decreased survival.[21,37,55,66,75]

Traditionally, corticosteroids, often combined with cyclophosphamide or other cytotoxic agents, have been used for treatment, but there is no evidence that they have a beneficial effect. There was initial enthusiasm for using interferon-γ, but recent controlled studies have shown no definite benefit to this therapy, except possibly in patients with early disease.[103,115,120] There is evidence that the antifibrotic agent pirfenidone may have beneficial effects in some cases.[9] Other newer therapies that aim to interrupt fibrogenesis at various levels are being developed and are yet to be tested. There is evidence that acetylcysteine may be beneficial in some cases.[32a,67]

Pathologic Features

The diagnostic features of UIP are summarized in Table 3–4. At low magnification, a strikingly non-uniform interstitial fibrosing process with associated architectural derangement is seen.[5,18,59] There is a heterogeneous, patchwork pattern of lung involvement whereby scarred areas of parenchyma are juxtaposed next to islands of normal lung, or areas with different abnormalities (honeycomb change and mild alveolar septal fibrosis, for example) occur side by side without intervening transition zones (Fig. 3–1). In addition to this *spatial variability*, there is evidence of *temporal variability* with areas of active, ongoing fibrosis (*fibroblast foci*, see later on) coexisting with areas of inactive collagen-type scarring (Fig. 3–2). Fibroblast foci are key findings, not only for establishing the diagnosis, but also for understanding pathogenesis.

The fibrosis in UIP is usually extensive by the time the patient is biopsied. In some areas there is only mild widening of alveolar septa by collagen deposition without destruction of alveolar septal integrity. More characteristically, however, there is architectural distortion by the fibrosis in the form of either plump interstitial scars or areas of honeycomb change. The scars are irregularly shaped and of varying sizes. They are composed of dense collagen deposition often combined with mild chronic inflammation containing lymphocytes and occasional plasma cells (Fig. 3–3). Elastic fibers are increased in the scarred areas as well.[108] Typically, the areas of alveolar septal fibrosis

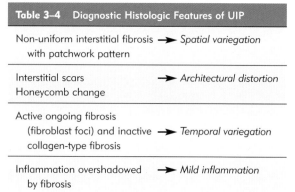

Table 3–4 Diagnostic Histologic Features of UIP		
Non-uniform interstitial fibrosis with patchwork pattern	➤	*Spatial variegation*
Interstitial scars Honeycomb change	➤	*Architectural distortion*
Active ongoing fibrosis (fibroblast foci) and inactive collagen-type fibrosis	➤	*Temporal variegation*
Inflammation overshadowed by fibrosis	➤	*Mild inflammation*

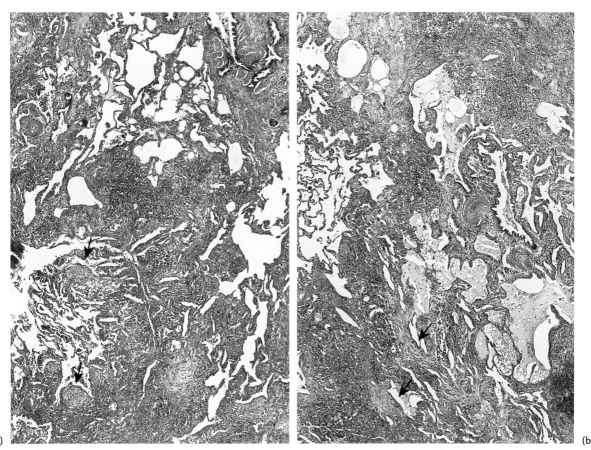

Figure 3–1 UIP. Low magnification view showing the characteristic patchwork pattern of lung involvement. **(a)** Foci of relatively normal lung (top and lower left) alternate with areas of prominent interstitial fibrosis. Lightly staining areas of fibroblast proliferation (fibroblast foci) are also present (arrows). **(b)** Prominent honeycomb change adjacent to a small island of normal lung (left mid) is seen in this field. Small fibroblast foci (arrows) are present near the bottom.

and the interstitial scars alternate with areas of relatively normal interstitium, a pattern of involvement described as 'patchwork'.[59] Not surprisingly, vascularity is decreased in the areas of greatest fibrosis, although increased vascular density has been noted in areas of mild fibrosis.[33,106] Subtle increase in smooth muscle cells in the interstitium away from the airways has been detected by immunohistochemical techniques.[96]

Areas of end-stage honeycomb lung are found in most biopsies of UIP and may be extensive (Fig. 3–4).[6,58,59] They are characterized by enlarged, restructured airspaces with thickened fibrotic walls. The spaces are lined by plump cuboidal or ciliated columnar cells, at least some of which represent the ingrowth of bronchiolar epithelium along alveolar ducts or directly into the alveoli through the bronchioloalveolar canals of Lambert, a process termed by some 'bronchiolar metaplasia' (Fig. 3–5a). Squamous metaplasia occasionally

occurs in this epithelial lining, but it is not prominent. Inspissated mucus, usually containing macrophages or neutrophils, often fills the honeycomb spaces. Hyperplasia of smooth muscle that normally surrounds alveolar ducts and respiratory bronchioles is a common associated feature (Fig. 3–5b).[62,97] Florid examples have been termed 'muscular cirrhosis' or 'bronchiolar emphysema', and they are characterized by clusters of disoriented smooth muscle bundles, sometimes having a stellate arrangement and often replacing a small bronchiole.

In addition to collagen deposition and end-stage scarring, small areas of active fibrosis (fibroblast foci) are identifiable. This mixture of remote, inactive fibrosis and current, ongoing disease is the essence of temporal variability that is key to diagnosing UIP (Fig. 3–6). The fibroblast foci are characterized by small aggregates of spindle-shaped cells within the interstitium that are arranged with their long axis parallel to the long axis

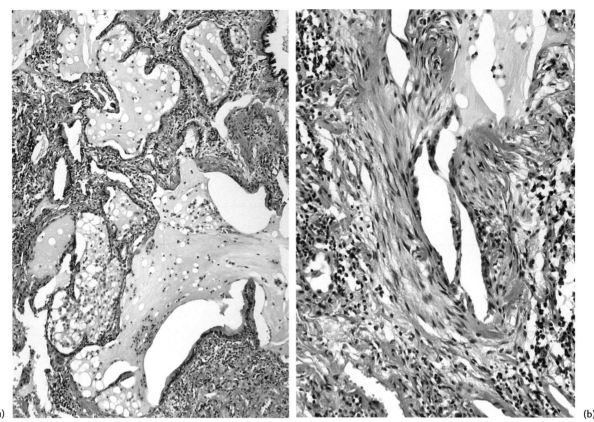

(a) (b)

Figure 3–2 UIP. (a) Closer view of honeycomb change from Figure 3–1b. There are enlarged airspaces containing a mucinous exudate and surrounded by fibrosis and chronic inflammation. Many of the spaces are lined by bronchiolar type epithelium. **(b)** Higher magnification of a fibroblast focus from Figure 3–1b showing the spindle-shaped fibroblasts and myofibroblasts with their long axis arranged parallel to the alveolar septa. This coexistence of active fibrosis and collagen-type fibrosis with scarring typifies the temporal variability that is characteristic of UIP.

of the alveolar septa (Fig. 3–7). They are present within lightly staining myxoid appearing stroma and are easily visible at low magnification. Decreased vascularity has been noted within them by CD34 staining.[30,33,106] The luminal surface of the fibroblast foci is covered by hyperplastic alveolar lining epithelium. Ultrastructural and immunohistochemical techniques have demonstrated that the spindle-shaped cells comprise a mixture of myofibroblasts and fibroblasts.[57,71] Various substances have been identified in the fibroblast foci, including fibronectin, integrin, tenascin, versican, decorin, various metalloproteinases and their tissue inhibitors, beta catenin and cyclin D1, and interleukin-18 (IL-18) receptors.[14,23,40,44,68,70,71,98,116,126] Fibroblast foci are thought to originate from the organization and subsequent incorporation of intraalveolar exudates into the interstitium.[12,16,40,70,71] Ultrastructurally, epithelial necrosis and alveolar collapse similar to changes in

organizing DAD (see Chapter 2) have been observed, and the evidence suggests that fibroblast foci represent sites of acute lung injury.[87] The spectrum of fibrotic changes apparent at the light microscopic level in UIP is reflected in collagen polymorphism noted by immunohistochemical and biochemical techniques.[13,114,117] Type III and type VI collagen are associated with fibroblast foci while type I collagen is localized to the later stages of fibrosis.

Prominent hobnail-shaped or low cuboidal epithelial cells line much of the thickened interstitium in UIP. Ultrastructurally, these cells mostly represent type 2 pneumocytes or their precursors, although some may be derived from bronchiolar lining cells.[60] They may show marked irregularity in size or shape and often contain prominent nucleoli or other features of cytologic atypia. Intranuclear tubular inclusions can be found occasionally by electron microscopy.[61] Sometimes,

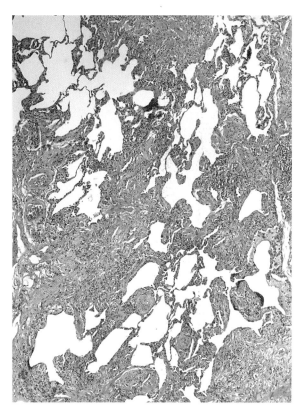

Figure 3–3 UIP. Architectural distortion caused by interstitial scarring in UIP. Note the irregular collagen-type fibrosis that widens and distorts alveolar septa. The scars alternate with areas of normal lung.

amorphous eosinophilic material resembling Mallory hyaline in hepatocytes is present in their cytoplasm (Fig. 3–8).[40,127] Similar material can also be found in cases of AIP and asbestosis. By immunohistochemical techniques, cytokines and other substances, including transforming growth factor beta (TGFβ_1), tumor necrosis factor alpha (TNFα), platelet-derived growth factor (PDGF-β), insulin-like growth factor (IGF-I), interleukin-1 receptor antagonist, monocyte chemoattractant protein-1, tissue factor, hepatocyte-derived growth factor, ENA-78, and endothelin-1, have been identified within the hyperplastic epithelial cells.[26,41,45,52,54,57,63,85,111,123,125] Staining has also been described for Δnp63, p53, p21, beta catenin, thioredoxin, and cyclin D-1,[22,23,72,90,102] as well as for multiple metalloproteinases, their tissue inhibitors,[44,111,116] and laminin 5λ chain.[76] Staining has also been noted for manganese superoxide dismutase and catalase.[73]

Although UIP is a predominantly fibrosing process, some inflammation is present in most cases. The inflammation is usually mild and composed of small lymphocytes and occasional plasma cells (Fig. 3–9). The lymphocytes may form small nodular aggregates, sometimes with germinal centers, and they have been shown by immunohistologic techniques to represent mainly B cells.[17] Lymphoid follicles with germinal centers tend to be more prominent in cases associated with rheumatoid arthritis. By electron microscopy, scattered macrophages, mast cells, neutrophils, and eosinophils can be found in the interstitium in addition to lymphocytes and plasma cells, but they usually are not numerous.[12,25,29] Mast cells appear to be present in increased numbers in UIP, and evidence of activation and degranulation has been noted.[50,57] Neither epithelioid histiocytes nor granulomas are ordinarily found in UIP. Sometimes, prominent inflammation is present in the honeycomb areas, but it is always overshadowed by the fibrosis and scarring. Significant inflammation is not seen in areas of lung lacking fibrosis, and this is an important point in distinguishing UIP from cases of NSIP (see later on) and other cellular interstitial processes.

Vascular changes are common in the scarred areas and include intimal proliferation and medial thickening of muscular pulmonary arteries. These findings reflect pulmonary hypertension that likely results from destruction of the distal capillary bed. Evidence of endothelial damage may be seen as well.[29]

The accumulation of macrophages within alveolar spaces frequently accompanies the characteristic interstitial changes in UIP, especially in cigarette smokers (see DIP-like reactions later on). These cells may form tight clusters or they may be loosely dispersed, and they are distributed unevenly from area to area. Small foci resembling eosinophilic pneumonia are also occasionally seen, but are always a minor component, being overshadowed by the other features of UIP.[131] When intra-alveolar macrophage accumulation is prominent, DIP/respiratory bronchiolitis interstitial lung disease (RBILD) enters the differential diagnosis (see text following). The presence of marked alteration of the interstitium by fibrosis and scarring with distinct temporal variability is the most important distinguishing feature. DIP/RBILD, in contrast, is both temporally and spatially uniform.

Sometimes, severe acute lung injury in the form of DAD is superimposed on otherwise typical UIP. This situation is referred to as acute exacerbation of IPF and is discussed in Chapter 2. BOOP can also complicate UIP.[89] Patients with this finding often have subacute symptoms that respond to corticosteroid therapy.

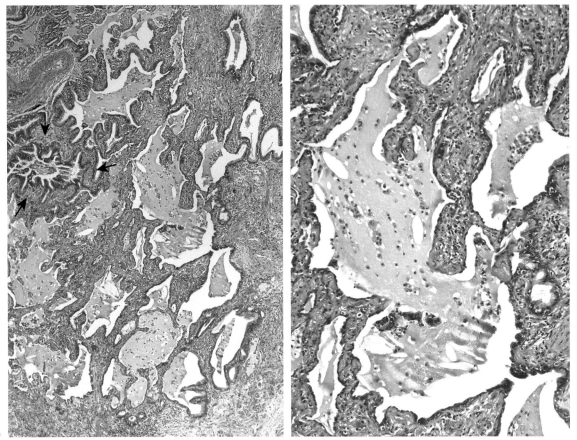

(a)   (b)

Figure 3–4 Honeycomb change in UIP. (a) Note the enlarged, irregular airspaces within background scarring. A mucinous exudate fills most of the airspaces. The process emanates from around a normal bronchiole (arrows) that is identified by the surrounding smooth muscle bundles. **(b)** At higher magnification the intraluminal mucinous exudate is better appreciated. Most of the spaces are lined by flattened epithelium in this example, although focally there is bronchiolar-type epithelium.

Relationship of Pathologic Findings and Prognosis

UIP is a progressive fibrosing disease, and the diagnosis itself is associated with a poor prognosis. In the past, pathologists were asked to grade 'cellularity' or extent of fibrosis as markers of prognosis. That practice related to the fact that other forms of idiopathic interstitial pneumonia were lumped with UIP under the category of IPF. It is now known that the degree of cellularity is fairly constant and low in UIP, but more cellular forms of idiopathic interstitial pneumonia such as DIP and NSIP are associated with a better prognosis. Therefore, the correct classification of the idiopathic interstitial pneumonia supersedes grading of cellularity or fibrosis. Complex grading systems have been devised, however, that quantitate a variety of clinical, physiologic, and pathologic findings, and some have been shown to correlate with prognosis.[19,20,51,66] In general, they are not practical in routine diagnoses. The one pathologic finding that has been related to prognosis and is easily recognizable is the extent of fibroblast foci. Several studies have shown a worse prognosis with greater number of fibroblast foci.[35,56,65,93]

Pathogenesis

For many years UIP was thought to begin with an inflammatory reaction in the alveoli (alveolitis) followed by release of a number of cytokines and a subsequent cascade of events leading to fibroblast activation and the development of fibrosis. This theory has been largely abandoned since it has become clear that therapy with anti-inflammatory agents is ineffectual and inflammation is not the main histologic finding.

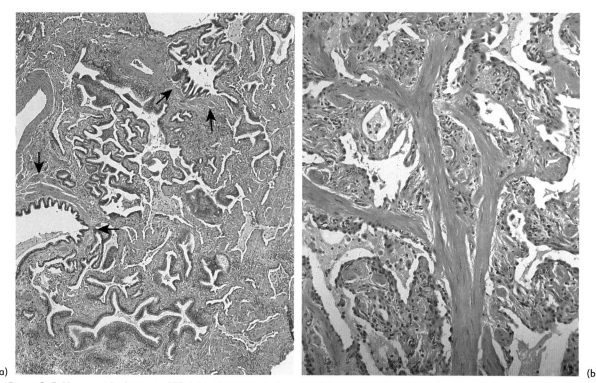

Figure 3–5 Honeycomb change in UIP. (a) In this example there is striking proliferation of bronchiolar epithelium along fibrotic and distorted alveolar walls. Note the residual normal bronchioles (arrows) identified by the adjacent bronchiolar smooth muscle bundles. **(b)** Smooth muscle hyperplasia is prominent in this area of honeycomb change.

Rather than inflammation, fibroblast foci appear to be central in the development of fibrosis in UIP.[110] They have been shown by electron microscopy and immunohistochemistry to represent sites of acute lung injury, and thus they are considered to be the initial abnormality in UIP.[12,70,71,87] Occurrence of fibroblast foci in widely separated areas of lung over many years can explain the slowly progressive and relentless downhill course. The specific cause of the acute injury remains an enigma, however, and future research will need to focus on this question. Clearly, genetic predisposition is important. Mutations in surfactant protein C genes have been demonstrated in familial cases,[21] although they are rare in sporadic cases.[76] Other theories have suggested autoimmune origin, imbalance of oxidative-antioxidant systems, viral infections (Epstein-Barr virus, other herpes viruses, HTLV-1, hepatitis C virus), and gastroesophageal reflux.[34,64,81,100,101,109,119,121,124]

Numerous studies have suggested that the fibrosing process is abnormal in UIP rather than representing a 'normal' reaction to the acute lung injury, and it is considered by some to represent a form of abnormal

wound healing.[28,31,110,121,129] Decreased apoptosis of myofibroblasts as well as increased response to fibrogenic cytokines has been described in some studies,[83,84] although others have noted increased apoptosis.[105] Increased contractibility of fibroblasts has also been reported.[82] An imbalance between synthesis and degradation of extracellular matrix molecules has been noted.[111] Aberrant angiogenesis possibly related to an imbalance of angiogenic and angiostatic chemokines may play a role.[30,33,106] The role of various other chemokines is the subject of ongoing investigation.[24]

There is some evidence that the alveolar epithelial proliferation in UIP may also be abnormal.[22,23] Increased apoptosis has been noted in normal and hyperplastic epithelium.[10,102] Dysregulated interactions between epithelial and mesenchymal components has been postulated.[22,23] The epithelial proliferation may have a role in myofibroblast differentiation.[130] Oxidant stress may play a role in disease progression.[32a,67]

These various theories of pathogenesis are important for developing treatment strategies. Most new therapy options are aimed at interrupting the fibrosis at varying

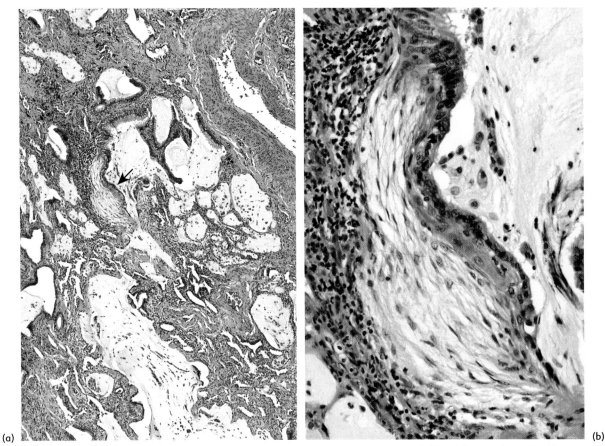

(a)

(b)

Figure 3–6 Temporal variability in UIP. (a) End-stage honeycomb change is present in this field and there is also a fibroblast focus (arrow). The fibroblast focus is shown at higher magnification in **(b).** Note the hyperplastic alveolar epithelium overlying the fibroblast focus and the parallel arrangement of the spindle-shaped cells.

stages. Blocking of oxidant-mediated reactions is another approach.[32a,67]

Differential Diagnosis

UIP must be differentiated from the other idiopathic interstitial pneumonias (see later on and Tables 3–2 and 3–3). Differentiation from the fibrosing variant of NSIP can be difficult and is important since NSIP is associated with a better prognosis and may respond to corticosteroid therapy. Briefly, NSIP is a temporally uniform fibrosing lesion that lacks significant architectural distortion (scarring and honeycomb change). Fibroblast foci are inconspicuous to absent as well.

When fibroblast foci are prominent, the lesion must be distinguished from other processes containing proliferating fibroblasts, mainly AIP and BOOP (see Chapter 2). The presence or absence of temporal heterogeneity

and architectural distortion are important differentiating findings. Of course, the intraluminal rather than interstitial location of fibrosis in BOOP and the diffuse rather than focal fibroblast proliferation in AIP are key findings. Knowledge of the clinical findings should help in difficult cases.

Another condition that can be confused with UIP is Langerhans cell histiocytosis (eosinophilic granuloma) (see Chapter 15), especially when fibrosis is prominent and diagnostic aggregates of Langerhans cells are not numerous. This disease should be suspected in young persons and when there are patchy, stellate-shaped peribronchiolar scars with large areas of intervening normal lung. Respiratory bronchiolitis (see later on) is an invariable accompanying feature.

When intraalveolar macrophages are prominent, DIP/RBILD enters the differential diagnosis. Distinguishing features of these conditions are discussed further on.

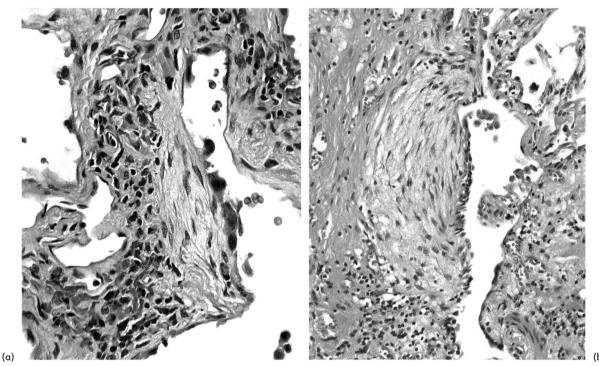

(a) (b)

Figure 3–7 Fibroblast foci in UIP. (a) This fibroblast focus is present in an alveolar septum that is mildly thickened by chronic inflammation and fibrosis. (b) This fibroblast focus is present in an area of dense collagen-type fibrosis.

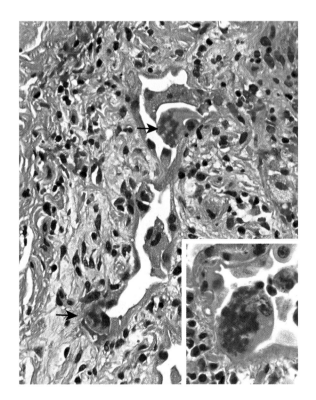

Figure 3–8 Mallory hyaline in UIP. Two alveolar lining cells (arrows) are seen that contain typical amorphous, deeply eosinophilic material in their cytoplasm. In this example they are present in an area of significant collagen-type fibrosis. Inset is a higher magnification of Mallory hyaline from another area.

DESQUAMATIVE INTERSTITIAL PNEUMONIA/RESPIRATORY BRONCHIOLITIS INTERSTITIAL LUNG DISEASE

Terminology

Desquamative interstitial pneumonia (DIP) was first described in 1965 by Liebow et al,[142] who recognized that it had a significantly better prognosis than UIP, with which it had been lumped. Subsequently, there was considerable debate as to whether it represented an early, 'cellular' form of UIP rather than a separate entity. As diagnostic features of UIP were refined, it became clear that DIP was different pathologically as well as clinically, and it is currently accepted as a separate entity. Respiratory bronchiolitis (RB, see also Chapter 16) was described in 1974 by Niewoehner et al[146] as a manifestation of cigarette smoking and was considered

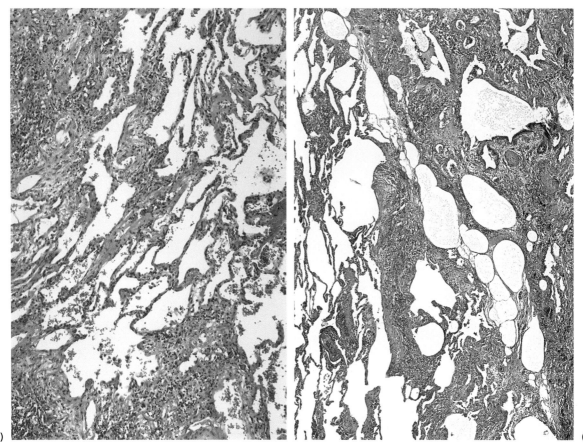

(a)

(b)

Figure 3–9 Mild interstitial inflammation in UIP. Scattered chronic inflammatory cells are seen in the interstitium along with patchy collagen-type fibrosis in **(a)**. Denser lymphoid infiltrates are seen in **(b)**. In both examples, however, the inflammatory infiltrate is overshadowed by the fibrosis and architectural distortion.

to be an incidental finding of little clinical consequence. In 1987, Myers et al[145] recognized that some cases of RB had clinical features of interstitial lung disease, and the process in that situation was subsequently termed respiratory bronchiolitis interstitial lung disease (RBILD).[151] Overlapping histologic features between RBILD and DIP have been noted since its description, and many authors consider the two entities to represent different ends of a spectrum of the same disease, with RBILD diagnosed when the changes are confined to peribronchiolar parenchyma and DIP when the changes are diffuse.[4,140,144,148] This distinction is not easy, however, since the appearance may vary from slide to slide. Some investigators suggest that the presence of diffuse changes in one low magnification field is sufficient to diagnose DIP.[149] Given the similar histologic changes, an identical pathogenesis, and similar clinical features, we feel that RBILD and DIP represent the same entity. We prefer the term RBILD, since DIP is a misnomer

based on the initial incorrect perception that the intraalveolar macrophages were type 2 pneumocytes that had desquamated from the alveolar septa. For the purpose of this discussion, the entities will be combined under the term 'DIP/RBILD', and for diagnosis the reader can choose which name he or she prefers. The term 'smoking-related interstitial lung disease' has been suggested for these diseases, although that term also includes cases of Langerhans cell histiocytosis, and it is thus not practical.[144,148]

Many of Liebow et al's original patients with DIP as well as those in subsequent reports had significant associated interstitial fibrosis, yet fibrosis is not considered a major feature of RBILD. The question, therefore, arises how to classify those lesions with significant interstitial fibrosis that otherwise resemble DIP/RBILD. NSIP (see later on) is characterized by relatively uniform interstitial fibrosis and/or inflammation, and it can have associated intraalveolar macrophage accumulation. Therefore, many cases that used to be diagnosed as DIP may be better diagnosed as NSIP.

Another question that may be posed, since interstitial fibrosis and inflammation are not prominent features of DIP/RBILD, is whether this condition should even be considered a type of interstitial lung disease. The current rationale is that these patients have clinical and radiographic features of interstitial lung disease as well as mild interstitial changes histologically. Consideration may be given in the future, however, if diagnostic features are better defined, to moving DIP/RBILD from the idiopathic interstitial pneumonia category to the category of bronchiolar/small airway disease.

Clinical Features

Patients with DIP/RBILD present with an insidious onset of dyspnea, often with cough, but usually without systemic symptoms.[18,137,142,145,149,151] Middle-aged adults are most often affected, with a mean age of onset in the fifth decade, about 10 years earlier than patients with UIP. There is a slight male predominance, as in UIP. Overall, about 90% of patients are cigarette smokers, and in some series 100% cigarette smoking is reported.[18,144,145,147,151] Cases diagnosed as DIP tend to have a less uniform smoking history than do RBILD.[137] Radiographically, bilateral ground glass opacities and centrilobular nodules are the most common CT findings. Little difference has been noted in cases diagnosed separately as DIP or RBILD,[139,147,149] although some reported cases of DIP have more evidence of fibrosis.[137] Occasionally the chest radiograph is normal. Most patients respond favorably to corticosteroid therapy, and complete recovery can occur. Recurrences have been described after many years.[143] Mortality is lower than in UIP, with some series reporting none and others noting deaths in up to 32% of patients.[18,92,137,149,151,180] Prognosis depends on criteria used for diagnosis and whether cases with a significant fibrosis are accepted. More recent series include only cases of DIP with mild interstitial fibrosis, and have noted higher survival rates, with figures approaching 100% for both DIP and RBILD.[92,137,180] Although there are rare case reports of RBILD progressing to end-stage fibrosis, it is likely that those cases represent other interstitial pneumonias with associated RB.[150]

Pathologic Features

The main histologic finding in DIP/RBILD is the presence of increased numbers of macrophages within alveolar spaces.[1,18,142] The process involves small bronchioles and peribronchiolar airspaces in RBILD (Fig. 3–10) and is more diffuse in DIP, although, as mentioned, there are no quantitative criteria for distinguishing these entities (Fig. 3–11). The alveolar macrophages possess bland, round nuclei and occasionally are multinucleated (Fig. 3–12). Their cytoplasm is abundant and usually contains coarsely granular golden brown pigment that stains weakly with Prussian blue. Ultrastructurally, numerous lysosomes and phagolysosomes are seen in the cell cytoplasm, and many contain elongated, needle-shaped inclusions that represent aluminum silicates originating from cigarette smoke (see Fig. 16–14).[135,145] The appearance differs from the foamy change characteristic of macrophages that accumulate distal to bronchial obstruction. Cytoplasmic pigmentation may be absent in those few cases of DIP occurring in non-smokers, and the macrophages in those cases contain eosinophilic cytoplasm. Occasionally, eosinophils may be admixed with the macrophages, but these cells are not numerous.

Sometimes, peculiar round or oval 'blue bodies' are present within alveolar macrophages in DIP/RBILD (Fig. 3–13).[141] These structures either occur within, or are surrounded by, macrophages, and are large, round, and laminated, measuring 15 to 20 µm in diameter. They stain pale blue or gray in hematoxylin and eosin, are periodic acid–Schiff (PAS)-positive, and contain iron and calcium. Blue bodies are not a specific diagnostic feature of DIP/RBILD and may be found in other disorders in which alveolar macrophages accumulate. They should not be confused with inhaled or aspirated exogenous material.

Mild interstitial fibrosis may occur in peribronchiolar interstitium in RBILD and more diffusely in DIP (Fig. 3–14). It is usually not severe, however, and is always overshadowed by the airspace macrophage accumulation. Alveolar epithelial hyperplasia may be seen along the thickened alveolar septa. Significant architectural distortion (scarring and honeycomb change) is not a feature, however, and fibroblast foci are usually not seen.

DIP-Like Reactions and the Differential Diagnosis of DIP/RBILD

After the description of DIP, it became clear that intra-alveolar accumulation of pigmented macrophages can be found in a variety of circumstances other than DIP. Most often it is found in subpleural parenchyma of cigarette smokers in association with nonspecific

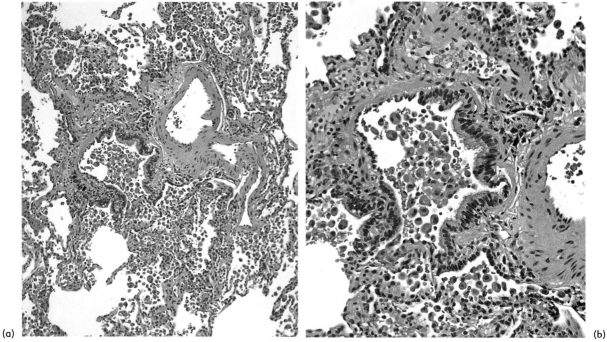

Figure 3–10 DIP/RBILD. In this example at low magnification **(a)** the intraluminal macrophage accumulation is seen to be present mainly within a respiratory bronchiole and peribronchiolar airspaces but it spares the more distal lung. **(b)** is a higher magnification from the same field, showing the pigmented macrophages within a respiratory bronchiole. This type of localized reaction can be diagnosed as RBILD.

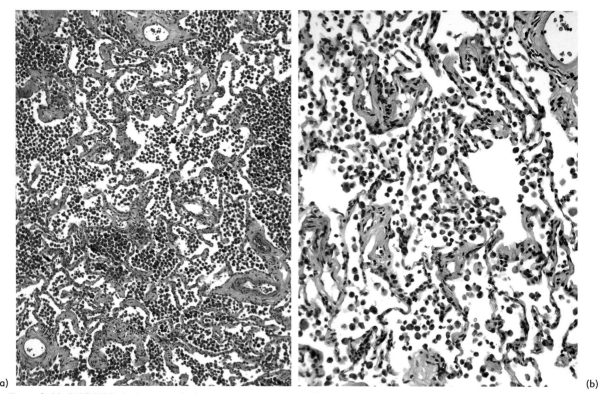

Figure 3–11 DIP/RBILD. In this example there is an extensive and diffuse intraalveolar accumulation of macrophages with lightly pigmented cytoplasm. Sheets of macrophages are present in **(a)** and there is mild associated alveolar septal fibrosis. In another area **(b)** there is less dense and more evenly dispersed macrophages with minimal fibrosis. If the entire biopsy has this diffuse pattern of involvement, the changes can be classified as DIP.

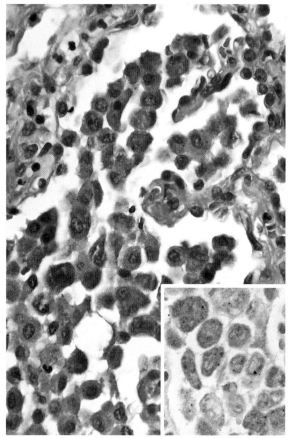

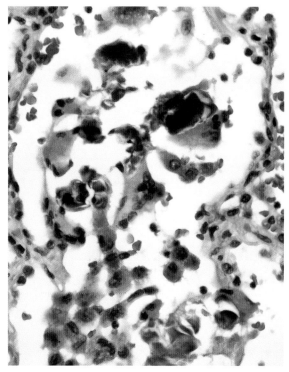

Figure 3–13 Blue bodies in DIP. Note the laminated, gray–blue structures present within macrophage cytoplasm.

Figure 3–12 Higher magnification view of macrophages in DIP/RBILD, showing the typical light yellow–brown cytoplasmic pigmentation. Note also the associated mild alveolar septal fibrosis and alveolar pneumocyte hyperplasia. The inset is a Prussian blue iron stain showing uneven light green–blue staining of cell cytoplasm.

interstitial scarring (Fig. 3–15).[136] This finding is common, especially in lobectomy specimens performed for lung cancer, and should not be misinterpreted as DIP. Intraalveolar macrophage accumulation is also common in various interstitial lung disorders, most notably UIP and Langerhans cell histiocytosis. This nonspecific macrophage accumulation has been termed DIP-like reaction to emphasize the similarity to DIP. Given our current state of knowledge about DIP and the fact that the term is a misnomer, it may be better to simply describe the findings as nonspecific intraalveolar macrophage accumulation. The process should be distinguished from the accumulation of macrophages containing foamy cytoplasm that is characteristic of changes occurring distal to bronchial obstruction

(postobstructive changes). The latter is invariably accompanied by significant chronic and sometimes acute inflammation in both airspaces and interstitium.

The presence of intraalveolar macrophage accumulation in cigarette smokers with UIP can cause confusion with DIP/RBILD (Fig. 3–16), and the distinction of UIP and DIP/RBILD is important since prognosis and treatment are so different. The differentiation is not difficult if the spatially and temporally varied interstitial fibrosis characteristic of UIP is recognized. Similarly, intraalveolar macrophage accumulation commonly accompanies cases of NSIP, and may be prominent. As mentioned earlier, some of these cases may have been classified as DIP in the past. The differentiation of DIP and NSIP makes little difference clinically since treatment and prognosis are similar, but we prefer to classify cases with prominent alveolar septal fibrosis and/or inflammation as NSIP. The exclusion of cases with significant fibrosis from the category of DIP likely accounts for the excellent prognosis reported in some series.[139,180]

Alveolar macrophage accumulation is usually present in cases of Langerhans cell histiocytosis (see Chapter

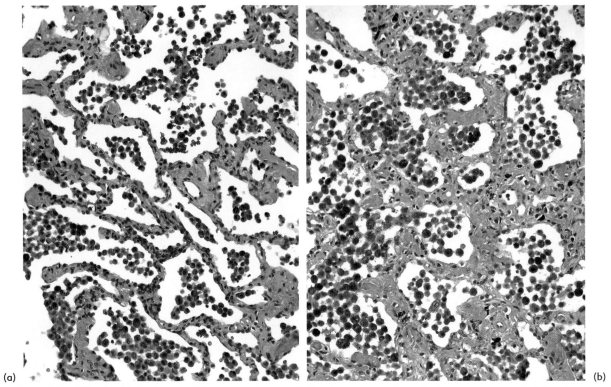

(a)   (b)

Figure 3–14 DIP. (a) Mild alveolar septal fibrosis was the main finding in this case. (b) Focally, however, more marked fibrosis was seen that was temporally uniform without fibroblast foci. If this degree of interstitial fibrosis was extensive, the case would be better diagnosed as NSIP with intraalveolar macrophage accumulation.

15), and it can be striking. Finding the characteristic nodules of Langerhans cells establishes the correct diagnosis and is usually not difficult. In longstanding, 'burned out' cases, stellate-shaped interstitial scars in peribronchiolar parenchyma may be prominent as well.

It should be remembered that RB is present in virtually all cigarette smokers, and it can be a striking finding (see Chapter 16). There are no reliable histologic features that distinguish RB from RBILD on biopsy specimens, and the diagnosis of DIP/RBILD therefore requires clinical evidence of interstitial lung disease.[138]

Pathogenesis

The role of cigarette smoking in the pathogenesis of DIP/RBILD is widely accepted and relates to the fact that all reported patients with RBILD, 98% of persons in whom RB is an incidental finding,[138] and over 90% of patients with DIP in most series are cigarette smokers. In the few patients lacking a smoking history, inhalation of dusts or fumes has been implicated.

ACUTE INTERSTITIAL PNEUMONIA (HAMMAN–RICH DISEASE)

Terminology

AIP is a rapidly progressive and histologically distinct form of interstitial pneumonia.[157,158] It is identical clinically and pathologically to the cases described by Hamman and Rich in 1944[153] and is therefore synonymous with *Hamman–Rich disease*. The disease affects previously healthy individuals, and an inciting event causing the illness cannot be identified. Most patients develop the acute respiratory distress syndrome (ARDS, see Chapter 2), and the disease is therefore sometimes referred to as *idiopathic ARDS*. The underlying pathologic findings resemble organizing DAD (see Chapter 2), and the term *idiopathic DAD* is sometimes used as well. The term acute interstitial pneumonia should be reserved for cases of unknown etiology, and should not be used for examples of organizing DAD occurring in immunocompromised persons or in clinical settings in which the etiology is known.

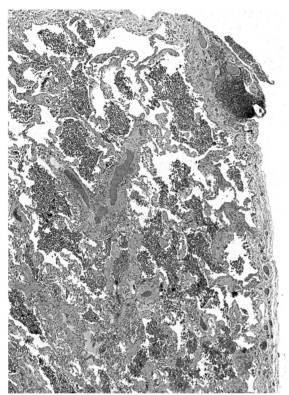

Figure 3–15 Nonspecific intraalveolar macrophage accumulation (DIP-like reaction). Note the large numbers of pigmented macrophages within alveolar spaces. There is also mild associated alveolar septal fibrosis and emphysematous changes. This field is from a lobectomy specimen that was removed for cancer. The patient had no signs or symptoms of diffuse interstitial lung disease.

AIP is an uncommon form of idiopathic interstitial pneumonia, and there are relatively few reported cases. The small number of published cases can be explained in part by the fact that most examples in the past were lumped under the category of UIP or IPF, and the clinicopathologic features were only recently well defined.

Clinical Features

Most patients present with severe dyspnea occurring over several days, usually accompanied by fever.[157,158] An antecedent flu-like syndrome characterized by myalgias, arthralgias, fever, chills, and malaise is common. Bilateral ground glass opacification and/or consolidation are present on CT examinations,[152,154,155,159] and respiratory failure requiring mechanical ventilation (ARDS, see Chapter 2) rapidly ensues.

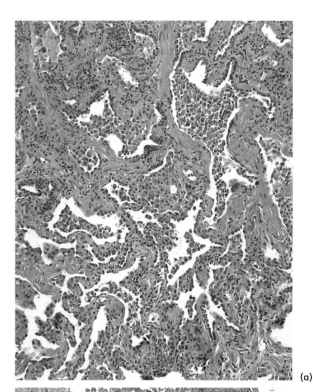

(a)

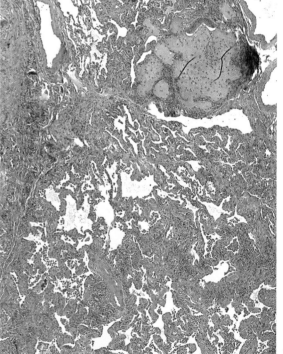

(b)

Figure 3–16 Nonspecific intraalveolar macrophage accumulation in UIP. (a) One focus of alveolar septal fibrosis and intraalveolar macrophage accumulation. If the entire biopsy had this appearance, a diagnosis of DIP/RBILD would be warranted. However, at low magnification **(b)**, the typical spatially variegated appearance of UIP with architectural distortion (note honeycomb change at top) is seen.

The mean age of reported patients is 54 years, although the disease occurs over a wide age range, and can affect both children and the elderly.[161] In fact, young adults (mean age, 28 years) were predominantly affected in one series.[157] Patients, by definition, have no known underlying disease. The course is usually fulminant and rapidly progressive, with mortality rates greater than 70% in most series,[157,161] although one recent report of eight cases noted only a 12.5% mortality rate.[160] Most deaths occur within 1 to 2 months. Corticosteroids are generally used for therapy, although there is little evidence of a beneficial effect. Importantly, those few patients who do survive have only mild residual pulmonary functional defects. Recurrences can occur, however, and chronic lung disease has been noted in some survivors, although it is possible that the latter individuals had an unrecognized preexistent chronic lung disease.[161]

Pathologic Features

Pathologically, AIP closely resembles the organizing stage of DAD (see Chapter 2). The most striking histologic feature is interstitial fibroblast proliferation with mild associated chronic inflammation (Fig. 3–17). The alveolar septa are widened by oval- to spindle-shaped fibroblasts and myofibroblasts admixed with scattered lymphocytes or plasma cells (Fig. 3–18). Alveolar epithelial hyperplasia usually accompanies the other changes, and cytologic atypia and squamous metaplasia are common in bronchiolar epithelium (Fig. 3–19). Residual alveolar spaces vary in size and shape, and in places are reduced to narrow slits. Remnants of hyaline membranes are present in a few areas but are usually not prominent. Thrombi in various stages of organization may be seen in small pulmonary arteries. By electron microscopy, epithelial and endothelial necrosis identical to that described in cases of DAD is seen.[156,157] As in DAD, collapse of alveoli and apposition of their walls contribute to the light microscopic appearance of fibrosis.

Differential Diagnosis

The presence of extensive fibrosis in AIP explains why early investigators included this disorder with other

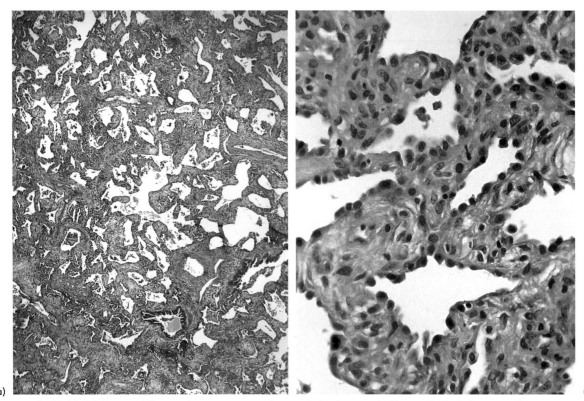

(a)　　　　　　　　　　　　　　　　　　　　　　　　　　　　　　　　　　　　(b)

Figure 3–17 AIP. (a) There is diffuse, uniform-appearing widening of alveolar septa by fibrosis. **(b)** At higher magnification the fibrosis is composed of oval- to spindle-shaped fibroblasts along with prominent alveolar pneumocyte hyperplasia.

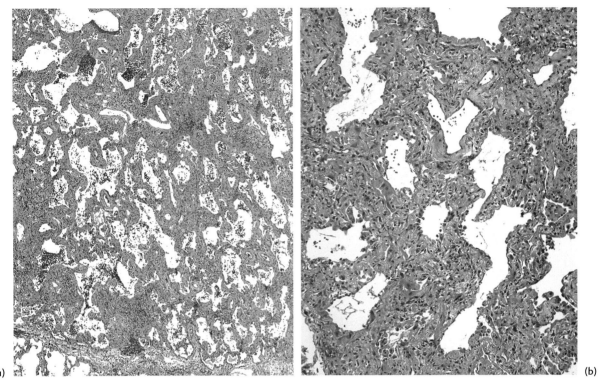

(a)   (b)

Figure 3–18 AIP. (a) In this example at low magnification the alveolar septal thickening appears more cellular. **(b)** At higher magnification evidence of alveolar collapse is seen along with the fibroblast proliferation and alveolar pneumocyte hyperplasia. Note the irregularity in size and shape of residual alveolar spaces.

more common forms of interstitial fibrosis, especially UIP. If the appearance of the fibrosis and its extent are taken into consideration, however, these disorders can be easily and reliably distinguished (see Tables 3–2 and 3–3). In AIP, the fibrosis is diffuse and characterized by proliferation of fibroblasts with relatively little collagen deposition. The appearance thus is *temporally uniform*, and reflects onset in the recent past at one finite time. Whereas fibrosis is also extensive in UIP, it is patchy (patchwork pattern), characterized mostly by collagen deposition and often accompanied by areas of honeycomb change. Small foci of fibroblast proliferation (fibroblast foci) occur in UIP, but they are widely scattered and over-shadowed by large areas of collagen deposition. The appearance, therefore, is *temporally variegated* with both active fibrosis and inactive scarring, and reflects ongoing lung injury occurring in small foci over a long period of time. In difficult cases, of course, a knowledge of the clinical history should help, since the onset in UIP is insidious compared with acute in AIP, and patients with AIP almost invariably require ventilator therapy. The distinction of AIP from UIP is important because, although the prognosis is poor in

both, the length of survival is much shorter in AIP than in UIP (months versus years). Moreover, those few patients who survive an episode of AIP can expect to recover pulmonary function almost completely, whereas the changes in UIP are not reversible.

AIP must also be distinguished from BOOP (see Chapter 2 and Tables 3–2 and 3–3). Although both are temporally uniform and characterized by prominent fibroblast proliferation, the process in BOOP is a patchy, peribronchiolar airspace (intraluminal) lesion, compared with a diffuse interstitial lesion in AIP. Additionally, other features of acute lung injury (thrombi, epithelial metaplasias with atypia, and hyaline membrane remnants) are common in AIP but are not seen in BOOP. Knowledge of the clinical situation should help in difficult cases since patients with AIP usually manifest respiratory failure requiring mechanical ventilation, while respiratory failure is uncommon in BOOP. The differentiation is important because BOOP has a considerably better prognosis. Occasionally, foci of BOOP can be found in otherwise typical AIP (so-called mixed acute lung injury pattern, see Chapter 2). The prognosis in such cases is that of AIP, not BOOP.

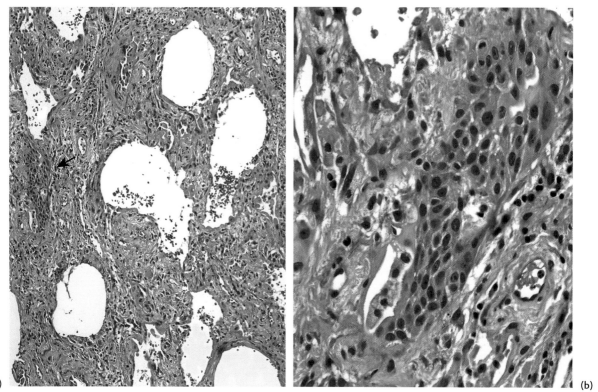

(a)   (b)

Figure 3–19 AIP. (a) Small foci of residual hyaline membrane formation are seen in this example. Also, there is focal squamous metaplasia (arrow) that is shown at higher magnification in **(b)**.

NONSPECIFIC INTERSTITIAL PNEUMONIA/FIBROSIS

NSIP was initially described in 1994 to encompass those interstitial inflammatory and fibrosing lesions that do not fulfill diagnostic criteria for UIP, DIP/RBILD, or AIP.[172] At that time, the diagnosis was considered a descriptive term rather than a specific disease, and it included cases related to underlying connective tissue diseases, hypersensitivity pneumonia, slowly resolving acute lung injury, drug reactions, and poorly sampled UIP or BOOP, in addition to cases of unknown etiology. The term has evolved over the years, however, and currently is used for a disease of unknown etiology.

Clinical Features

Dyspnea and cough occurring over several months are the most common complaints, and, occasionally, systemic symptoms such as fever are present.[168,172] The disease usually affects adults in their early to mid fifties,

although there is a wide age range, and cases also occur in children. In contrast to UIP, most series report an equal gender distribution or a female predominance.[15,164,166,168,174,176] Underlying connective tissue diseases are present in some patients, and, in fact, NSIP is the most common interstitial pneumonia associated with collagen vascular disease.[163,165,173,177,179] By definition, however, NSIP is not diagnosed in immunocompromised persons. Radiographically, bilateral ground glass opacities constitute the most common finding.[162,170,171,174] Interstitial reticular markings are also common. Honeycomb change is not a prominent feature.

The prognosis of NSIP is considerably better than that of UIP, although probably not as good as the 11% mortality rate reported by Katzenstein and Fiorelli in the original article.[172] Subsequent reports have noted mortality rates ranging from 0% to as high as 63%, with most between 11% and 40%. Five-year survival rates range from 76% to 90%.[15,55,75,92,164,166,168,176–178,180] Several investigators have noted a relationship of prognosis to extent of fibrosis, with the best prognosis in cellular forms of the disease and the worst prognosis in fibrotic forms.[55,92,172,180] Most patients respond favorably to corticosteroid therapy.

Pathologic Features

A temporally uniform interstitial inflammatory and fibrosing process containing varying proportions of inflammation and fibrosis is characteristic of NSIP. The *cellular variant* is characterized by a predominance of interstitial chronic inflammation containing small lymphocytes and occasional plasma cells (Figs 3–20 and 3–21). Fibrosis in the form of collagen deposition may be present to some degree but is overshadowed by the inflammation (Fig. 3–22). Alveolar pneumocyte hyperplasia usually accompanies the interstitial changes and is often prominent. The process may be patchy and is often bronchiolocentric in distribution with intervening areas of normal lung.

In the *fibrosing variant* of NSIP, interstitial fibrosis is predominant and there is little associated inflammation (Fig. 3–23). The fibrosis is characterized by collagen deposition with few fibroblasts (Fig. 3–24). The underlying lung architecture is maintained, with minimal, if any, honeycomb change. Fibroblast foci are described in up to 20% of cases, but they are inconspicuous and never numerous, and the process appears uniform in distribution.[172]

Small areas of BOOP are found in nearly half the cases. They are always focal, however, and overshadowed by the interstitial process. Increased numbers of macrophages are frequently found within alveolar spaces. The macrophages often contain abundant foamy cytoplasm, but in cigarette smokers they contain golden yellow to brown pigment. Although occasional poorly formed granulomas in peribronchiolar interstitium were observed in the initial report, their presence should preclude NSIP and suggest hypersensitivity pneumonia (see Chapter 6) instead.

Differential Diagnosis

The fibrosing variant of NSIP can be difficult to differentiate from UIP since fibrosis is a prominent feature of both. Their distinction is important, however, since treatment and prognosis are different. As summarized

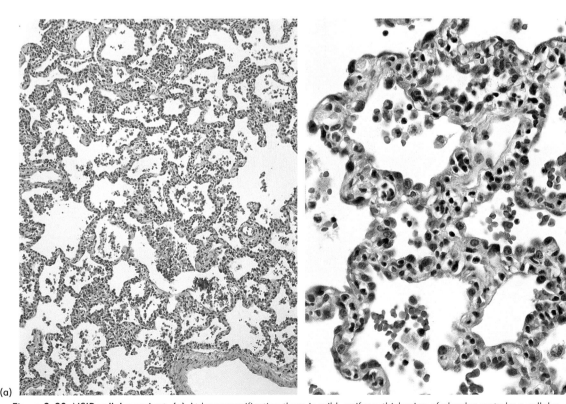

(a)   (b)

Figure 3–20 NSIP, cellular variant. (a) At low magnification there is mild, uniform thickening of alveolar septa by a cellular infiltrate. **(b)** At higher magnification the alveolar septa are thickened by chronic inflammatory cells and mild alveolar pneumocyte hyperplasia. There is no significant collagen deposition.

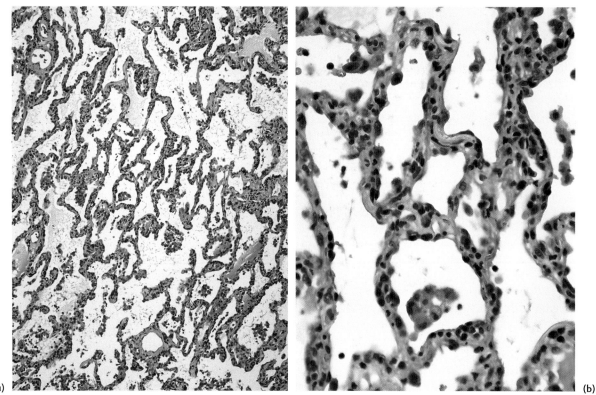

(a)

(b)

Figure 3–21 NSIP, cellular variant. (a) Low magnification view showing uniform thickening of the alveolar septa by a cellular infiltrate. **(b)** Higher magnification showing mild collagen deposition in addition to the inflammation. Plasma cells are prominent in this case.

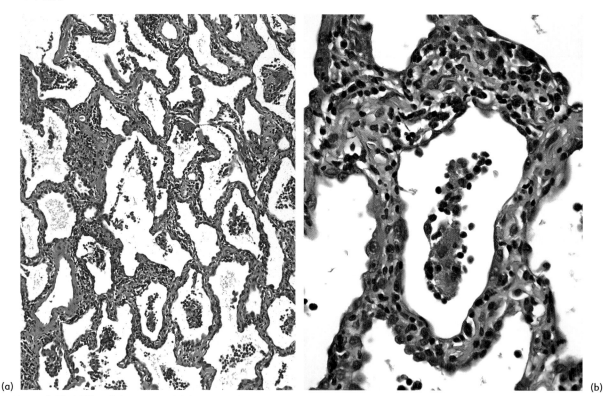

(a)

(b)

Figure 3–22 NSIP, cellular variant. (a) Low magnification view showing collagen deposition in addition to the prominent cellular infiltrate. **(b)** Higher magnification showing a mixture of collagen and chronic inflammatory cells that are thickening alveolar septa. There are also scattered intraalveolar macrophages and a focal proteinaceous exudate present in alveolar spaces.

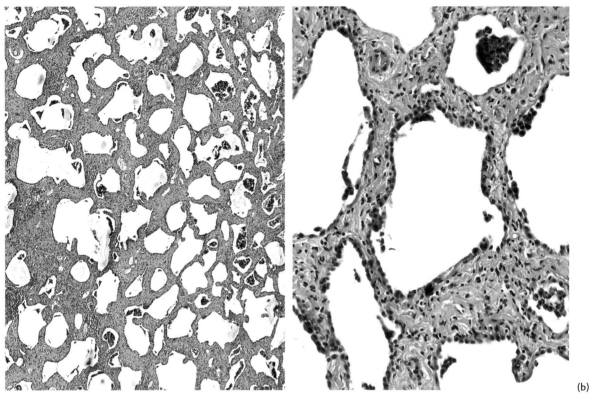

(a)   (b)

Figure 3–23 NSIP, fibrosing variant. (a) Low magnification view showing prominent uniform thickening of alveolar septa by collagen. **(b)** At higher magnification the alveolar septal thickening is due mainly to collagen deposition with mild inflammation. Alveolar pneumocyte hyperplasia is also prominent.

in Table 3–5, the patchwork pattern of parenchymal involvement that is typical of UIP is not seen in NSIP. Likewise, honeycomb change and interstitial scars as well as fibroblast foci are usually absent in NSIP, and, if present, are focal and inconspicuous. One source of difficulty is the fact that NSIP-like areas (areas of uniform appearing alveolar septal collagen deposition with mild inflammation) can be seen in otherwise typical cases of UIP (Fig. 3–25).[59] This observation should not be surprising since, after all, NSIP is a nonspecific

form of interstitial reaction. Just like an intraalveolar accumulation of macrophages (DIP-like reaction) can be found in conditions other than DIP (UIP, Langerhans cell histiocytosis, etc.), NSIP-like areas of fibrosis are common in conditions other than NSIP (especially UIP). The correct diagnosis is established by recognizing the overall pattern rather than focusing on one area. The presence of NSIP-like areas in otherwise typical UIP cases likely explains the reports of NSIP and UIP occurring in biopsies from different lobes of the same patient and also explains the observation that the disease in those cases behaves like UIP.[167,175]

When intraalveolar macrophages are prominent, DIP/RBILD enters the differential diagnosis, since the macrophages often contain light brown–yellow pigment characteristic of cigarette smokers' macrophages. There are no well-established criteria to separate such cases from NSIP, and the differentiation makes little difference clinically. We prefer the diagnosis of NSIP when the interstitial fibrosis and inflammation are prominent, and restrict the diagnosis of DIP/RBILD to cases with minimal interstitial abnormality.

Table 3–5 Contrasting Features of Fibrosing NSIP and UIP

	Fibrosing NSIP	UIP
Patchwork pattern	Absent	Characteristic
Architectural distortion (honeycomb change, interstitial scars)	Minimal to absent	Characteristic
Fibroblast foci	Few to absent	Characteristic

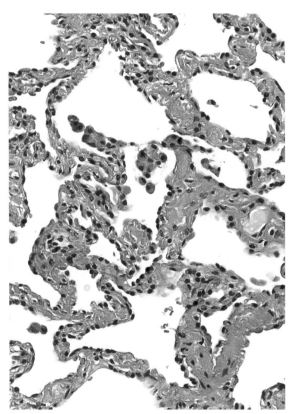

Figure 3–24 Fibrosing NSIP. In this example the alveolar septal thickening is due almost entirely to collagen with minimal inflammation. Alveolar macrophages are focally numerous.

Hypersensitivity pneumonia enters the differential diagnosis of the cellular variant of NSIP, especially when the changes are accentuated around bronchioles.[181] It should be excluded clinically in all such cases. NSIP has been reported following ARDS, and in this situation likely represents slowly resolving DAD.[169,172] Other potential causes should also be excluded clinically, including drug toxicity and collagen vascular diseases, for example.

OTHER IDIOPATHIC INTERSTITIAL PNEUMONIAS

Morphologic variants of idiopathic interstitial pneumonia have been recently described as 'bronchiolocentric interstitial pneumonia',[185] 'centrilobular fibrosis',[183] and 'airway centered interstitial pneumonia',[182] and appear to be related entities. They are characterized by mild peribronchiolar interstitial fibrosis associated with extension of bronchiolar epithelium along thickened alveolar septa (microscopic honeycomb change) (Fig. 3–26). Inflammation is not a prominent feature, although intraalveolar foamy macrophages and mucous plugging may be observed. The cases are encountered over a wide age range, with a reported mean age of 46 to 58 years. A female predominance was noted in some series. Prognosis is not good, with mortality rates of 33% to 40%, although it is better than UIP. Whether this lesion represents a separate form of interstitial pneumonia is not clear. Similar findings can be seen in a variety of otherwise typical interstitial lung diseases, including UIP, NSIP, DIP, RB, and hypersensitivity pneumonia, however, and it is likely that the lesion is a reaction pattern resulting from bronchiolar injury in a variety of settings.[184] Mucous plugging with foamy macrophages and cholesterol clefts is prominent in some cases and suggests that prior infection may be etiologic. Some investigators have suggested aspiration in the etiology.[183]

Prominent pleural fibrosis has been described in some patients with interstitial fibrosis and termed 'idiopathic pleuroparenchymal fibroelastosis'.[183a] Whether this lesion is a variant of UIP with pleural fibrosis, a primary inflammatory pleural disease with secondary parenchymal involvement, or a truly separate clinicopathologic entity is not clear. The pleural changes are somewhat similar to apical pulmonary cap (see Chapter 16), except that they are diffuse rather than localized.

It should be remembered that not all interstitial inflammatory and fibrosing processes can be classified into a named category of idiopathic interstitial pneumonia, and a descriptive diagnosis of 'unclassifiable interstitial fibrosis', 'interstitial fibrosis with honeycomb change', or 'honeycomb change' may be necessary. For example, some biopsies consist entirely of honeycomb lung without other diagnostic features. Sometimes, interstitial fibrosis is seen that resembles fibrosing NSIP except for the presence of prominent honeycomb change and thus does not fit with a specific entity. Some biopsies are too small and contain only peripheral subpleural lung parenchyma that is not sufficient for definitive diagnosis.

BIOPSY DIAGNOSES IN THE IDIOPATHIC INTERSTITIAL PNEUMONIAS

As mentioned earlier, diagnosis of the idiopathic interstitial pneumonias is facilitated by clinical input both to confirm that the patient has interstitial lung disease and to be certain that an etiology has not been identified.

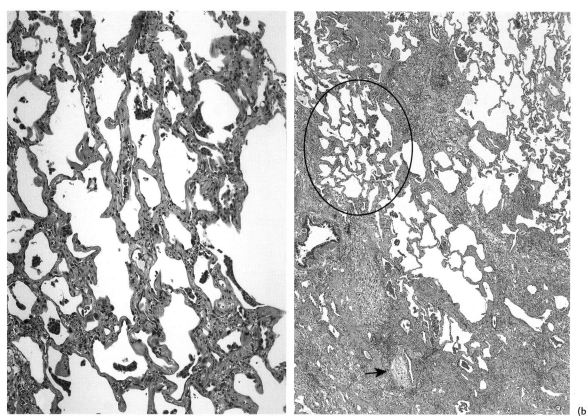

Figure 3–25 NSIP-like areas in UIP. (a) An area of uniform alveolar septal thickening by collagen-type fibrosis and mild chronic inflammation can be seen. The appearance would fit with the fibrosing variant of NSIP if the entire biopsy had this appearance. However, at low magnification **(b)** the typical variegated appearance of UIP is appreciated. A small NSIP-like area is seen between the scarred areas of parenchyma in the upper left (circle). Note the fibroblast in an area of scarring (arrow).

The ATS/ERS consensus statement advocates diagnosing cases as a 'pattern' (UIP pattern, DIP pattern, NSIP pattern, DAD pattern, RB pattern, BOOP pattern, LIP pattern) to avoid reliance on clinical findings. This approach, however, inappropriately minimizes the significance of the pathologic diagnosis and it encourages indecisiveness. While clinical input is needed for certain diseases (DIP/RBILD, AIP, IPF, idiopathic BOOP), the pathologic entities of RB, DAD, UIP, and BOOP, for example, can be diagnosed from the pathologic findings alone. Moreover, for changes resembling NSIP, a descriptive diagnosis such as 'cellular chronic interstitial pneumonia' is more practical and understandable than 'NSIP pattern'. When alveolar macrophages are more extensive than occurs in RB, the diagnosis of 'intra-alveolar macrophage accumulation' is more appropriate than 'DIP pattern'. If strict pathologic criteria are followed for diagnosing LIP (see Chapter 9), there is no need to diagnose 'LIP pattern', since no other entities fit with this appearance. It seems superfluous to add 'pattern' to what already is a discrete histologic finding. Moreover, a similar approach using 'patterns' is not utilized for other analogous situations, either in the lung (for example, one does not diagnose 'non-necrotizing granuloma pattern' in sarcoidosis, or 'eosinophilic pneumonia pattern' in chronic eosinophilic pneumonia), or in other organ systems (one does not diagnose 'chronic dermatitis pattern', or 'chronic hepatitis pattern'). Our approach to diagnosing these various entities is summarized in Table 3–6. In the right clinical setting when appropriate history is known, the diseases can be diagnosed directly. It should be remembered that the histologic features of UIP are often so characteristic that it can be diagnosed with minimal clinical input.

HONEYCOMB LUNG

Honeycomb lung refers to a distinct alteration of lung parenchyma that results from scarring. It is an end-stage

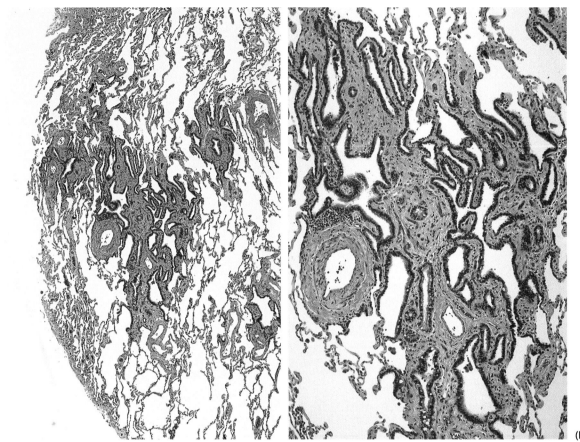

(a) (b)

Figure 3–26 Bronchiolocentric interstitial pneumonia. (a) Low magnification view showing the presence of interstitial scarring and microscopic honeycomb change occurring around a bronchiole. Note the intervening areas of normal interstitium. **(b)** Higher magnification showing the typical restructured airspaces lined by bronchiolar-type epithelium.

and irreversible lesion, and it can result from a variety of interstitial inflammatory and fibrosing processes.[186,189] It has a characteristic gross appearance, with relatively uniformly sized cysts ranging from several millimeters to one or more centimeters in diameter that are set in a background of dense scarring (Fig. 3–27). The cyst walls are composed of firm, thick, fibrous tissue, and the overall appearance is reminiscent of a honeycomb produced by honeybees. Honeycomb areas are usually most prominent in subpleural lung parenchyma and at the lung bases. Traction bronchiectasis is a frequent accompanying finding radiographically. Although usually associated with a diffuse interstitial process, occasionally honeycomb areas are isolated findings in the peripheral lung that have little clinical significance. Most examples of honeycomb lung take many years to develop, although it can evolve in as rapidly as a few weeks in patients with DAD or AIP (Fig. 3–28). The lesion in this situation differs microscopically from

classic honeycomb change (see later on) and may be related in part to barotrauma from the mechanical ventilation.

Microscopically, as discussed earlier in the section on UIP, honeycomb lung is characterized by enlarged airspaces surrounded by collagen-type fibrosis and lined by bronchiolar or hyperplastic alveolar epithelium (see Figs 3–4 and 3–5). The process is always centered around a bronchiole which is identified by the presence of regularly arranged peribronchiolar smooth muscle bundles. Mucin, containing variable numbers of inflammatory cells, often fills the abnormal spaces. The honeycomb spaces in end-stage DAD differ in that their walls contain less collagen and they are usually lined by alveolar pneumocytes rather than bronchiolar epithelium.

Honeycomb change can be recognized microscopically before it is apparent grossly or radiographically (so-called *microscopic honeycomb change*). Microscopic

Table 3–6   Biopsy Diagnosis of Idiopathic Interstitial Pneumonias

Disease	Clinical and Radiographic Input Needed for Diagnosis	Pathologic Diagnosis	
		Clinical History Not Provided	Clinical History Known
IPF/UIP	Not in classic cases, but may help to confirm the diagnosis in difficult cases	'UIP'	'UIP'
NSIP	Yes, to exclude drug toxicity, hypersensitivity pneumonia, immunocompromise, other etiologies	'Chronic interstitial pneumonia' ('cellular' or 'with fibrosis')	'NSIP' ('cellular' or 'fibrotic' variant)
DIP/RBILD	Yes, to exclude nonspecific intraalveolar macrophage accumulation (DIP-like reaction) and to differentiate from incidental RB	'Intraalveolar macrophage accumulation', 'RB'	'RBILD/DIP'
AIP	Yes, to exclude multiple potential causes of DAD	'Organizing DAD'	'AIP'

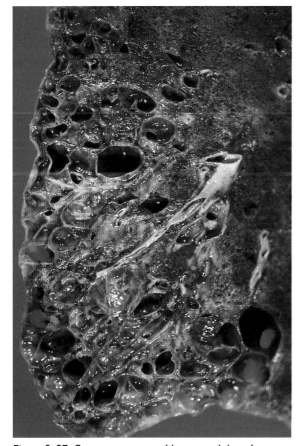

Figure 3–27 Gross appearance of honeycomb lung from a case of UIP. Note the enlarged airspaces with thick walls that are present at the lung base and periphery.

honeycomb change is a characteristic feature of UIP, as previously mentioned. In its earliest stage it is characterized by growth of bronchiolar epithelium along thickened alveolar septa adjacent to bronchioles, with the formation of small cysts containing inspissated mucin.

The pathogenesis of honeycomb change is related to the combination of parenchymal collapse in areas of previous lung injury and collagen deposition.[16,87,156] The development of associated bronchiolectasis due to traction from adjacent scarring also contributes to the morphologic derangement, as does loss of the elastic fiber framework.[46,190]

The gross and microscopic appearances of end-stage honeycomb lung are nonspecific as regards etiology, and one can determine the cause only by the examination of earlier biopsy material, the careful correlation of clinical and radiographic data, or the detection of a more active and informative area of disease elsewhere in the biopsy.[189] A diverse group of diseases or processes can lead to honeycomb lung, as listed in Table 3–7.[186,188]

Table 3–7   Pulmonary Disorders Leading to Honeycomb Lung

Idiopathic interstitial pneumonia (AIP, UIP, DIP)
Diffuse alveolar damage
Inorganic dust exposure (asbestosis)
Interstitial granulomatous diseases (infections, hypersensitivity pneumonia, sarcoidosis, berylliosis)
Eosinophilic granuloma

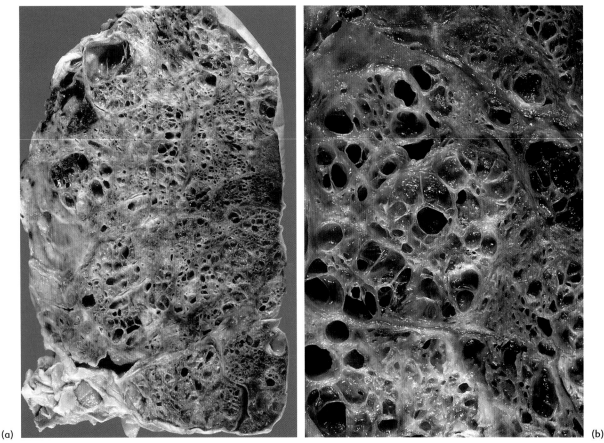

(a)

(b)

Figure 3–28 Honeycomb lung from a patient with DAD for 6 weeks following an episode of trauma and sepsis. (a) Cross-section of lung showing diffuse cystic appearance. (b) Closer view demonstrating the thick walls surrounding most of the cysts.

The idiopathic interstitial pneumonias, especially UIP and AIP, are important precursors of honeycomb lung. Similarly, DAD due to a variety of causes may also evolve into honeycomb lung (see Chapter 2). Certain pneumoconioses, especially asbestosis or other fibrogenic dust-related diseases, may cause a similar picture (see Chapter 5). Granulomatous diseases, including both infectious disorders (such as miliary tuberculosis) and noninfectious disorders (such as sarcoidosis, hypersensitivity pneumonia, or berylliosis), may be the initiating event. Rare examples of Langerhans cell histiocytosis evolve into honeycomb lung (see Chapter 15).[188]

The extensive scar formation and reparative activity in lungs with interstitial fibrosis and honeycomb areas are associated with an increased risk of developing peripheral pulmonary carcinomas and likely explain the observed increase in lung cancer in patients with UIP.[7,47,187] The tumors may be multifocal.

REFERENCES

General

1. American Thoracic Society/European Respiratory Society International Multidisciplinary Consensus Classification of the Idiopathic Interstitial Pneumonias. Am J Respir Crit Care Med 165:277, 2002.
2. Green FHY: Overview of pulmonary fibrosis. Chest 122:334S, 2002.
3. Gross TJ, Hunninghake GW: Idiopathic pulmonary fibrosis. N Engl J Med 345:517, 2001.
4. Katzenstein A-LA, Myers JL: Idiopathic pulmonary fibrosis. Clinical relevance of pathologic classification. Am J Respir Crit Care Med 157:1301, 1998.
5. Katzenstein A-LA, Myers JL: Nonspecific interstitial pneumonia and the other idiopathic interstitial pneumonias: Classification and diagnostic criteria. Am J Surg Pathol 24:1, 2000.
6. Liebow AA: Definition and classification of interstitial pneumonias in human pathology. Prog Respir Res 8:1, 1975.

Usual Interstitial Pneumonia

7. Akira T, Katsura H, Sawabe M, Kida K: A clinical study of idiopathic pulmonary fibrosis based on autopsy studies in elderly patients. Intern Med 42:483, 2003.

8. American Thoracic Society: Idiopathic pulmonary fibrosis: Diagnosis and treatment. International consensus statement. American Thoracic Society (ATS), and the European Respiratory Society (ERS). Am J Respir Crit Care Med 161:646, 2000.

9. Azuma A, Nukiwa T, Tsuboi E, et al: Double blind, placebo-controlled trial of pirfenidone in patients with idiopathic pulmonary fibrosis. Am J Respir Crit Care Med 171:1040, 2005.

10. Barbas-Filho JV, Ferreira MA, Sesso A, Kairalla RA, Carvalho CRR, Capelozzi VL: Evidence of type II pneumocyte apoptosis in the pathogenesis of idiopathic pulmonary fibrosis (IPF)/usual interstitial pneumonia (UIP). J Clin Path 54:132, 2001.

11. Barzo P: Familial idiopathic fibrosing alveolitis. Eur J Respir Dis 66:350, 1985.

12. Basset F, Ferrans FJ, Soler P, et al: Intraluminal fibrosis in interstitial lung disorders. Am J Pathol 122:443, 1986.

13. Bateman E, Turner-Warwick M, Haslam PL, Adelmann-Grill BC: Cryptogenic fibrosing alveolitis: Prediction of fibrogenic activity from immunohistochemical studies of collagen types in lung biopsy specimens. Thorax 38:93, 1983.

14. Bensadoun ES, Burke AK, Hogg JC, Roberts CR: Proteoglycan deposition in pulmonary fibrosis. Am J Respir Crit Care Med 154:1819, 1996.

15. Bjoraker JA, Ryu JH, Edwin MK, et al: Prognostic significance of histopathologic subsets in idiopathic pulmonary fibrosis. Am J Respir Crit Care Med 157:199, 1998.

16. Burkhardt A: Alveolitis and collapse in the pathogenesis of pulmonary fibrosis. Am Rev Respir Dis 140:513, 1989.

17. Campbell DA, Poulter LW, Janossy G, DuBois RM: Immunohistological analysis of lung tissue from patients with cryptogenic fibrosing alveolitis suggesting local expression of immune hypersensitivity. Thorax 40: 405, 1985.

18. Carrington CB, Gaensler EA, Coutu RE, et al: Natural history and treated course of usual and desquamative interstitial pneumonia. N Engl J Med 298:801, 1978.

19. Cherniack RM, Colby TV, Flint A, et al: Quantitative assessment of lung pathology in idiopathic pulmonary fibrosis. The BAL Cooperative Group Steering Committee. Am Rev Respir Dis 144:892, 1991.

20. Cherniack RM, Colby TV, Flint A, et al: Correlation of structure and function in idiopathic pulmonary fibrosis. Am J Respir Crit Care Med 151:1180, 1995.

21. Chibar R, Shih F, Baga M, et al: Nonspecific interstitial pneumonia and usual interstitial pneumonia with mutation in surfactant protein C in familial pulmonary fibrosis. Mod Pathol 17:973, 2004.

22. Chilosi M, Poletti V, Murer B, et al: Abnormal re-epithelialization and lung remodeling in idiopathic pulmonary fibrosis: The role of ΔN-p63. Lab Invest 82:1335, 2002.

23. Chilosi M, Poletti V, Zamo A, et al: Aberrant Wnt/β-catenin pathway activation in idiopathic pulmonary fibrosis. Am J Pathol 162:1495, 2003.

24. Choi ES, Jakubzick C, Carpenter KJ, et al: Enhanced monocyte chemoattractant protein-3/CC chemokine ligand-7 in usual interstitial pneumonia. Am J Respir Crit Care Med 170:508, 2004.

25. Coalson JJ: The ultrastructure of human fibrosing alveolitis. Virchows Arch [Pathol Anat] 395:181, 1982.

26. Coker RK, Laurent GJ, Jeffery PK, et al: Localisation of transforming growth factor β_1 and β_3 mRNA transcripts in normal and fibrotic human lung. Thorax 56:549, 2001.

27. Collard HR, King TE Jr, Bartelson BB, et al: Changes in clinical and physiologic variables predict survival in idiopathic pulmonary fibrosis. Am J Respir Crit Care Med 168:538, 2003.

28. Cook DN, Brass DM, Schwartz DA: A matrix for new ideas in pulmonary fibrosis. Am J Respir Cell Mol Biol 27:122, 2002.

29. Corrin B, Dewar A, Rodriguez-Roisin R, Turner-Warwick M: Fine structural changes in cryptogenic fibrosing alveolitis and asbestosis. J Pathol 147:107, 1985.

30. Cosgrove GP, Brown KK, Schiemann WP, et al: Pigment epithelium-derived factor in idiopathic pulmonary fibrosis: A role in aberrant angiogenesis. Am J Respir Crit Care Med 170:242, 2004.

31. Crystal RG, Bitterman PB, Mossman B, Schwarz MI: Future research directions in idiopathic pulmonary fibrosis. Am J Respir Crit Care Med 166:236, 2002.

32. Crystal RG, Fulmer JD, Roberts WC, et al: Idiopathic pulmonary fibrosis. Clinical, histologic, radiographic, physiologic, scintigraphic, cytologic and biochemical aspects. Ann Intern Med, 85:769, 1976.

32a. Demedts M, Behr J, Buhl R, et al: High-dose acetylcysteine in idiopathic pulmonary fibrosis. N Engl J Med 353:2229, 2005.

33. Ebina M, Shimizukawa M, Shibata N, Kimura Y: Heterogeneous increase of CD34-positive alveolar capillaries in idiopathic pulmonary fibrosis. Am J Respir Crit Care Med 169:1203, 2004.

34. Egan JJ, Woodcock AA, Stewart JP: Viruses and idiopathic pulmonary fibrosis. Eur Respir J 10:1433, 1997.

35. Flaherty KR, Colby TV, Travis WD, et al: Fibroblastic foci in usual interstitial pneumonia: Idiopathic versus collagen vascular disease. Am J Respir Crit Care Med 167:1410, 2003.

36. Flaherty KR, King TE Jr, Raghu G, et al: Idiopathic interstitial pneumonia: What is the effect of a multidisciplinary approach to diagnosis? Am J Respir Crit Care Med 170:904, 2004.

37. Flaherty KR, Mumford JA, Murray S, et al: Prognostic implications of physiologic and radiographic changes in idiopathic interstitial pneumonia. Am J Respir Crit Care Med 168:543, 2003.

38. Flaherty KR, Thwaite EL, Kazerooni EA, et al: Radiological versus histological diagnosis in UIP and NSIP: Survival implications. Thorax 58:143, 2003.

39. Flaherty KR, Toews GB, Travis WD, Colby TV: Clinical significance of histological classification of idiopathic interstitial pneumonia. Eur Respir J 19:275, 2002.

40. Fukuda Y, Basset F, Ferrans VJ, Yamanaka N: Significance of early intraalveolar fibrotic lesions and integrin expression in lung biopsy specimens from patients with idiopathic pulmonary fibrosis. Hum Pathol 26:53, 1995.

41. Giaid A, Michel RP, Stewart DJ, et al: Expression of endothelin-1 in lungs of patients with cryptogenic fibrosing alveolitis. Lancet 341:1550, 1993.

42. Guerry-Force ML, Muller NL, Wright JL, et al: A comparison of bronchiolitis obliterans with organizing pneumonia, usual interstitial pneumonia, and small airways disease. Am Rev Respir Dis 135:705, 1987.

43. Harmon KR, Witkop CJ, White JG, et al: Pathogenesis of pulmonary fibrosis: Platelet-derived growth factor precedes structural alterations in the Hermansky-Pudlak syndrome. J Lab Clin Med 123:617, 1994.

44. Hayashi T, Stetler-Stevenson WG, Fleming MV, et al: Immunohistochemical study of metalloproteinases and their tissue inhibitors in the lungs of patients with diffuse alveolar damage and idiopathic pulmonary fibrosis. Am J Pathol 149:1241, 1996.

45. Homma S, Nagaoka I, Abe H, et al: Localization of platelet-derived growth factor and insulin-like growth factor I in the fibrotic lung. Am J Respir Crit Care Med 152:2084, 1995.

46. Honda T, Ota H, Arai K, et al: Three-dimensional analysis of alveolar structure in usual interstitial pneumonia. Virchows Arch 441:47, 2002.

47. Hubbard R, Venn A, Lewis S, Britton J: Lung cancer and cryptogenic fibrosing alveolitis: A population-based cohort study. Am J Respir Crit Care Med 161:5, 2000.

48. Hunninghake GW, Lynch DA, Galvin JR, et al: Radiologic findings are strongly associated with a pathologic diagnosis of usual interstitial pneumonia. Chest 124:1215, 2003.

49. Hunninghake GW, Zimmerman MB, Schwartz DA, et al: Utility of a lung biopsy for the diagnosis of idiopathic pulmonary fibrosis. Am J Respir Crit Care Med 164:193, 2001.

50. Hunt LW, Colby TV, Weiler DA, et al: Immunofluorescent staining for mast cells in idiopathic pulmonary fibrosis: Quantification and evidence for extracellular release of mast cell tryptase. Mayo Clin Proc 67:941, 1992.

51. Hyde DM, King TE Jr, McDermott T, et al: Idiopathic pulmonary fibrosis. Quantitative assessment of lung pathology. Comparison of a semiquantitative and a morphometric histopathologic scoring system. Am Rev Respir Dis 146:1042, 1992.

52. Imokawa S, Sato A, Hayakawa H, Kotani M, Urano T, Takada A: Tissue factor expression and fibrin deposition in the lungs of patients with idiopathic pulmonary fibrosis and systemic sclerosis. Am J Respir Crit Care Med 156:631, 1997.

53. Irving WL, Day S, Johnston IDA: Idiopathic pulmonary fibrosis and hepatitis C virus infection. Am Rev Respir Dis 148:1683, 1993.

54. Iyonaga K, Motohira T, Saita N, et al: Monocyte chemoattractant protein-1 in idiopathic pulmonary fibrosis and other interstitial lung diseases. Hum Pathol 25:455, 1994.

55. Jegal Y, Kim DS, Shim TS, et al: Physiology is a stronger predictor of survival than pathology in fibrotic interstitial pneumonia. Am J Respir Crit Care Med 171:639, 2005.

56. Kaarteenaho-Wiik R, Tani T, Sormunen R, Soini Y, Virtanen I, Pääkö P: Tenascin immunoreactivity as a prognostic marker in usual interstitial pneumonia. Am J Respir Crit Care Med 154:511, 1996.

57. Kapanci Y, Desmouliere A, Pache J-C, et al: Cytoskeletal protein modulation in pulmonary alveolar myofibroblasts during idiopathic pulmonary fibrosis. Possible role of transforming growth factor beta and tumor necrosis factor alpha. Am J Respir Crit Care Med 152:2163, 1995.

58. Katzenstein A-LA, Myers JL, Prophet WD, et al: Bronchiolitis obliterans and usual interstitial pneumonia. A comparative clinicopathologic study. Am J Surg Pathol 106:373, 1986.

59. Katzenstein A-LA, Zisman DA, Litzky LA, Nguyen BT, Kotloff RM: Usual interstitial pneumonia: Histologic study of biopsy and explant specimens. Am J Surg Pathol 261:1567, 2002.

60. Kawanami O, Ferrans VJ, Crystal RG: Structure of alveolar epithelial cells in patients with fibrotic lung disorders. Lab Invest 46:39, 1982.

61. Kawanami O, Ferrans VJ, Fulmer JD, Crystal RG: Nuclear inclusions in alveolar epithelium of patients with fibrotic lung disorders. Am J Pathol 94:301, 1979.

62. Kay JM, Kahana LM, Rihal C: Diffuse smooth muscle proliferation of the lungs with severe pulmonary hypertension. Hum Pathol 27:969, 1996.

63. Keane MP, Belperio JA, Burdick MD, et al: ENA-78 is an important angiogenic factor in idiopathic pulmonary fibrosis. Am J Respir Crit Care Med 164:2239, 2001.

64. Kelly BG, Lok SS, Hasleton PS, Egan JJ, Stewart JP: A rearranged form of Epstein-Barr virus DNA is associated with idiopathic pulmonary fibrosis. Am J Respir Crit Care Med 166:510, 2002.

65. King TE, Schwarz MJ, Brown K, et al: Idiopathic pulmonary fibrosis: Relationship between histopathologic features and mortality. Am J Respir Crit Care Med 164:1025, 2001.

66. King TE, Tooze JA, Schwarz MI, et al: Predicting survival in idiopathic pulmonary fibrosis: Scoring system and survival model. Am J Respir Crit Care Med 164:1171, 2001.

67. Kinnula VL, Fattman CL, Tan RJ, Oury TD: Oxidative stress in pulmonary fibrosis: A possible role for redox modulatory therapy. Am J Respir Crit Care Med 172:417, 2005.

68. Kitasato Y, Hoshino T, Okamoto M, et al: Enhanced expression of interleukin-18 and its receptor in

idiopathic pulmonary fibrosis. Am J Respir Cell Mol Biol 31:619, 2004.

69. Kondoh Y, Taniguchi H, Kawabata Y, Yokoi T, Suzuki K, Takagi K: Acute exacerbation in idiopathic pulmonary fibrosis: Analysis of clinical and pathologic findings in three cases. Chest 103:1808, 1993.

70. Kuhn C III, Boldt J, King TE, et al: An immunohistochemical study of architectural remodeling and connective tissue synthesis in pulmonary fibrosis. Am Rev Respir Dis 140:1693, 1989.

71. Kuhn C, McDonald JA: The roles of the myofibroblast in idiopathic pulmonary fibrosis: Ultrastructural and immunohistochemical features of sites of active extracellular matrix synthesis. Am J Pathol 138:1257, 1991.

72. Kuwano K, Kunitake R, Kawasaki M, et al: p21$^{Wa1/Cip1/Sdi1}$ and p53 expression in association with DNA strand breaks in idiopathic pulmonary fibrosis. Am J Respir Crit Care Med 154:477, 1996.

73. Lakari E, Pääkö P, Pietarinen-Runtti P, Kinnula VL: Manganese superoxide dismutase and catalase are coordinately expressed in the alveolar region in chronic interstitial pneumonias and granulomatous diseases of the lung. Am J Respir Crit Care Med 161:615, 2000.

74. Lappi-Blanco E, Kaarteenaho-Wiik R, Salo S, et al: Laminin-5 γ_2 chain in cryptogenic organizing pneumonia and idiopathic pulmonary fibrosis. Am J Respir Crit Care Med 169:27, 2004.

75. Latsi PI, du Bois RM, Nicholson AG, et al: Fibrotic idiopathic interstitial pneumonia: The prognostic value of longitudinal functional trends. Am J Respir Crit Care Med 168:531, 2003.

76. Lawson WE, Grant SW, Ambrosini V, et al: Interstitial lung disease: Genetic mutations in surfactant protein C are a rare cause of sporadic cases of IPF. Thorax 59:977, 2004.

77. Lee H-L, Ryu JH, Wittmer MH, et al: Familial idiopathic pulmonary fibrosis. Clinical features and outcome. Chest 127:2034, 2005.

78. Lynch DA, Godwin JD, Safrin S, et al: High-resolution computed tomography in idiopathic pulmonary fibrosis: Diagnosis and prognosis. Am J Respir Crit Care Med 172:488, 2005.

79. Marshall RP, Puddicombe A, Cookson WOC, Laurent GJ: Adult familial cryptogenic fibrosing alveolitis in the United Kingdom. Thorax 55:143, 2000.

80. Martinez FJ, Safrin S, Weycker D, et al: The clinical course of patients with idiopathic pulmonary fibrosis. Ann Intern Med 142:963, 2005.

81. Matsuyama W, Kawabata M, Mizoguchi A, et al: Influence of human T lymphotrophic virus type I on cryptogenic fibrosing alveolitis – HTLV-I associated fibrosing alveolitis: Proposal of a new clinical entity. Clin Exp Immunol 133:397, 2003.

82. Miki H, Mio T, Nagai S, et al: Fibroblast contractility: Usual interstitial pneumonia and nonspecific interstitial pneumonia. Am J Respir Crit Care Med 162:2259, 2000.

83. Moodley YP, Caterina P, Scaffidi AK, et al: Comparison of the morphological and biochemical changes in normal human lung fibroblasts and fibroblasts derived from lungs of patients with idiopathic pulmonary fibrosis during FasL-induced apoptosis. J Pathol 202:486, 2004.

84. Moodley YP, Misso NLA, Scaffidi AK, et al: Inverse effects of interleukin-6 on apoptosis of fibroblasts from pulmonary fibrosis and normal lung. Am J Respir Cell Mol Biol 29:490, 2003.

85. Mori M, Morishita H, Nakamura H, et al: Hepatoma-derived growth factor is involved in lung remodeling by stimulating epithelial growth. Am J Respir Cell Mol Biol 10:1165, 2003.

86. Muller N, Colby TV: Idiopathic interstitial pneumonias: High-resolution CT and histologic findings. Radiographics 17:1016, 1997.

87. Myers J, Katzenstein A: Epithelial necrosis and alveolar collapse in the pathogenesis of usual interstitial pneumonia. Chest 94:1309, 1988.

88. Nadrous HF, Myers JL, Decker PA, Ryu JH: Idiopathic pulmonary fibrosis in patients younger than 50 years. Mayo Clin Proc 80:37, 2005.

89. Nagata N, Nagatomo H, Yoshii C, Nikaido Y, Kido M: Features of idiopathic pulmonary fibrosis with organizing pneumonia. Respiration 64:331, 1997.

90. Nakashima N, Kuwano K, Maeyama T, et al: The p-53-Mdm2 association in epithelial cells in idiopathic pulmonary fibrosis and non-specific interstitial pneumonia. J Clin Pathol 58:583, 2005.

91. Nicholson AG, Addis BJ, Bharucha H, et al: Inter-observer variation between pathologists in diffuse parenchymal lung disease. Thorax 59:500, 2004.

92. Nicholson AG, Colby TV, Dubois RM, Hansell DM, Wells AU: The prognostic significance of the histologic pattern of interstitial pneumonia in patients presenting with the clinical entity of cryptogenic fibrosing alveolitis. Am J Respir Crit Care Med 162:2213, 2000.

93. Nicholson AG, Fulford LG, Colby TV, et al: The relationship between individual histologic features and disease progression in idiopathic pulmonary fibrosis. Am J Respir Crit Care Med 166:173, 2002.

94. Nishimura K, Kitaichi M, Izumi T, et al: Usual interstitial pneumonia: Histologic correlation with high-resolution CT. Radiology 182:337, 1992.

95. Nishiyama O, Taniguchi H, Kondoh Y, et al: Familial idiopathic pulmonary fibrosis: Serial high-resolution computed tomography findings in 9 patients. J Comput Assist Tomogr 28:443, 2004.

96. Ohta K, Mortenson RL, Clark RAF, et al: Immunohisto-chemical identification and characterization of smooth muscle-like cells in idiopathic pulmonary fibrosis. Am J Respir Crit Care Med 152:1659, 1995.

97. Ovenfors C-O, Dahlgren S, Ripe E, Ost A: Muscular hyperplasia of the lung. A clinical, radiographic, and histopathologic study. AJR Am J Roentgenol 135:703, 1980.

98. Pääkö P, Kaarteenaho-Wiik R, Pollänen R, Soini Y: Tenascin mRNA expression at the foci of recent injury

in usual interstitial pneumonia. Am J Respir Crit Care Med 161:967, 2000.

99. Peckham RM, Shorr AF, Helman DL: Potential limitations of clinical criteria for the diagnosis of idiopathic pulmonary fibrosis/cryptogenic fibrosing alveolitis. Respiration 71:165, 2004.

100. Peltoniemi M, Kaarteenaho-Wiik R, Säily M, et al: Expression of glutaredoxin is highly cell specific in human lung and is decreased by transforming growth factor-β in vitro and in interstitial lung diseases in vivo. Hum Pathol 35:1000, 2004.

101. Petkova DK, Clelland CA, Ronan JE, Lewis S, Knox AJ: Reduced expression of cyclooxygenase (COX) in idiopathic pulmonary fibrosis and sarcoidosis. Histopathology 43:381, 2003.

102. Plataki M, Koutsopoulos AV, Darivianaki K, et al: Expression of apoptotic and antiapoptotic markers in epithelial cells in idiopathic pulmonary fibrosis. Chest 127:266, 2005.

103. Raghu G, Brown KK, Bradford WZ, et al: A placebo-controlled trial of interferon gamma-1b in patients with idiopathic pulmonary fibrosis. N Engl J Med 350:125, 2004.

104. Raghu G, Mageto YN, Lockhart D, Schmidt RA, Wood DE, Godwin JD: The accuracy of the clinical diagnosis of new-onset idiopathic pulmonary fibrosis and other interstitial lung disease: A prospective study. Chest 116:1168, 1999.

105. Ramos C, Montano M, Garcia-Alvarez J, et al: Fibroblasts from idiopathic pulmonary fibrosis and normal lungs differ in growth rate, apoptosis, and tissue inhibitor of metalloproteinases expression. Am J Respir Cell Mol Biol 24:591, 2001.

106. Renzoni EA, Walsh DA, Salmon M, et al: Interstitial vascularity in fibrosing alveolitis. Am J Respir Crit Care Med 167:438, 2003.

107. Riha RL, Duhig EE, Clark RH, Slaughter RE, Zimmerman PV: Survival of patients with biopsy-proven usual interstitial pneumonia and nonspecific interstitial pneumonia. Eur Respir J 19:114, 2002.

108. Rozin GF, Gomes MM, Parra ER, et al: Collagen and elastic system in the remodeling process of major types of idiopathic interstitial pneumonia (IIP). Histopathology 46:413, 2005.

109. Saleh D, Barnes PJ, Giaid A: Increased production of the potent oxidant peroxynitrite in the lungs of patients with idiopathic pulmonary fibrosis. Am J Respir Crit Care Med 155:1763, 1997.

110. Selman M, King TE, Pardo A: Idiopathic pulmonary fibrosis: Prevailing and evolving hypotheses about its pathogenesis and implications for therapy. Ann Intern Med 134:136, 2001.

111. Selman M, Ruiz V, Cabrera S, et al: TIMP-1, -2, -3, and -4 in idiopathic pulmonary fibrosis. A prevailing nondegradative lung microenvironment? Am J Physiol Lung Cell Mol Physiol 279:L562, 2000.

112. Smith DR, Kunkel SL, Standiford TJ, et al: Increased interleukin-1 receptor antagonist in idiopathic

pulmonary fibrosis. Am J Respir Crit Care Med 151:1965, 1995.

113. Southcott AM, Jones KP, Li D, et al: Interleukin-8: Differential expression in lone fibrosing alveolitis and systemic sclerosis. Am J Respir Crit Care Med 151:1604, 1995.

114. Specks U, Nerlich A, Colby TV, et al: Increased expression of type VI collagen in lung fibrosis. Am J Respir Crit Care Med 151:1956, 1995.

115. Strieter RM, Starko KM, Enelow RI, et al: Effects of interferon-γ 1b on biomarker expression in patients with idiopathic pulmonary fibrosis. Am J Respir Crit Care Med 170:133, 2004.

116. Suga M, Iyonaga K, Okamoto T, et al: Characteristic elevation of matrix metalloproteinase activity in idiopathic interstitial pneumonias. Am J Respir Crit Care Med 162:1949, 2000.

117. Takiya C, Peyrol S, Cordier J-F, Grimaud J-A: Connective matrix organization in human pulmonary fibrosis. Collagen polymorphism analysis in fibrotic deposits by immunohistological methods. Virchows Arch [Cell Pathol] 44:223, 1983.

118. Tang Y-W, Johnson JE, Browning PJ, et al: Herpesvirus DNA is consistently detected in lungs of patients with idiopathic pulmonary fibrosis. J Clin Microbiol 41:2633, 2003.

119. Tazelaar HD, Viggiano RW, Pickersgill J, Colby TV: Interstitial lung disease in polymyositis and dermatomyositis. Clinical features and prognosis as correlated with histologic findings. Am Rev Respir Dis 141:727, 1990.

120. Teirstein AS: The elusive goal of therapy for usual interstitial pneumonia. N Engl J Med 350:2, 2004.

121. Thannickal VJ, Toews GB, White ES, Lynch JP, Martinez FJ: Mechanisms of pulmonary fibrosis. Annu Rev Med 55:395, 2004.

122. Thomas AQ, Lane K, Phillips J, et al: Heterozygosity for a surfactant protein C gene mutation associated with usual interstitial pneumonitis and cellular nonspecific interstitial pneumonitis in one kindred. Am J Respir Crit Care Med 165:1322, 2002.

123. Tiitto L, Kaarteenaho-Wiik R, Sormunen R: Expression of the thioredoxin system in interstitial lung disease. J Pathol 201:363, 2003.

124. Tobin RW, Pope CE, Pellegrini CA, et al: Increased prevalence of gastroesophageal reflux in patients with idiopathic pulmonary fibrosis. Am J Respir Crit Care Med 158:1804, 1998.

125. Uh S-T, Inoue Y, King TE, et al: Morphometric analysis of insulin-like growth factor-I localized in lung tissues of patients with idiopathic pulmonary fibrosis. Am J Respir Crit Care Med 158:1626, 1998.

126. Wallace WAH, Howie SEM, Lamb D, Salter DM: Tenascin immunoreactivity in cryptogenic fibrosing alveolitis. J Pathol 175:415, 1995.

127. Warnock M, Press M, Churg A: Further observations on cytoplasmic hyaline in the lung. Hum Pathol 11:59, 1980.

128. Wells AU, Cullinan P, Hansell DM, et al: Fibrosing alveolitis associated with systemic sclerosis has a better prognosis than lone cryptogenic fibrosing alveolitis. Am J Respir Crit Care Med 149:1583, 1994.

129. White ES, Lazar MH, Thannickal VJ: Pathogenic mechanisms in usual interstitial pneumonia/idiopathic pulmonary fibrosis. J Pathol 201:343, 2003.

130. Willis BC, Liebler JM, Luby-Phelps K, et al: Induction of epithelial-mesenchymal transition in alveolar epithelial cells by transforming growth factor-β 1: potential role in idiopathic pulmonary fibrosis. Am J Pathol 166:1321, 2005.

131. Yousem SA: Eosinophilic pneumonia-like areas in idiopathic usual interstitial pneumonia. Mod Pathol 13:1280, 2000.

132. Yousem SA, Colby TV, Carrington CB: Lung biopsy in rheumatoid arthritis. Am Rev Resp Dis 131:770, 1985.

Desquamative Interstitial Pneumonia/Respiratory Bronchiolitis Interstitial Lung Disease

133. Abraham JL, Hertzberg MA: Inorganic particulates associated with desquamative interstitial pneumonia. Chest 80S:67S, 1981.

134. Bedrossian CWM, Kuhn C III, Luna MA, et al: Desquamative interstitial pneumonia-like reaction accompanying pulmonary lesions. Chest 72:166, 1977.

135. Brody A, Craighead J: Cytoplasmic inclusions in pulmonary macrophages of cigarette smokers. Lab Invest 32:125, 1975.

136. Cottin V, Streichenberger N, Gamondes J-P, et al: Respiratory bronchiolitis in smokers with spontaneous pneumothorax. Eur Respir J 12:702, 1998.

137. Craig PJ, Wells AU, Doffman S, et al: Desquamative interstitial pneumonia, respiratory bronchiolitis and their relationship to smoking. Histopathology 45:275, 2004.

138. Fraig M, Shreesha U, Savici D, Katzenstein A-LA: Respiratory bronchiolitis: A clinicopathologic study in current smokers, ex-smokers, and never-smokers. Am J Surg Pathol 26:647, 2002.

139. Hartman TE, Primack SL, Kang E-Y, et al: Disease progression in usual interstitial pneumonia compared with desquamative interstitial pneumonia: Assessment with serial CT. Chest 110:378, 1996.

140. Heyneman LE, Ward S, Lynch DA, et al: Respiratory bronchiolitis, respiratory bronchiolitis-associated interstitial lung disease, and desquamative interstitial pneumonia: Different entities or part of the spectrum of the same disease process? AJR Am J Roentgenol 173:1617, 1999.

141. Koss MN, Johnson FB, Hochholzer L: Pulmonary blue bodies. Hum Pathol 12:258, 1981.

142. Liebow AA, Steer A, Billingsley JG: Desquamative interstitial pneumonia. Am J Med 39:369, 1965.

143. Lipworth B, Woodcock A, Addis B, Turner-Warwick M: Late relapse of desquamative interstitial pneumonia. Am Rev Respir Dis 136:1253, 1987.

144. Moon J, du Bois RM, Colby TV, Hansell DM, Nicholson AG: Clinical significance of respiratory bronchiolitis on open lung biopsy and its relationship to smoking related interstitial lung disease. Thorax 54:1009, 1999.

145. Myers JL, Veal CF Jr, Shin MS, Katzenstein A-LA: Respiratory bronchiolitis causing interstitial lung disease. A clinicopathologic study of six cases. Am Rev Respir Dis 135:880, 1987.

146. Niewoehner D, Kleinerman J, Rice D: Pathologic changes in the peripheral airways of young cigarette smokers. N Engl J Med 291:755, 1974.

147. Park JS, Brown KK, Tuder, RM, et al: Respiratory bronchiolitis-associated interstitial lung disease: Radiologic features with clinical and pathologic correlation. J Comput Assist Tomogr 26:13, 2002.

148. Ryu JH, Colby TV, Hartman TE, Vassallo R: Smoking-related interstitial lung diseases: A concise review. Eur Respir J 17:122, 2001.

149. Ryu JH, Myers JL, Capizzi SA, et al: Desquamative interstitial pneumonia and respiratory bronchiolitis-associated interstitial lung disease. Chest 127:178, 2005.

150. Sadikot RT, Johnson J, Loyd JE, Christman JW: Respiratory bronchiolitis associated with severe dyspnea, exertional hypoxemia and clubbing. Chest 117:282, 2000.

151. Yousem SA, Colby TV, Gaensler EA: Respiratory bronchiolitis-associated interstitial lung disease and its relationship to desquamative interstitial pneumonia. Mayo Clin Proc 64:1373, 1989.

Acute Interstitial Pneumonia (Hamman–Rich Disease)

152. Akira M: Computed tomography and pathologic findings in fulminant forms of idiopathic interstitial pneumonia. J Thorac Imag 14:76, 1999.

153. Hamman L, Rich A: Acute diffuse interstitial fibrosis of the lung. Bull Johns Hopkins Hosp 74:177, 1944.

154. Ichikado K, Johkoh T, Ikezoe J, et al: Acute interstitial pneumonia: High-resolution CT findings correlated with pathology. AJR Am J Roentgenol 168:333, 1997.

155. Ichikado K, Suga M, Müller NL: Acute interstitial pneumonia: Comparison of high-resolution computed tomography findings between survivors and nonsurvivors. Am J Respir Crit Care Med 165:1551, 2002.

156. Katzenstein A-LA: Pathogenesis of "fibrosis" in interstitial pneumonia. An electron microscopic study. Hum Pathol 16:1015, 1985.

157. Katzenstein A-LA, Myers JL, Mazur MT: Acute interstitial pneumonia. A clinicopathologic, ultrastructural, and cell kinetic study. Am J Surg Pathol 10:256, 1986.

158. Olsen J, Colby T, Elliott C: Hamman-Rich syndrome revisited. Mayo Clin Proc 65:1538, 1990.

159. Primack SL, Hartman TE, Ikezoe J, et al: Acute interstitial pneumonia: Radiographic and CT findings in nine patients. Radiology 188:817, 1993.

160. Quefatieh A, Stone CH, DiGiovine B, et al: Low hospital mortality in patients with acute interstitial pneumonia. Chest 124:554, 2003.

161. Vourlekis JS, Brown KK, Cool CD, et al: Acute interstitial pneumonitis: Case series and review of the literature. Medicine (Baltimore) 79:369, 2000.

Nonspecific Interstitial Pneumonia

162. Akira M, Inoue G, Yamamoto S, Sakatani M: Non-specific interstitial pneumonia: Findings on sequential CT scans of nine patients. Thorax 55:854, 2000.
163. Bouros D, Wells AU, Nicholson AG, et al: Histopathologic subsets of fibrosing alveolitis in patients with systemic sclerosis and their relationship to outcome. Am J Respir Crit Care Med 165:1581, 2002.
164. Cottin V, Donsbeck A-V, Revel D, Loire R, Cordier J-F: Nonspecific interstitial pneumonia: Individualization of a clinicopathologic entity in a series of 12 patients. Am J Respir Crit Care Med 158:1286, 1998.
165. Cottin V, Thivolet-Béjui F, Reynaud-Gaubert M, et al: Interstitial lung disease in amyopathic dermatomyositis, dermatomyositis and polymyositis. Eur Respir J 22:245, 2003.
166. Daniil ZD, Gilchrist FC, Nicholson AG, et al: A histologic pattern of nonspecific interstitial pneumonia is associated with a better prognosis than usual interstitial pneumonia in patients with cryptogenic fibrosing alveolitis. Am J Respir Crit Care Med 160:899, 1999.
167. Flaherty KR, Travis WD, Colby TV, et al: Histopathologic variability in usual and nonspecific interstitial pneumonias. Am J Respir Crit Care Med 164:1722, 2001.
168. Fujita J, Yamadori I, Suemitsu I, et al: Clinical features of non-specific interstitial pneumonia. Respir Med 93:113, 1999.
169. Ishioka S, Nishisaka T, Maeda A, Hiyama K, Yamakido M: A case of group II non-specific interstitial pneumonia developed during corticosteroid therapy after acute respiratory distress syndrome. Respirology 4:283, 1999.
170. Jokoh T, Müller NL, Colby TV, et al: Nonspecific interstitial pneumonia: Correlation between thin-section CT findings and pathologic subgroups in 55 patients. Radiology 225:199, 2002.
171. Katoh T, Andoh T, Mikawa K, et al: Computed tomographic findings in non-specific interstitial pneumonia. Respirology 3:69, 1998.
172. Katzenstein A, Fiorelli R: Non-specific interstitial pneumonia/fibrosis. Histologic patterns and clinical significance. Am J Surg Pathol 18:136, 1994.
173. Kim D-S, Yoo B, Lee J-S, et al: The major histopathologic pattern of pulmonary fibrosis in scleroderma is nonspecific interstitial pneumonia. Sarcoidosis Vasc Diffuse Lung Dis 19:121, 2002.
174. Kim TS, Lee KS, Chung MP: Nonspecific interstitial pneumonia with fibrosis: High-resolution CT and pathologic findings. AJR Am J Roentgenol 171:1645, 1998.
175. Monaghan H, Wells AU, Colby TV, et al: Prognostic implications of histologic patterns in multiple surgical lung biopsies from patients with idiopathic interstitial pneumonias. Chest 125:522, 2004.
176. Nagai S, Kitaihi M, Itoh H, Nishimura K, Izumi T, Colby TV: Idiopathic nonspecific interstitial pneumonia/fibrosis: Comparison with idiopathic pulmonary fibrosis and BOOP. Eur Resp J 12:1010, 1998.
177. Nakamura Y, Chida K, Suda T, et al: Nonspecific interstitial pneumonia in collagen vascular diseases: Comparison of the clinical characteristics and prognostic significance with usual interstitial pneumonia. Sarcoidosis Vasc Diffuse Lung Dis 20:235, 2003.
178. Park JS, Lee KS, Kim JS, et al: Nonspecific interstitial pneumonia with fibrosis: Radiographic and CT findings in seven patients. Radiology 195:645, 1995.
179. Tansey D, Wells AU, Colby TV, et al: Variations in histological patterns of interstitial pneumonia between connective tissue disorders and their relationship to prognosis. Histopathology 44:585, 2004.
180. Travis WD, Matsui K, Moss, J, Ferrans VJ: Idiopathic nonspecific interstitial pneumonia: Prognostic significance of cellular and fibrosing patterns: Survival comparison with usual interstitial pneumonia and desquamative interstitial pneumonia. Am J Surg Pathol 24:19, 2000.
181. Vourlekis JS, Schwarz MI, Cool CD, et al: Nonspecific interstitial pneumonitis as the sole histologic expression of hypersensitivity pneumonitis. Am J Med 112:490, 2002.

Other Idiopathic Interstitial Pneumonias

182. Churg A, Myers J, Suarez T, et al: Airway-centered interstitial fibrosis: A distinct form of aggressive diffuse lung disease. Am J Surg Pathol 28:62, 2004.
183. de Carvalho M-EP, Kairalla RA, Capelozzi VL, et al: Centrilobular fibrosis: A novel histological pattern of idiopathic interstitial pneumonia. Pathol Res Pract 198:577, 2002.
183a. Frankel SK, Cool CD, Lynch DA, Brown KK: Idiopathic pleuroparenchymal fibroelastosis. Description of a novel clinicopathologic entity. Chest 126:2007, 2004.
184. Fukuoka J, Franks TJ, Colby TV, et al: Peribronchiolar metaplasia: A common histologic lesion in diffuse lung disease and a rare cause of interstitial lung disease: Clinicopathological features of 15 cases. Am J Surg Pathol 29:948, 2005.
185. Yousem SA, Dacic S: Idiopathic bronchiolocentric interstitial pneumonia. Mod Pathol 15:1148, 2002.

Honeycomb Lung

186. Genereux GP: The end-stage lung. Radiology 116:279, 1975.
187. Meyer EC, Liebow AA: Relationship of interstitial pneumonia, honeycombing and atypical epithelial proliferation to cancer of the lung. Cancer 18:322, 1965.
188. Powers M, Askin F, Cresson D: Pulmonary eosinophilic granuloma. Twenty-five year follow-up. Am Rev Respir Dis 129:503, 1984.
189. Primack SL, Hartman TE, Hansell DM, Muller NL: End-stage lung disease: CT findings in 61 patients. Radiology 189:681, 1993.
190. Westcott JL, Cole SR: Traction bronchiectasis in end-stage pulmonary fibrosis. Radiology 161:665, 1986.

PATHOLOGY OF DRUG-INDUCED LUNG DISEASE

Jeffrey L. Myers and Ola El-Zammar

Numerous drugs may adversely affect the lung.[5,6,12] The recognition of drug-induced pulmonary toxicity is difficult because the clinical, radiographic, and pathologic features are often nonspecific, and the affected patients frequently have complex illnesses in which a variety of unrelated pulmonary complications may occur. Clinical considerations in the differential diagnosis usually include (1) recrudescence of the primary illness; (2) opportunistic infection; and (3) iatrogenic disease resulting from radiation therapy, oxygen administration, drugs, or a combination of these.[11,12] Lung biopsies are frequently obtained in this setting. The diagnosis of drug toxicity requires a high index of suspicion as well as the vigorous exclusion of other potential causes of the patient's respiratory illness. The aim of this chapter is to provide for the pathologist a practical and easy-to-use guide to the tissue diagnosis of drug-induced lung disease. A limited number of tissue reactions have been described in cases of drug-induced lung disease and are summarized in Table 4–1. The following sections review the reactions reported for each drug and describe relevant clinical features and risk factors when known. Morphologic features are discussed in detail only when they have not been addressed in other chapters. Several excellent reviews of drug-induced lung disease are available.[1–14]

CYTOTOXIC DRUGS

Cytotoxic drugs compose the largest, and probably the most important, group of drugs associated with lung toxicity (Table 4–2).[5,10,14] They include mainly those agents used in the chemotherapy of malignant neoplasms, although some cytotoxic agents are also used in the treatment of non-neoplastic diseases.

Table 4–1　Pulmonary Manifestations of Drug Toxicity: Tissue Reactions and Associated Drugs

Chronic interstitial pneumonia (amiodarone,[339,343,344,350] BCNU,[50,51,59] busulfan,[21] chlorambucil,[20,22] cocaine,[441,445,446] cyclophosphamide,[27,32,33] docetaxel,[173,190,191,196] fludarabine,[135,142,143,145,163] fluoxetine hydrochloride [Prozac],[393] gemcitabine,[120,157] gold salts,[257,282,290] hydroxycarbamide [hydroxyurea],[148] imatinib,[181,194,198] infliximab,[264] interferon-α,[295,298-300,304-306] melphalan,[23,43] methotrexate,[126,130,134,137,138,146,153,156,161] methyl-CCNU,[46,53] nilutamide,[489,506] nitrofurantoin,[219,221,235,239] phenytoin,[382,386] pindolol,[363] procarbazine,[178] quinidine sulfate,[347] sirolimus,[79] statins,[483,491,497] sulfasalazine,[230,241,243] ticlopidine,[501,505] tocainide,[321,349] tryptophan,[449,451,455,460-464] uracil mustard,[25] venlafaxine[391])

Diffuse alveolar damage (amiodarone,[324,339] amitriptyline,[395,397] azathioprine,[123,128,150,169] BCNU,[55,57,58,61,64] bleomycin,[88,96] busulfan,[18,26,28,29,31,35] carbamazepine,[388] CCNU,[47,48,65] cocaine,[427] colchicine,[6] cyclophosphamide,[17,39,41,42] cytosine arabinoside,[119] deferoxamine mesylate,[487] docetaxel,[176,191,193] fludarabine,[142] gemcitabine,[121,139,154,155,157] gold salts,[259,266] hexamethonium,[358,364] infliximab,[264] interferon-α,[295,299] interferon-γ,[303,314] melphalan,[40] methotrexate,[122,124,129,131,160-162] mitomycin,[75,89,104,105] nitrofurantoin,[215] penicillamine,[250] procarbazine,[182] sirolimus,[98] statins,[491,503] streptokinase,[488,499] sulfasalazine,[209,217,227] sulfathiazole,[216] teniposide,[174] vinblastine,[185] zinostatin[76,109])

Bronchiolitis obliterans–organizing pneumonia (amiodarone,[8,339,343,344,350] bleomycin,[80,102,111] carbamazepine,[381] chlorozotocin,[44] cocaine,[443] cromolyn sodium,[480] cyclophosphamide,[36] gold salts,[255,269,272] hexamethonium,[365] hydroxycarbamide [hydroxyurea],[147] interferon-α,[306,308] mecamylamine,[366] methotrexate,[127,136] mitomycin,[85] nilutamide,[506] nitrofurantoin,[204] phenytoin,[385] sirolimus,[95,97,100,107] statins,[491,503] sulfasalazine,[214,244] tocainide,[345] venlafaxine[391])

Obliterative bronchiolitis (CCNU,[67] penicillamine[254,274,291])

Eosinophilic pneumonia (acetaminophen,[263] ampicillin,[233] AVC [vaginal] cream,[211] bleomycin,[87,116] carbamazepine,[387] chlorpropamide,[484] cocaine,[427] cromolyn sodium,[508] fludarabine,[166] imipramine,[405] infliximab,[280] interferon-α,[302] mephenesin,[509] minocycline,[232] nabumetone,[272] naproxen,[249,275] nitrofurantoin,[206] para-aminosalicylic acid,[245] phenylbutazone,[288] procarbazine,[175] prontosil,[212] propranolol,[369] pyrimethamine,[209] sulfasalazine,[205,227,238,240,242] tetracycline,[218] trazodone[401])

Hypersensitivity pneumonia (docetaxel,[193] fluoxetine hydrochloride,[393] hydroxycarbamide [hydroxyurea],[158] methotrexate,[129,132,153,162] nitrofurantoin,[228] paclitaxel,[179,197] statins,[498] sulfasalazine,[225] venlafaxine[391])

Pulmonary hemorrhage (amphotericin B,[246] anticoagulants,[486,510] cocaine,[438,439] cyclophosphamide,[38] haloperidol,[396] hydralazine,[354] mitomycin,[78,99] nitrofurantoin,[200,203] penicillamine,[253,267,268,285] propylthiouracil,[514] sirolimus,[101,107] streptokinase,[479,502] sulfonamides,[213] urokinase[479,502])

Pulmonary hypertension (aminorex,[467,469,476] cocaine,[434,448] methamphetamine,[511] mitomycin,[78,89,99] phentermine–fenfluramine,[468,470,471,474,475] tryptophan[462])

Pulmonary edema (albuterol,[372] buprenorphine,[418] chlordiazepoxide,[400] cocaine,[420,427] codeine,[415] cytosine arabinoside,[119,141,165] epinephrine,[485] ethchlorvynol,[390,392,398,400] haloperidol,[396] heroin,[414,416] hydrochlorothiazide,[355,359,362] isoxsuprine,[374] lidocaine,[330] magnesium sulfate,[373] methadone,[408,412] methotrexate,[124] mitomycin,[89] nalbuphine,[417] naloxone,[411,413] nifedipine,[507] paraldehyde,[399,402] penicillin,[222] propoxyphene,[407] propranolol,[357,368] radiocontrast material,[496] ritodrine,[377] salbutamol,[380] salicylates,[260] sulindac,[283] terbutaline[376,377])

Pulmonary venoocclusive disease (BCNU,[56] bleomycin,[56,90,92] gemcitabine,[168] mitomycin,[114] zinostatin[76,109])

Granulomatous inflammation (acebutolol,[370] BCG,[493,504,513] cocaine,[424] cromolyn sodium,[480] etanercept,[251,279,293] fluoxetine hydrochloride [Prozac],[393] interferon-α,[297,301,307,310,311,313] methotrexate,[137,161] nitrofurantoin,[228] procarbazine,[178] venlafaxine[391])

Alkylating Agents

Alkylating agents represent a chemically diverse group of drugs that have in common the ability to form covalent linkages (alkylation) with DNA components. Busulfan and cyclophosphamide are the most commonly cited causes of drug-induced lung disease in this group, while chlorambucil, melphalan, and uracil mustard are responsible for only a handful of cases.

Busulfan

Busulfan has been used extensively in the treatment of chronic myelogenous leukemia and was the first

Table 4–2   Pulmonary Reactions to Cytotoxic Drugs

Drug	Tissue Reactions
Alkylating Agents	
Busulfan	DAD,[18,26,28,29,31,35] CIP[21] ossification,[30] PAP[15]
Cyclophosphamide	DAD,[17,39,41,42] CIP[27,32,33] UIP,[27] BOOP,[36] hemorrhage,[38] DIP-like reaction[33]
Chlorambucil	UIP,[22] CIP[20]
Melphalan	CIP,[23,43] DAD[40]
Uracil mustard	CIP[25]
Nitrosoureas	
BCNU	DAD,[55,57,58,61,64] CIP,[50,51,59] PVOD,[56] pleural fibrosis[49–51,66]
CCNU	DAD,[47,48,65] obliterative bronchiolitis[67]
Methyl-CCNU	UIP[46,53]
Chlorozotocin	BOOP[44]
Cytotoxic Antibiotics	
Bleomycin	DAD,[88,96] pleural fibrosis,[96] EP,[87,116] BOOP,[80,102,111] PVOD[56,90,92]
Mitomycin	DAD,[75,89,104,105] BOOP,[85] edema,[89] hemorrhage,[78,99] hypertension,[78,89,99] PVOD,[114] pleuritis[104]
Zinostatin	DAD,[76,109] PVOD[76,109]
Sirolimus	BOOP,[95,97,100,107] interstitial pneumonia,[79] granulomas,[71,101] hemorrhage,[101,107] DAD,[98] alveolar proteinosis[71]
Antimetabolites	
Methotrexate	CIP (+ granulomas),[126,130,134,137,138,146,153,156,161] HP,[129,132,153,162] BOOP (+ granulomas),[127,136] DAD,[122,124,129,131,160–162] edema[124]
Hydroxycarbamide (hydroxyurea)	HP,[158] BOOP,[147] CIP,[148] DIP[172]
Fludarabine	CIP,[135,142,143,145,163] EP,[166] DAD,[142] organizing pneumonia[142]
Gemcitabine	DAD,[121,139,154,155,157] NSIP,[120,157] PVOD[168]
Cytosine arabinoside	Edema,[119,141,165] DAD[119]
Azathioprine	DAD[123,128,150,169]
Miscellaneous	
Docetaxel	CIP,[173,190,191,196] DAD,[176,191,193] HP[193]
Paclitaxel	HP[179,197]
Vinblastine	DAD[185]
Procarbazine	CIP (+ granulomas),[178] EP,[175] DAD[182]
Teniposide (VM-26)	DAD[174]
Imatinib	CIP,[181,194,198] PAP,[195] pleural effusion[180]

Abbreviations: DAD = diffuse alveolar damage; CIP = nonspecific chronic interstitial pneumonia; DIP = desquamative interstitial pneumonia; PAP = pulmonary alveolar proteinosis; UIP = usual interstitial pneumonia; BOOP = bronchiolitis obliterans–organizing pneumonia; PVOD = pulmonary venoocclusive disease; EP = eosinophilic pneumonia; HP = hypersensitivity pneumonia.

chemotherapeutic agent reported to cause lung disease.[35] Pulmonary toxicity occurs in about 4% of patients, usually in those who have received a total dose of at least 500 mg.[5] Latent periods have ranged from 1 month to 12 years, with a mean of 3.5 years and a median of 3 years. Melphalan and uracil mustard may potentiate the toxic effects of busulfan therapy.[1] Busulfan may also sensitize patients to the effects of

thoracic irradiation.[1] The prognosis for patients with busulfan-induced lung disease is poor, and most die of their lung disease within 6 months.[1]

Organizing *diffuse alveolar damage* (DAD) (see Chapter 2) is the most common manifestation of busulfan lung toxicity and is associated with bronchiolar and alveolar epithelial atypia.[18,26,28,29,31,35] Cytopathic changes include cytomegaly, nuclear pleomorphism,

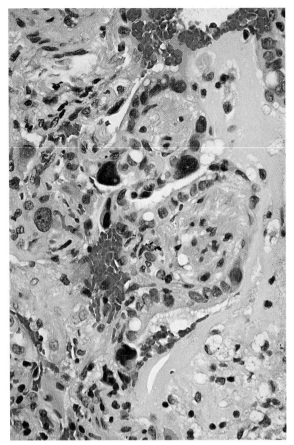

Figure 4–1 Busulfan toxicity. Enlarged, hyperchromatic and pleomorphic nuclei are seen along bronchiolar epithelium in this transbronchial biopsy specimen. Elsewhere the biopsy showed DAD.

and prominent nucleoli (Fig. 4–1).[21,29] Cytologic atypia may occur without clinical, radiographic, or pathologic evidence of lung disease and is not by itself diagnostic of pulmonary toxicity.[26] It has also been described in a variety of extrapulmonary sites, including urinary bladder, breast, pancreas, and uterine cervix.[21,29] Ultrastructural studies of busulfan lung toxicity have demonstrated intranuclear tubular inclusions in type 2 cells.[24,31] Similar intranuclear inclusions have also been identified in patients with bleomycin-induced lung disease but may be seen in other reactive processes as well as certain neoplasms.

A nonspecific type of *chronic interstitial pneumonia* (CIP) is a less common manifestation of busulfan toxicity and has been reported only in individuals who have received large doses of the drug over relatively long periods of time.[21] *Pulmonary ossification* and *pulmonary alveolar proteinosis* (see Chapter 16) have both been reported as possible complications of busulfan therapy.[15,30] The former has been reported in a single patient and may represent a chance association between busulfan therapy and idiopathic diffuse pulmonary ossification. Pulmonary alveolar proteinosis has been reported in only a few patients, all of whom had other potential explanations for their lung disease, and none recovered despite discontinuation of busulfan therapy.[15] A *fibrinous alveolar exudate* was described by Heard and Cooke in autopsies of busulfan-treated patients.[26] A similar exudate was seen in a leukemic patient who had never received busulfan, however, making it unlikely that the alveolar exudate represented a manifestation of busulfan toxicity. *Adenocarcinoma* of the lung has also been reported in a patient who had taken busulfan, but the tumor was an incidental autopsy finding that was probably unrelated to busulfan therapy.[34]

Cyclophosphamide

Most patients with cyclophosphamide-induced lung disease were being treated for underlying malignancies and were receiving other cytotoxic drugs. A few were taking prednisone and cyclophosphamide for non-neoplastic diseases, including glomerulonephritis and Wegener's granulomatosis.[5,17,33] Lung toxicity as a consequence of lone cyclophosphamide is rare, and results in two distinct patterns: early-onset pneumonitis that is reversible and may respond to steroids, and late-onset pneumonitis with pleural thickening and a chronically progressive course.[32] No relationship between duration of therapy or total drug dose and pulmonary complications has been established. Chemotherapeutic regimens that include a combination of cyclophosphamide and carmustine (BCNU) may be associated with an increased risk of lung toxicity in patients undergoing autologous bone marrow transplantation for breast carcinoma.[41] Latent periods are unpredictable and have ranged from 2 weeks to 13 years. One patient developed pulmonary edema within minutes of receiving a second intravenous dose of cyclophosphamide.[5] Most of the patients with well-documented drug toxicity have recovered or remained stable with discontinuation of therapy, although three patients with late-onset pneumonitis died of respiratory failure.[32] Fatal interstitial pneumonia has been reported in one patient receiving ifosfamide, a structural isomer of cyclophosphamide.[16]

Organizing DAD is the most common manifestation of cyclophosphamide-induced lung disease.[17,39,41,42] A CIP sometimes resembling usual interstitial pneumonia (UIP) occurs less frequently and is well-documented in only three patients who received prolonged treatment with cyclophosphamide.[27,32,33] In one case, pigmented macrophages were prominent within some alveolar spaces, thus imparting a desquamative interstitial pneumonia (DIP)-like appearance to the process.[33]

Bronchiolitis obliterans–organizing pneumonia (BOOP) (see Chapter 2) has been reported in one patient who developed lung disease after 5 months of combination chemotherapy with bleomycin, cyclophosphamide, vincristine, and prednisone.[36] Patchy acute *alveolar hemorrhage* has been noted in autopsies of patients receiving high-dose intermittent cyclophosphamide as a single agent.[38] Pulmonary hemorrhage was seen in more than half of patients dying within the first month of therapy and may have been related to thrombocytopenia. Interestingly, this same series found no evidence of cyclophosphamide-induced interstitial pneumonia, and atypia of bronchial epithelium was seen in only a single case.

Chlorambucil

Chlorambucil has only rarely been implicated as a cause of drug-induced lung disease.[5,20,22,170] Most reported patients were taking chlorambucil as a single agent, while some were receiving combination chemotherapy that included methotrexate, fluorouracil, vincristine, and prednisone in addition to chlorambucil.[170] No relationship between total drug dose and pulmonary toxicity has emerged, and latent periods have ranged from 2 months to almost 5 years. Half of the reported patients have survived with discontinuation of therapy.

CIP appears to be the most common pathologic finding in chlorambucil-induced lung toxicity.[20,22] Some cases resemble UIP, while a nonspecific CIP occurs less commonly and may be associated with evidence of organizing pneumonia.[20,22] Ultrastructural studies have confirmed the presence of a CIP but have not demonstrated any specific findings.[20]

Melphalan

Pulmonary toxicity to melphalan has been well documented in only a few patients.[19,23,37,40,43] Respiratory side effects occurred 2 to 16 months after initiating therapy. Two patients died from respiratory failure, one had progressive disease, and two responded partially or completely to discontinuation of melphalan therapy. CIP was seen in two patients, and organizing DAD was present in two others, both of whom died.[23,40,43] Taetle et al emphasized the presence of associated atypical hyperplasia of alveolar lining cells and atypia and squamous metaplasia of bronchiolar epithelium.[40]

Epithelial atypia was also documented in autopsies of melphalan-treated patients who lacked clinical or morphologic evidence of drug toxicity.[40] Thus, melphalan is similar to busulfan in that it may cause cytologic atypia without significant associated lung disease.

Nitrosoureas

The nitrosoureas include carmustine (BCNU), lomustine (CCNU), semustine (methyl-CCNU), and chlorozotocin. All have been associated with pulmonary toxicity, but BCNU accounts for the vast majority of cases.

Carmustine (BCNU)

BCNU is one of the most convincingly proven pulmonary toxins in humans, mainly because it is often used as a single agent in treating patients with primary brain neoplasms, a population at relatively low risk for developing other types of lung disease. It is also one of the few agents for which there is a direct relationship between total cumulative dose and lung toxicity.[5,45,70] The overall incidence of lung toxicity is 20–30%, but the incidence approaches 50% in patients who have received cumulative doses of 1.5 g/m^2 or more.[45] Pulmonary toxicity may occur at lower doses in patients being treated with cyclophosphamide-containing combination chemotherapy or in patients who have received thoracic irradiation.[41,49,57] Preexisting lung disease and a history of cigarette smoking have also been associated with an increased risk of BCNU-induced lung disease.[45] The prognosis reported in earlier series was poor, with mortality rates of greater than 90%, but earlier detection and treatment may result in improved survival.[52,69]

Delayed lung toxicity has been described in survivors of childhood brain tumors who were treated with BCNU either as a single agent or in combination with vincristine and/or craniospinal irradiation.[50,59,60,66] Symptoms related to late toxicity may not occur until as many as 12 years after treatment.[59,60] Long-term follow-up indicates that delayed toxicity occurs in the majority of patients treated with BCNU in childhood, with an associated mortality of nearly 40% after survivals ranging from 8 to 20 years after treatment.[60] Patients who receive BCNU before the age of 5 years may be at greatest risk for developing fatal delayed pulmonary toxicity.[60]

Acute and *organizing DAD* is the most common manifestation of BCNU-induced lung disease.[55,57,58,61,64] Bronchoalveolar lavage (BAL) has been reported in a single patient with acute toxicity and showed a lymphocytosis with a diminished ratio of CD4:CD8 cells.[54] No specific features have been noted by electron microscopy.[50,58] CIP has been reported less commonly and may be accompanied by cytologic atypia.[51] Delayed toxicity is characterized by changes similar to *nonspecific interstitial pneumonia with fibrosis* (NSIP, see Chapter 3), involving predominantly the upper lung zones and peripheral subpleural parenchyma bilaterally.[50,59] Unilateral upper lobe involvement has also been described.[62] Necrotizing granulomatous reactions and 'angiitis' have been reported in several patients but are unlikely to represent manifestations of BCNU toxicity.[64]

Pulmonary venoocclusive disease (see Chapter 8) has been described in two patients who had received BCNU as a single agent for primary brain tumors.[56] In both, the insidious onset of dyspnea developed several months after chemotherapy was completed. The total doses received were 550 and 953 mg/m^2, and both patients died within 4 months.

Pleural disease has accompanied the pulmonary parenchymal abnormalities in a minority of patients, including those with delayed toxicity.[49–51,66] It is characterized by nonspecific fibrosis of visceral pleura and subpleural pulmonary parenchyma associated with chronic inflammation and bleb formation. These changes may be associated with pneumothorax in a small number of patients.[49,51,66,68]

Other Nitrosoureas

Only a few examples of *lomustine* (CCNU)-induced pulmonary toxicity have been reported, and most of these patients had received other potentially toxic drugs, including cyclophosphamide and busulfan.[47,48,65,67] DAD with hyaline membranes was the most common autopsy finding.[47,48,65] Obliterative bronchiolitis has been reported in one patient.[67]

Semustine (methyl-CCNU) and *chlorozotocin* are rarely associated with pulmonary toxicity.[44,46,53] UIP has been reported in two patients who had received 1.1 g and 4.1 g of semustine over 12- and 25-month periods, respectively.[46,53] Both of these patients were cigarette smokers, which may imply an increased risk of developing semustine-induced pulmonary toxicity.[46] BOOP has been described in one patient who received chlorozotocin.[44]

Cytotoxic Antibiotics

The cytotoxic antibiotics are a chemically heterogeneous group of antineoplastic agents derived from bacterial cultures. Three (bleomycin, mitomycin, and zinostatin) have been associated with pulmonary toxicity.

Rapamycin (Sirolimus), a new immunosuppressive drug with macrolide structure that is used in the context of solid-organ transplantation, has also been shown to cause pulmonary toxicity.

Bleomycin

Bleomycin has been more extensively studied as a cause of lung disease than has any other pharmacologic agent. This is due to multiple factors, including its widespread use in treating a variety of neoplasms, recognition of pulmonary toxicity as the dose-limiting toxicity in humans, and its utility in animal models of lung disease. The incidence of clinically significant pulmonary toxicity ranges from 3% to 5%.[5,81,91] Although pulmonary toxicity has been reported at doses as low as 20 units, the risk of pulmonary complications increases after a total cumulative dose of 400 to 450 units.[5,81,91] Other risk factors for developing bleomycin-induced lung disease include (1) age over 70 years, (2) prior or concomitant thoracic irradiation, (3) high levels of inspired oxygen during general anesthesia, (4) smoking, (5) renal dysfunction, and (6) previous exposure to bleomycin within 6 months of reinstituting therapy.[5,81,91,110] Bleomycin-containing combination chemotherapy that includes cyclophosphamide (i.e. BACOP) or high-dose cisplatin may carry an added risk of pulmonary side effects.[72,74] Granulocyte colony-stimulating factor may also exacerbate pulmonary toxicity in patients treated with bleomycin-containing multiagent regimens.[93] Some examples of suspected drug toxicity in patients receiving multiagent chemotherapy for malignant lymphoma may result from multiple pulmonary thromboemboli.[84]

The pulmonary manifestations of bleomycin toxicity are varied. Most patients present with the insidious onset of dyspnea and cough associated with diffuse interstitial infiltrates on chest radiographs. Open lung biopsies and autopsies in this group have consistently shown a spectrum of histopathologic features consistent with *DAD* (Fig. 4–2).[88,96] The pathologic changes have shown a predilection for the lower lobes and subpleural parenchyma.[95] Alveolar hemorrhage may be an associated finding.[88] Although some cases have been classified as UIP, it is likely that many represent examples of organizing DAD with honeycomb change.[73,96] Electron microscopic descriptions have confirmed the presence of DAD.[24,73,82] A variety of nuclear alterations have been described, including nucleolar fibrillar centers, an increase in the number of nuclear bodies, and intranuclear tubular inclusions.[24,82] *Pleural fibrosis* has been associated with organizing

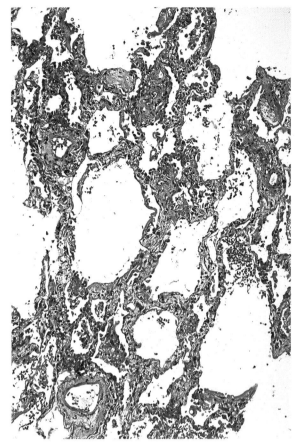

Figure 4–2 Bleomycin toxicity characterized by acute DAD. There is alveolar septal thickening and patchy hyaline membrane formation.

DAD in some patients.[96] Pleural blebs have also been described and may explain the rare examples of pneumothorax and pneumomediastinum in patients with underlying bleomycin lung disease.[115] The prognosis for patients with bleomycin-induced DAD is poor, and nearly all die of rapidly progressive respiratory failure within 3 months of onset.

Eosinophilic pneumonia is an uncommon manifestation of bleomycin-induced lung disease that has been reported in six patients, all of whom were receiving combination chemotherapy containing other cytotoxic agents.[87,116] Three of the six reported patients were asymptomatic. Peripheral eosinophilia occurred in two. There were diffuse infiltrates found on radiographs in four patients, while two had localized nodular densities. Three were treated with corticosteroids, and all recovered. Pathologically, the changes were identical to those seen in eosinophilic pneumonia of any etiology. An associated *eosinophilic pleuritis* was present in

one case.[116] Electron microscopy confirmed the light microscopic findings of eosinophilic pneumonia.[87]

BOOP is another uncommon tissue reaction in bleomycin-induced lung disease (Fig. 4–3).[80,102,111] There may be associated eosinophilia in some cases; indeed, both the clinical and histologic features may overlap with those described in patients with eosinophilic pneumonia.[108] Reported patients had complex illnesses and were receiving bleomycin-containing combination chemotherapy for osteosarcoma, metastatic carcinoma, or metastatic germ cell tumors.[80,88,102,108,111] Chest radiographs in some patients showed asymptomatic lung nodules that were thought to represent pulmonary metastases.[80,102,111] Most patients recovered after discontinuation of bleomycin therapy. A few patients received additional chemotherapy without recurrent lung toxicity.[108]

Pulmonary venoocclusive disease has been attributed to bleomycin toxicity in five patients.[56,90,92] Several patients had either multiple pulmonary lesions, including DAD, thromboemboli, infarcts, or evidence of left-sided heart failure, making it difficult to assess the significance of the vascular alterations.[56,91] Others had received combination chemotherapy containing mitomycin, which has also been implicated as a cause of vascular lesions.[90]

Mitomycin

Mitomycin causes pulmonary toxicity in about 8% of patients.[77,103,113] Unlike bleomycin, there are no well-defined risk factors for developing pulmonary toxicity, although most affected patients have received a total cumulative dose of at least 30 mg/m^2.[113] Combination chemotherapy containing mitomycin and vinca alkaloids carries an increased risk of pulmonary toxicity.[5,85] Early recognition of respiratory side effects is important because complete recovery can occur following discontinuation of the drug. Steroids may also have a beneficial effect in this condition.[77] The overall mortality is about 50%.

Pathologic details are available for only a limited number of cases of suspected mitomycin toxicity.[75,77,78,83,85,89,99,104,105] Most patients appear to have had varying stages of *DAD*.[75,89,90,104,105] DAD was associated with a *fibrinous pleuritis* in one patient.[104]

BOOP is a less common manifestation of mitomycin-induced lung disease.[85] Most of the reported patients had received other potentially toxic drugs, including vinca alkaloids, cyclophosphamide, and bleomycin, but the chronology of their illnesses implicated mitomycin as the most likely cause.

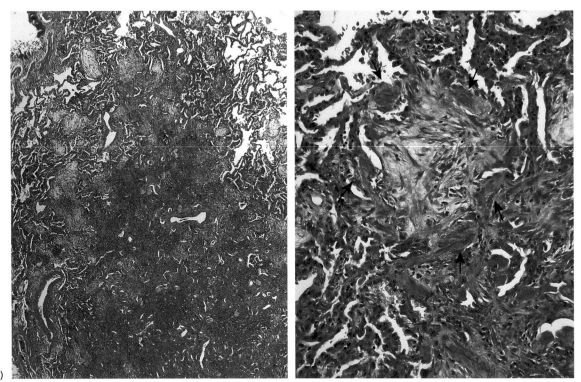

(a) (b)

Figure 4–3 Bleomycin toxicity characterized by BOOP. (a) Low magnification showing the peribronchiolar airspace filling by fibroblast plugs. **(b)** The typical intraluminal active fibrosis is better seen at higher magnification. Smooth muscle bundles of the involved alveolar duct are seen surrounding the fibrosis (arrows).

Pulmonary edema and *diffuse alveolar hemorrhage* have been described in mitomycin-treated patients who develop an unusual syndrome of thrombotic micro-angiopathy.[5,78,89,99] Respiratory complications occur in a minority of these patients and have been precipitated in some by blood transfusions.[5,89] A variety of pulmonary vascular alterations have also been described in these patients and likely represent manifestations of *pulmonary hypertension*. A single example of *pulmonary venoocclusive disease* has also been reported in this condition.[114] Unusual angiomatoid malformations affecting alveolar septal capillaries without other morphologic indications of pulmonary hypertension have been illustrated in one case.[78]

Zinostatin (Neocarzinostatin)

DAD has been described in two patients receiving zinostatin.[76,109] There were associated vascular alterations suggestive of pulmonary venoocclusive disease, including venous thrombosis, endothelial hypertrophy, and thickening of muscular arteries and arterioles.

Sirolimus

Sirolimus, also known as rapamycin, is a new immuno-suppressive drug with macrolide structure that inhibits T-lymphocyte proliferation induced by cytokine stimulation. It is increasingly used in solid-organ transplantation, either by itself or along with calcineurin inhibitors (cyclosporine and tacrolimus) to limit nephrotoxicity of the latter drugs. The incidence of sirolimus-associated pulmonary toxicity is unknown. It has been mainly reported in renal and cardiac transplant recipients, and rarely in liver transplant recipients.[94] In most cases, toxicity is dose-dependent and has been documented in patients receiving at least 5 mg daily, or in patients with serum concentrations greater than 15 ng/ml.[98] Onset occurs from 3 weeks to 12 months following initiation of therapy. Symptoms typically include dry cough, progressive dyspnea, fatigue, and weakness; fever and hemoptysis are less commonly present.[101,107] Bilateral interstitial infiltrates, alveolar consolidation, and nodular opacities are the most common radiographic abnormalities.[100,101] Discontinuation of the drug, with steroid treatment in some cases, leads to prompt clinical improvement, whereas radiographic abnormalities may take several months to resolve. Rare fatalities have been reported.[95,98]

BOOP is the most common pathologic finding in sirolimus-associated pulmonary toxicity.[95,97,100,107] It was reported in seven of 29 cardiac transplant recipients who were switched from a calcineurin inhibitor to sirolimus, and it seems to occur most often from 1 to 3 years following transplantation.[95] A chronic interstitial pneumonia with varying amounts of associated organizing pneumonia has also been reported.[79,100,101] Loosely formed non-necrotizing granulomas may be associated with the organizing pneumonia.[79,101] *Alveolar hemorrhage*, as evidenced by hemosiderin-laden macrophages on BAL or biopsy, was reported in four patients.[101,107] One case of *DAD* was documented at autopsy in a heart transplant recipient, who died 14 days after administration of a loading dose and had blood concentrations between 20 and 24 ng/ml.[98] One report described a pediatric liver transplant recipient who developed diffuse pneumonitis with alveolar proteinosis and well-formed granulomas, in addition to posttransplant lymphoproliferative disorder, 9 months after initiation of sirolimus.[71]

Antimetabolites

Antimetabolites are structural analogues of metabolites normally required for cell function and replication. Seven members of this group – methotrexate, hydroxycarbamide (hydroxyurea), fludarabine, gemcitabine, cytosine arabinoside, mercaptopurine, and azathioprine – have been associated with lung toxicity.

Methotrexate

Methotrexate was first recognized as a potential pulmonary toxin in 1969.[130] Since then, numerous cases of suspected methotrexate-induced lung disease have been reported. The incidence of drug-induced lung disease is difficult to ascertain but is probably between 5% and 10%.[5,137,140,161] No definite risk factors have been identified, and there is no relationship between total cumulative dose and toxicity.[5,137,140] Bleomycin may potentiate methotrexate toxicity in patients receiving combination chemotherapy.[160] Rarely, lung disease can occur after discontinuation of methotrexate therapy.[132] Most patients have enjoyed complete recovery, with a lower than 10% mortality.

Most patients present with a subacute febrile illness occurring within 3 to 4 months of initiating therapy.

Peripheral eosinophilia is seen in about a third of patients, and diffuse pulmonary infiltrates are the most common radiographic finding.[5,146] This group is interesting because many have recovered despite continuous therapy or rechallenge with methotrexate. This latter feature argues for an idiosyncratic reaction and suggests that etiologic agents other than methotrexate may contribute to the development of this lesion. An unusual response to viral infection has been proposed in some cases.

Most lung biopsies in patients with methotrexate toxicity have shown a distinctive *CIP* characterized by a nodular interstitial infiltrate consisting of lymphocytes, plasma cells, histiocytes, and occasional multinucleated giant cells (Fig. 4–4).[126,130,134,137,138,146,153,156,161] Eosinophils are present in about half, and there may be associated poorly formed non-necrotizing granulomas. BAL has shown a marked lymphocytosis with a reversed CD4:CD8 ratio in some cases, although neutrophilia has also been described.[117,146,153] Nearly all patients with this lesion have recovered from their lung disease, although progression may occur rarely.[156]

Changes resembling *hypersensitivity pneumonitis* are less commonly found in methotrexate toxicity and overlap with the above-described CIP.[129,132,153,162] Reported patients were receiving low-dose therapy for either rheumatoid arthritis or psoriasis, and all recovered rapidly with discontinuation of methotrexate. Steroids were also given in some patients. Lung biopsies in these instances usually show a combination of patchy CIP with a bronchiolocentric distribution and small, poorly formed granulomas. Eosinophils may be present but are usually not a conspicuous finding.

BOOP has been described as an additional manifestation of methotrexate toxicity and may also be associated with the presence of poorly formed non-necrotizing granulomas.[127,136] This complication has been reported in patients receiving relatively low doses of methotrexate for rheumatoid arthritis or mycosis fungoides. Peripheral eosinophilia was present in some cases. Improvement or recovery occurred after the drug was discontinued.

DAD is an uncommon manifestation of methotrexate toxicity that has been reported following intrathecal, as well as parenteral, administration of methotrexate.[122,124,129,131,160,161,162] Organizing DAD has been associated with honeycomb change in some cases.[122,161] *Pulmonary edema* leading to acute respiratory failure and death has also been reported after intrathecal methotrexate administration.[124] In these patients, pulmonary edema has occasionally been associated with patchy alveolar hemorrhage, and has also been

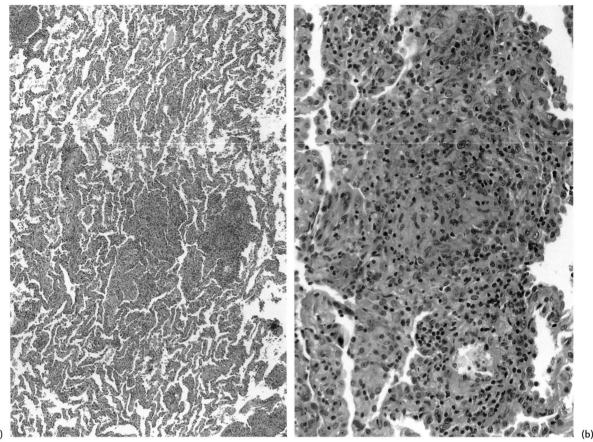

(a)   (b)

Figure 4–4 Methotrexate toxicity. (a) Low magnification showing a cellular CIP with patchy nodular areas. **(b)** At higher magnification, the nodular areas are seen to consist of a mixture of epithelioid histiocytes and chronic inflammatory cells.

superimposed on the distinctive CIP described previously.[152]

Hydroxycarbamide (hydroxyurea)

Hydroxycarbamide is a ribonucleotide reductase inhibitor used in the treatment of myeloproliferative disorders, sickle cell anemia, and psoriasis. Pulmonary toxicity has been reported rarely, and only in patients with an underlying myeloproliferative disorder. Patients present with fever, dry cough, dyspnea, and bilateral interstitial infiltrates, usually within 3 to 12 weeks of drug initiation. One report described a patient who presented after 2 years.[181] The majority have responded to discontinuation of hydroxycarbamide, with or without steroids.

Pathologic changes are described in only four cases. *Hypersensitivity pneumonia* and *DIP* were noted on surgical biopsies, nonspecific interstitial fibrosis with hyperplasia of type 2 pneumocytes on transbronchial biopsy, while *BOOP* was described in an autopsy specimen.[147,148,158,172] The latter patient died of acute respiratory failure 5 days after initiation of treatment with hydroxycarbamide, interferon-α, and oral cytarabine.[147]

Fludarabine

Fludarabine is a purine analogue with activity in chronic lymphocytic leukemia and non-Hodgkin's lymphoma. Its cytotoxic action is mediated by inhibition of DNA synthesis. It can produce a sustained lymphopenia, with a marked decrease in CD4 cells, and an increased risk of opportunistic infection.[118] Pulmonary toxicity was reported in 8.6% of patients receiving fludarabine in one report.[142] There was no correlation with dose or duration of therapy. Previous chemotherapy regimens that include alkylating agents may be associated with an increased risk of lung toxicity.[118] Patients with chronic lymphocytic leukemia appear to be more likely to develop pulmonary toxicity than patients with other diagnoses.[142] Radiation, preexisting

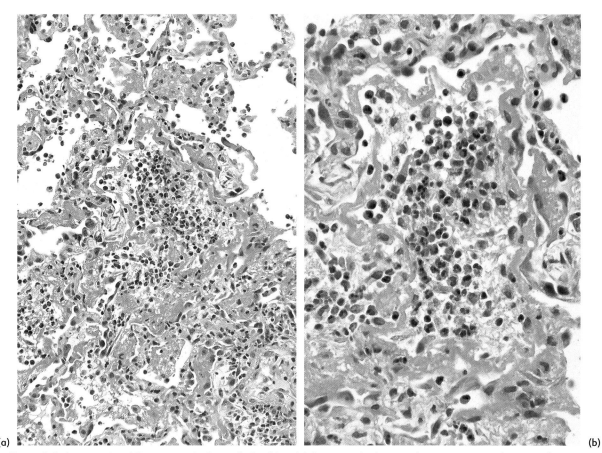

Figure 4–5 Acute eosinophilic pneumonia due to fludarabine. (a) Prominent hyaline membranes are seen at low magnification, along with numerous intraalveolar eosinophils which are better illustrated at higher magnification **(b)**.

lung disease, and intrapulmonary malignancy are other reported potentiating factors for lung toxicity. Latent periods have ranged from 2 days after the first cycle to 6 weeks after the last cycle.[142] Fever, dyspnea, dry cough, and hypoxemia are the most common presenting complaints. Most patients improved with steroids or withdrawal of fludarabine. Death from respiratory failure is rare.[142]

CIP with fibrosis appears to be the most common pathologic finding in fludarabine-induced lung toxicity.[135,142,143,145,163] *Organizing pneumonia* and *DAD* have been described less frequently.[142] *Eosinophilic pneumonia* (Fig. 4–5) with peripheral eosinophilia also has been reported, although the diagnosis was based on BAL and peripheral blood findings without lung biopsy.[166]

Gemcitabine

Gemcitabine is an analogue of the nucleoside deoxycytidine. Its antitumor activity is derived from substitution for deoxycytidine in tumor DNA. Its pulmonary toxicity has been attributed to capillary leak syndrome analogous to that of Ara-C, another substituted nucleoside.[157] Risk factors include increased age, pulmonary neoplasm, and prior history of radiotherapy.[139] Pulmonary toxicity of gemcitabine may be enhanced by the coadministration of anti-microtubule agents, such as the taxanes and vinca alkaloids.[144,149] No relationship to dose has been demonstrated.

The onset of toxicity has ranged from as early as the first dose to as late as the twelfth, with a median of five doses. Most patients present with low-grade fever, dry cough, dyspnea on exertion, and hypoxemia. Reticulonodular infiltrates are typically seen on chest radiographs.[139] Ground glass infiltrates, thickened septal lines, and reticular opacities have been described on chest computed tomography (CT).[125] There is generally a brisk response to steroids, although fatalities have been reported.[120,121,139,154–156,164,167,168] Severe pulmonary toxicity with acute respiratory distress syndrome has been described in up to 5% of patients with extrapulmonary tumors, and 13.8% of patients with lung cancer.[121]

Pathologic findings are reported in only a few cases, most of which are from autopsies. *DAD* is the most common manifestation.[121,139,154,155,157] *NSIP* occurs less frequently.[120,157] *Pulmonary venoocclusive disease* has been reported in one patient who died after repeated administration of gemcitabine.[168]

Other Antimetabolites

Pulmonary toxicity occurs in 10–15% of patients undergoing high-dose *cytarabine* (cytosine arabinoside; ara-C) therapy for acute leukemia.[119,165] Affected patients usually develop symptoms within 2 weeks of initiating therapy, and the risk of pulmonary toxicity increases with the increasing number of doses. The changes are reversible in some patients, but nearly half succumb to respiratory failure.[119,165] Autopsies have shown pulmonary edema in most patients, characterized by an acellular proteinaceous airspace exudate.[119,141,165] DAD has also been described.[119] A single example of *mercaptopurine*-induced lung disease has been reported, but the pathologic changes were not detailed.[5] Rare examples of acute and organizing DAD have been attributed to *azathioprine* toxicity.[123,128,150,169]

Miscellaneous Cytotoxic Drugs

Taxanes

The taxanes include *paclitaxel* and *docetaxel*. They inhibit tumor growth by disrupting microtubule formation, similar to the vinca alkaloids, and they are active against various solid tumors, including breast, lung, prostate, bladder, ovary, and head and neck.

Pulmonary toxicity induced by *docetaxel* is more common than that induced by paclitaxel and has a less favorable prognosis, with a significant number of fatalities.[176,191,193,196] The risk factors for docetaxel toxicity are not known. It does not appear to be dose-related. However, toxicity is increased when docetaxel is combined with gemcitabine, thalidomide, estramustine, or thoracic irradiation.[173,176,189,191] Most patients present between the first and eighth cycle.

CIP with fibrosis is the most commonly reported pathologic finding.[173,190,191,196] DAD has also been reported.[176,191,193] Hypersensitivity pneumonia with lymphohistiocytic interstitial infiltrates and poorly formed granulomas was described in one case, while an increased eosinophil count on BAL was seen in another.[184,193]

Paclitaxel is lipid-soluble and is delivered intravenously in an oil-based preparation, cremophor (polyoxyethylated castor oil). As a consequence of the cremophor, paclitaxel administration may be associated with a type of hypersensitivity or anaphylactoid reaction which can occur within minutes. Most patients are premedicated with a combination of steroids and antihistamines to minimize this complication.[192]

The incidence of pulmonary toxicity with paclitaxel is lower than that with docetaxel. In 71 patients with non-small cell lung cancer enrolled in a randomized trial where 35 patients received docetaxel and 36 patients received paclitaxel, pulmonary toxicity was seen in seven patients (20%) treated with docetaxel compared to one patient (3%) treated with paclitaxel. The patients presented with bilateral interstitial pulmonary infiltrates, progressive fatigue, and hypoxia in the absence of fever.[177] A cellular CIP associated with poorly formed granulomas resembling hypersensitivity pneumonia was described in two cases.[179,197] In one patient, there was an increased lymphocyte count (36%) on BAL, and the patient's lymphocytes demonstrated a positive migration test when exposed to paclitaxel.[179] Both patients responded to steroid therapy.

Vinca alkaloids

Vinblastine and *vindesine*, members of the vinca alkaloid group, have been associated with a distinctive clinical syndrome characterized by the sudden onset of dyspnea and airway obstruction within hours of drug administration.[185,186,188] This syndrome appears to be especially common when these drugs are used in conjunction with mitomycin, occurring in as many as 5.5% of patients receiving this therapy.[188] Open lung biopsy has been reported in a single case and showed organizing DAD.[185] The overall prognosis is good, and the majority have recovered after discontinuation of therapy.

Others

Procarbazine lung toxicity is rare and has occurred only in individuals receiving combination chemotherapy for Hodgkin's disease.[175,178,182,183,187] The prognosis is excellent, and all but a single patient recovered with discontinuation of therapy. The main change reported in lung biopsies is a CIP resembling that seen with methotrexate hypersensitivity.[178] Poorly formed non-necrotizing granulomas accompany the interstitial pneumonia in some cases.[178] A tissue reaction resembling eosinophilic pneumonia has also been associated with procarbazine administration.[175] Acute and organizing

DAD was described in one patient who died with evidence of procarbazine toxicity.[182]

Teniposide (VM-26) has been associated with DAD in one patient.[174]

Imatinib mesylate (Gleevec) is a specific tyrosine kinase receptor inhibitor used for the treatment of chronic myelogenous leukemia, Philadelphia chromosome-positive acute lymphoblastic leukemia, and gastrointestinal stromal tumors. Pulmonary toxicity is rare and has been infrequently reported, mostly in letters and correspondence. Patients presented between 10 days and 11 months after initiation of therapy, and symptoms included dyspnea on exertion, dry cough, and hypoxia. All patients responded favorably to discontinuation of the drug, with or without steroid therapy. CIP is the most commonly described pathologic finding, and it was associated with an eosinophilic infiltrate in one case.[181,194,198] Interstitial pneumonia has also been described in a patient with underlying idiopathic pulmonary fibrosis.[197a] Pulmonary alveolar proteinosis was described in one patient, who improved after therapeutic lung lavage.[195] Pleural effusions were additionally noted in three pediatric patients.[180]

NONCYTOTOXIC DRUGS

The list of noncytotoxic drugs associated with pulmonary toxicity is growing and includes a wide range of therapeutic agents. In the following discussion these drugs are categorized into groups based mainly on pharmacologic action and therapeutic indications. The various drugs and related reactions are summarized in Tables 4–3 and 4–4.

Antimicrobials

The most important antimicrobial agent associated with lung toxicity is nitrofurantoin, although a number of others have also been associated with pulmonary toxicity.

Nitrofurantoin

Nitrofurantoin is responsible for more reported cases of pulmonary toxicity than any other drug. The actual incidence of lung toxicity is low, however, and the large number of reported cases is more a reflection of the drug's popularity.[6,219,223,237] Elderly women are most commonly affected. Two distinct syndromes, an acute and a chronic reaction, have been described. The acute reaction occurs in about 90% of patients.[6,219,223,237] In these individuals, fever, dyspnea, and cough usually

develop within 2 weeks of initiating therapy, although symptoms may occur as early as several hours following a single dose in patients previously exposed to nitrofurantoin. Diffuse interstitial infiltrates are the usual radiographic abnormality.[6,219,237] Peripheral eosinophilia occurs in about two-thirds of these patients and is more common with succeeding episodes of lung toxicity. Nearly all will recover after discontinuation of therapy. Tissue biopsy is rarely needed to establish the diagnosis, and therefore few pathologic descriptions of acute nitrofurantoin toxicity are available. Eosinophilic pneumonia has long been considered the underlying lesion in most patients, but no biopsy-proven case has been reported. Nitrofurantoin toxicity differs from eosinophilic pneumonia, however, in that the peripheral eosinophilia tends to be less pronounced, chest radiographs usually show interstitial opacities in a bibasilar distribution rather than migratory airspace opacities, and the symptoms and radiographic abnormalities have resolved within minutes or hours of antihistamine injections in patients rechallenged with nitrofurantoin.[219,231,237] It seems likely, therefore, that the lesion represents a type I hypersensitivity response in which pulmonary edema is the underlying pulmonary abnormality. Other uncommonly reported manifestations of acute pulmonary toxicity include DAD (two cases),[215] a DIP-like reaction (one case),[219] a cellular interstitial pneumonia with poorly formed nonnecrotizing granulomas resembling hypersensitivity pneumonia (one case),[228] and diffuse alveolar hemorrhage (three cases).[200,203] These latter tissue reactions are unusual in that most have been associated with rapidly progressive respiratory failure, and the majority of reported patients have died.

About 10% of patients with nitrofurantoin-induced lung disease present with the insidious onset of dyspnea and cough occurring after months to years of therapy. The clinical and radiographic features of this chronic nitrofurantoin reaction are nonspecific and mimic the idiopathic chronic interstitial pneumonias.[6,219,221,235,237,239] Peripheral eosinophilia is less common than with the acute form but occurs in as many as 44% of patients.[219] Low titers of antinuclear autoantibodies are present in the majority of patients and will revert to normal after nitrofurantoin is discontinued. A reversible lupus-like syndrome is associated with pulmonary toxicity in some of these individuals.[236] Recognition of chronic nitrofurantoin toxicity is important because most patients will improve, and many will recover after nitrofurantoin therapy is terminated. Lung biopsies are frequently done in this

Table 4–3 Pulmonary Reactions to Noncytotoxic Drugs. I: Antimicrobials, Anti-inflammatory Drugs, Antiarrhythmics, Antihypertensives

Drug	Tissue Reactions
Antimicrobials	
Nitrofurantoin	DAD,[215] hemorrhage,[200,203] HP,[228] DIP,[201,219] EP,[206] UIP,[219,221,235,239] GIP,[228] BOOP[204]
Sulfasalazine	EP,[205,227,238,240,242] CIP,[205,217,230,243] DIP,[241] BOOP,[214,244] HP[225]
Sulfonamides (Prontosil, sulfadimethoxine, AVC [vaginal] cream)	EP[211,212]
Sulfathiazole [oral]	DAD[216]
Unspecified sulfonamides	Hemorrhage with capillaritis[213]
Amphotericin B plus leukocyte transfusion	Hemorrhage[246]
Penicillin	Edema[222]
Ampicillin	EP[233]
Pyrimethamine	EP[209]
Tetracycline	EP[218]
Minocycline	EP[232]
Para-aminosalicylic acid	EP[245]
Anti-inflammatory Drugs	
Gold salts	DAD,[259,266] CIP,[257,282,290] BOOP,[261,269,273] chronic bronchiolitis[276,277]
Penicillamine	Obliterative bronchiolitis,[254,274,291] follicular bronchiolitis,[254] hemorrhage,[253,267,268,285] DAD[250]
Infliximab	DAD,[264] CIP,[264] organizing pneumonia,[264] EP[280]
Etanercept	Granulomatous pneumonia,[251,279,293] vasculitis[251]
Naproxen	EP[249,275]
Nabumetone	EP[272]
Phenylbutazone	EP[288]
Salicylates	Edema[260]
Colchicine	DAD[6]
Acetaminophen	EP[263]
Interferons	
Interferon-α	CIP,[295,298–300,304–306] granulomas,[297,301,307,310,311,313] DAD,[295,299] BOOP,[306,308] EP,[302] pleural effusion[312]
Interferon-γ	DAD[303,314]
Antiarrhythmics	
Amiodarone	CIP (+ foam cells),[339,343,344,350] pleuritis,[328] BOOP,[8,339,343,344,350] DAD (+ foam cells)[324,339]
Tocainide	DIP,[326] CIP,[321,349] BOOP[345]
Lidocaine	Edema[330]
Quinidine sulfate	CIP[347]
Antihypertensives	
Hydrochlorothiazide	Edema[355,359,362]
Propranolol	Edema,[357,368] EP[369]
Pindolol	UIP[363]
Acebutolol	Granulomas with eosinophils[370]
Hexamethonium	DAD,[358,364] BOOP[365]
Mecamylamine	BOOP[366]
Hydralazine	Hemorrhage[354]
Captopril	Eosinophilia[367]

Abbreviations: DAD = diffuse alveolar damage; HP = hypersensitivity pneumonia; DIP = desquamative interstitial pneumonia; BOOP = bronchiolitis obliterans–organizing pneumonia; EP = eosinophilic pneumonia; CIP = nonspecific chronic interstitial pneumonia; UIP = usual interstitial pneumonia; GIP = giant cell interstitial pneumonia.

Table 4–4 Pulmonary Reactions to Noncytotoxic Drugs. II: Tocolytic Agents, Anticonvulsants, Psychotherapeutic Drugs, Opioids, Cocaine, Tryptophan, Miscellaneous

Drug	Tissue Reactions
Tocolytic Agents (ritodrine, terbutaline, albuterol, isoxsuprine, magnesium sulfate)	Edema[371–380]
Anticonvulsants	
Phenytoin (Dilantin)	BOOP,[385] CIP,[386] LIP,[382] vasculitis[389]
Carbamazepine	EP,[387] BOOP,[381] DAD[388]
Psychotherapeutic Drugs	
Haloperidol	Edema,[396] hemorrhage[396]
Sedative-hypnotics (chlordiazepoxide, paraldehyde, ethclorvynol)	Edema[390,392,394,398–400,402]
Amitriptyline (Elavil)	DAD[395,397]
Imipramine	EP[405]
Trazodone	EP[401]
Fluoxetine hydrochloride (Prozac)	HP,[393] granulomas[393]
Venlafaxine	HP,[391] organizing pneumonia[391]
Opioids	
Agonists (morphine, methadone, propoxyphene, codeine, buprenorphine, heroin)	Edema,[414,416] bronchiectasis[406,419]
Antagonists (nalbuphine, naloxone)	Edema[411,413,417]
Cocaine	DAD,[427] EP,[427] hemorrhage,[438,439] BOOP,[443] airway stenosis,[447] CIP,[441,445,446] foreign body (cellulose) granulomas,[424] airway-centered fibrosis,[423] hypertension,[434,448] capillaritis,[444] edema[435,442]
Anorexigens	
Phentermine–fenfluramine, dexfenfluramine	Pulmonary hypertension[468,470,471,474, 475]
Aminorex	Pulmonary hypertension[467,469,476]
Miscellaneous	
Tryptophan	CIP,[449,451,455,461–464] pulmonary hypertension[462]
Methamphetamine	Pulmonary hypertension[511]
Statins (pravastatin, lovastatin, simvastatin)	CIP,[483,491] HP,[498] NSIP,[497] BOOP,[491,503] DAD,[491,503] eosinophilic pleural effusion[494]
Anticoagulants (warfarin, heparin)	Hemorrhage[486,510]
Thrombolytic agents (streptokinase, urokinase)	Hemorrhage,[479,502] DAD[488,499]
Ticlopidine	CIP[501,505]
Nilutamide	CIP,[489,506] BOOP[506]
Chlorpropamide	EP[484]
Cromolyn sodium	EP,[508] granulomas with BOOP[480]
Mephenesin	EP[509]
Methysergide	Pleural fibrosis[490,492]
Pergolide	Pleural fibrosis[482]
Bromocriptine, mesulergine	Pleural fibrosis[500]
BCG	Granulomas[493,504,513]
Nifedipine	Edema[507]
Radiocontrast material	Edema[496]
Epinephrine	Edema[485]
Propylthiouracil	Hemorrhage[514]
Deferoxamine mesylate	DAD[487]

Abbreviations: BOOP = bronchiolitis obliterans–organizing pneumonia; CIP = nonspecific chronic interstitial pneumonia; EP = eosinophilic pneumonia; DAD = diffuse alveolar damage; HP = hypersensitivity pneumonia

group, and the pathologist may be the first to suggest the diagnosis.

Histologically, the majority of patients with chronic nitrofurantoin toxicity have a CIP that may be difficult to distinguish from UIP.[219,221,235,239] Eosinophils may or may not be present but are rarely conspicuous. Immunofluorescence has been reported in a few cases and has shown no evidence of immune complex deposition.[221] Likewise, ultrastructural studies have shown no specific changes.[221] Less common patterns of chronic lung injury in nitrofurantoin toxicity include DIP,[201] giant cell interstitial pneumonia,[228] and BOOP.[204] Eosinophilic pneumonia has been reported as a manifestation of chronic pulmonary toxicity in one patient.[206]

Sulfasalazine, 5-Aminosalicylate, and Other Sulfonamides

Sulfasalazine is a poorly absorbed sulfonamide that has been used extensively in the treatment of inflammatory bowel disease. Pulmonary toxicity is uncommon, with fewer than 50 well-documented cases in the literature.[199,205,214,217,223,225,230,240–244] Pulmonary toxicity has also been attributed to 5-aminosalicylate (mesalamine), the clinically active moiety in sulfasalazine.[205,234] Most patients with sulfasalazine toxicity develop symptoms within 6 months of initiating therapy, although latent periods of as long as 8 years have been reported.[205] There appears to be no relationship between lung toxicity and duration of therapy, total cumulative dose, or daily maintenance dose. Allergies to other sulfonamides or aspirin may predispose patients to pulmonary side effects. All but three patients have survived after discontinuation of therapy.[205] Corticosteroids have been used in some patients as well. The few reported examples of 5-aminosalicylate-induced lung disease have also recovered with cessation of the drug alone or after steroid therapy.[205]

Eosinophilic pneumonia is thought to be the underlying pathologic lesion in most patients with sulfasalazine toxicity, most of whom present with cough, dyspnea, eosinophilia, and peripheral lung opacities.[205,227,238,240,242] An open lung biopsy in one case showed changes of eosinophilic pneumonia, and BAL showed increased numbers of eosinophils in others.[205,240,242] Pleural effusion with eosinophilia is uncommon and may occur as an isolated finding or in combination with pulmonary parenchymal disease.[205,217]

CIP has been reported in other cases, although this diagnosis has usually been made on transbronchial biopsy specimens.[205,217,230,243] Eosinophilia has not been noted in these cases. In one patient there were associated poorly formed non-necrotizing granulomas resembling those seen in hypersensitivity pneumonia.[225] Changes of DIP and BOOP have been reported less commonly, although some affected patients failed to respond to discontinuation of the drug, suggesting that sulfasalazine may not have been directly responsible for their lung diseases.[214,241,244] CIP and BOOP have also been described in patients with 5-aminosalicylate toxicity.[205]

One reported fatality from sulfasalazine toxicity occurred in a woman who died of progressive respiratory failure over a period of 4 weeks.[209] An autopsy revealed bilateral pulmonary thromboemboli as well as organizing DAD, and it is uncertain to what extent sulfasalazine contributed to her lung disease. Presumed DAD has been reported in two additional patients, one who died of progressive respiratory disease and another who recovered after high-dose corticosteroid therapy.[217,227]

Most reports of toxicity due to other sulfonamides appeared prior to 1970, suggesting that they may have been related to older-generation sulfa drugs.[212,213,21] Eosinophilic pneumonia has been reported following therapy with AVC [vaginal] cream and other sulfonamides that are no longer available for clinical use (*prontosil* and *sulfadimethoxine*).[211,212] Pulmonary hemorrhage with capillaritis has been reported in one patient who was receiving an unspecified sulfonamide.[212] DAD has been described in a patient who received an oral preparation of *sulfathiazole*, another sulfa drug that is no longer used.[216]

Amphotericin B

Diffuse lung infiltrates have been reported in as many as two-thirds of severely neutropenic patients who are treated with a combination of amphotericin B and leukocyte transfusion, although it is uncertain to what extent this represents a direct complication of drug therapy.[208,246] Institution of amphotericin therapy at or shortly after the time at which leukocyte transfusions begin appears to increase the risk of developing this complication, and the reactions are most severe in patients who receive amphotericin infusions within 4 hours of leukocyte transfusion.[246] About one-third of patients have died as a result of their respiratory disease. Diffuse alveolar hemorrhage is the underlying lesion in those patients for whom lung biopsy or autopsy results are available.[246]

Other Antimicrobials

Rare cases of pulmonary toxicity have occurred with other antimicrobial agents. *Nalidixic acid* is used primarily for chronic urinary tract infections, and, in one patient, caused a respiratory illness resembling acute nitrofurantoin toxicity.[207] Pathologic descriptions of pulmonary reactions to *penicillin* have been limited to examples of large airway edema occurring as part of a generalized anaphylactic response.[222] One case of eosinophilic pneumonia due to *ampicillin* has been reported.[233] *Pyrimethamine*-containing antimalarial agents have been implicated in some biopsy-proven cases of eosinophilic pneumonia.[209] Clinical evidence of eosinophilic pneumonia has also been reported with *tetracycline, minocycline,* and *para-aminosalicylic acid* (PAS), an antituberculous drug that has been largely replaced by more effective agents.[218,232,245]

Anti-inflammatory Drugs

Numerous drugs, such as gold, penicillamine, aspirin, a growing number of aspirin-like drugs (i.e. nonsteroidal anti-inflammatory agents), and biologic response modifiers (infliximab, etanercept), are used to treat rheumatoid arthritis and related inflammatory conditions. Several have been implicated as causes of drug-induced lung disease.[6,294]

Gold

A number of serious side effects are associated with gold therapy, including proteinuria, blood dyscrasias, skin rash, mucositis, and drug-induced lung disease. Pulmonary toxicity is uncommon, occurring in about 1% of patients.[6,287,294] There are no well-defined risk factors, although patients with certain major histocompatibility complex haplotypes have an increased risk of developing lung toxicity.[278] Most individuals present with the acute onset of respiratory symptoms within 2 to 6 months of initiating therapy, and nearly one-third have associated mucocutaneous toxicity.[6] Peripheral eosinophilia occurs in about one-fourth of cases. Nearly all reported patients have recovered or improved after discontinuation of gold therapy. Corticosteroid therapy has been used in some cases. Only two fatalities have been reported and neither was clearly attributable to drug-induced lung disease.[261,269]

Most tissue reactions that have been associated with gold toxicity are similar to manifestations of rheumatoid lung disease, and therefore it can be difficult in a given case to identify a specific cause.[292,294] Organizing DAD and a nonspecific CIP are the most commonly described lung reactions.[257,259,266,282,290] BOOP has also been described and is usually associated with a CIP.[255,269,273] Chronic bronchiolitis may also occur and is characterized by a peribronchiolar infiltrate of chronic inflammatory cells.[276,277] A granulomatous bronchiolitis resembling hypersensitivity pneumonia has been described in one patient.[265] This change was seen several months after withdrawal of gold salts and after reinstitution of penicillamine therapy, however, and was probably unrelated to gold therapy. Tissue eosinophilia has been reported in a single transbronchial biopsy but was more likely related to that patient's history of asthma than to gold toxicity.[266]

Ultrastructural studies of biopsies and BAL specimens have shown gold-containing lysosomes (i.e. aurosomes) in some examples of pulmonary toxicity.[269,277,284] Gold has been identified within alveolar macrophages of patients who lack evidence of lung disease, however, and may be present for as long as 2 years after withdrawal of therapy.[256]

Penicillamine

Pulmonary complications occur in well under 1% of patients receiving penicillamine.[6,274,294] The interval from initiation of therapy to onset of respiratory side effects has ranged from 18 days to 7 years (mean, 15 months). No risk factors have been identified, and there is no apparent relationship between lung toxicity and duration of therapy, total cumulative dose, or daily maintenance dose.[6,294]

Several different clinicopathologic syndromes have been attributed to penicillamine. The most commonly reported is a rapidly progressive form of obstructive airways disease in which *obliterative bronchiolitis* (*constrictive bronchiolitis obliterans,* see Chapter 16) is the usual pathologic finding.[254,274,291] This lesion is characterized by luminal narrowing and/or obstruction by a dense peribronchiolar infiltrate of mononuclear inflammatory cells associated with epithelial necrosis and accompanied by varying degrees of fibrosis. In some cases the submucosal infiltrate is associated with prominent lymphoid follicles and resembles *follicular bronchiolitis.*[254] Whether these airway changes truly represent a manifestation of drug-induced lung disease or whether they are related to the underlying rheumatoid disease is difficult to assess. Regardless, the prognosis of this complication is poor, with death due to progressive lung disease occurring in half the patients.

A 'pulmonary–renal' syndrome characterized by hemoptysis and hematuria has been reported as a possible complication of penicillamine therapy in patients with underlying Wilson's disease, primary biliary cirrhosis, rheumatoid arthritis, and scleroderma.[6,253,267,268,285,294] All had taken relatively high daily maintenance doses ranging from 1 to 3.5 g, and all developed respiratory symptoms after 1.5 to 7 years of therapy. Nearly half of the reported patients succumbed to their illness, while the others recovered with aggressive therapy, including immunosuppressive agents and plasmapheresis. Autopsies have shown diffuse alveolar hemorrhage with no evidence of vasculitis.[285] Immunofluorescence was negative in the one case tested.[285] A crescentic glomerulonephritis with variable immunofluorescence findings is seen in the kidneys.[253,285]

Several patients who were being treated for rheumatoid arthritis developed dyspnea and diffuse lung infiltrates 3 weeks to 12 months after initiating penicillamine therapy.[6,250,252] Peripheral eosinophilia was present in nearly half, and all improved or recovered after discontinuation of therapy. Biopsy specimens have not been examined during the acute illness in these patients. Organizing DAD was found at autopsy in one patient who died abruptly of a cerebrovascular accident during a 2-week hospitalization for an *adult respiratory distress syndrome* (ARDS)-like illness.[250] Whether this represented a manifestation of penicillamine toxicity or was related to some other process is unclear.

Biologic response modifiers

Infliximab is a neutralizing chimeric human/murine monoclonal antibody with specificity and high affinity for tumor necrosis factor alpha (TNFα). It is effective in patients with rheumatoid arthritis, Crohn's disease, and the arthritis symptoms associated with inflammatory bowel disease and psoriasis. Infection is the main reported complication of infliximab therapy. Tuberculosis occurred within a mean of 12 weeks of initiating treatment in one series, of which 31% had pulmonary involvement.[262] One case of pulmonary aspergillosis has also been reported, which occurred 5 days after beginning treatment and resulted in death.[289]

Infliximab is thought to be synergistic in the development of methotrexate pneumonitis. Three patients receiving methotrexate developed fever, dyspnea, fatigue, and bilateral interstitial infiltrates from 1 to 4 weeks after the addition of infliximab.[264] All patients responded rapidly to steroids. Pathologic findings included DAD, cellular interstitial pneumonia, and changes suggestive of organizing pneumonia.[264]

One recent report described eosinophilic pneumonia in a patient who developed fever, arthralgias, myalgias, leukocytosis, and ARDS following two infusions of infliximab administered 15 months apart. Serum human anti-chimeric antibodies against the murine-binding portion of infliximab were present, and the changes were thought to represent an unusually severe delayed hypersensitivity reaction to infliximab.[280] Eosinophilic pleural effusion has also been reported.[248]

Etanercept is a dimeric fusion protein that binds specifically to TNFα rendering it biologically inactive. It is used in rheumatoid arthritis and juvenile arthritis. Concerns regarding etanercept have focused on infectious complications and the induction of autoimmune phenomena, including development of autoantibodies (ANA, ANCA). Tuberculosis has been reported in some patients after a median interval of 11.5 months following receipt of the drug.[271] A systemic non-necrotizing granulomatous process involving the skin and the lung was reported in another patient in whom *Mycobacterium avium-intracellulare* was recovered from a BAL specimen.[279]

There are only a few reports of etanercept-associated lung injury. An unusual granulomatous pneumonia was reported in four patients who developed dyspnea, dry cough, and ground glass infiltrates.[293] All had rheumatoid arthritis, three had rheumatoid arthritis-associated UIP, and two had been receiving methotrexate. Symptoms occurred from 1 week to 3 months after institution of etanercept. All patients had resolution of symptoms and pulmonary infiltrates following steroid treatment. Necrotizing pulmonary nodules and vasculitis were reported in one patient.[251]

Other Anti-inflammatory Drugs

A number of nonsteroidal anti-inflammatory drugs, including *naproxen*, *ibuprofen*, *phenylbutazone*, *sulindac*, *fenoprofen*, *nabumetone*, and *apazone* (azapropazone), have been responsible for rare cases of pulmonary toxicity.[247,249,258,272,275,283,286,288] One report suggests that naproxen may have a synergistic effect when used in combination with gold salts.[270] Pathologic descriptions are limited, but the lesions in some cases appear to represent examples of eosinophilic pneumonia.[249,270,272,275,288] Pulmonary edema has also been described.[283] Most patients recover after therapy is discontinued. Corticosteroids have been used in some cases as well.

Salicylate-induced pulmonary toxicity is limited to patients with salicylate intoxication, occurring most commonly in those with salicylate levels of 40 mg/dl or greater.[6,260,294] Affected patients present with clinical and radiographic evidence of pulmonary edema, although tissue documentation has not been reported. Some authors have emphasized that the hemodynamic profiles in these patients are consistent with ARDS, raising the possibility that the underlying pathologic lesion is DAD. Most patients recover with a reduction in serum salicylate levels and supportive measures.

DAD has been attributed to *colchicine* in one patient who died of rapidly progressive respiratory failure after an intentional overdose.[6] Eosinophilic pneumonia has been described in one patient who developed dyspnea, fever, and a skin rash 5 days after taking a nonprescription *acetaminophen*-containing preparation.[263] Lymphocyte stimulation testing indicated that acetaminophen was the likely causal agent.

Interferons

Interferons are naturally occurring cytokines produced as a reaction to many stimuli, especially viral infections. *Interferon-α* is synthesized by recombinant DNA technology and is approved for the treatment of chronic hepatitis B and C, as well as chronic myelogenous leukemia, hairy cell leukemia, multiple myeloma, non-Hodgkin's lymphoma, and melanoma. There are reports of severe pulmonary toxicity during therapy with interferon-α alone or in combination with ribavirin, as well as with pegylated interferon-α in combination with ribavirin. The Chinese herbal medicine Sho-Sai-Koto has been shown to increase the risk of pulmonary toxicity.[306,309] Toxicity usually develops from 2 to 12 weeks after starting therapy.[298,299] Clinical presentation includes dyspnea, dry cough, hypoxemia, a restrictive pattern on pulmonary function testing, along with bilateral diffuse lung infiltrates. Interferon toxicity is generally dose-dependent and related to duration of treatment. The overall incidence of pulmonary toxicity is less than 1% for conventional doses of standard interferon, and 5.7% for high-dose standard interferon and pegylated interferon. Pegylation of interferon provides higher levels due to prolonged half-life. The majority of patients have prompt improvement after discontinuation of treatment, with or without corticosteroids. Deaths have been reported rarely.[295,299]

A cellular CIP with or without fibrosis is the most commonly reported pathologic finding in interferon-α toxicity.[295,298–300,304–306] Increased numbers of lymphocytes with decreased CD4:CD8 ratio have been reported in BAL fluid.[304,305] Noncaseating granulomas resembling sarcoidosis have been described occasionally.[297,301,307,310,311,313] Symptoms and radiologic findings resolved spontaneously in some cases, and after steroid treatment in others. Most patients were receiving ribavirin in addition to interferon-α. Severe exacerbation of asthma was described in two patients treated with interferon-α for chronic hepatitis.[296] It was suggested that stimulation of the T-helper subset TH-1 by interferon-α may be involved in the development of both sarcoidosis and asthma.[296,301] DAD was seen in two patients who developed fever, dry cough and dyspnea 2 and 5 weeks after institution of interferon-α, and both patients died despite steroid therapy.[295,299] BOOP, pleural effusion, and eosinophilic pneumonia have also been reported.[302,306,308,312]

Interferon-γ is used for the treatment of chronic granulomatous disease, malignant osteopetrosis, and various malignancies. It has also been used in idiopathic pulmonary fibrosis. Its effect is mediated by a reduction in the transcription of genes for the production of transforming growth factor beta (TGFβ) and connective tissue growth factor. Significant adverse effects have been reported only infrequently, and DAD is the most common pathologic finding. One report described respiratory failure leading to death in four of 10 patients with advanced UIP treated with interferon-γ.[303] This event occurred 7 to 90 days after initiation of treatment, and all patients were taking or had recently been taking relatively high doses of prednisone. The clinical presentation was increasing dyspnea, fever, and rapidly progressive hypoxemia. Chest radiography revealed new alveolar opacities. Pathologic analysis in two patients showed DAD in addition to UIP.[303] Pneumonitis has also been reported in patients receiving recombinant interferon-γ as maintenance therapy for small cell lung cancer, and DAD was demonstrated at autopsy in one patient.[314]

Antiarrhythmic Drugs

Amiodarone

Amiodarone is used for the treatment of tachyarrhythmias that are refractory to other therapy. The reported incidence of respiratory side effects has varied widely, but appears to be between 5% and 10%.[325,327,333,334,338] Although neither duration of therapy nor total cumulative dose correlates with the risk of lung toxicity, daily maintenance doses of 400 mg or greater are associated with an incidence of respiratory complications ranging from 5% to 15%.[315,322,325]

Toxicity can also occur in patients who are exposed to low doses (200 mg daily), although the incidence is lower, ranging between 0.1% and 0.5%.[322,344] Individuals older than 60 years of age may also be more likely to develop lung toxicity.[315,329] Most patients present with the insidious onset of dyspnea and a dry cough within months of initiating therapy. In rare cases, toxicity may develop within days to weeks of the initiation of therapy.[319] Constitutional complaints such as low-grade fever and malaise are common, and about one-third of patients present with an acute febrile illness that mimics an infectious pneumonia.[327,333,334,338] Chest roentgenograms typically show diffuse interstitial infiltrates, although a wide range of abnormalities has been reported, including localized airspace opacities.[333–335,338] CT scans show a combination of peripheral high-attenuation opacities and nonspecific infiltrates associated with increased attenuation in the liver and/or spleen.[335,348] Most patients will recover from their lung disease after discontinuation of the drug.[324,332,333,338] Recovery has also occurred in some patients who were treated with corticosteroid therapy while being maintained on amiodarone. ARDS has developed in some patients with presumed amiodarone-associated lung injury after pulmonary angiography, open heart surgery, pneumonectomy, and other surgical procedures requiring general anesthesia.[332,340,351,352]

Several different types of tissue reactions have been attributed to amiodarone toxicity. The most common is a nonspecific CIP associated with the accumulation of intraalveolar *foamy macrophages* (Fig. 4–6).[334,338,339] The foamy macrophages contain finely vacuolated clear cytoplasm, and they may be present within alveolar septa as well as alveolar spaces. Foamy macrophages are increased in areas corresponding to regions of high attenuation on CT scans.[348] Nonspecific *pleural inflammation* is an accompanying feature in some cases and has been associated with pleural effusion.[328] Ultrastructurally the vacuolated appearance of the macrophages is due to the presence of distinctive cytoplasmic lamellar inclusions (Fig. 4–7). The inclusions are round, oval, or irregular in shape and are composed of closely spaced concentrically or haphazardly arranged lamellae surrounded by an electron-dense rim of amorphous material.[324,334,336,338,339] They may be seen within endothelial cells, interstitial cells, and alveolar lining cells in addition to alveolar macrophages. The inclusions often resemble surfactant lamellar bodies and sometimes can be distinguished only by their location within cells other than type 2 pneumocytes. Foamy macrophages and cytoplasmic

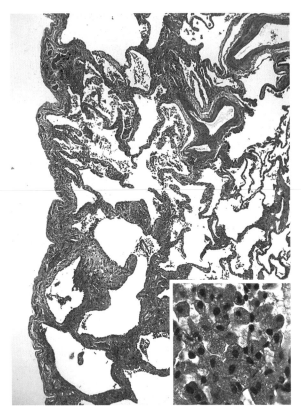

Figure 4–6 Amiodarone toxicity. CIP with fibrosis is seen at low magnification. Note the numerous intraalveolar macrophages present in the airspaces in the upper left portion of the photograph. The inset is a higher magnification, showing the characteristic foamy cytoplasm of the intraalveolar macrophages.

lamellar inclusions are frequently found in nontoxic patients and, therefore, indicate exposure but are not by themselves diagnostic of drug-induced lung disease.[319,336,338,339]

BOOP is a less common manifestation of amiodarone toxicity and is often associated with a CIP.[8,339,343,344,350] DAD is seen in a minority of patients, in whom it is accompanied by the presence of foamy intraalveolar macrophages.[324,339] The mortality in this group of patients approaches 50%.

BAL can be a useful technique for evaluating patients with possible amiodarone toxicity, although its precise role remains controversial.[316,318,323,331,336–338,341,342] As in tissue biopsies, foamy alveolar macrophages are common but do not reliably distinguish toxic from nontoxic patients.[336,341,342] Increased numbers of neutrophils and lymphocytes, specifically T-suppressor–cytotoxic cells, are important markers of pulmonary

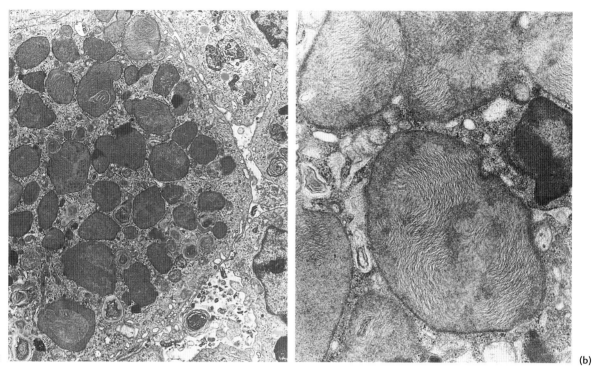

(a)   (b)

Figure 4–7 Ultrastructure of the foamy macrophages in amiodarone toxicity. (a) Numerous round-to-oval membrane-bound inclusions are seen in the macrophage cytoplasm. **(b)** Higher magnification of the inclusions shows the characteristic closely spaced concentrically arranged lamellae surrounded by an electron-dense rim of amorphous material.

toxicity, although normal differential cell counts occur in as many as a third of toxic patients.[318,323,331,338,341,342] Direct quantitative assays of BAL for phospholipid content and specific phospholipids are investigational tools that may eventually prove useful in routine clinical diagnosis.[338,341] Leukocyte migration inhibition assays of peripheral blood lymphocytes and detection of anti-amiodarone antibodies may also prove useful in the recognition of amiodarone toxicity.[317,341,346]

Other Antiarrhythmic Drugs

Tocainide is a lidocaine analogue used for the treatment of life-threatening ventricular arrhythmias. Pulmonary toxicity is rare, occurring in less than 1% of treated patients, and has been well characterized in only six patients.[321,326,345,349] All were taking 600 to 1600 mg of tocainide per day and developed respiratory symptoms 2 to 14 months after the initiation of therapy. Open lung biopsies in two and transbronchial biopsies in another were reported to show CIP.[321,326,349] The changes closely resembled UIP in one patient.[326] Transbronchial biopsies in a fourth patient showed BOOP.[345] All recovered after discontinuation of tocainide. Corticosteroids were used in some patients.

A clinical syndrome resembling pulmonary edema has been reported in one patient after topical anesthesia with *lidocaine*.[330] No biopsy was obtained. A single instance of *quinidine sulfate*-induced lung toxicity has been reported and was associated with a mild NSIP on transbronchial biopsy.[347]

Antihypertensive Drugs

Several drugs used in the treatment of systemic hypertension have been associated with pulmonary toxicity. Rare examples of pulmonary reactions following *hydrochlorothiazide* administration have been reported.[6,355,356,359,362] Nearly all the patients were women who developed shortness of breath within minutes or hours of a single dose. Some had histories of previous adverse reactions to hydrochlorothiazide. Chest radiographs show diffuse interstitial and airspace opacities compatible with pulmonary edema. The prognosis is excellent, and nearly all patients have recovered within several days. No tissue diagnosis has been reported.

Pulmonary edema is also an uncommon reaction to *propranolol* and usually results from acute left ventricular failure.[357,368] A syndrome resembling eosinophilic pneumonia has also been described as a manifestation of propranolol toxicity.[369] Propranolol has also been incriminated as a cause of interstitial lung disease with BAL lymphocytosis, but no pathologic descriptions are available.[353] Examples of UIP and nonclassifiable granulomatous inflammation with eosinophils have been attributed to *pindolol* and *acebutolol*, respectively, in one patient each.[363,370] A form of rapidly progressive obstructive airways disease has been reported in one patient receiving *practolol*, a beta blocker no longer in clinical use.[360] Transbronchial biopsies were nondiagnostic, and the nature of the lesion was unclear.

Pulmonary toxicity, a well-documented complication of *hexamethonium* therapy, is mainly of historic interest, since the drug is no longer used.[358,364,365] Respiratory symptoms occurred 4 to 15 months (mean, 9 months) after initiation of therapy, and the mortality rate was high. Some patients were also taking hydralazine. Acute and organizing DAD was the main pathologic finding in most cases, while changes of BOOP were found in a few.[358,364,365] BOOP has also been described in one patient receiving *mecamylamine*.[366]

Hydralazine is one of nearly 50 drugs reported to cause a lupus-like syndrome.[354] It is similar to other causes of drug-induced lupus in that the most common intrathoracic manifestation of toxicity is pleuropericarditis. The diagnosis is usually made clinically, and a lung biopsy is rarely obtained. Clinical and radiographic evidence of DAD has been reported in a few patients, some of whom were also receiving anticoagulants.[354] All recovered with steroids and discontinuation of hydralazine, or withdrawal from hydralazine alone.

Captopril has caused one reported example of parenchymal lung disease.[367] The patient developed a skin rash, peripheral eosinophilia, and interstitial upper lobe opacities within days of restarting therapy with captopril. Transbronchial biopsy was not diagnostic of a specific lesion but did document the presence of eosinophils within alveolar septa.

Tocolytic Agents

Pulmonary edema has been documented with various tocolytic agents, including the beta-adrenergic agonists *ritodrine*, *terbutaline*, and *albuterol*, as well as *isoxsuprine* and *magnesium sulfate*.[6,371–380] The incidence of lung toxicity in patients receiving tocolytic drugs is variable but has been as high as 5% in some series. Twin

pregnancies, concurrent administration of glucocorticoids, and volume overload may be associated with an increased incidence of pulmonary complications.[371,376,378] Symptoms usually appear 1 to 4 days after initiating therapy and can occur either before or after delivery. Nearly all recover after discontinuation of therapy and institution of supportive measures.

Anticonvulsants

Phenytoin (Dilantin) is a rare cause of pulmonary toxicity.[6,385,386,389] Reported patients usually developed an acute febrile illness with an associated skin rash 1 week to 3 months after initiation of therapy. Peripheral eosinophilia was present in all patients, and elevated liver function tests were found in the majority. Transbronchial biopsy showed BOOP with occasional eosinophils in one case and a CIP resembling lymphoid interstitial pneumonia (see Chapter 9) in two others.[382,385,386] BAL in the latter two patients showed marked lymphocytosis.[382,386] Most patients recovered after withdrawal from phenytoin. A necrotizing vasculitis affecting small- and medium-sized pulmonary vessels was found in one individual who died of pulmonary complications.[389] The vasculitis was associated with prominent tissue eosinophilia and resembled the changes of allergic angiitis and granulomatosis (Churg–Strauss disease, see Chapter 8).

Carbamazepine (Tegretol)-induced pulmonary toxicity is also rare.[381,383,387,388] Pathologic findings include eosinophilic pneumonia, BOOP, and DAD.[381,387,388] Withdrawal from carbamazepine therapy and treatment with steroids usually results in complete recovery.

Psychotherapeutic Drugs

Pulmonary edema has been described rarely in patients receiving various antipsychotic drugs, although pathologic confirmation is lacking.[6,403] Most cases have been associated with the so-called neuroleptic malignant syndrome, an acute febrile reaction characterized by altered consciousness, muscular rigidity, and autonomic dysfunction.[403] Pulmonary edema occurs in fewer than half of these patients.[6,403] A combination of pulmonary edema and intraalveolar hemorrhage has also been described in a patient receiving *haloperidol* who died of rapidly progressive respiratory failure.[396] Pulmonary edema has also been related to sedative-hypnotic drugs such as *chlordiazepoxide* (Librium), *paraldehyde*, and *ethchlorvynol* (Placidyl) and usually occurs after overdosage or intravenous injection.[390,392,394,398–400,402]

Tricyclic antidepressants have only rarely caused pulmonary complications.[401,404] ARDS has been reported rarely in patients after *amitriptyline* overdose, and autopsies have shown acute and organizing DAD in these patients.[395,397] A clinical syndrome resembling eosinophilic pneumonia has been described with *desipramine, imipramine,* and *nomifensine* therapy, but tissue documentation has not been reported.[401,405] More recently, one example of so-called acute eosinophilic pneumonia with BAL eosinophilia has been described following an overdose with *trazodone,* a newer-generation heterocyclic antidepressant.[401]

Fluoxetine hydrochloride (Prozac) has been implicated as a cause of lung disease in only a single patient.[393] The affected patient developed respiratory symptoms 4 months after starting therapy. BAL demonstrated a marked lymphocytosis. Transbronchial lung biopsy showed changes resembling those seen in hypersensitivity pneumonia, including a nonspecific CIP with scattered granulomas and multinucleated giant cells. Foamy alveolar macrophages were also described but may have reflected distal airway obstruction due to bronchiolitis rather than a drug-related phospholipidosis. Ultrastructural studies were not illustrated but were reported to show intracytoplasmic membrane-bound lamellar inclusions similar to those described in amiodarone toxicity.[393]

Venlafaxine (Effexor) has been reported to cause pulmonary toxicity and heart failure simultaneously in two patients. One of these patients died, while the other recovered with steroid treatment. Open lung biopsy in the patient who survived showed chronic interstitial pneumonitis with non-necrotizing granulomas. Autopsy in the other patient revealed organizing pneumonia.[391]

Opioids

A syndrome of pulmonary edema following accidental or intentional intoxication has been well documented with several opioid agonists, including *morphine, methadone, propoxyphene, codeine,* and *heroin.*[6,406-410,412-416,419] Pulmonary edema has also been reported following sublingual administration of *buprenorphine* and parenteral administration of the opioid antagonists *nalbuphine* and *naloxone.*[411,413,417,418] The onset of pulmonary edema usually occurs within several hours of drug use but may be delayed for as long as 24 hours. The changes are usually reversible, and most patients survive with supportive care. Descriptions of pathologic changes are available for only a limited number of

cases and have confirmed the presence of pulmonary edema.[407,414,416] Evidence of superimposed aspiration pneumonia is seen in some patients.[414] Immunofluorescent staining of heroin-induced pulmonary edema has shown granular deposits of IgM, IgG, and C3 along alveolar septa, although no ultrastructural evidence of immune complex deposition was demonstrated.[416]

Bronchiectasis is a potential complication of heroin-induced pulmonary edema.[406,419] Affected patients usually present with chronic respiratory complaints dating to an episode of acute pulmonary edema. Aspiration of gastric contents may be a contributing factor in some patients.[410,419] The changes may stabilize or partially improve with discontinuation of heroin use.[406]

Cocaine

Cocaine is a stimulant drug derived from the leaves of *Erythroxylon coca.*[420,429] Cocaine has been used in various forms since the late sixteenth century and is now one of the most frequently abused illicit drugs in the United States.[420] Cocaine can be self-administered by a variety of routes utilizing parenteral and inhalational methods. Freebase ('crack') cocaine, derived from alkaline extraction of cocaine hydrochloride, has become the most commonly abused form and is usually self-administered by smoking. Pulmonary complications can occur with any route of drug administration. Pneumothorax, pneumomediastinum, pneumopericardium, and bullous emphysema are uncommon complications that likely result from maneuvers performed during drug administration rather than drug-induced morphologic abnormalities.[420,429,430,432,437] When smoked together with tobacco, cocaine appears to have an additive effect on bronchial injury and on increased lung iron content caused by tobacco.[431]

'Crack lung' refers to a syndrome of acute respiratory distress associated with diffuse lung infiltrates following heavy smoking of freebase cocaine.[421,425,427,429,433,435,437,438,440,442,443] Acute noncardiogenic pulmonary edema, pulmonary hemorrhage, and pulmonary infiltrates with eosinophilia have been reported and comprise the spectrum of crack lung syndrome. Symptoms develop within 1 to 48 hours of cocaine use and usually include cough and dyspnea.[420,427] Cough productive of black sputum is seen in as many as 40% of patients and is due to the presence of pigmented alveolar macrophages, a common finding in heavy smokers of crack cocaine.[428,436] Hemoptysis, fever, and chest pain also are common complaints.[420,427] Associated peripheral, BAL, and/or tissue eosinophilia occur in a minority of patients.[420,427,433,438,440,442] Severity of the illness is variable, ranging from progressive respiratory failure requiring mechanical ventilation to a more self-limited form that resolves within 12 to 24 hours of drug cessation. Corticosteroids may be beneficial in some patients, particularly those with associated eosinophilia.[440]

DAD is the most frequently described finding in lung biopsies from patients with acute crack lung syndrome (Fig. 4–8).[427] Associated findings include the presence of eosinophils and evidence of alveolar hemorrhage in the form of hemosiderin-laden macrophages. In cases with eosinophilia, the changes resemble those described in acute eosinophilic pneumonia. Interstitial and intracellular IgE deposition have been documented by immunofluorescence studies in some cases and are of uncertain significance.[427] Diffuse alveolar hemorrhage may be the only finding in some patients,[438] and acute capillaritis is identified rarely.[444] BOOP has been described in one patient.[443] Thermal injury of large

airways can result from ignition of inhaled vapors and may lead to scarring and airway stenosis.[447]

Chronic cocaine abuse is associated with various histologic abnormalities, including evidence of recurrent alveolar hemorrhage, pulmonary edema, nonspecific CIP, and medial hypertrophy of small muscular arteries.[422,439] It is unclear the extent to which these changes correlate with clinically significant respiratory disease, but they may explain the pulmonary function abnormalities seen in some patients.[445,446] Airway-centered interstitial fibrosis was described in a cigarette smoker with a history of cocaine use.[423] Progressive interstitial pneumonia has been described in one patient who died 10 months after developing respiratory symptoms following an episode of prolonged crack cocaine smoking.[441] Lung biopsy showed an unusual CIP with numerous histiocytes and abundant birefringent particles of crystalline silica. The patient had no history of occupational dust exposure, and the authors concluded that the silica may have been a

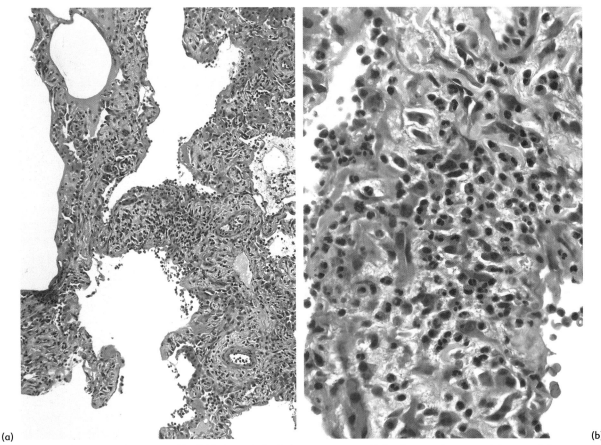

(a)   (b)

Figure 4–8 Crack lung characterized by DAD that is in both the acute stage with hyaline membranes and the organizing stage with interstitial fibroblast proliferation (a). Focally there is a cellular interstitial infiltrate containing numerous eosinophils (b).

contaminant of inhaled crack cocaine. Foreign body granulomas associated with cellulose-like particles have been described in one additional patient, who self-administered cocaine by nasal insufflation.[424] Interstitial and perivascular collections of pigmented macrophages containing refractile polarizable material were noted in another case, which mimicked sarcoidosis clinically, although the well-formed non-necrotizing granulomas characteristic of sarcoidosis were not present.[426] Pulmonary hypertension has been described after both inhalational and intravenous cocaine use.[434,448]

Tryptophan

Ingestion of tryptophan, an essential amino acid usually sold as a nonprescription food supplement, has been linked to the *eosinophilia–myalgia syndrome* (EMS).[450,452,456,458-460,465] EMS first appeared in the fall of 1989 and was quickly traced to a specific manufacturer of tryptophan powder. Prompt recall of tryptophan-containing products by the Food and Drug Administration led to an early end to the epidemic, which is now largely of historical interest only. Epidemiological studies indicated that minor modifications of the manufacturing process had apparently resulted in contaminated lots of tryptophan, although a specific causal agent has not been identified.[459] Risk factors for developing EMS included female sex, older age, and greater total dose of contaminated tryptophan products.[456]

EMS is characterized by peripheral eosinophilia and generalized myalgias, frequently associated with arthralgias and skin rash.[450,454,456,458] Respiratory complaints, most commonly cough and dyspnea, have been noted in the majority of patients and can occur without other manifestations of EMS.[449,451,453,457,461-464] Pulmonary hypertension occurs in some patients. Chest radiographs are abnormal in most patients with respiratory symptoms and typically show diffuse interstitial opacities and/or pleural effusions. Most patients recover with tryptophan discontinuation and corticosteroid therapy, although death from respiratory failure and persistent pulmonary hypertension has been described.[451,458,462]

Tryptophan-induced lung disease is characterized by a combination of CIP, vascular and perivascular inflammation, and eosinophilia (Fig. 4–9).[449,451,455,461-464] Hypertensive pulmonary arteriopathy comprising medial hypertrophy and intimal fibroelastosis is seen in some cases. Ultrastructural studies have confirmed the presence of vasculitis and interstitial pneumonia.[463]

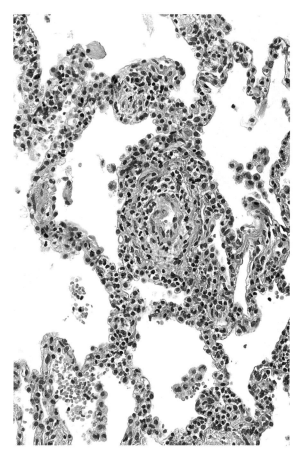

Figure 4–9 L-tryptophan toxicity characterized by a cellular CIP with prominent perivascular inflammation.

Immunophenotypic analysis has demonstrated a preponderance of cytotoxic-suppressor T lymphocytes within areas of interstitial and perivascular inflammation.[464] Neither immunofluorescence nor ultrastructural studies have shown any evidence of immune complex-mediated disease.[463]

Anorexigens

Fenfluramine is a sympathomimetic amine that produces an anorexic action through the activation of serotonin pathways in the brain. *Phentermine* is a noradrenergic agent that interferes with the pulmonary clearance of serotonin. The combination of these drugs (*fen-phen*) is associated with fewer side effects. The main pulmonary complication is pulmonary hypertension, which has been reported after treatment with fenfluramine or phentermine alone, or in combination. The d-isomer of fenfluramine, dexfenfluramine, also increases the risk of pulmonary hypertension, particularly when patients receive high doses for more than 3 months.[466] Symptoms, mainly dyspnea on exertion, have occurred from 27 days to 23 years following drug intake.[473] Prognosis is poor, with 1- and 3-year survivals of 50% and 17%, respectively, in one study.[472]

Most of the available pathologic data are from autopsy studies. The pulmonary hypertension associated with anorexigens is morphologically indistinguishable from primary (idiopathic) pulmonary hypertension (see Chapter 13). Plexiform lesions are present in most cases, in addition to medial and intimal hypertrophy. Rare cases resembling thrombotic arteriopathy have also been reported.[468,470,471,474,475]

Aminorex, an appetite-suppressing drug structurally related to amphetamine that is no longer available for therapeutic use, may have been responsible for an 'epidemic' of pulmonary hypertension that occurred in the late 1960s and early 1970s in Europe.[467,469,476] Biopsies and autopsies in affected patients showed the same range of changes seen in primary pulmonary hypertension, including medial hypertrophy and intimal fibrosis as well as plexiform and angiomatoid lesions, and rare examples of thrombotic pulmonary arteriopathy were also reported.[469]

Miscellaneous Noncytotoxic Drugs

Statins (3-hydroxy-3-methyl-glutaryl coenzyme A reductase inhibitors) are the most frequently prescribed lipid-lowering drugs. Their therapeutic indications have been recently extended to the treatment of osteoporosis. The most frequent side effects are cataracts, myopathy, rhabdomyolysis, and elevation of hepatic enzyme levels.[497] A few systemic adverse effects, such as pseudo-polymyositis, and lupus-like syndromes have been reported. Pulmonary side effects are rare, and have been reported with *pravastatin, lovastatin,* and *simvastatin.* Symptoms are often insidious in onset and include dyspnea, cough, myalgias, and sometimes fever. They are frequently delayed for years, with intervals ranging from 6 months to 6 years after starting the drug. Pathologic findings include CIP, hypersensitivity pneumonia, NSIP, BOOP, and DAD.[483,491,497,498,503] Ultrastructural analysis in the case of NSIP revealed unusual intralysosomal lamellar inclusions in type 2 pneumonocytes, interstitial histiocytes, and endothelial cells.[497]

Eosinophilic pleural effusion with positive ANA and antihistone antibodies has also been reported.[494]

Clinically significant pulmonary hemorrhage is a rare complication of anticoagulation with either *warfarin* or *heparin*, occurring in well under 1% of patients.[486,510]

DAD has been confirmed at autopsy in one patient, and BAL specimens have shown abnormally increased numbers of hemosiderin-filled macrophages.[486,510] Nearly all patients have recovered after complete or partial reversal of anticoagulation. Spontaneous pulmonary hemorrhage has also occurred after thrombolytic therapy with *streptokinase* and *urokinase*.[479,502] Intravenous and intrapleural instillation of thrombolytic agents can also result in DAD.[488,499] Two cases of steroid-responsive interstitial lung disease have been reported with *ticlopidine*, an inhibitor of platelet activation, although tissue confirmation is lacking.[501,505]

Nilutamide, a nonsteroidal antiandrogen not yet available for routine clinical usage in the United States, has been linked to a syndrome of CIP.[477,489,506,512] Pulmonary toxicity occurs in about 1% of patients, usually after total doses of at least 10 to 15 g. Latent periods have ranged from 10 days to 8 months, with a mean of about 4 months.[506] Dyspnea is the most common complaint, frequently accompanied by fever and cough. BAL typically demonstrates a lymphocytosis with a decreased CD4:CD8 ratio.[477,506] Neutrophilia and/or eosinophilia occur in a minority of patients.[506,512] Transbronchial (two cases) and open (one case) lung biopsies have been illustrated in three patients, and showed nonspecific CIP in all cases, with associated BOOP in one.[489,506] The prognosis of nilutamide-induced lung disease is excellent, and all patients have recovered after drug cessation alone, a reduction in drug dose, or a combination of drug cessation and corticosteroids.

Rare examples of presumed eosinophilic pneumonia have been reported following *chlorpropamide* therapy, although tissue confirmation is lacking.[484] Clinical evidence of eosinophilic pneumonia has also been reported in patients receiving *cromolyn sodium* and *mephenesin*.[508,509] A combination of granulomatous inflammation and bronchiolitis obliterans has been reported with the former drug as well.[480]

Pleuritis and pleural fibrosis have been reported with ergot derivatives, including *methysergide* and *pergolide*.[482,490,492] Symptoms usually begin 6 months to 3 years after initiation of therapy, although latent periods of as long as 6 years have been reported.[492] Most patients recover with discontinuation of therapy. *Bromocriptine* and its congener, *mesulergine*, are chemically related to methysergide and have also caused adverse pleuropulmonary reactions.[495,500] Pleural biopsies in some cases have shown fibrosis and nonspecific chronic inflammation.[500] The majority of patients have recovered after termination of therapy.

Pulmonary complications occur in 1–3% of patients after intravesical *Bacille Calmette-Guérin* (BCG) immunotherapy.[513] Lung biopsies show well-formed necrotizing or non-necrotizing granulomas.[493,504,513] Acid-fast bacilli have been identified only rarely, and most are thought to represent a noninfectious hypersensitivity reaction. Intrapulmonary granulomas have also been reported after intralesional BCG therapy for solid tumors and can mimic the radiographic appearance of pulmonary metastases.[478]

Other miscellaneous drug reactions include rare examples of pulmonary edema after *nifedipine* (a calcium channel blocker), intravenous administration of *radiocontrast material* (diatrizoate meglumine), and *epinephrine* overdose.[485,496,507] DAD has been described in one patient who developed an ANCA-associated vasculitic syndrome 2 weeks after starting *propylthiouracil* treatment for Graves' disease.[514] Intravenous administration of *deferoxamine mesylate*, a chelating agent useful in reducing iron overload, can cause a syndrome of acute respiratory failure associated with DAD.[487] *Methamphetamine*, an illicit drug, has been associated with pulmonary hypertension in one patient.[511]

REFERENCES

General
1. Allen J: Drug-induced eosinophilic lung disease. Clin Chest Med 25:77, 2004.
2. Camus P, Bonniaud P, Fanton A, et al: Drug-induced and iatrogenic infiltrative lung disease. Clin Chest Med 25:479, 2004.
3. Cleverley J, Screaton N, Hiorns M, et al: Drug-induced lung disease: High-resolution CT and histological findings. Clin Radiol 57:292, 2002.
4. Cooper J Jr: Drug-induced lung disease. Adv Intern Med 42:231,1997.
5. Cooper J Jr, White D, Matthay R: Drug-induced pulmonary disease. Part 1: Cytotoxic drugs. Am Rev Respir Dis 133:321, 1986.
6. Cooper J, White D, Matthay R: Drug-induced pulmonary disease. Part 2: Noncytotoxic drugs. Am Rev Respir Dis 133:488, 1986.
7. Costabel U, Uzaslan E, Guzman J: Bronchoalveolar lavage in drug-induced lung disease. Clin Chest Med 25:25, 2004.
8. Epler G: Drug-induced bronchiolitis obliterans organizing pneumonia. Clin Chest Med 25:89, 2004.
9. Flieder D, Travis W: Pathologic characteristics of drug-induced lung disease. Clin Chest Med 25:37, 2004.
10. Foucher P, Biour M, Blayac J: Drugs that may injure the respiratory system. Eur Respir J 10:265, 1997.
11. Lock B, Eggert M, Cooper J Jr. Infiltrative lung disease due to noncytotoxic agents. Clin Chest Med 25:47, 2004.
12. Rossi S, Erasmus J, McAdams H, et al: Pulmonary drug toxicity: Radiologic and pathologic manifestations. Radiographics 20:1245, 2000.
13. Smith G: The histopathology of pulmonary reactions to drugs. Clin Chest Med 11:95, 1990.
14. Vander N, Stover D: Chemotherapy-induced lung disease. Clin Pulm Med 11:84, 2004.

Alkylating Agents
15. Aymard J, Gyger M, Lavallee R, et al: A case of pulmonary alveolar proteinosis complicating chronic myelogenous leukemia. A peculiar pathologic aspect of busulfan lung? Cancer 53:954, 1984.
16. Baker W, Fistel S, Jones R, Weiss R: Interstitial pneumonitis associated with ifosfamide therapy. Cancer 65:2217, 1990.
17. Burke D, Stoddart J, Ward M, Simpson C: Fatal pulmonary fibrosis occurring during treatment with cyclophosphamide. Br Med J 285:696, 1982.
18. Burns W, McFarland W, Matthews M: Busulfan-induced pulmonary disease. Report of a case and review of the literature. Am Rev Respir Dis 101:408, 1970.
19. Codling B, Chakera T: Pulmonary fibrosis following therapy with melphalan for multiple myeloma. J Clin Pathol 25:668, 1972.
20. Cole S, Myers T, Klatsky A: Pulmonary disease with chlorambucil therapy. Cancer 41:455, 1978.
21. Feingold M, Koss L: Effects of long-term administration of busulfan. Arch Intern Med 124:66, 1969.
22. Godard P, Marty J, Michel P: Interstitial pneumonia and chlorambucil. Chest 76:471, 1979.
23. Goucher G, Rowland V, Hawkins J: Melphalan-induced pulmonary interstitial fibrosis. Chest 77:805, 1980.
24. Gyorkey F, Gyorkey P, Sinkovics J: Origin and significance of intranuclear tubular inclusions in type II pulmonary alveolar epithelial cells of patients with bleomycin and busulfan toxicity. Ultrastruct Pathol 1:211, 1980.
25. Hankins D, Sanders S, MacDonald F, Drage C: Pulmonary toxicity recurring after a six week course of busulfan therapy and after subsequent therapy with uracil mustard. Chest 73:415, 1978.
26. Heard B, Cooke R: Busulphan lung. Thorax 23:187, 1968.
27. Karim F, Ayash R, Allam C, Salem P: Pulmonary fibrosis after prolonged treatment with low-dose cyclophosphamide. Oncology 40:174, 1983.
28. Kirschner R, Esterly J: Pulmonary lesions associated with busulfan therapy of chronic myelogenous leukemia. Cancer 27:1074, 1971.
29. Koss L, Melamed M, Mayer K: The effect of busulfan on human epithelia. Am J Clin Pathol 44:385, 1965.
30. Kuplic J, Higley C, Niewoehner D: Pulmonary ossification associated with long-term busulfan therapy in chronic myeloid leukemia. Am Rev Respir Dis 106:759, 1972.

31. Littler W, Kay J, Hasleton P, Heath D: Busulphan lung. Thorax 24:639, 1969.

32. Malik SW, Myers JL, DeRemee RA: Lung toxicity associated with cyclophosphamide use. Two distinct patterns. Am J Respir Crit Care Med 154:1851, 1996.

33. Mark G, Lehimgar-Zadeh A, Ragsdale B: Cyclophosphamide pneumonitis. Thorax 33:89, 1978.

34. Min K, Gyorkey F: Interstitial pulmonary fibrosis, atypical epithelial changes and bronchiolar cell carcinoma following busulfan therapy. Cancer 22:1027, 1968.

35. Oliner H, Schwartz R, Rubio F, Dameshek W: Interstitial pulmonary fibrosis following busulfan therapy. Am J Med 31:134, 1961.

36. Patel A, Shah P, Rhee H, et al.: Cyclophosphamide therapy and interstitial pulmonary fibrosis. Cancer 38:1542, 1976.

37. Schallier D, Impens N, Warson F, et al: Additive pulmonary toxicity with melphalan and busulfan. Chest 84:492, 1983.

38. Slavin R, Millan J, Mullins G: Pathology of high dose intermittent cyclophosphamide therapy. Hum Pathol 6:693, 1975.

39. Spector J, Zimbler H, Ross J: Early-onset cyclophosphamide-induced interstitial pneumonitis. JAMA 242:2852, 1979.

40. Taetle R, Dickman P, Feldman P: Pulmonary histopathologic changes associated with melphalan therapy. Cancer 42:1239, 1978.

41. Todd N, Peters W, Ost A, et al: Pulmonary drug toxicity in patients with primary breast cancer treated with high-dose combination chemotherapy and autologous bone marrow transplantation. Am Rev Respir Dis 147:1264, 1993.

42. Topilow A, Rothenberg S, Cottrell T: Interstitial pneumonia after prolonged treatment with cyclophosphamide. Am Rev Respir Dis 108:114, 1973.

43. Westerfield B, Michalski J, McCombs C, Light R: Reversible melphalan-induced lung damage. Am J Med 68:767, 1980.

Nitrosoureas

44. Ahlgren J, Smith F, Kerwin D, et al: Pulmonary disease as a complication of chlorozotocin chemotherapy. Cancer Treat Rep 65:223, 1981.

45. Aronin P, Mahaley M, Rudnick S, et al: Prediction of BCNU pulmonary toxicity in patients with malignant gliomas. An assessment of risk factors. N Engl J Med, 303:183, 1980.

46. Block M, Lachowiez R, Rios C, Hirschl S: Pulmonary fibrosis associated with low-dose adjuvant methyl-CCNU. Med Pediatr Oncol 18:256, 1990.

47. Cordonnier C, Vernant J, Mital P, et al: Pulmonary fibrosis subsequent to high doses of CCNU for chronic myeloid leukemia. Cancer 51:1814, 1983.

48. Dent R: Fatal pulmonary toxic effects of lomustine. Thorax 37:627, 1982.

49. Durant J, Norgard M, Murad T, et al: Pulmonary toxicity associated with bischloroethylnitrosourea (BCNU). Ann Intern Med 90:191, 1979.

50. Hasleton P, O'Driscoll B, Lynch P, et al: Late BCNU lung: A light and ultrastructural study on the delayed effect of BCNU on the lung parenchyma. J Pathol 164:31, 1991.

51. Holoye P, Jenkins D, Greenberg S: Pulmonary toxicity in long-term administration of BCNU. Cancer Treat Rep 60:1691, 1976.

52. Kalaycioglu M, Kavuru M, Tuason L, Bolwell B: Empiric prednisone therapy for pulmonary toxic reaction after high-dose chemotherapy containing carmustine (BCNU). Chest 107:482, 1995.

53. Lee W, Moore R, Wampler G: Interstitial pulmonary fibrosis as a complication of prolonged methyl-CCNU therapy. Cancer Treat Rep 62:1355, 1978.

54. Lena H, Desrues B, Le Coz A, et al: Severe diffuse interstitial pneumonitis induced by carmustine (BCNU). Chest 105:1602, 1994.

55. Litam J, Dail D, Spitzer G, et al: Early pulmonary toxicity after administration of high-dose BCNU. Cancer Treat Rep 65:39, 1981.

56. Lombard C, Churg A, Winokur S: Pulmonary veno-occlusive disease following therapy for malignant neoplasms. Chest 92:871, 1987.

57. Melato M, Tuveri G: Pulmonary fibrosis following low-dose 1,3-bis(2-chloroethyl)-1-nitrosourea (BCNU) therapy. Cancer 45:1311, 1980.

58. Mitsudo S, Greenwald E, Banerji B, Koss L: BCNU (2,3-bis-(2-chloroethyl)-1-nitrosourea) lung. Drug-induced pulmonary changes. Cancer 54:751, 1984.

59. O'Driscoll B, Hasleton P, Taylor P, et al: Active lung fibrosis up to 17 years after chemotherapy with carmustine (BCNU) in childhood. N Engl J Med 323:378, 1990.

60. O'Driscoll B, Kalra S, Gattamaneni H, Woodcock A: Late carmustine lung fibrosis. Age at treatment may influence severity and survival. Chest 107:1355, 1995.

61. Patten G, Billi J, Rotman H: Rapidly progressive, fatal pulmonary fibrosis induced by carmustine. JAMA 244:687, 1980.

62. Patterson D, Wiemann M, Lee T, Byron W Jr: Carmustine toxicity presenting as a lobar infiltrate. Chest 104:315, 1993.

63. Ryan B, Walters T: Pulmonary fibrosis: A complication of 1,3-bis(2-chloroethyl)-1-nitrosourea (BCNU) therapy. Cancer 48:909, 1981.

64. Selker R, Jacobs S, Moore P, et al: 1,3-bis(2-chloroethyl)-1-nitrosourea (BCNU)-induced pulmonary fibrosis. Neurosurgery 7:560, 1980.

65. Stone M, Richardson M: Pulmonary toxicity of lomustine. Cancer Treat Rep 71:786, 1987.

66. Taylor P, O'Driscoll B, Gattamaneni H, Woodcock A: Chronic lung fibrosis following carmustine (BCNU) chemotherapy: Radiological features. Clin Radiol 44:299, 1991.

67. Vats T, Trueworthy R, Langston C: Pulmonary fibrosis associated with lomustine (CCNU): A case report. Cancer Treat Rep 66:1881, 1982.

68. Weinstein A, Diener-West M, Nelson D, Pakuris E: Pulmonary toxicity of carmustine in patients treated for malignant glioma. Cancer Treat Rep 70:943, 1986.

69. Weiss R, Poster D, Penta J: The nitrosoureas and pulmonary toxicity. Cancer Treat Rev 8:111, 1981.

70. Wolff S, Phillips G, Herzig G: High-dose carmustine with autologous bone marrow transplantation for the adjuvant treatment of high-grade gliomas of the central nervous system. Cancer Treat Rep 71:183, 1987.

Cytotoxic Antibiotics

71. Avitzur Y, Jimenez-Rivera C, Fecteau A, et al : Interstitial granulomatous pneumonitis associated with sirolimus in a child after liver transplantation. J Pediatr Gastroenterol Nutr 37:91, 2003.

72. Bauer K, Skarin A, Balikian J, et al: Pulmonary complications associated with combination chemotherapy programs containing bleomycin. Am J Med 74:557, 1983.

73. Bedrossian C, Luna M, MacKay B, Lichtiger B: Ultrastructure of pulmonary bleomycin toxicity. Cancer 32:44, 1973.

74. Blayney D, Goldberg D, Leong L, et al: High-risk germ cell tumors in men. High response rate and severe toxicity with cisplatin, vinblastine, bleomycin, and etoposide. Cancer 71:2351, 1993.

75. Buzdar A, Legha S, Luna M, et al: Pulmonary toxicity of mitomycin. Cancer 45:236, 1980.

76. Calvo D, Legha S, McKelvey E, et al: Zinostatin-related pulmonary toxicity. Cancer Treat Rep 65:165, 1981.

77. Chang A, Kuebler J, Pandya K, et al: Pulmonary toxicity induced by mitomycin C is highly responsive to glucocorticoids. Cancer 57:2285, 1986.

78. Chang-Poon V, Hwang W, Wong A, et al: Pulmonary angiomatoid vascular changes in mitomycin C-associated hemolytic-uremic syndrome. Arch Pathol Lab Med 109:877, 1985.

79. Chhajed PN, Dickenmann M, Bubendorf L, et al: Patterns of pulmonary complications associated with sirolimus. Respiration, In press, 2005.

80. Cohen M, Austin J, Smith-Vaniz A, et al: Nodular bleomycin toxicity. Am J Clin Pathol 92:101, 1989.

81. Comis R: Bleomycin pulmonary toxicity: Current status and future directions. Semin Oncol 19:S64, 1992.

82. Daskal Y, Gyorkey F, Gyorkey P, Busch H: Ultrastructural study of pulmonary bleomycin toxicity. Cancer Res 36:1267, 1976.

83. Garewal H, Brooks R, Jones S, Miller T: Treatment of advanced breast cancer with mitomycin C combined with vinblastine or vindesine. J Clin Oncol 1:772, 1983.

84. Glenn L, Armitage J, Goldsmith J, et al: Pulmonary emboli in patients receiving chemotherapy for non-Hodgkin's lymphoma. Chest 94:589, 1988.

85. Gunstream S, Seidenfeld J, Sobonya R, McMahon L: Mitomycin-associated lung disease. Cancer Treat Rep 67:301, 1983.

86. Henry MT, Newstead CG. Sirolimus: Another cause of drug-induced interstitial pneumonitis. Transplantation 72:773, 2001.

87. Holoye P, Luna M, MacKay B, Bedrossian C: Bleomycin hypersensitivity pneumonitis. Ann Intern Med 88:47, 1978.

88. Iacovino J, Leitner J, Abbas A, et al: Fatal pulmonary reaction from low doses of bleomycin. An idiosyncratic tissue response. JAMA 235:1253, 1976.

89. Jolivet J, Giroux L, Laurin S, et al: Microangiopathic hemolytic anemia, renal failure, and noncardiogenic pulmonary edema: A chemotherapy-induced syndrome. Cancer Treat Rep 67:429, 1983.

90. Joselson R, Warnock M: Pulmonary veno-occlusive disease after chemotherapy. Hum Pathol 13:88, 1983.

91. Jules-Elysee K, White D: Bleomycin-induced pulmonary toxicity. Clin Chest Med 11:1, 1990.

92. Knight B, Rose A: Pulmonary veno-occlusive disease after chemotherapy. Thorax 40:847, 1985.

93. Lei K, Leung W, Johnson P: Serious pulmonary complications in patients receiving recombinant granulocyte-stimulating factor during BACOP chemotherapy for aggressive non-Hodgkin's lymphoma. Br J Cancer 70:1009, 1994.

94. Lennon A, Finan K, Fitzgerald M X, et al: Interstitial pneumonitis associated with sirolimus (Rapamycin) therapy after liver transplantation. Transplantation 72:1166, 2001.

95. Lindenfeld JA, Simon SF, Zamora MR, et al: BOOP is common in cardiac transplant recipients switched from a calcineurin inhibitor to sirolimus. Am J Transplant 5:1392, 2005.

96. Luna M, Bedrossian C, Lichtiger B, Salem P: Interstitial pneumonitis associated with bleomycin therapy. Am J Clin Pathol 58:501, 1972.

97. Mahalati K, Murphy D, West M. Bronchiolitis obliterans and organizing pneumonia in renal transplant recipients. Transplantation 69:1531, 2000.

98. Manito N, Kaplinsky E, Bernat R, et al. Fatal interstitial pneumonitis associated with sirolimus therapy in a heart transplant recipient. J Heart Lung Transplant 23:780, 2004.

99. McCarthy J, Staats B: Pulmonary hypertension, hemolytic anemia, and renal failure. A mitomycin-associated syndrome. Chest 89:608, 1986.

100. McWilliams T, Levvey B, Russell P, et al: Interstitial pneumonitis associated with sirolimus: A dilemma for lung transplantation. J Heart Lung Transplant 22:210, 2003.

101. Morelon E, Stern M, Israel-Biet D, et al: Characteristics of sirolimus-associated interstitial pneumonitis in renal-transplant patients. Transplantation 72:787, 2001.

102. Nachman J, Baum E, White H, Cruissi F: Bleomycin-induced pulmonary fibrosis mimicking recurrent metastatic disease in a patient with testicular carcinoma: Case report of the CT scan appearance. Cancer 47:236, 1981.

103. Niell H, Griffin J, West W, Neely C: Combination chemotherapy with mitomycin C, methotrexate, cisplatin, and vinblastine in the treatment of non-small cell lung cancer. Cancer 54:1260, 1984.

104. Orwoll E, Kiessling P, Patterson J: Interstitial pneumonia from mitomycin. Ann Intern Med 89:352, 1978.

105. Ozols R, Hogan W, Ostchega Y, Young R: MVP (mitomycin, vinblastine, and progesterone): A second-line regimen in ovarian cancer with a high incidence of pulmonary toxicity. Cancer Treat Rep 67:721, 1983.

106. Perez-Guerra F, Harkleroad L, Walsh R, Costanzi J: Acute bleomycin lung. Am Rev Respir Dis 106:909, 1972.

107. Pham PT, Pham PC, Danovitch G, et al: Sirolimus-associated pulmonary toxicity. Transplantation 27:1215, 2004.

108. Santrach P, Askin F, Wills R, et al: Nodular form of bleomycin-related pulmonary injury in patients with osteogenic sarcoma. Cancer 64:806, 1989.

109. Seltzer S, Griffin T, D'Orsi C, et al: Pulmonary reaction associated with neocarzinostatin therapy. Cancer Treat Rep 62:1271, 1978.

110. Sleijfer S: Bleomycin-induced pneumonitis. Chest 120:617, 2001.

111. Trump D, Bartel E, Pozniak M: Nodular pneumonitis after chemotherapy for germ cell tumors. Ann Intern Med 109:431, 1988.

112. Van Barneveld P, Sleijfer D, Van der Mark T, et al: Natural course of bleomycin-induced pneumonitis. A follow-up study. Am Rev Respir Dis 135:48, 1987.

113. Verweij J, Van Zanten T, Souren T, et al: Prospective study on the dose relationship of mitomycin C-induced interstitial pneumonitis. Cancer 60:756, 1987.

114. Waldhorn R, Tsou E, Smith F, Kerwin D: Pulmonary veno-occlusive disease associated with microangiopathic hemolytic anemia and chemotherapy of gastric adenocarcinoma. Med. Pediatr Oncol 12:394, 1984.

115. White D, Stover D: Severe bleomycin-induced pneumonitis. Clinical features and response to corticosteroids. Chest 86:723, 1984.

116. Yousem S, Lifson J, Colby T: Chemotherapy-induced eosinophilic pneumonia. Relation to bleomycin. Chest 88:103, 1985.

Antimetabolites

117. Akoun G, Gauthier-Rahman S, Mayaud C, et al: Leukocyte migration inhibition in methotrexate-induced pneumonitis. Evidence for an immunologic cell-mediated mechanism. Chest 91:96, 1987.

118. Anaissie EJ, Kontoyiannis D, O'Brien S, et al: Infections in patients with chronic lymphocytic leukemia treated with fludarabine. Ann Intern Med 129:559, 1998.

119. Andersson B, Luna M, Yee C, et al: Fatal pulmonary failure complicating high-dose cytosine arabinoside therapy in acute leukemia. Cancer 65:1079, 1990.

120. Attar E, Ervin T, Janicek M, et al: Acute interstitial pneumonitis related to gemcitabine. J Clin Oncol 18:697, 2000.

121. Barlesi F, Villani P, Doddoli C, et al: Gemcitabine-induced severe pulmonary toxicity. Fundam Clin Pharmacol 18:85, 2004.

122. Bedrossian C, Miller W, Luna M: Methotrexate-induced diffuse interstitial pulmonary fibrosis. South Med J 72:313, 1979.

123. Bedrossian C, Sussman J, Conklin R, Kahan B: Azathioprine-associated interstitial pneumonitis. Am J Clin Pathol 82:148, 1984.

124. Bernstein M, Sobel D, Wimmer R: Noncardiogenic pulmonary edema following injection of methotrexate into the cerebrospinal fluid. Cancer 50:866, 1982.

125. Boiselle P, Marvin M, Huberman M: Gemcitabine pulmonary toxicity: CT features. J Comput Assist Tomogr 24:977, 2000.

126. Cannon GW: Methotrexate pulmonary toxicity. Rheum Dis Clin North Am 23:917, 1997.

127. Cannon G, Ward J, Clegg D, et al: Acute lung disease associated with low-dose pulse methotrexate therapy in patients with rheumatoid arthritis. Arthritis Rheum 26:1269, 1983.

128. Carmichael D, Hamilton D, Evans D, et al: Interstitial pneumonitis secondary to azathioprine in a renal transplant patient. Thorax 38:951, 1983.

129. Carson C, Cannon G, Egger M, et al: Pulmonary disease during the treatment of rheumatoid arthritis with low dose pulse methotrexate. Semin Arthritis Rheum 16:186, 1987.

130. Clarysse A, Cathey W, Cartwright G, Wintrobe M: Pulmonary disease complicating intermittent therapy with methotrexate. JAMA 209:1861, 1969.

131. Dai MS, Ho CL, Chen YC, et al: Acute respiratory distress syndrome following intrathecal methotrexate administration: A case report and review of literature. Ann Hematol 79:696, 2000.

132. Elsasser S, Dalquen P, Soler M, Perruchoud A: Methotrexate-induced pneumonitis: Appearance four weeks after discontinuation of treatment. Am Rev Respir Dis 140:1089, 1989.

133. Engelbrecht, J, Calhoon S, Scherrer J: Methotrexate pneumonitis after low-dose therapy for rheumatoid arthritis. Arthritis Rheum 26:1275, 1983.

134. Everts C, Westcott J, Bragg D: Methotrexate therapy and pulmonary disease. Radiology 107:539, 1973.

135. Garg S, Garg M, Basmaji N. Multiple pulmonary nodules: An unusual presentation of fludarabine pulmonary toxicity: Case report and review of literature. Am J Hematol 70:241, 2002.

136. Goldman G, Moschella S: Severe pneumonitis occurring during methotrexate therapy. Arch Dermatol 103:194, 1971.

137. Goodman T, Polisson R: Methotrexate: Adverse reactions and major toxicities. Rheum Dis Clin North Am 20:513, 1994.

138. Green L, Schattner A, Berkenstadt H: Severe reversible interstitial pneumonitis induced by low dose methotrexate: Report of a case and review of the literature. J Rheumatol 15:110, 1988.

139. Gupta N, Ahmed I, Steinberg H, et al: Gemcitabine-induced pulmonary toxicity. Case report and review of the literature. Am J Clin Oncol 25:96, 2002.

140. Hargreaves M, Mowat A, Benson M: Acute pneumonitis

associated with low dose methotrexate treatment for rheumatoid arthritis: Report of five cases and review of published reports. Thorax 47:628, 1992.

141. Haupt H, Hutchins G, Moore G: Ara-C lung: Noncardiogenic pulmonary edema complicating cytosine arabinoside therapy of leukemia. Am J Med 70:256, 1981.

142. Helman DL, Byrd JC, Ales NC, et al: Fludarabine-related pulmonary toxicity: A distinct clinical entity in chronic lymphoproliferative syndromes. Chest 122:785, 2002.

143. Hochster H, Oken M, Winter J, et al: Phase I study of fludarabine plus cyclophosphamide in patients with previously untreated low-grade lymphoma: Results and long-term follow-up – a report from the Eastern Cooperative Oncology Group. J Clin Oncol 18:987, 2000.

144. Hosoe S, Komuta K, Shibata K, et al: Gemcitabine and vinorelbine followed by docetaxel in patients with advanced non small cell lung cancer: A multi-institutional phase II trial of non-platinum sequential triplet combination chemotherapy. Br J Cancer 88:342, 2003.

145. Hurst PG, Habib MP, Garewal H, et al: Pulmonary toxicity associated with fludarabine monophosphate. Invest New Drugs 5:207, 1987.

146. Imokawa S, Colby TV, Leslie KO, et al: Methotrexate pneumonitis: Review of the literature and histopathological findings in nine patients. Eur Respir J 15:373, 2000.

147. Kalambokis G, Stefanou D, Arkoumani E, et al: Fulminant bronchiolitis obliterans organizing pneumonia following 2 d of treatment with hydroxyurea, interferon-alpha and oral cytarabine ocfosfate for chronic myelogenous leukemia. Eur J Haematol 73:67, 2004.

148. Kavuru MS, Gadsden T, Lichtin A, et al. Hydroxyurea-induced acute interstitial lung disease. South Med J 87:767, 1994.

149. Kouroussis C, Mavroudis D, Kakolyris S, et al: High incidence of pulmonary toxicity of weekly docetaxel and gemcitabine in patients with non-small cell lung cancer: Results of a dose-finding study. Lung Cancer 44:363, 2004.

150. Krowka M, Breuer R, Kehoe T: Azathioprine-associated pulmonary dysfunction. Chest 83:696, 1983.

151. Larfars G, Uden-Blohme AM, Samuelsson J: Fludarabine, as well as 2-chlorodeoxyadenosine, can induce eosinophilia during treatment of lymphoid malignancies. Br J Haematol 94:709, 1996.

152. Lascari A, Strano A, Johnson W, Collins J: Methotrexate-induced sudden fatal pulmonary reaction. Cancer 40:1393, 1977.

153. Leduc D, De Vuyst P, Lheureux P, et al: Pneumonitis complicating low-dose methotrexate therapy for rheumatoid arthritis. Discrepancies between lung biopsy and bronchoalveolar lavage findings. Chest 104:1620, 1993.

154. Maniwa K, Tanaka E, Inoue T, et al: An autopsy case of

acute pulmonary toxicity associated with gemcitabine. Intern Med 42:1022, 2003.

155. Marruchella A, Fiorenzano G, Merizzi A, et al: Diffuse alveolar damage in a patient treated with gemcitabine. Eur Respir J 11:504, 1998.

156. Nesbit M, Krivit W, Heyn R, Sharp H: Acute and chronic effects of methotrexate on hepatic, pulmonary, and skeletal systems. Cancer 37:1048, 1976.

157. Pavlakis N, Bell DR, Millward MJ, et al: Fatal pulmonary toxicity resulting from treatment with gemcitabine. Cancer 80:286, 1997.

158. Sandhu HS, Barnes PJ, Hernandez P: Hydroxyurea-induced hypersensitivity pneumonitis: A case report and literature review. Can Respir J 7:491, 2000.

159. Searles G, McKendry R: Methotrexate pneumonitis in rheumatoid arthritis: Potential risk factors. Four case reports and a review of the literature. J Rheumatol 14:1164, 1987.

160. Shapiro C, Yeap B, Godleski J, et al: Drug-related pulmonary toxicity in non-Hodgkin's lymphoma. Comparative results with three different treatment regimens. Cancer 68:699, 1991.

161. Sostman H, Matthay R, Putman C, Smith G: Methotrexate-induced pneumonitis. Medicine (Baltimore) 55:371, 1976.

162. St Clair E, Rice J, Snyderman R: Pneumonitis complicating low-dose methotrexate therapy in rheumatoid arthritis. Arch Intern Med 145:2035, 1985.

163. Stoica GS, Greenberg HE, Rossoff LJ: Corticosteroid responsive fludarabine pulmonary toxicity. Am J Clin Oncol 25:340, 2002.

164. Tempero M, Brand R: Fatal pulmonary toxicity resulting from treatment with gemcitabine. Cancer 82:1800, 1998.

165. Tham R, Peters W, de Bruine F, Willemze R: Pulmonary complications of cytosine-arabinoside therapy: Radiographic findings. AJR Am J Roentgenol 149:23, 1987.

166. Trojan A, Meier R, Licht A: Eosinophilic pneumonia after administration of fludarabine for the treatment of non-Hodgkin's lymphoma. Ann Hematol 81:535, 2002.

167. Vander Els N, Miller V: Successful treatment of gemcitabine toxicity with a brief course of oral corticosteroid therapy. Chest 114:1779, 1998.

168. Vansteenkiste JF, Bomans P, Verbeken EK, et al: Fatal pulmonary veno-occlusive disease possibly related to gemcitabine. Lung Cancer 31:83, 2001.

169. Weisenburger D: Interstitial pneumonitis associated with azathioprine therapy. Am J Clin Pathol 69:181, 1978.

170. White D, Orenstein M, Godwin T, Stover D: Chemotherapy-associated pulmonary toxic reactions during treatment for breast cancer. Arch Intern Med 144:953, 1984.

171. White D, Rankin J, Stover D, et al: Methotrexate pneumonitis. Bronchoalveolar lavage findings suggest an immunologic disorder. Am Rev Respir Dis 139:18, 1989.

172. Wong CC, Brown D, Howling SJ, et al. Hydroxyurea-induced pneumonitis in a patient with chronic idiopathic myelofibrosis after prolonged drug exposure. Eur J Haematol 71:388, 2003.

Miscellaneous Cytotoxic Drugs

173. Behrens RJ, Gulley JL, Dahut WL: Pulmonary toxicity during prostate cancer treatment with docetaxel and thalidomide. Am J Ther 10:228, 2003.
174. Commers J, Foley J: Pulmonary hyaline membrane disease occurring in the course of VM-26 therapy. Cancer Treat Rep 63:2093, 1979.
175. Dohner V, Ward H, Standord R: Alveolitis during procarbazine, vincristine, and cyclophosphamide therapy. Chest 62:636, 1972.
176. Dunsford ML, Mead GM, Bateman AC, et al: Severe pulmonary toxicity in patients treated with a combination of docetaxel and gemcitabine for metastatic transitional cell carcinoma. Ann Oncol 10:943, 1999.
177. Esteban E, Gonzalez de Sande L, Fernandez Y, et al : Prospective randomized phase II study of docetaxel versus paclitaxel administered weekly in patients with non-small-cell lung cancer previously treated with platinum-based chemotherapy. Ann Oncol. 14:1640, 2003.
178. Farney R, Morris A, Armstrong J, Hammer S: Diffuse pulmonary disease after therapy with nitrogen mustard, vincristine, procarbazine, and prednisone. Am Rev Respir Dis 115:135, 1977.
179. Fujimori K, Yokoyama A, Kurita Y, et al: Paclitaxel-induced cell-mediated hypersensitivity pneumonitis: Diagnosis using leukocyte migration test, bronchoalveolar lavage and transbronchial lung biopsy. Oncology 55:340, 1998.
180. Goldsby R, Pulsipher M, Adams R, et al: Unexpected pleural effusions in 3 pediatric patients treated with STI-571. J Pediatr Hematol Oncol 24:694, 2002.
181. Grimson P, Goldstein D, Schneeweiss J, et al: Corticosteroid-responsive interstitial pneumonitis related to imatinib mesylate with successful rechallenge, and potential causative mechanisms. Intern Med J 35:136, 2005.
182. Horton L, Chappell A, Powell D: Diffuse interstitial pulmonary fibrosis complicating Hodgkin's disease. Br J Dis Chest 71:44, 1977.
183. Jones S, Moore M, Blank N, Castellino R: Hypersensitivity to procarbazine (Matulane) manifested by fever and pleuropulmonary reaction. Cancer 29:498, 1972.
184. Karacan O, Eyuboglu FO, Akcay S, et al. Acute interstitial pneumopathy associated with docetaxel hypersensitivity. Onkologie 27:563, 2004.
185. Konits P, Aisner J, Sutherland J, Wiernik P: Possible pulmonary toxicity secondary to vinblastine. Cancer 50:2771, 1982.
186. Kris M, Pablo D, Gralla R, et al: Dyspnea following vinblastine or vindesine administration in patients receiving mitomycin plus vinca alkaloid combination therapy. Cancer Treat Rep 68:1029, 1984.
187. Lewis L: Procarbazine associated alveolitis. Thorax 39:206, 1984.
188. Luedke D, McLaughlin T, Daughaday C, et al: Mitomycin C and vindesine associated pulmonary toxicity with variable clinical expression. Cancer 55:542, 1985.
189. Mauer AM, Masters GA, Haraf DJ, et al: Phase I study of docetaxel with concomitant thoracic radiation therapy. J Clin Oncol 16:159, 1998.
190. Merad M, Le Cesne A, Baldeyrou P, et al: Docetaxel and interstitial pulmonary injury. Ann Oncol 8:191, 1997.
191. Morris MV, Santamauro J, Shia J, et al: Fatal respiratory failure associated with treatment of prostate cancer using docetaxel and estramustine. Urology 60:1111, 2002.
192. Ramanathan RK, Reddy VV, Holbert JM, et al: Pulmonary infiltrates following administration of paclitaxel. Chest 110:289, 1996.
193. Read WL, Mortimer JE, Picus J: Severe interstitial pneumonitis associated with docetaxel administration. Cancer 94:847, 2002.
194. Rosado M, Donna E, Ahn Y: Imatinib mesylate-induced interstitial pneumonitis. J Clin Oncol 21:3171, 2003.
195. Wagner U, Staats P, Moll R, et al: Imatinib-associated pulmonary alveolar proteinosis. Am J Med 115:674, 2003.
196. Wang GS, Yang KY, Perng RP: Life-threatening hypersensitivity pneumonitis induced by docetaxel (taxotere). Br J Cancer 85:1247, 2001.
197. Wong P, Leung AN, Berry GJ, et al: Paclitaxel-induced hypersensitivity pneumonitis. Radiographic and CT findings. AJR Am J Roentgenol 176:718, 2001.
197a. Yamasawa H, Sugiyama Y, Bando M, Ohno S. Drug-induced pneumonitis associated with imatinib mesylate in a patient with idiopathic pulmonary fibrosis. Respir, in press, 2006.
198. Yokoyama T, Miyazawa K, Kurakawa E, et al: Interstitial pneumonia induced by imatinib mesylate: pathologic study demonstrates alveolar destruction and fibrosis with eosinophilic infiltration. Leukemia 18:645, 2004.

Antimicrobials

199. Auerbuch M, Halpern Z, Hallak A, et al: Sulfasalazine pneumonitis. Am J Gastroenterol 80:343, 1985.
200. Auerbuch S, Yungbluth P: Fatal pulmonary hemorrhage due to nitrofurantoin. Arch Intern Med 140:271, 1980.
201. Bone R, Wolfe J, Sobonya R, et al: Desquamative interstitial pneumonia following long-term nitrofurantoin therapy. Am J Med 60:697, 1976.
202. Brutinel W, Martin W: Chronic nitrofurantoin reaction associated with T-lymphocyte alveolitis. Chest 89:150, 1986.
203. Bucknall C, Adamson M, Banham S: Non fatal pulmonary haemorrhage associated with nitrofurantoin. Thorax 42:474, 1987.
204. Cameron R, Kolbe J, Wilsher M, et al: Bronchiolitis obliterans organising pneumonia associated with the use of nitrofurantoin. Thorax 55:249, 2000.

205. Camus P, Piard F, Ashcroft T, et al: The lung in inflammatory bowel disease. Medicine (Baltimore) 72:151, 1993.

206. Carrington C, Addington W, Goff A, et al: Chronic eosinophilic pneumonia. N Engl J Med 280:787, 1969.

207. Dan M, Aderka D, Topilsky M, et al: Hypersensitivity pneumonitis induced by nalidixic acid. Arch Intern Med 146:1423, 1986.

208. Dana B, Durie B, White R, Huestis D: Concomitant administration of granulocyte transfusions and amphotericin B in neutropenic patients: Absence of significant pulmonary toxicity. Blood 57:90, 1981.

209. Davidson A, Bateman C, Shovlin C, et al: Pulmonary toxicity of malaria prophylaxis. Br Med J 297:1240, 1988.

210. Davies D, MacFarlane A: Fibrosing alveolitis and treatment with sulphasalazine. Gut 15:185, 1974.

211. Donlan C, Scutero J: Transient eosinophilic pneumonia secondary to use of a vaginal cream. Chest 67:232, 1975.

212. Fiegenberg D, Weiss H, Kirshman H: Migratory pneumonia with eosinophilia associated with sulfonamide administration. Arch Intern Med 120:85, 1967.

213. French A: Hypersensitivity in the pathogenesis of the histopathologic changes associated with sulfonamide chemotherapy. Am J Pathol 22:679, 1946.

214. Gabazza E, Taguchi O, Yamakami T, et al: Pulmonary infiltrates and skin pigmentation associated with sulfasalazine. Am J Gastroenterol 87:1654, 1992.

215. Geller M, Dickie H, Kass D, et al: The histopathology of acute nitrofurantoin-associated pneumonitis. Ann Allergy 37:275, 1976.

216. Gessler C: Deaths from sulfonamides. A clinical and pathological study, with report of three cases. South Med J 37:365, 1944.

217. Hamadeh M, Atkinson J, Smith L: Sulfasalazine-induced pulmonary disease. Chest 101:1033, 1992.

218. Ho D, Tashkin D, Bein M, Sharma O: Pulmonary infiltrates with eosinophilia associated with tetracycline. Chest 76:33, 1979.

219. Holmberg L, Boman G: Pulmonary reactions to nitrofurantoin. 447 cases reported to the Swedish Adverse Drug Reaction Committee 1966–1976. Eur J Respir Dis 62:180, 1981.

220. Israel H, Diamond P: Recurrent pulmonary infiltration and pleural effusion due to nitrofurantoin sensitivity. N Engl J Med 166:1024, 1962.

221. Israel K, Brashear R, Sharma H, et al: Pulmonary fibrosis and nitrofurantoin. Am Rev Respir Dis 108:353, 1973.

222. James L, Austen K: Fatal systemic anaphylaxis in man. N Engl J Med 270:597, 1964.

223. Jick S, Jick H, Walker A, Hunter J: Hospitalizations for pulmonary reactions following nitrofurantoin use. Chest 96:512, 1989.

224. Jones G, Malone D: Sulphasalazine induced lung disease. Thorax 27:713, 1972.

225. Kolbe J, Caughey D, Rainer S: Sulphasalazine-induced sub-acute hyper-sensitivity pneumonitis. Respir Med 88:149, 1994.

226. Kursh E, Mostyn E, Persky L: Nitrofurantoin pulmonary complications. J Urol 113:392, 1975.

227. Leino R, Liippo K, Ekfors T: Sulfasalazine-induced reversible hypersensitivity pneumonitis and fatal fibrosing alveolitis: Report of two cases. J Intern Med 229:553, 1991.

228. Magee F, Wright J, Chan N, et al: Two unusual pathological reactions to nitrofurantoin: Case reports. Histopathology 10:701, 1986.

229. Meyer M, Meyer R: Nitrofurantoin-induced pulmonary hemorrhage in a renal transplant recipient receiving immunosuppressive therapy: Case report and review of the literature. J Urol 152:938, 1994.

230. Moseley R, Barwick K, Dobuler K, DeLuca V Jr: Sulfasalazine-induced pulmonary disease. Dig Dis Sci 30:901, 1985.

231. Murray M, Kronenberg R: Pulmonary reactions simulating cardiac pulmonary edema caused by nitrofurantoin. N Engl J Med 273:1185, 1965.

232. Oddo M, Liaudet L, Lepori M, et al: Relapsing acute respiratory failure induced by minocycline. Chest 123:2146, 2003.

233. Poe R, Condemi J, Weinstein S, Schuster R: Adult respiratory distress syndrome related to ampicillin sensitivity. Chest 77:449, 1980.

234. Reinoso M, Schroeder K, Pisani R: Lung disease associated with orally administered mesalamine for ulcerative colitis. Chest 101:1469, 1992.

235. Rosenow E, DeRemee R, Dines D: Chronic nitrofurantoin pulmonary reaction. Report of five cases. N Engl J Med 279:1258, 1968.

236. Selroos O, Edgren J: Lupus-like syndrome associated with pulmonary reaction to nitrofurantoin. Report of three cases. Acta Med Scand 197:125, 1975.

237. Sovijarvi A, Lemola M, Stenius B, Idanpaan-Heikkila J: Nitrofurantoin-induced acute, subacute and chronic pulmonary reactions. A report of 66 cases. Scand J Respir Dis 58:41, 1977.

238. Storch I, Sachar D, Katz S: Pulmonary manifestations of inflammatory bowel disease. Inflamm Bowel Dis 9:104, 2003.

239. Strandberg I, Wengle B, Fagrell B: Chronic interstitial pneumonitis with fibrosis during long-term treatment with nitrofurantoin. Acta Med Scand 196:483, 1974.

240. Sullivan S: Sulfasalazine lung. Desensitization to sulfasalazine and treatment with acrylic coated 5-ASA and azodisalicylate. J Clin Gastroenterol 9:461, 1987.

241. Teague W, Sutphen J, Fechner R: Desquamative interstitial pneumonitis complicating inflammatory bowel disease of childhood. J Pediatr Gastroenterol Nutr 4:663, 1985.

242. Valcke Y, Pauwels R, Van der Straeten M: Bronchoalveolar lavage in acute hypersensitivity pneumonitis caused by sulfasalazine. Chest 92:572, 1987.

243. Wang K, Bowyer B, Fleming C, Schroeder K: Pulmonary infiltrates and eosinophilia associated with sulfasalazine. Mayo Clin Proc 59:343, 1984.

244. Williams T, Eidus L, Thomas P: Fibrosing alveolitis, bronchiolitis obliterans, and sulfasalazine therapy. Chest 81:766, 1982.

245. Wold D, Zahn D: Allergic (Loffler's) pneumonitis occurring during antituberculous chemotherapy. Report of three cases. Am Rev Tuberc 74:445, 1956.

246. Wright D, Robichaud K, Pizzo P, Deisseroth A: Lethal pulmonary reactions associated with the combined use of amphotericin B and leukocyte transfusions. N Engl J Med 304:1185, 1981.

Anti-inflammatory Drugs

247. Albazzaz M, Harvey J, Hoffman J, Siddorn J: Alveolitis and haemolytic anaemia induced by azapropazone. Br Med J (Clin Res Ed) 293:1537, 1986.

248. Baig I, Storch I, Katz S: Infliximab induced eosinophilic pleural effusion in inflammatory bowel diseases. Am J Gastroenterol 97:S177, 2002.

249. Buscaglia A, Cowden F, Brill H: Pulmonary infiltrates associated with naproxen. JAMA 25:65, 1984.

250. Camus P, Degat O, Justrabo E, Jeannin L: D-Penicillamine-induced severe pneumonitis. Chest 81:376, 1982.

251. Cunnane G, Warnock M, Fye KH, et al: Accelerated nodulosis and vasculitis following etanercept therapy for rheumatoid arthritis. Arthritis Rheum 47:445, 2002.

252. Davies D, Jones J: Pulmonary eosinophilia caused by penicillamine. Thorax 35:957, 1983.

253. Derk CT, Jimenez SA: Goodpasture-like syndrome induced by D-penicillamine in a patient with systemic sclerosis: Report and review of the literature. J Rheumatol 30:1616, 2003.

254. Epler G, Snider G, Gaensler E, et al: Bronchiolitis and bronchitis in connective tissue disease. A possible relationship to the use of penicillamine. JAMA 242:528, 1979.

255. Fort J, Scovern H, Abruzzo J: Intravenous cyclophosphamide and methylprednisolone for the treatment of bronchiolitis obliterans and interstitial fibrosis associated with crysotherapy. J Rheumatol 15:850, 1988.

256. Garcia J, Munim A, Nugent K, et al: Alveolar macrophage gold retention in rheumatoid arthritis. J Rheumatol 14:435, 1987.

257. Geddes D, Brostoff J: Pulmonary fibrosis associated with hypersensitivity to gold salts. Br Med J 1:1444, 1976.

258. Goodwin S, Glenny R: Nonsteroidal anti-inflammatory drug-associated pulmonary infiltrates with eosinophilia. Arch Intern Med 152:1521, 1992.

259. Gould P, McCormack P, Palmer D: Pulmonary damage associated with sodium aurothio-malate therapy. J Rheumatol 4:252, 1977.

260. Heffner J, Sahn S: Salicylate-induced pulmonary edema. Clinical features and prognosis. Ann Intern Med 95:405, 1981.

261. Holness L, Tenenbaum J, Cooter N, Grossman R: Fatal bronchiolitis obliterans associated with chrysotherapy. Ann Rheum Dis 42:593, 1983.

262. Keane J, Gershon S, Wise R, et al: Tuberculosis associated with infliximab, a tumor necrosis factor alpha-neutralizing agent. N Engl J Med 345:1098, 2001.

263. Kondo K, Inoue Y, Hamada H, et al: Acetaminophen-induced eosinophilic pneumonia. Chest 104:291, 1993.

264. Kramer N, Chuzhin Y, Kaufman LD, et al: Methotrexate pneumonitis after initiation of infliximab therapy for rheumatoid arthritis. Arthritis Rheum 47:670, 2002.

265. Lahdensuo A, Mattila J, Vilppula A: Bronchiolitis in rheumatoid arthritis. Chest 85:705, 1984.

266. Levinson M, Lynch J III, Bower J: Reversal of progressive, life-threatening gold hypersensitivity pneumonitis by corticosteroids. Am J Med 71:908, 1981.

267. Louie S, Gamble C, Cross C: Penicillamine associated pulmonary hemorrhage. J Rheumatol 13:963, 1986.

268. Matloff D, Kaplan M: D-Penicillamine-induced Goodpasture's-like syndrome in primary biliary cirrhosis – successful treatment with plasmapheresis and immunosuppressives. Gastroenterology 78:1046, 1980.

269. McCormick J, Cole S, Lahirir B, et al: Pneumonitis caused by gold salt therapy: Evidence for the role of cell-mediated immunity in its pathogenesis. Am Rev Respir Dis 122:145, 1980.

270. McFadden R, Fraher L, Thompson J: Gold-naproxen pneumonitis. A toxic drug interation? Chest 96:216, 1989.

271. Mohan AK, Cote TR, Block JA, et al. Tuberculosis following the use of etanercept, a tumor necrosis factor inhibitor. Clin Infect Dis 39:295, 2004.

272. Morice A, Atherton A, Gleeson F, Stewart S: Pulmonary fibrosis associated with nabumetone. Postgrad Med J 67:1021, 1991.

273. Morley T, Komansky H, Adelizzi R, Giudice J: Pulmonary gold toxicity. Eur J Respir Dis 65:627, 1984.

274. Murphy K, Atkins C, Offer R, et al: Obliterative bronchiolitis in two rheumatoid arthritis patients treated with penicillamine. Arthritis Rheum 24:557, 1981.

275. Nader D, Schillaci R: Pulmonary infiltrates with eosinophilia due to naproxen. Chest 83:280, 1983.

276. O'Duffy J, Luthra H, Unni K, Hyatt R: Bronchiolitis in a rheumatoid arthritis patient receiving auranotin. Arthritis Rheum 29:556, 1986.

277. Paakko P, Sutinen S, Anttila S, et al: Bronchiolo-alveolitis with pulmonary basal lamina injury in rheumatoid patient during gold treatment. Pathol Res Pract 183:46, 1988.

278. Partanen J, Van Assendelft A, Koskimies S, et al: Patients with rheumatoid arthritis and gold-induced pneumonitis express two high-risk major histocompatibility complex patterns. Chest 92:277, 1987.

279. Peno-Green L, Lluberas G, Kingsley T, et al. Lung injury linked to etanercept therapy. Chest 122:1858, 2002.

280. Riegert-Johnson DL, Godfrey, JA, Myers J, et al: Delayed hypersensitivity reaction and acute respiratory distress syndrome following infliximab infusion. Inflamm Bowel Dis 8:186, 2002.

281. Scharf J, Nahir M, Kleinhaus U, Barzilai D: Diffuse pulmonary injury associated with gold therapy. JAMA 237:2412, 1977.

282. Scott D, Bradby G, Aitman T, et al: Relationship of gold and penicillamine therapy to diffuse interstitial lung disease. Ann Rheum Dis 40:136, 1981.

283. Smith F, Lindberg P: Life-threatening hypersensitivity to sulindac. JAMA 244:269, 1980.

284. Smith W, Ball G: Lung injury due to gold treatment. Arthritis Rheum 23:351, 1980.

285. Sternlieb I, Bennett B, Scheinberg I: D-Penicillamine induced Goodpasture's syndrome in Wilson's disease. Ann Intern Med 82:673, 1975.

286. Takimoto C, Lynch D, Stulbarg M: Pulmonary infiltrates associated with sulindac therapy. Chest 97:230, 1990.

287. Tomioka R, King TE. Gold-induced pulmonary disease: Clinical features, outcome, and differentiation from rheumatoid lung disease: Am J Respir Crit Care Med 155:1011, 1997.

288. Thurston J, Marks P, Trapnell D: Lung changes associated with phenylbutazone treatment. Br Med J 2:1422, 1976.

289. Warris A, Bjorneklett A, Gaustad P: Invasive pulmonary aspergillosis associated with infliximab therapy. N Engl J Med 344:1099, 2001.

290. Winterbauer R, Wilske K, Wheelis R: Diffuse pulmonary injury associated with gold treatment. N Engl J Med 294:919, 1976.

291. Wolfe F, Schurle D, Lin J, et al: Upper and lower airway disease in penicillamine-treated patients with rheumatoid arthritis. J Rheumatol 10:406, 1983.

292. Yousem S, Colby T, Carrington C: Lung biopsy in rheumatoid arthritis. Am Rev Respir Dis 131:770, 1985.

293. Yousem SA, Dacic S. Pulmonary lymphohistiocytic reactions temporally related to etanercept therapy. Mod Pathol 18:651, 2005.

294. Zitnik R, Cooper J: Pulmonary disease due to antirheumatic agents. Clin Chest Med 11:139, 1990.

Interferons

295. Abi-Nassif S, Mark E, Fogel R, et al: Pegylated interferon and ribavirin induced interstitial pneumonitis with ARDS. Chest 124:406, 2003.

296. Bini E, Weinshel E: Severe exacerbation of asthma: A new side-effect of interferon alpha in patients with asthma and chronic hepatitis C. Mayo Clin Proc 74:367, 1999.

297. Butnor KJ: Pulmonary sarcoidosis induced by interferon-α therapy. Am J Surg Pathol 29:976, 2005.

298. Chin K, Tabata C, Sataka N, et al: Pneumonitis associated with natural and recombinant interferon alfa therapy for chronic hepatitis C. Chest 105:939, 1994.

299. Fuhrmann V, Kramer L, Bauer E, et al: Severe interstitial pneumonitis secondary to pegylated interferon alpha-2b and ribavirin treatment of hepatitis C infection. Dig Dis Sci 49:1966, 2004.

300. Harris J, Bines S, Das Gupta T: Therapy of disseminated malignant melanoma with recombinant alpha 2b-interferon and piroxicam: Clinical results with a report of an unusual response-associated feature (vitiligo) and unusual toxicity (diffuse pulmonary interstitial fibrosis). Med Pediatr Oncol 22:103, 1994.

301. Hoffmann RM, Jung M, Motz R, et al: Sarcoidosis associated with interferon alpha therapy for chronic hepatitis C. J Hepatol 28:1058, 1998.

302. Hoffman SD, Hammadeh R, Shah N: Eosinophilic pneumonitis secondary to pegylated interferon alpha-2b and/or ribavirin therapy. Am J Gastroenterol 98:S152, 2003.

303. Honoré I, Nunes H, Groussard O, et al: Acute respiratory failure after interferon-γ therapy of end-stage pulmonary fibrosis. Am J Respir Crit Care Med 167:953, 2003.

304. Ishizaki T, Sasaki F, Ameshima S, et al: Pneumonitis during interferon and/or herbal drug therapy in patients with chronic active hepatitis. Eur Respir J 9:2691, 1996.

305. Kamisako T, Adachi Y, Chihara J, et al: Interstitial pneumonitis and interferon-alfa. Br Med J 306:896, 1993.

306. Kumar K, Russo M, Borczuk A, et al: Significant pulmonary toxicity associated with interferon and ribavirin therapy for hepatitis C. Am J Gastroenterol 97:2432, 2002.

307. Nakajima M, Kubota Y, Miyashita N, et al : Recurrence of sarcoidosis following interferon-alpha therapy for chronic hepatitis C. Intern Med 35:376, 1996.

308. Ogata K, Koga T, Yagawa K: Interferon-related bronchiolitis obliterans organizing pneumonia. Chest 106:612, 1994.

309. Okanoue T, Sakamoto S, Itoh Y, et al: Side-effects of high dose interferon therapy for chronic hepatitis C. J Hepatol 25:283, 1996.

310. Rubinowitz AN, Naidich DP, Alinsonorin C: Interferon-induced sarcoidosis. J Comput Assist Tomogr 27:279, 2003.

311. Tahan V, Ozseker F, Guneylioglu D, et al: Sarcoidosis after use of interferon for chronic hepatitis C. Report of a case and review of the literature. Dig Dis Sci 48:169, 2003.

312. Takeda A, Ikegame K, Kimura Y, et al: Pleural effusion during interferon treatment for chronic hepatitis C. Hepatogastroenterology 47:1431, 2000.

313. Teragawa H, Hondo T, Takahashi K, et al: Sarcoidosis after interferon therapy for chronic active hepatitis C. Intern Med 35:19, 1996.

314. Van Zandwijk N, Groen HJM, Postmus PE, et al: Role of recombinant interferon-gamma maintenance in responding patients with small cell lung cancer. A randomised phase III study of the EORTC Lung Cancer Cooperative Group. Eur J Cancer 33:1759, 1997.

Antiarrhythmic Drugs

315. Adams G, Kenoe R, Lesch M, Glassroth J: Amiodarone-induced pneumonitis. Assessment of risk factors and possible risk reduction. Chest 93:254, 1988.

316. Akoun G, Cadranel J, Blanchette G, et al: Bronchoalveolar lavage cell data in amiodarone-associated pneumonitis. Evaluation in 22 patients. Chest 99:1177, 1991.

317. Akoun G, Gauthier-Rahman S, Liote H, et al: Leukocyte migration inhibition in amiodarone-associated pneumonitis. Chest 94:1050, 1988.

318. Akoun G, Gauthier-Rahman S, Milleron B, et al: Amiodarone-induced hypersensitivity pneumonitis. Chest 85:133, 1984.

319. Ashrafian H, Davey P: Is amiodarone an underrecognized cause of acute respiratory failure in the ICU? Chest 120:275, 2001.

320. Bedrossian CW, Warren CJ, Ohar J, et al: Amiodarone pulmonary toxicity: cytopathology, ultrastructure, and immunocytochemistry. Ann Diagn Pathol 1:47, 1997.

321. Braude A, Downar E, Chamberlain D, Rebuck A: Tocainide-associated interstitial pneumonitis. Thorax 37:309, 1982.

322. Camus P, Martin WJ 2nd, Rosenow EC 3rd: Amiodarone pulmonary toxicity. Clin Chest Med 25:65, 2004.

323. Coudert B, Bailly F, Lombard J, et al: Amiodarone pneumonitis. Bronchoalveolar lavage findings in 15 patients and review of the literature. Chest 102:1005, 1992.

324. Dean P, Groshart K, Porterfield J, et al: Amiodarone-associated pulmonary toxicity. A clinical and pathologic study of eleven cases. Am J Clin Pathol 87:7, 1987.

325. Dusman R, Stanton M, Miles W, et al: Clinical features of amiodarone-induced pulmonary toxicity. Circulation 82:51, 1990.

326. Feinberg L, Travis W, Ferrans V, et al: Pulmonary fibrosis associated with tocainide: Report of a case with literature review. Am Rev Respir Dis 141:505, 1990.

327. Fraire A, Guntupalli K, Greenberg S, et al: Amiodarone pulmonary toxicity: A multidisciplinary review of current status. South Med J 86:67, 1993.

328. Gonzalez-Rothi R, Hannan S, Hood I, Franzini D: Amiodarone pulmonary toxicity presenting as bilateral exudative pleural effusions. Chest 92:179, 1987.

329. Herre J, Sauve M, Malone P, et al: Long-term results of amiodarone therapy in patients with recurrent sustained ventricular tachycardia or ventricular fibrillation. J Am Coll Cardiol 13:442, 1989.

330. Howard J, Mohsenifar Z, Simons S: Adult respiratory distress syndrome following administration of lidocaine. Chest 81:644, 1982.

331. Israel-Biet D, Venet A, Caubarrere I, et al: Bronchoalveolar lavage in amiodarone pneumonitis. Cellular abnormalities and their relevance to pathogenesis. Chest 91:214, 1987.

332. Kay G, Epstein A, Kirklin J, et al: Fatal postoperative amiodarone pulmonary toxicity. Am J Cardiol 62:490, 1988.

333. Kennedy J: Clinical aspects of amiodarone pulmonary toxicity. Clin Chest Med 11:119, 1990.

334. Kennedy J, Myers J, Plumb V, Fulmer J: Amiodarone pulmonary toxicity. Clinical, radiologic, and pathologic correlations. Arch Intern Med 147:50, 1987.

335. Kuhlman J, Teigen C, Ren H, et al: Amiodarone pulmonary toxicity: CT findings in symptomatic patients. Radiology 177:121, 1990.

336. Liu F, Cohen R, Downar E, et al: Amiodarone pulmonary toxicity: Functional and ultrastructural evaluation. Thorax 41:100, 1986.

337. Martin W II, Osborn M, Douglas W: Amiodarone pulmonary toxicity. Assessment by bronchoalveolar lavage. Chest 88:630, 1985.

338. Martin W II, Rosenow E III: Amiodarone pulmonary toxicity. Recognition and pathogenesis. Chest 93:1067 (Pt 1) and 1242 (Pt 2), 1988.

339. Myers J, Kennedy J, Plumb V: Amiodarone lung: Pathologic findings in clinically toxic patients. Hum Pathol 18:349, 1987.

340. Nalos P, Kass R, Gang E, et al: Life-threatening postoperative pulmonary complications in patients with previous amiodarone pulmonary toxicity undergoing cardiothoracic operations. J Thorac Cardiovasc Surg 93:904, 1987.

341. Nicolet-Chatelain G, Prevost M, Escamilla R, Migueres J: Amiodarone-induced pulmonary toxicity. Immunoallergologic tests and bronchoalveolar lavage phospholipid content. Chest 99:363, 1991.

342. Ohar J, Jackson F, Dettenmeier P, et al: Bronchoalveolar lavage cell count and differential are not reliable indicators of amiodarone-induced pneumonitis. Chest 102:999, 1992.

343. Oren S, Turkot S, Golzman B: Amiodarone-induced bronchiolitis obliterans organizing pneumonia (BOOP). Respir Med 90:167, 1996.

344. Ott MC, Khoor A, Leventhal JP, et al: Pulmonary toxicity in patients receiving low-dose amiodarone. Chest 123:646, 2003.

345. Perlow G, Jain B, Pauker S, et al: Tocainide-associated interstitial pneumonitis. Ann Intern Med 94:489, 1981.

346. Pichler W, Schindler L, Staubli M, et al: Anti-amiodarone antibodies: Detection and relationship to the development of side effects. Am J Med 85:197, 1988.

347. Poukkula A, Paakko P: Quinidine-induced reversible pneumonitis. Chest 106:304, 1994.

348. Ren H, Kuhlman J, Hruban R, et al: CT-pathology correlation of amiodarone lung. J Comput Assist Tomogr 14:760, 1990.

349. Stein M, Demarco T, Gamsu G, et al: Computed tomography: Pathologic correlation in lung disease due to tocainide. Am Rev Respir Dis 137:458, 1988.

350. Valle JM, Alvarez D, Antunez J, et al: Bronchiolitis obliterans organizing pneumonia secondary to amiodarone: A rare aetiology. Eur Respir J 8:470, 1995.

351. Van Mieghem W, Coolen L, Malysse I, et al: Amiodarone and the development of ARDS after lung surgery. Chest 105:1642, 1994.

352. Wood D, Osborn M, Rooke J, Holmes D Jr: Amiodarone pulmonary toxicity: Report of two cases associated with rapidly progressive fatal adult respiratory distress syndrome after pulmonary angiography. Mayo Clin Proc 60:601, 1985.

Antihypertensive Drugs
353. Akoun G, Milleron B, Mayaud C, Tholoniat D: Provocation test coupled with bronchoalveolar lavage in diagnosis of propranolol-induced hypersensitivity pneumonitis. Am Rev Respir Dis 139:247, 1989.
354. Bass B: Hydralazine lung. Thorax 36:695, 1981.
355. Bell R, Lippmann M: Hydrochlorothiazide-induced pulmonary edema. Report of a case and review of the literature. Arch Intern Med 139:817, 1979.
356. Biron P, Dessureault J, Napke E: Acute allergic interstitial pneumonitis induced by hydrochlorothiazide. Can Med Assoc J 145:28, 1991.
357. Desai S, Pierce E Jr, Fleming T: Severe hypertension, propranolol, and acute pulmonary edema. Crit Care Med 15:799, 1987.
358. Doniach I, Morrison B, Steiner R: Lung changes during hexamethonium therapy for hypertension. Br Heart J 16:101, 1954.
359. Dorn M, Walker B: Noncardiogenic pulmonary edema associated with hydrochlorothiazide therapy. Chest 79:482, 1981.
360. Erwteman T, Braat M, Van Aken W: Interstitial pulmonary fibrosis: A new side effect of practolol. Br Med J 2:297, 1977.
361. Finley T, Aronow A, Cosentino A, Golde D: Occult pulmonary hemorrhage in anticoagulated patients. Am Rev Respir Dis 112:23, 1975.
362. Kounis N, Nikolaou S, Zavras G, Siablis D: Severe acute interstitial pulmonary edema from Moduretic® (amiloride plus hydrochlorothiazide). Ann Allergy 57:417, 1986.
363. Musk A, Pollard J: Pindolol and pulmonary fibrosis. Br Med J 2:581, 1979.
364. Perry H Jr, O'Neal R, Thomas W: Pulmonary disease following chronic chemical ganglionic blockade. A clinical and pathologic study. Am J Med 22:37, 1957.
365. Petersen A, Dodge M, Helwig F: Pulmonary changes associated with hexamethonium therapy. Arch Intern Med 103:285, 1959.
366. Rokseth R, Storstein O: Pulmonary complications during mecamylamine therapy. Acta Med Scand 167:23, 1960.
367. Schatz P, Mesologites D, Hyun J, et al: Captopril-induced hypersensitivity lung disease. An immune-complex-mediated phenomenon. Chest 95:685, 1989.
368. Sloand E, Thompson T: Propranolol-induced pulmonary edema and shock in a patient with pheochromocytoma. Arch Intern Med 144:173, 1984.
369. Thompson R, Grennan D: Acebutolol induced hypersensitivity pneumonitis (letter). Br Med J (Clin Res Ed) 286:894, 1983.
370. Wood G, Bolton R, Muers M, Losowsky M: Pleurisy and pulmonary granulomas after treatment with acebutolol. Br Med J 285:936, 1982.

Tocolytic Agents
371. Bloss J, Hankins G, Gilstrap L, Hauth J: Pulmonary edema as a delayed complication of ritodrine therapy. A case report. J Reprod Med 32:469, 1987.
372. Clesham G: Beta adrenergic agonists and pulmonary oedema in preterm labour. Br Med J 308:260, 1994.
373. Elliott J, O'Keeffe D, Greenberg P, Freeman R: Pulmonary edema associated with magnesium sulfate and betamethasone administration. Am J Obstet Gynecol 134:717, 1979.
374. Guernsey B, Villarreal Y, Snyder M, Gabert H: Pulmonary edema associated with the use of betamimetic agents in preterm labor. Am J Hosp Pharmacol 38:1942, 1981.
375. Gupta R, Foster S, Romano P, Thomas H III: Acute pulmonary edema associated with the use of oral ritodrine for premature labor. Chest 95:479, 1989.
376. Jacobs M, Knight A, Arias F: Maternal pulmonary edema resulting from betamimetic and glucocorticoid therapy. Obstet Gynecol 56:56, 1980.
377. Mabie W, Pernoll M, Witty J, Biswas M: Pulmonary edema induced by betamimetic drugs. South Med J 76:1354, 1983.
378. Nimrod C, Rambihar V, Fallen E, et al: Pulmonary edema associated with isoxsuprine therapy. Am J Obstet Gynecol 148:625, 1984.
379. Pisani R, Rosenow E III: Pulmonary edema associated with tocolytic therapy. Ann Intern Med 110:714, 1989.
380. Whitehead M, Mander A, Hertogs K, et al: Acute congestive cardiac failure in a hypertensive woman receiving salbutamol for premature labour. Br Med J 2:1221, 1980.

Anticonvulsants
381. Banka R, Ward M: Bronchiolitis obliterans and organising pneumonia caused by carbamazepine and mimicking community acquired pneumonia. Postgrad Med J 78:621, 2002.
382. Chamberlain D, Hyland R, Ross D: Diphenylhydantoin-induced lymphocytic interstitial pneumonia. Chest 90:458, 1986.
383. Cullinan S, Bower G: Acute pulmonary hypersensitivity to carbamazepine. Chest 68:580, 1975.
384. Mahatma M, Haponik E, Nelson S, et al: Phenytoin-induced acute respiratory failure with pulmonary eosinophilia. Am J Med 87:93, 1989.
385. Michael J, Rudin M: Acute pulmonary disease caused by phenytoin. Ann Intern Med 95:452, 1981.
386. Munn N, Baughman R, Ploysongsang Y, et al: Bronchoalveolar lavage in acute drug-hypersensitivity pneumonitis probably caused by phenytoin. South Med J 77:1594, 1984.
387. Stephan W, Parks R, Tempest B: Acute hypersensitivity pneumonitis associated with carbamazepine therapy. Chest 74:463, 1978.
388. Wilschut F, Cobben N, Thunnissen F, et al: Recurrent respiratory distress associated with carbamazepine overdose. Eur Respir J 10:2163, 1997.

389. Yermakov V, Hitti I, Sutton A: Necrotizing vasculitis associated with diphenylhydantoin: Two fatal cases. Hum Pathol 13:182, 1983.

Psychotherapeutic Drugs

390. Conces D Jr, Kreipke D, Tarver R: Pulmonary edema induced by intravenous ethchlorvynol. Am J Emerg Med 4:549, 1986.
391. Drent M, Singh S, Gorgels A, et al: Drug-induced pneumonitis and heart failure simultaneously associated with venlafaxine. Am J Respir Crit Care Med 167:958, 2003.
392. Glauser F, Smith W, Caldwell A, et al: Ethchlorvynol (Placidyl)-induced pulmonary edema. Ann Intern Med 84:46, 1976.
393. Gonzalez-Rothi R, Zander D, Ros P: Fluoxetine hydrochloride (Prozac)-induced pulmonary disease. Chest 107:1763, 1995.
394. Li C, Gefter W: Acute pulmonary edema induced by overdosage of phenothiazines. Chest 101:102, 1992.
395. Lindstrom F, Flodmark O, Gustafsson B: Respiratory distress syndrome and thrombotic, non-bacterial endocarditis after amitriptyline overdose. Acta Med Scand 202:203, 1977.
396. Mahutte C, Nakasato S, Light R: Haloperidol and sudden death due to pulmonary edema. Arch Intern Med 142:1951, 1982.
397. Marshall A, Moore K: Pulmonary disease after amitriptyline overdosage. Br Med J 1:716, 1973.
398. Miller K, Sahn S: Bilateral exudative pleural effusions following intravenous ethchlorvynol administration. Chest 95:464, 1989.
399. Mountain R, Ferguson S, Fowler A, Hyers T: Noncardiac pulmonary edema following administration of parenteral paraldehyde. Chest 82:371, 1982.
400. Richman S, Harris R: Acute pulmonary edema associated with Librium abuse. A case report. Radiology 103:57, 1972.
401. Salerno S, Strong J, Roth B, Sakata V: Eosinophilic pneumonia and respiratory failure associated with a trazodone overdose. Am J Respir Crit Care Med 152:2170, 1995.
402. Sinal S, Crowe J: Cyanosis, cough, and hypotension following intravenous administration of paraldehyde. Pediatrics 57:158, 1976.
403. Smego R, Durack D: The neuroleptic malignant syndrome. Arch Intern Med 142:1183, 1982.
404. Varnell R, Godwin J, Richardson M, Vincent J: Adult respiratory distress syndrome from overdose of tricyclic antidepressants. Radiology 170:667, 1989.
405. Wilson I, Gambill J, Sandifer M: Loeffler's syndrome occurring during imipramine therapy. Am J Psychol 119:892, 1963.

Opioids

406. Banner A, Rodriquez J, Sunderrajan E, et al: Bronchiectasis: A cause of pulmonary symptoms in heroin addicts. Respiration 37:232, 1979.

407. Bogartz L, Miller W: Pulmonary edema associated with propoxyphene intoxication. JAMA 215:259, 1971.
408. Goldman A, Enquist R: Methadone pulmonary edema. Chest 63:275, 1973.
409. Katz S, Aberman A, Frand U, et al: Heroin pulmonary edema. Evidence for increased pulmonary capillary permeability. Am Rev Respir Dis 106:472, 1972.
410. Light R, Dunham T: Severe slowly resolving heroin-induced pulmonary edema. Chest 67:61, 1975.
411. Prough D, Roy R, Bumgarner J, Shannon G: Acute pulmonary edema in healthy teenagers following conservative doses of intravenous naloxone. Anesthesiology 60:485, 1984.
412. Schaaf J, Spivack M, Rath G, Snider G: Pulmonary edema and adult respiratory distress syndrome following methadone abuse. Am Rev Respir Dis 107:1047, 1973.
413. Schwartz J, Koenigsberg M: Naloxone-induced pulmonary edema. Ann Emerg Med 16:1294, 1987.
414. Siegel H: Human pulmonary pathology associated with narcotic and other addictive drugs. Hum Pathol 3:55, 1972.
415. Sklar J, Timms R: Codeine-induced pulmonary edema. Chest 72:230, 1977.
416. Smith W, Glauser F, Dearden L, et al: Deposits of immunoglobulin and complement in the pulmonary tissue of patients with "heroin lung." Chest 73:471, 1978.
417. Stadnyk A, Grossman R: Nalbuphine-induced pulmonary edema. Chest 90:773, 1986.
418. Thammakumpee G, Sumpatanukule P: Noncardiogenic pulmonary edema induced by sublingual buprenorphine. Chest 106:306, 1994.
419. Warnock M, Ghahremani G, Rattenborg C, et al: Pulmonary complication of heroin intoxication. JAMA 219:1051, 1972.

Cocaine

420. Albertson T, Walby W, Derlet R: Stimulant-induced pulmonary toxicity. Chest 108:1140, 1995.
421. Allred R, Ewer S: Fatal pulmonary edema following intravenous "freebase" cocaine use. Ann Emerg Med 10:441, 1981.
422. Baily M, Fraire A, Greenberg S, et al: Pulmonary histopathology in cocaine abusers. Hum Pathol 25:203, 1994.
423. Churg A, Myers J, Suarez T, et al: Airway-centered interstitial fibrosis: A distinct form of aggressive diffuse lung disease. Am J Surg Pathol 28:62, 2004.
424. Cooper C, Bai T, Heyderman B, Corrin B: Cellulose granulomas in the lungs of a cocaine sniffer. Br Med J 286:2021, 1983.
425. Cucco R, Yoo O, Cregler L, Chang J: Nonfatal pulmonary edema after "freebase" cocaine smoking. Am Rev Respir Dis 136:179, 1987.
426. Dicpinigaitis PV, Jones JG, Frymus MM, et al: "Crack" cocaine-induced syndrome mimicking sarcoidosis. Am J Med Sci 317:416, 1999.

427. Forrester J, Steele A, Waldron J, Parsons P: Crack lung: An acute pulmonary syndrome with a spectrum of clinical and histopathologic findings. Am Rev Respir Dis 142:462, 1990.

428. Greenebaum E, Copeland A, Grewal R: Blackened bronchoalveolar lavage fluid in crack smokers. A preliminary study. Am J Clin Pathol 100:481, 1993.

429. Haim D, Lippmann M, Goldberg S, Walkenstein M: The pulmonary complications of crack cocaine. A comprehensive review. Chest 107:233, 1995.

430. Heffner J, Harley R, Schabel S: Pulmonary reactions from illicit substance abuse. Clin Chest Med 11:151, 1990.

431. Janjua T, Bohan A, Wesselius L: Increased lower respiratory tract iron concentrations in alkaloidal ("crack") cocaine users. Chest 119:422, 2001.

432. Khalsa M, Tashkin D, Perrochet B: Smoked cocaine: Patterns of use and pulmonary consequences. J Psychoactive Drugs 24:265, 1992.

433. Kissner D, Lawrence W, Selis J, Flint A: Crack lung: Pulmonary disease caused by cocaine abuse. Am Rev Respir Dis 136:1250, 1987.

434. Kleerup EC, Wong M, Marques-Magallanes JA, et al: Acute effects of intravenous cocaine on pulmonary artery pressure and cardiac index in habitual crack smokers. Chest 111:30, 1997.

435. Kline J, Hirasuna J: Pulmonary edema after freebase cocaine smoking – not due to an adulterant. Chest 97:1009, 1990.

436. Klinger J, Bensadoun E, Corrao W: Pulmonary complications from alveolar accumulation of carbonaceous material in a cocaine smoker. Chest 101:1171, 1992.

437. Meisels I, Loke J: The pulmonary effects of free-base cocaine: A review. Cleve Clin J Med 60:325, 1993.

438. Murray R, Albin R, Mergner W, Criner G: Diffuse alveolar hemorrhage temporally related to cocaine smoking. Chest 93:427, 1988.

439. Murray R, Smialek J, Golle M, Albin R: Pulmonary artery medial hypertrophy in cocaine users without foreign particle microembolization. Chest 96:1050, 1989.

440. Nadeem S, Nasir N, Israel R: Loffler's syndrome secondary to crack cocaine. Chest 105:1599, 1994.

441. O'Donnell A, Mappin F, Sebo T, Tazelaar H: Interstitial pneumonitis associated with "crack" cocaine abuse. Chest 100:1155, 1991.

442. Oh P, Balter M: Cocaine induced eosinophilic lung disease. Thorax 47:478, 1992.

443. Patel R, Dutta D, Schonfeld S: Free-base cocaine use associated with bronchiolitis obliterans organizing pneumonia. Ann Intern Med 107:186, 1987.

444. Perez G, Bragado F, Gil A, et al: Pulmonary hemorrhage and antiglomerular basement membrane antibody-mediated glomerulonephritis after exposure to smoked cocaine (crack): A case report and review of the literature. Pathol Int 47:692, 1997.

445. Susskind H, Weber D, Volkow N, Hitzemann R: Increased lung permeability following long-term use of free-base cocaine (crack). Chest 100:903, 1991.

446. Tashkin D, Khalsa M-E, Gorelick D, et al: Pulmonary status of habitual cocaine smokers. Am Rev Respir Dis 145:92, 1992.

447. Taylor R, Bernard G: Airway complications from free-basing cocaine. Chest 95:476, 1989.

448. Yakel DL Jr, Eisenberg MJ: Pulmonary artery hypertension in chronic intravenous cocaine users. Am Heart J 130:398, 1995.

Tryptophan

449. Banner A, Borochovitz D: Acute respiratory failure caused by pulmonary vasculitis after L-tryptophan ingestion. Am Rev Respir Dis 143:661, 1991.

450. Belongia E, Hedberg C, Gleich G, et al: An investigation of the cause of the eosinophilia-myalgia syndrome associated with tryptophan use. N Engl J Med 323:357, 1990.

451. Campagna A, Blanc P, Criswell L, et al: Pulmonary manifestations of the eosinophilia-myalgia syndrome associated with tryptophan ingestion. Chest 101:1274, 1992.

452. Carr L, Ruther E, Berg P, Lehnert H: Eosinophilia-myalgia syndrome in Germany: An epidemiologic review. Mayo Clin Proc 69:620, 1994.

453. Catton C, Elmer J, Whitehouse A, et al: Pulmonary involvement in the eosinophilia-myalgia syndrome. Chest 99:327, 1991.

454. Culpepper R, Williams R, Mease P, et al: Natural history of the eosinophilia-myalgia syndrome. Ann Intern Med 115:437, 1991.

455. Herrick M, Chang Y, Horoupian D, et al: L-tryptophan and the eosinophilia-myalgia syndrome: Pathologic findings in eight patients. Hum Pathol 22:12, 1991.

456. Jayeno A, Gleich G: The eosinophilia-myalgia syndrome: Lessons from Germany. Mayo Clin Proc 69:702, 1994.

457. Read C, Clauw D, Weir C, et al: Dyspnea and pulmonary function in the L-tryptophan-associated eosinophilia-myalgia syndrome. Chest 101:1282, 1992.

458. Sack K, Criswell L: Eosinophilia-myalgia syndrome: The aftermath. South Med J 85:878, 1992.

459. Sidransky H: Eosinophilia-myalgia syndrome: A recent syndrome serving as an alert to new diseases ahead. Mod Pathol 7:806, 1994.

460. Slutsker L, Hoesly F, Miller L, et al: Eosinophilia-myalgia syndrome associated with exposure to tryptophan from a single manufacturer. JAMA 264:213, 1990.

461. Strumpf I, Drucker R, Anders K, et al: Acute eosinophilic pulmonary disease associated with the ingestion of L-trytophan-containing products. Chest 99:8, 1991.

462. Tazelaar H, Myers J, Drage C, et al: Pulmonary disease associated with L-tryptophan-induced eosinophilic myalgia syndrome. Clinical and pathologic features. Chest 97:1032, 1990.

463. Tazelaar H, Myers J, Strickler J, et al: Tryptophan-induced lung disease: An immunophenotypic, immunofluorescent, and electron microscopic study. Mod Pathol 6:56, 1993.

464. Travis W, Kalafer M, Robin H, Luibel F: Hypersensitivity pneumonitis and pulmonary vasculitis with eosinophilia in a patient taking an L-tryptophan preparation. Ann Intern Med 112:301, 1990.

465. Varga J, Uitto J, Jimenez S: The cause and pathogenesis of the eosinophilia-myalgia syndrome. Ann Intern Med 116:140, 1992.

Anorexigens

466. Abenhaim L, Moride Y, Brenot F, et al: Appetite-suppressant drugs and the risk of primary pulmonary hypertension. N Engl J Med 335:609, 1996.

467. Gurtner H: Aminorex and pulmonary hypertension. A review. Cor Vasa 27:160, 1985.

468. Horton MR, Tuder RM: Primary pulmonary arterial hypertension presenting as diffuse micronodules on CT. Crit Rev Comput Tomogr 45:335, 2004.

469. Kay J: Dietary pulmonary hypertension. Thorax 49:S33, 1994.

470. Mark E, Palatas, Chang H, et al: Fatal pulmonary hypertension associated with short-term use of fenfluramine and phentermine. N Engl J Med 337:602, 1998.

471. McMurray J, Bloomfield P, Miller HC: Irreversible pulmonary hypertension after treatment with fenfluramine. Br Med J 292:239,1986.

472. Rich S, Shillington A, McLaughlin V: Comparison of survival in patients with pulmonary hypertension associated with fenfluramine to patients with primary pulmonary hypertension. Am J Cardiol 92:1366, 2003.

473. Simonneau G, Fartoukh M, Sitbon O, et al : Primary pulmonary hypertension associated with the use of fenfluramine derivatives. Chest 114:195S, 1998.

474. Strother J, Fedullo P, Yi ES: Complex vascular lesions at autopsy in a patient with phentermine-fenfluramine use and rapidly progressing pulmonary hypertension. Arch Pathol Lab Med 123:539, 1999.

475. Tomita T, Zhao Q: Autopsy findings of heart and lungs in a patient with primary pulmonary hypertension associated with use of fenfluramine and phentermine. Chest 121:649, 2002.

476. Widgren S: Pulmonary hypertension related to aminorex intake. Histologic, ultrastructural, and morphometric studies of 37 cases in Switzerland. Curr Top Pathol 64:1, 1977.

Miscellaneous Noncytotoxic Drugs

477. Akoun G, Liote H, Liote F, et al: Provocation test coupled with bronchoalveolar lavage in diagnosis of drug (Nilutamide)-induced hypersensitivity pneumonitis. Chest 97:495, 1990.

478. Au F, Webber B, Rosenberg S: Pulmonary granulomas induced by BCG. Cancer 41:2209, 1978.

479. Awadh N, Ronco J, Bernstein V, et al: Spontaneous pulmonary hemorrhage after thrombolytic therapy for acute myocardial infarction. Chest 106:1622, 1994.

480. Burgher L, Kass I, Schenken J: Pulmonary allergic granulomatosis: A possible drug reaction in a patient receiving cromolyn sodium. Chest 66:84, 1974.

481. Chin K, Tabata C, Satake N, et al: Pneumonitis associated with natural and recombinant interferon alfa therapy for chronic hepatitis C. Chest 105:939, 1994.

482. Danoff SK, Grasso ME, Terry PB, et al: Pleuropulmonary disease due to pergolide use for restless legs syndrome. Chest 120:313, 2001.

483. De Groot R, Willems L, Dijkman J: Interstitial lung disease with pleural effusion caused by simvastin. J Intern Med 239:361,1996.

484. Diffee J III, Hayes J, Montesi S, et al: Chlorpropamide-induced pulmonary infiltration and eosinophilia with multisystem toxicity. J Tenn Med Assoc 79:82, 1986.

485. Ersoz N, Finestone S: Adrenaline-induced pulmonary oedema and its treatment. Report of two cases. Br J Anaesth 43:709, 1971.

486. Finley T, Aronow A, Cosentino A, Golde D: Occult pulmonary hemorrhage in anticoagulated patients. Am Rev Respir Dis 112:23, 1975.

487. Freedman M, Grisaru D, Olivieri N, et al: Pulmonary syndrome in patients with thalassemia major receiving intravenous deferoxamine infusions. Am J Dis Child 144:565, 1990.

488. Frye M, Jarratt M, Sahn S: Acute hypoxemic respiratory failure following intrapleural thrombolytic therapy for hemothorax. Chest 105:1595, 1994.

489. Gomez, J-L, Dupont A, Cusan L, et al: Simultaneous liver and lung toxicity related to nonsteroidal antiandrogen nilutamide (Anandron): A case report. Am J Med 92:563, 1992.

490. Graham J: Cardiac and pulmonary fibrosis during methysergide therapy for headache. Am J Med Sci 254:1, 1967.

491. Hill C, Zeitz C, Kirkham B: Dermatomyositis with lung involvement in a patient treated with simvastatin. Aust N Z J Med 25:745, 1995.

492. Hindle W, Posner E, Sweetnam M, et al: Pleural effusion and fibrosis during treatment with methysergide. Br Med J 1:605, 1970.

493. Israel-Biet D, Venet A, Sandron D, et al: Pulmonary complications of intravesical Bacille Calmette-Guerin immunotherapy. Am Rev Respir Dis 135:763, 1987.

494. Khosla R, Butman A, Hammer D: Simvastatin-induced lupus erythematosus. South Med J 91:873, 1998.

495. Kinnunen E, Viljanen A: Pleuropulmonary involvement during bromocriptine treatment. Chest 94:1034, 1988.

496. Kozlowski C, Koffel M: Noncardiogenic pulmonary edema associated with intravenous radiocontrast administration. Chest 102:620, 1992.

497. Lantuejoul S, Brambilla E, Brambilla C, et al: Statin-induced fibrotic nonspecific interstitial pneumonia. Eur Respir J 19:577, 2002.

498. Liebhaber M, Wright R, Gelberg H, et al: Polymyalgia, hypersensitivity pneumonitis and other reactions in patients receiving HMG-CoA reductase inhibitors. Chest 115:886, 1999.

499. Martin T, Sandblom R, Johnson R: Adult respiratory distress syndrome following thrombolytic therapy for pulmonary embolism. Chest 83:151, 1983.

500. McElvaney N, Wilcox P, Churg A, Fleetham J: Pleuropulmonary disease during bromocriptine treatment of Parkinson's disease. Arch Intern Med 148:2231, 1988.

501. Nakamura R, Imamura T, Onitsuka H, et al: Interstitial pneumonia induced by ticlopidine. Circ J 66:773, 2002.

502. Nathan P, Torres A, Smith A, et al: Spontaneous pulmonary hemorrhage following coronary thrombolysis. Chest 101:1150, 1992.

503. Nizami I, Kissner D, Visscher D, Dubaybo BA: Idiopathic bronchiolitis obliterans with organizing pneumonia. An acute and life-threatening syndrome. Chest 108:271, 1995.

504. Palayew M, Briedis D, Libman M, et al: Disseminated infection after intravesical BCG immunotherapy. Detection of organisms in pulmonary tissue. Chest 104:307, 1993.

505. Persoz C, Cornella F, Kaeser P, et al: Ticlopidine-induced interstitial pulmonary disease: A case report. Chest 119:1963, 2001.

506. Pfitzenmeyer P, Foucher P, Piard F, et al: Nilutamide pneumonitis: A report on eight patients. Thorax 47:622, 1992.

507. Prigogine T, Waterlot Y, Gottignies P, et al: Acute nonhemodynamic pulmonary edema with nifedipine in primary pulmonary hypertension. Chest 100:563, 1991.

508. Repo U, Nieminen P: Pulmonary infiltrates with eosinophilia and urinary symptoms during disodium cromoglycate treatment. A case report. Scand J Respir Dis 57:1, 1976.

509. Rodman T, Fraimow W, Myerson R: Loffler's syndrome: Report of a case associated with administration of mephenesin carbamate (Tolseram). Ann Intern Med 48:668, 1958.

510. Santalo M, Domingo P, Fontcuberta J, et al: Diffuse pulmonary hemorrhage associated with anticoagulant therapy. Eur J Respir Dis 69:114, 1986.

511. Schaiberger P, Kennedy T, Miller F, et al: Pulmonary hypertension associated with long-term inhalation of "crack" methamphetamine. Chest 104:614, 1993.

512. Seigneur J, Trechot P, Hubert J, Lamy P: Pulmonary complications of hormone treatment in prostate carcinoma. Chest 93:1106, 1988.

513. Smith R, Alexander R, Aranda C: Pulmonary granulomata. A complication of intravesical administration of Bacillus Calmette-Guerin for superficial bladder carcinoma. Cancer 71:1846, 1993.

514. Stankus S, Johnson N: Propylthiouracil-induced hypersensitivity vasculitis presenting as respiratory failure. Chest 102:1595, 1992.

PNEUMOCONIOSIS

Pneumoconiosis is defined as a non-neoplastic reaction of the lungs, excluding asthma, bronchitis, and emphysema, to inhaled mineral or organic dust.[5] *Occupational* or *environmental lung disorder* is a broader concept that also includes reactions resulting from exposure to fumes, gases, and other irritants.[2–4] Many of these injurious agents cause histologic reactions such as diffuse alveolar damage (DAD) or hypersensitivity pneumonia, which are considered elsewhere in this monograph. Broad coverage and detailed descriptions of occupational lung disorders in general are available in several excellent texts.[1–5] This chapter focuses on the major pneumoconioses that are likely to be encountered by the surgical pathologist. It is meant to be a practical overview, but is by no means all-inclusive.

The reaction of the lung to any dust will vary with the properties of the dust (*fibrogenic* or *inert*), the size of the inspired particles, the length of exposure, individual susceptibility of the host, and many other factors.[2,3,5] The admixture of several types of dust may cause a different reaction than would be expected from one type of dust alone. The histologic response in the lung following chronic exposure to mineral dust can be divided into several general categories, which are summarized in Table 5–1. *Inert dusts* usually produce a nonpalpable interstitial aggregate of dust-filled macrophages known as a 'dust macule'. This type of reaction is often associated with an abnormal chest radiograph but has little accompanying functional deficit. *Fibrogenic dusts* can cause hyaline nodules or stellate areas of fibrosis, peribronchiolar fibrosis, diffuse interstitial fibrosis with or without noncaseating or foreign body granulomas, and large fibrous or cavitary masses (progressive massive fibrosis). An intraalveolar exudative reaction resembling pulmonary alveolar proteinosis (see Chapter 15) may occur following acute heavy exposure to silica.

Table 5–1 Common Pulmonary Reactions to Inorganic Dust Exposure

Histologic Reaction	Etiologic Dust	Disease
Dust macule	Coal dust	Coal workers' pneumoconiosis
	Iron/Iron oxides	Siderosis
Concentric hyaline nodules	Silica	Nodular silicosis
Stellate interstitial nodules	Silica plus inert dust	Mixed dust fibrosis
Diffuse interstitial fibrosis	Asbestos	Asbestosis
	Cobalt	Hard metal pneumoconiosis
	Silica (rarely)	Silicosis
Peribronchiolar fibrosis	Asbestos	
Granulomas		
Sarcoid-like	Beryllium	Berylliosis
Foreign body	Talc	Talc pneumoconiosis
Pulmonary alveolar proteinosis	Silica	Acute silicosis

Handling of Specimens

In general, if a pneumoconiosis is suspected clinically, a portion of tissue should be retained for analytical studies. The tissue may be frozen, but formalin-fixed tissue is also satisfactory. Fixatives containing mercuric or chromate compounds, however, should be avoided. Sodium cacodylate, commonly used as a buffer in glutaraldehyde fixatives, also should not be used, because it contains arsenic, which may contaminate the specimen. It should be remembered that the majority of pneumoconioses can be reliably diagnosed by light microscopy alone, and the most important step for the surgical pathologist is to ensure that *adequate tissue is maintained for routine histologic study.* Many analytic techniques can be performed on tissue not only embedded in paraffin blocks but also present on microscopic slides, and, therefore, small biopsy specimens should probably be entirely submitted for light microscopy.

DIAGNOSTIC METHODS FOR PNEUMOCONIOSIS

Clinical History

A complete and detailed clinical history is probably the most helpful factor in the diagnosis of pneumoconiosis and should include all past and present industrial or environmental exposure to dust and potentially toxic inhalants. Since there is usually a long latent period between exposure and development of pneumoconiosis, information needs to be obtained about all occupations, hobbies, or other potential sources of exposure that may have occurred at any time during the patient's life – not just in the recent past. Details should be provided regarding the precise mode and length of time of exposure and the nature of the substance inhaled. This information needs to be correlated along with the chest radiographic findings and results of pulmonary function tests.

Light Microscopy

Open lung biopsy, including video-assisted thoracoscopic methods, is the procedure of choice for diagnosing pneumoconioses, although success has been reported occasionally with transbronchial biopsies or percutaneous needle biopsies.[32,61,78,90] Analysis of alveolar macrophages obtained by bronchoalveolar lavage also may be productive in some cases.[6,32]

The usefulness of routine light microscopy in evaluating cases of suspected pneumoconiosis cannot be overemphasized. In most cases this technique can identify tissue reactions or particles that are associated with or suggestive of pneumoconiosis, such as interstitial fibrosis, granulomas, silicotic nodules, dust macules, ferruginous bodies, or talc fragments, for example. Of equal importance, it can document the absence of a tissue reaction indicative of a pneumoconiosis or detect changes that might suggest an alternative diagnosis. Special stains can aid light microscopic examination, such as the Prussian blue stain when searching for asbestos bodies and other iron-coated particles. The use of cross-polarizers may also help in some cases as a coarse screening procedure.[9,30] Close attention to light microscopic structural details of suspected inhaled particles will help both in identifying the material and in distinguishing it from an endogenous or otherwise insignificant substance.[2,55,128,139] For example, assessing the shape and appearance of the core of ferruginous bodies can suggest a specific mineral (see text following). Knowledge of the morphologic features of 'blue bodies' (see Chapter 1), corpora amylacea (see Chapter 1), or crystals common in sarcoidosis (see Chapter 6) will prevent mistaking these structures for inhaled agents of pneumoconiosis.

Analytic Techniques

A large number of analytic techniques can be used to examine tissue samples, although many are available only in research laboratories. The choice of a particular procedure will depend partly on its availability and partly on the specific question being posed.[2] Briefly, there are *bulk analytic techniques* that require destruction of the tissue and *microanalytic techniques* that can be performed on routine tissue sections. The latter are the most commonly available techniques. Since they can be applied to sections taken from routinely embedded paraffin blocks, they have the advantage that abnormal areas visualized under the microscope can be directly examined. They can also be applied to cells from bronchoalveolar lavage fluid. These microanalytic techniques employ both scanning and transmission electron microscopy and require an electron microscope equipped with an energy dispersive x-ray spectrometer.[7–9] This procedure yields mainly qualitative or semiquantitative results and usually does not detect elements lighter than sodium (such as beryllium). The bulk techniques (such as quantitative x-ray diffraction or atomic absorption spectroscopy, for example) are necessary for more precise quantitation of particles and for identification of light elements such as beryllium.

SILICOSIS

Free, or uncombined, silica (silicon dioxide) occurs in both crystalline and amorphous forms. Only the crystalline form, of which quartz is a major source,

Table 5–2   Diseases Associated with Silica Exposure

Disease	Latent Period	Pathologic Manifestation
Nodular silicosis		
Chronic	20+ years	Silicotic nodules
Accelerated	5–10 years	Silicotic nodules
Acute silicosis	1–3 years	Alveolar proteinosis
Mixed dust fibrosis	20+ years	Stellate interstitial fibrosis

is fibrogenic. *Silicosis* occurs as a reaction to inhaled crystalline silica. Exposure may be obvious and direct,[17,28,39] as in stonecutting, quarry work, or sandblasting, or it may occur when silica is a contaminant or an added component of other inspired dusts, such as asbestos, iron, coal dust, or clay.[39] In addition, exposure through trades, crafts, or even the household can lead to clinical disease.[18,20–22,39] Lung disease in some dental laboratory technicians may be a form of silicosis (see further on).[14] The classic pulmonary response to crystalline free silica is the formation of hyaline and collagenous nodules in the lung, but other reactions may also occur (Table 5–2).

Silica may be combined with a number of other elements, and the resultant minerals are termed *silicates*. These include asbestos, talc, mica, and kaolin, for example. This terminology is important, since the pathologic reactions to silica and silicates (see text following) are different.

Nodular Silicosis

Nodular, or 'pure', *silicosis* occurs in a *chronic form* after 20 or more years of exposure in occupations in which the respirable dust contains up to 30% quartz.[2,4,5,16,28,39] An *accelerated form* of the disease occurs after heavier exposure for 5 to 10 years.[5,16,39] The pathologic features of these disorders are the same and are characterized by the presence of small, discrete, hyalinized nodules, predominantly in the upper lobes of the lungs. Bronchopulmonary lymph nodes may contain similar lesions and often include a peripheral 'eggshell' type of calcification visible on chest radiographs. Silicotic nodules have also been described in the liver, spleen, bone marrow, and extrathoracic lymph nodes.[35]

Grossly, silicotic nodules are firm, discrete, rounded lesions that contain variable amounts of black pigment,

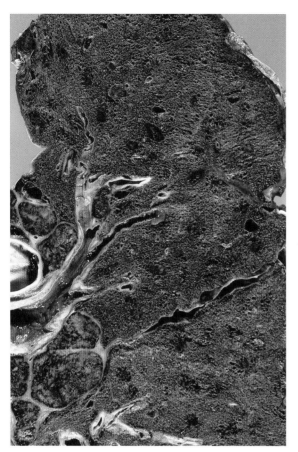

Figure 5–1 Gross appearance of nodular silicosis. There are scattered, well-demarcated, firm, black nodular lesions throughout the parenchyma of the upper lobe. Note also the enlarged, black peribronchial lymph nodes.

depending on whether there has been concomitant exposure to coal dust (Fig. 5–1).[2,5,39] The nodules tend to occur around respiratory bronchioles and small pulmonary arteries and in the subpleural and paraseptal areas. Progressive expansion causes obliteration of small airways and pulmonary vessels. Microscopically, silicotic nodules are composed of concentrically arranged, hyalinized, collagen bundles surrounded by variable numbers of dust-filled histiocytes (Fig. 5–2). In early nodules, fibroblasts and histiocytes are prominent, while acellular collagen lamellae predominate in older lesions (Fig. 5–3). Small, polarizable, doubly refractile, round or oval particles averaging 1 to 2 μm in diameter are often found within the nodules (see Fig. 5–3, *inset*). Their presence helps to confirm the diagnosis, but they may be absent in some cases, and they are not specific for silicosis.[16,30] Rarely, giant cells or granulomas occur

in the capsule of silicotic nodules, and their presence should raise the suspicion of associated mycobacterial infection (see later on). Likewise, central necrosis is unusual, and although it may result from ischemia, its presence should suggest a superimposed mycobacterial infection. The surrounding lung parenchyma may be largely unremarkable, although dust macules and pigment-laden macrophages are usually seen around small airways.

A nonspecific type of interstitial fibrosis has been noted occasionally in patients with chronic silicosis. Craighead and Vallyathan[17] described diffuse and localized pulmonary fibrotic lesions, usually without typical silicotic nodules, in autopsies of granite workers exposed to silica dust. Doubly refractile particles were not seen, but silica was identified by scanning electron microscopy and x-ray spectrometry. Interestingly, the chest radiographs in these patients did not show evidence of pneumoconiosis. Similar interstitial fibrosis has been described in foundry workers exposed to quartz admixed with cristobalite (another crystalline form of silica).[16] Nodular fibrosis and dust-filled macrophages without silicotic nodules have been reported in rush mat workers chronically exposed to dust containing 20–30% silica.[21]

Acute Silicosis

Acute silicosis is an unusual reaction caused by heavy exposure over a short period of time (1 to 3 years) to high levels of silica of small particle size.[13,16,37–39] Classically, it occurs in sandblasters, although non-occupational exposures such as inhalation of scouring powder have been reported rarely.[20] Histologically and ultrastructurally, the disease resembles *pulmonary alveolar proteinosis* (see Chapter 15) and is characterized by the filling of alveoli with an eosinophilic, granular, PAS-positive material.[16,25,38] Unlike ordinary pulmonary alveolar proteinosis, however, there are usually also interstitial inflammation and fibrosis or irregular hyaline scars as well as a variable amount of pigment. Silicotic nodules are poorly formed or absent in most cases, although they have been noted in a few.[16]

Complications of Silicosis

A variety of complications may result from silicosis.[2,4,5,16,39] Progressive massive fibrosis (PMF) is defined by the presence of nodular fibrosis that is greater than 1.0 cm in dimension. Usually there is a

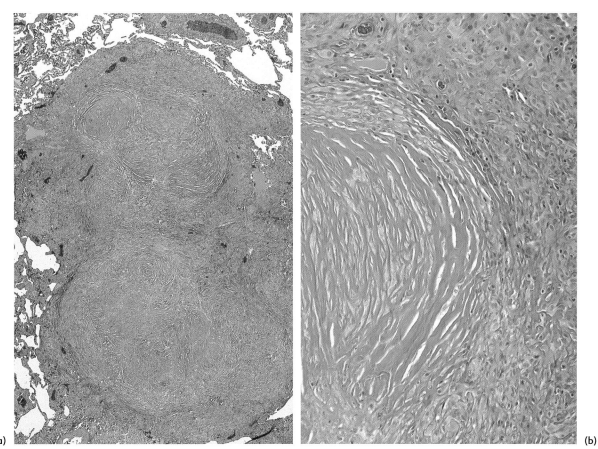

(a) (b)

Figure 5–2 Silicotic nodules. (a) At low magnification there are well-circumscribed collagenous nodules surrounded by a rim of histiocytes. **(b)** Higher magnification shows the lamellated appearance to the collagen bundles. Note the surrounding thick rim of histiocytes.

large amorphous mass of fibrous tissue that is composed of conglomerated nodules causing obliteration and contracture of lung parenchyma (Fig. 5–4). Typically the upper lobes are preferentially involved. This lesion also occurs in other pneumoconioses, including asbestosis, coal workers' pneumoconiosis, or mixed dust fibrosis, for example (see text following).[5,29] Central bronchial obstruction by fibrosis has been described as a rare complication of silicosis, and may be a variant of PMF.[27] The lesion shares some similarity with fibrosing mediastinitis (see Chapter 16).

Tuberculosis and nontuberculous mycobacteriosis are closely associated with silicosis and probably represent its most common complications.[11,16,33,36,39] These infections occur with both nodular and acute silicosis. They should be suspected clinically when there is rapid enlargement of small nodules or when nodules undergo cavitation. Histologically, the presence of necrosis

and/or granulomatous inflammation within silicotic nodules should suggest the diagnosis and stimulate a careful search of special stains for acid-fast bacilli.

In patients with rheumatoid arthritis, the silicotic nodule may show features resembling a rheumatoid nodule (*Caplan's syndrome*, see Chapter 7).[12,16] These nodules are characterized by central, acellular areas of necrosis surrounded by palisading histiocytes and a peripheral rim of lymphocytes and plasma cells. This lesion is identical to that occurring in coal workers with rheumatoid arthritis, as originally described by Caplan (see later on).[4,5] Other minerals may produce this reaction as well, such as asbestos, for example.[10]

An increased incidence of scleroderma has been noted in patients who are chronically exposed to silica, but this phenomenon remains unexplained.[16,39] Similarly, acute glomerulonephritis has been reported in association with accelerated silicosis.[16,19]

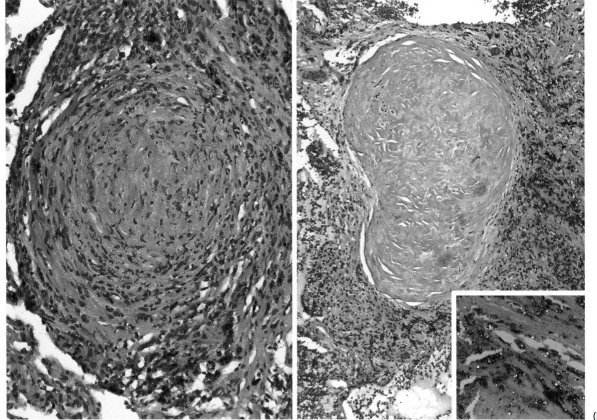

(a)   (b)

Figure 5–3 Silicotic nodules. (a) Early silicotic nodule characterized by numerous fibroblasts arranged in a lamellar configuration around the center. A thin layer of pigmented histiocytes is seen on the periphery. **(b)** Older nodule characterized by lamellated collagen bundles but very few cells. Note the surrounding layer of histiocytes. Inset shows the small, doubly refractile silica crystals in partially polarized light.

Pathogenesis

The pathogenesis of nodular silicosis has been studied in detail and appears to be related to the cytotoxic action of silica on alveolar macrophages.[16,18,28,31] These cells ingest the silica particles and die, perhaps liberating fibroblast-stimulating factors (interleukin 1, tumor necrosis factor alpha, transforming growth factor beta, platelet-derived growth factor, fibronectin, and so forth) which promote fibrosis.[16,18,34] A role for tissue mast cells has also been postulated.[24] There is also some evidence that silica interferes with the ability of macrophages to inhibit the growth of mycobacteria,[16,36] and this effect may explain the common association of tuberculosis with silicosis. In the acute form of silicosis, a direct toxic effect on alveolar type 2 cells, as well as on macrophages, may occur. A role for immunologic factors has long been postulated, but not proven, in silicosis.[16,19,28]

MIXED DUST FIBROSIS

Mixed dust fibrosis occurs when a mixture of silica and other less-fibrogenic dusts is inhaled. It affects foundry workers, arc welders, quarry workers, hematite miners, coal miners, pottery and ceramic workers, and boiler scalers, among others.[3–5,16,26] Cases have been described in African women who grind maize between rocks and are exposed to smoke in cooking huts (so-called hut lung).[23] *Siderosilicosis, anthracosilicosis,* and *slate worker's pneumoconiosis* are all examples of mixed dust pneumoconiosis.[2,15]

The clinical and radiographic features and the functional defects of mixed dust fibrosis are similar to those of silicosis except that the radiographic opacities tend to be more irregular.[2,16] Microscopically, however, the lesion differs in that silicotic nodules usually do not occur, presumably because the proportion of silica in

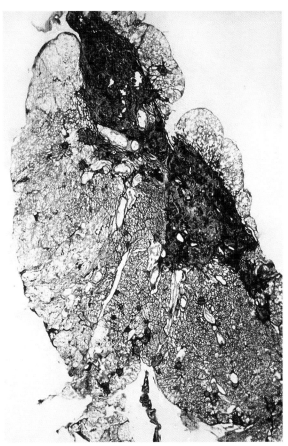

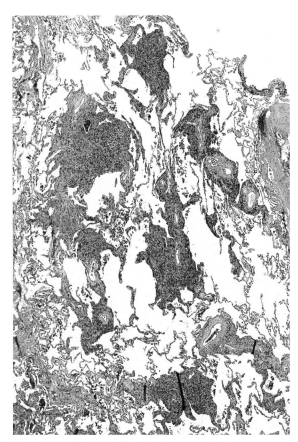

Figure 5–4 Progressive massive fibrosis. This Gough section of lung shows large confluent areas of scarring replacing portions of parenchyma. Note the small, round silicotic nodules present elsewhere in the parenchyma. (Courtesy of Dr Averill A Liebow.)

Figure 5–5 Mixed dust fibrosis. Low magnification view showing irregular, interstitial stellate-shaped cellular foci around respiratory bronchioles and alveolar ducts.

ASBESTOS-RELATED REACTIONS

the inspired dust is low. The characteristic histologic feature instead is patchy interstitial fibrosis that occurs predominantly in the area of respiratory bronchioles and adjacent small arteries but which may spread into the surrounding parenchyma in an irregular fashion (Fig. 5–5).[26] The fibrotic zones have a characteristic stellate shape and, at higher magnification, consist of a mixture of fibroblasts, collagen fibers, and dust-filled macrophages (Fig. 5–6). Large areas of uninvolved parenchyma are usually present between the fibrotic zones although dust macules may be prominent. Variable associated pigmentation is seen, depending on the nature of the associated inert dust (Fig. 5–7).[16] Often, the inert dust consists of iron oxides, which appear as yellow–brown deposits that stain positively with Prussian blue.

The term *asbestos* refers to a group of hydrated silicates, i.e. minerals composed of silica plus iron, magnesium, sodium, or other metals in varying combinations. A detailed description of the geologic and mineralogic features of asbestos and related compounds can be found elsewhere,[2,5] but, in general, two classes of asbestos fibers are commonly encountered: the *serpentine group* (of which chrysotile is the major type) and the *amphibole group* (of which amosite and crocidolite are the most important.)[47–49] Chrysotile is the type of asbestos used most frequently in industry. Special techniques such as energy-dispersive x-ray analysis, electron diffraction, or mass spectrometry are required for definitive fiber identification.[2,48,54] Chrysotile fibers are relatively soluble in lung fluids, and they are somewhat less likely to cause disease than are other forms

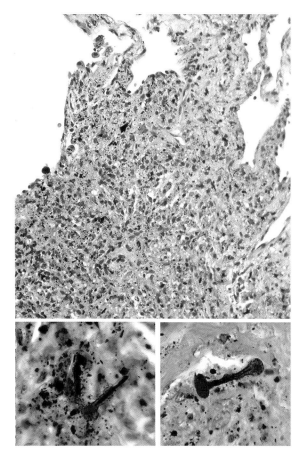

Figure 5–6 Mixed dust fibrosis. Higher magnification of the characteristic stellate-shaped interstitial infiltrate composed of histiocytes, fibroblasts, and pigment. Insets are higher magnifications showing the golden brown to black pigment containing ferruginous bodies. The ferruginous bodies differ from asbestos bodies in that they contain black rather than clear cores.

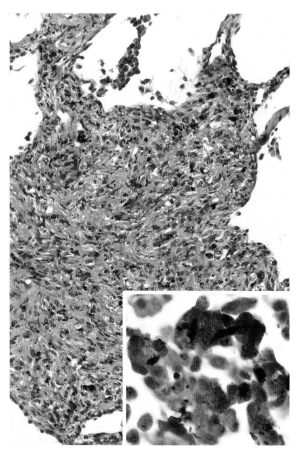

Figure 5–7 Black pigmentation is prominent in this example of mixed dust fibrosis. Inset is a higher magnification view showing a mixture of golden brown and black pigment in adjacent alveolar macrophages.

of asbestos. Also, because they may be dissolved, the fibers identified in tissue late after exposure may not be representative of every type of asbestos to which the patient has been exposed.[47–49,59]

Asbestos fibers are a type of fibrous particle that by definition have a length of at least three times their diameter.[5] They cause a more diffuse reaction in the lung than the compact particles of silica. They are also associated with a wider variety of reactions in the thorax, including the production of neoplasms, as summarized in Table 5–3.[42,50,54,83]

Asbestosis

Asbestosis is defined as interstitial pulmonary fibrosis caused by inhaled asbestos dust.[2,5,31,49,54,70,83] The

Table 5–3	Asbestos-Associated Reactions in the Thorax
Lung	**Pleura**
Interstitial fibrosis (*asbestosis*)	Plaques
Peribronchiolar fibrosis	Diffuse pleural fibrosis
Round atelectasis	Pleuritis with effusion
Carcinoma	Mesothelioma

interstitial fibrosis is preferentially distributed in the lower lobes (although upper lobe disease has been reported) and is frequently accompanied by pleural fibrosis and calcification.[40,42,54,74] The development of asbestosis requires heavy exposure to asbestos, and there is a threshold below which disease does not occur.[2,31] A latent period of 15 to 20 years following exposure is usually present, although the latency depends somewhat on exposure dose, with heavier exposure producing disease more quickly and smaller doses having a longer latency period.[31,70,97] Clinically, asbestosis resembles other chronic interstitial lung diseases in that patients manifest dyspnea, clubbing, restrictive pulmonary function defects, and bilateral interstitial opacities on chest radiographs.[42,68] Interstitial fibrosis can progress even after exposure has ceased – a phenomenon related, at least in part, to the persistence of asbestos fibers in the lungs.[2,5]

Occupational exposure to asbestos may be by direct handling or, more indirectly, by working in an area where asbestos is used by others, as well as by working with products in which asbestos is a component.[2,5,54] Nonoccupational and nonindustrial exposure may result from environmental or air pollution.[2,54] There are also reported cases of asbestosis acquired in the home from exposure to dust-contaminated work clothes.[67]

Pathologic Features

The interstitial fibrosis of asbestosis varies in appearance, but in many cases is indistinguishable from usual interstitial pneumonia (UIP, see Chapter 3).[2,70,98] Those cases are characterized by patchy, non-uniform alveolar septal fibrosis alternating with residual areas of normal lung (Fig. 5–8). Areas of end-stage honeycomb lung may be present, and active ongoing fibrosis (fibroblast foci) may be found in addition to collagen-type fibrosis. The interstitial fibrosis in other cases appears more uniform, with less architectural distortion, and fits with fibrosing nonspecific interstitial pneumonia (see Chapter 3). Changes resembling desquamative interstitial pneumonia (DIP) have been described in a few cases as well, but likely represent DIP-like reactions

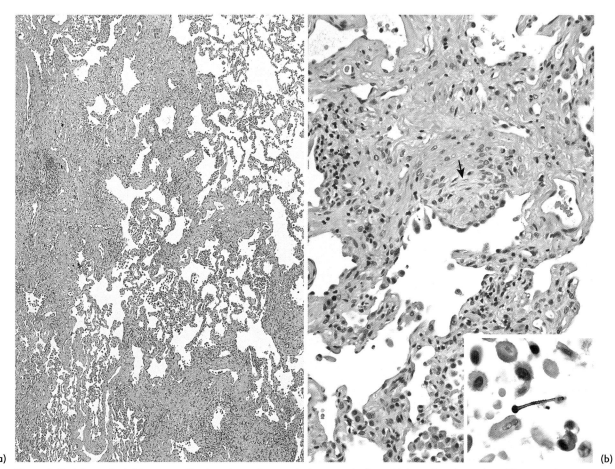

(a)   (b)

Figure 5–8 Asbestosis. (a) Low magnification photomicrograph shows patchy interstitial scarring alternating with areas of relatively normal lung. The appearance is similar to usual interstitial pneumonia. **(b)** At higher magnification a fibroblast focus (arrow) can be appreciated, and there is an intraalveolar asbestos body (inset). Note the clear core in the asbestos body.

(see Chapter 3) related to interstitial fibrosis.[2,54] Cytoplasmic accumulation within alveolar epithelial cells of amorphous eosinophilic material resembling Mallory, or alcoholic, hyalin may occur.[2,79] It is not a specific diagnostic feature, however, since it has also been described in other interstitial pneumonias and DAD (see Fig. 3–8). PMF, usually affecting the lower lobes, has been reported rarely.[5,29] Localized inflammatory lesions, including bronchiolitis obliterans–organizing pneumonia (BOOP) and granulomas, for example, have also been reported.[72] They most likely represent superimposed conditions, however, and should not be considered manifestations of asbestosis.

An early manifestation of asbestos exposure is peribronchiolar fibrosis.[2,41,44,54,95,98] It can be the only abnormality present or it can accompany the diffuse interstitial fibrosis of full-blown asbestosis. Whether the diagnosis of asbestosis can be made in biopsies showing only peribronchiolar fibrosis and asbestos bodies (but not diffuse interstitial fibrosis) is a controversial issue, but most authorities require the presence of diffuse interstitial fibrosis.[49,50] This type of small airways lesion is not specific for asbestos exposure, since it may occur in the absence of asbestos bodies.[47,95,96] Moreover, there is also no evidence that it necessarily progresses to diffuse interstitial fibrosis.

The diagnosis of asbestosis depends on identifying asbestos fibers or bodies (see text following) in lung tissue in addition to diffuse interstitial fibrosis.[2,49,50,54] Using light microscopy and ordinary 5-μm-thick sections, the demonstration of at least one asbestos body in a setting of diffuse pulmonary fibrosis is considered diagnostic of asbestosis.[54,92] Although asbestos bodies and uncoated fibers are an indication of exposure, it should be remembered that they are not per se (in the absence of interstitial fibrosis) an indication of disease (i.e. asbestosis).[46–49,54,59,65] Additionally, other forms of diffuse interstitial lung disease, including idiopathic pulmonary fibrosis, can occur in asbestos-exposed individuals.[49,68] Therefore, careful documentation of exposure history and knowledge of the clinical and radiographic manifestations are mandatory. Sometimes, analytic electron microscopy will also be needed to sort out difficult cases.[68,77]

Although the diagnosis of asbestosis usually requires an open lung biopsy, cutting needle[90] and transbronchial lung biopsies[61,78] have been reported to be diagnostic in some cases. Asbestos bodies can also be identified in bronchoalveolar lavage fluids and sputum, but in this situation they are more a marker of exposure than a criterion for diagnosing asbestosis.[58,63,86,87,89,91]

Asbestos Bodies and Fibers

Asbestos fibers can be identified in hematoxylin and eosin (H and E)-stained sections by the presence of a histologic marker, the *asbestos body*.[48,54,59,68,92] They are present mainly in lung parenchyma, but can be identified in hilar lymph nodes as well as in the omentum, mesentery, and pleural plaques if tissue digestion techniques are used.[62,64,74,82] Asbestos bodies are formed when the fibers become coated by minute iron particles, probably related to endogenous ferritin, and they may be found within cells or lying free (Fig. 5–9).[48,54] Since compounds other than asbestos (including fibrous glass, aluminum silicates, diatomaceous earth, and other materials) can become similarly coated, the term *ferruginous body* is used to include all such iron-coated particles.[128] With careful attention to structural detail, however, true asbestos bodies can be accurately identified histologically and separated from most other materials that produce ferruginous bodies.[2,54,55]

Asbestos bodies are characterized by a clear central core surrounded by a golden yellow coating with terminal bulbs or knobs that may have a diffusely beaded pattern (Fig. 5–10).[48,54] This clear core distinguishes asbestos bodies from other ferruginous bodies that contain black or brown cores (see Fig. 5–6, *insets*). Asbestos bodies are generally straight, but curved, and even branched, forms have been noted. They can vary in length from 10 to over 100 μm and in width from

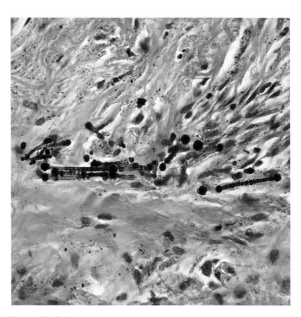

Figure 5–9 Asbestos bodies. Refractile-appearing, brown–yellow, elongated beaded structures with bulbous ends are present within scarred lung.

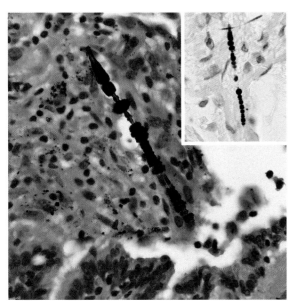

Figure 5–10 Asbestos bodies. At higher magnification the golden brown coating with beaded configuration is seen surrounding the characteristic central clear core. Inset is a Prussian blue iron stain that highlights the asbestos body. The clear core can still be appreciated.

1 to 6 μm. Rarely, oxalate crystals are deposited on their surface.[70] Iron stains are very helpful in demonstrating asbestos bodies, especially when they are inconspicuous in H and E-stained material (see Fig. 5–10, *inset*). Some investigators have found asbestos fibers as contaminants in paraffin blocks, although others have been unable to confirm this observation.[60,80]

Structures similar to asbestos bodies have been reported in tissues and bronchoalveolar lavage fluids from persons exposed to refractory ceramic fibers.[66] Refractory ceramic fibers have been used to replace asbestos in high-temperature insulations, and when coated with iron may mimic asbestos bodies. A careful exposure history should suggest the nature of the fibers, and the diagnosis can be confirmed by analytical electron microscopy.

Uncoated asbestos fibers are often present in addition to asbestos bodies, but, since they have a diameter of less than 1 μm, they are difficult to find by light microscopy. Darkfield microscopy may help in identifying these fibers, and they are well visualized by transmission or scanning electron microscopy.[76] Various studies have indicated that the uncoated asbestos fibers outnumber asbestos bodies by ratios ranging from 30:1 to 200:1.[2,52] They can be identified in pleural plaques and other extrapulmonary sites.[62,64,82] Definitive identification of fiber types requires x-ray or mass spectrometry with the analysis of elements present in the individual fibers.[2,54,64]

Population studies have indicated that asbestos exposure is widespread, as reflected by the frequent presence of asbestos bodies in lung fluids, sections, or extracts.[2,43,46–48,54,58,59,65,68,87,92] The exact prevalence varies with the efficacy of the laboratory technique, but small numbers of bodies have been found in 20% to almost 100% of the general population in assorted studies.[2] A quantitative measurement of asbestos bodies can be made by counting asbestos bodies in the sediment obtained after dissolving a weighed portion of lung, using bleach or another form of digestion.[2,54,69,72] By means of this technique, various investigators have demonstrated that asbestos workers usually have from 10,000 to 100,000 bodies per gram of lung tissue, patients with asbestosis have even higher values, and white-collar workers (environmental exposure) have under 100 – and generally under 50 – asbestos bodies per gram of lung.[2,54,59,93] Vollmer and Roggli[92] have devised a mathematical formula that appears to predict asbestos body concentration in the lung from counts in microscopic sections.

Other Reactions to Asbestos

A number of benign pleural reactions have been associated with asbestos exposure, including *hyaline plaques, diffuse pleural fibrosis,* and *fibrinous pleuritis* with effusion.[2,54,56,74,85] *Pleural plaques* are localized areas of hyalinized fibrosis, often containing foci of calcification that occur predominantly on the parietal pleura.[73] They are usually bilateral and most often are located on the posterior lower lobes and diaphragm. They are composed of thick collagen bundles, often arranged in parallel or showing a basket-weave pattern. Asbestos fibers have been identified in plaques as well as in anthracotic areas ('black spots') on the parietal pleura using analytic electron microscopy.[64] Asbestos bodies, however, are not found in routine sections of pleural plaques, although they have been demonstrated by the digestion-filtration technique.[74]

Diffuse pleural fibrosis is an uncommon complication of asbestos exposure and is characterized by extensive collagenous thickening that may encase the entire lung.[88] It must be distinguished from malignant mesothelioma, especially the sclerosing or desmoplastic variant. The presence of cytologically atypical cells or cellular foci of spindle-shaped cells within the areas of dense collagen deposition should suggest mesothelioma. In patients with *pleural effusion,* pleural biopsies show an active *pleuritis* with a chronic inflammatory cell infiltrate, fibroblast proliferation, a fibrinous or proteinaceous exudate, and prominent hyperplasia of mesothelial cells.[81] The latter cells may manifest considerable cytologic atypia and must be distinguished from malignant neoplasms. The fact that they occur only on the surface of the pleura without invasion into underlying stroma is a helpful feature.

Asbestos has been convincingly implicated in the production of neoplasms.[54,57] *Malignant mesothelioma*, both pleural and peritoneal, is probably the best-known example. Although there is evidence for a dose–response relationship in the production of interstitial fibrosis by asbestos, this phenomenon does not appear to be true for mesothelioma.[2,43,52–54,71,90] Interstitial fibrosis is usually not present in patients with pleural mesotheliomas, although asbestos bodies are commonly found in the lung.

The relationship of asbestos exposure to lung *carcinoma* has been difficult to prove because of the frequent presence of other carcinogens, especially cigarette smoke. There is evidence, however, that the combination of asbestos exposure and cigarette smoking leads to a greatly increased incidence of lung carcinoma compared with nonsmoking, non-asbestos-exposed individuals.[2,54,57] This increase may be due in part to enhanced accumulation of asbestos fibers in the airway mucosa of cigarette smokers.[51] Asbestos exposure alone appears to be associated with a smaller, but documented, increase in the incidence of lung carcinoma.[2] In several studies, these asbestos-associated carcinomas have had a lower lobe predominance,[2,54] a feature that is unusual for primary pulmonary cancer in the general population. From a legal standpoint, however, lung carcinoma is considered related to asbestos exposure only if there is also evidence of diffuse interstitial fibrosis (i.e. asbestosis).[2,50]

Round atelectasis is another finding that may be associated with asbestos exposure, and it is discussed in detail in Chapter 16.[75] Briefly, it represents a focus of thickened, fibrotic pleura that becomes invaginated into the lung, causing collapse of adjacent parenchyma. It produces a radiographic opacity that may mimic a neoplasm.

Pathogenesis of Asbestos-Related Diseases

Factors related to the development of asbestosis include preferential aerodynamic distribution of fibers within the lower lung fields and also production of fibrogenic factors by macrophages, as in other fibrotic lung diseases.[31,84] Phagocytosis of asbestos fibers by macrophages is thought to cause release of mediators that attract inflammatory cells and promote fibrosis. Additionally, release of oxidants may cause epithelial cell damage that promotes restructuring of lung parenchyma.[69] One hypothesis for the formation of pleural plaques involves repeated pleural injury by fibers protruding from the lung.[2] The increased incidence of carcinoma may be partly related to scarring and reparative phenomena in patients with asbestosis.

COAL WORKERS' PNEUMOCONIOSIS

Coal workers' pneumoconiosis (CWP) refers to the pulmonary reaction to inhaled coal dust, and it occurs in both *simple* and *complicated* forms.[101,102,104,105,108,109] Coal miners may develop several other types of pneumoconiosis as well, depending on the nature of the dusts to which they are exposed; silicosis or mixed dust fibrosis, for example, may develop when inhaled dust has a high silica content or when there is exposure to the sand used in mining operations.[100,102,108]

Coal dust is a complicated mixture of elemental carbon and various organic compounds, metals, and minerals. The respirable particles are angular in outline and range in size from submicroscopic to 10 µm. They vary from yellow–brown and translucent (bituminous coal) to dark and opaque (anthracite coal) when seen through the light microscope.[102]

Simple CWP

Simple CWP is characterized by the presence of dust macules and nodules that are usually most prominent in the upper lobes. Grossly, these lesions are characterized by discrete, patchy black collections of dust (Fig. 5–11). Macules are located around bronchioles and are not palpable, while nodules are more widely distributed, often in subpleural areas, and are palpable. Focal emphysema characterized by dilatation of adjacent airspaces is often associated with the dust deposition.[104] Whether this type of emphysema is different from the centrilobular emphysema related to cigarette smoking in the general population is a controversial issue.[102,104,105,107]

Microscopically, coal dust macules are characterized by an accumulation of dust-filled macrophages in the interstitium surrounding respiratory bronchioles

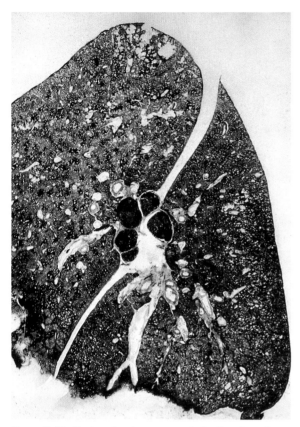

Figure 5–11 Coal workers' pneumoconiosis. Gough section showing black pigment deposition around respiratory bronchioles.

(Fig. 5–12). They usually appear stellate shaped because of extension of the cellular infiltrate into the surrounding alveolar septa. Fibrosis is minimal or absent. Coal nodules contain, in addition to dust-filled macrophages, a fibrous stroma with haphazardly arranged collagen bundles. The presence of these nodules is required to diagnose CWP, since dust macules may be found in urban dwellers with no mining exposure.

Little functional deficit can be attributed to the lesions of simple CWP, and radiographic changes may be minimal or absent.[106,109] Some of the reported abnormalities of pulmonary function in simple CWP, such as a mild increase in residual volume and other minor defects, may be related to industrial bronchitis. This lesion is an inflammatory process in the large airways that is a consequence of dust exposure. Industrial bronchitis accompanies CWP and other pneumoconioses, and histologically is not distinguishable from chronic bronchitis in the general public.[2,3]

Complicated CWP

Complicated CWP is characterized by the development of large, usually bilateral areas of fibrosis referred to as *progressive massive fibrosis* (PMF).[2,4,5,29,109] In contrast to simple CWP, PMF is often associated with pulmonary function abnormalities, including obstructive defects, abnormal diffusing capacity, and restrictive defects.[4,78]

PMF may be a feature of several different pneumoconiosis (see Fig. 5–4). When it occurs in CWP, large black masses that are round, oval, or stellate in configuration and often have a central cavity obliterate portions of the lung.[2,104] By definition, nodules or masses greater than 1 cm in diameter are designated PMF, but many lesions are much larger and may cross the lobar septa. Microscopically, PMF consists of irregular bundles of collagen between which dust is deposited. Varying numbers of lymphocytes and plasma cells are also present. Obliterated arteries, veins, and airways are seen in the center of the lesion and can be identified with elastic tissue stains. Blood vessels around the periphery are often destroyed by the chronic inflammatory cell infiltrate and fibrosis, and muscularization of pulmonary arterioles in adjacent lung parenchyma may be prominent.[103] Central necrosis may occur secondary to ischemia related to the vascular obliteration. Since granulomatous infections may also cause necrosis, however, special stains for mycobacteria and fungi should be carefully examined in such cases.

Other lesions may also be associated with CWP. Classic silicotic nodules occur occasionally, and ordinary infectious granulomas caused by mycobacteria or fungi can be found. *Caplan's nodules* are large (up to 5 cm in diameter) nodular lesions that occur in coal workers who have rheumatoid arthritis.[12,16] The nodules may precede or follow the clinical presentation of arthritis. They are identical to the nodules described in patients with silicosis and rheumatoid arthritis (see previous section). Microscopically, they resemble rheumatoid nodules, except that there is usually also associated dust accumulation.

The pathogenesis of PMF is not known, although the following factors appear to be associated with an increased risk of developing the lesion: (1) high total dust content of the lung, (2) the presence of silica in the inspired dust (usually in the form of quartz), and (3) tuberculosis.[5,102,104] The immunologic reactivity in the patient is also likely important in the pathogenesis of this condition.

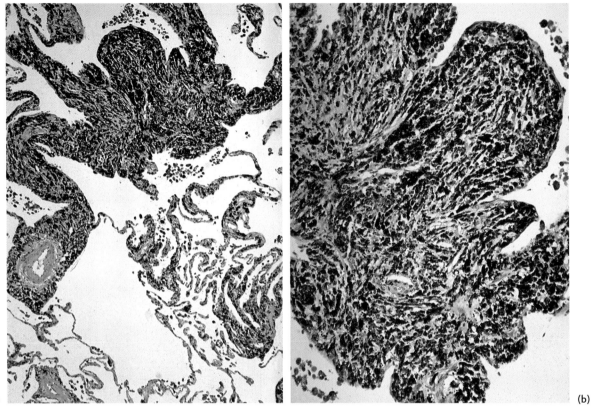

(a)

(b)

Figure 5–12 Coal workers' pneumoconiosis. (a) Low magnification showing a dust macule characterized by dust-filled histiocytes expanding the interstitium around a respiratory bronchiole. Note the adjacent focal emphysema. **(b)** Higher magnification showing the sheets of histiocytes containing black pigment that are present within the interstitium.

OTHER PNEUMOCONIOSES

Siderosis

Siderosis results from exposure to inert metallic iron or iron oxides and is characterized by the formation of dust macules similar to those seen in CWP (Fig. 5–13).[2,4,135] The macules in siderosis differ, however, in that they contain coarse, brown–black, irregular particles of iron oxides admixed with variable numbers of golden brown hemosiderin particles. In extensively involved lungs, this accumulation of iron oxide and hemosiderin imparts a striking rusty brown gross appearance (Fig. 5–14). The Prussian blue reaction is helpful in identifying the iron content of the dust microscopically, although it is perhaps endogenous hemosiderin (ferrugination of exogenous iron particles) – and not the inhaled iron or iron oxide – that is being stained.[2]

Siderosis is most often seen in iron workers, hematite miners, and welders, and is also known as *arc welder's lung* or *hematite lung*. When these individuals are also exposed to silica, a form of mixed dust fibrosis (*siderosilicosis*, see previous section) may result, in which there are characteristic patchy, stellate-shaped foci of fibrosis and dust (see Figs 5–5 and 5–6).

Berylliosis

Berylliosis is a systemic disease caused by exposure to beryllium or beryllium compounds.[113,122,130,132,144,149,150,163] Exposure usually occurs in the workplace, especially in the aerospace, computer, ceramics, electronics, and beryllium extraction and production industries, but nonoccupational exposures have also been described.[162] Rare cases have been reported in dental technicians.[148] The disease may present as an acute process or in a chronic form. *Acute berylliosis* produces DAD (see Chapter 2), and recovery is the usual outcome. *Chronic berylliosis* develops in a small number of individuals who manifest the acute syndrome, and

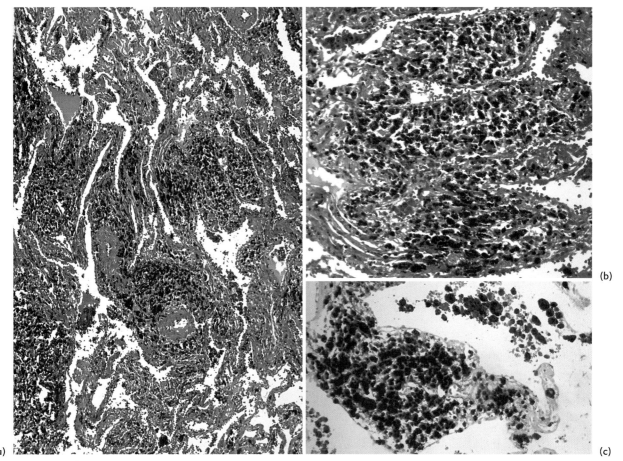

Figure 5–13 Siderosis. (a) Low magnification showing dust macules containing golden brown to black pigment. **(b)** Higher magnification better demonstrates the abundant brown to black pigmented macrophages within interstitium. **(c)** A Prussian blue iron stain is strongly positive in the macule.

it may also occur in patients without documented acute disease. The latent period from the last exposure to onset of disease may be as long as 15 years. Microscopically, chronic berylliosis is characterized by interstitial fibrosis, usually accompanied by noncaseating, 'sarcoid-like' granulomas. The changes may exactly mimic sarcoidosis, although granulomas are poorly formed or absent in some cases. Small hyaline nodules occasionally demonstrating central necrosis may also be seen.[2,150]

Definitive diagnosis, especially the differentiation from sarcoidosis, may be possible only by correlating the exposure history, clinical course, and radiographic findings.[143,175a] Tissue analysis by biochemical or physical means may be helpful. Beryllium is not readily demonstrated in tissue by microanalytic techniques, however, although new technologies utilizing electron probe x-ray analysis are being developed.[119,144]

Peripheral blood or bronchoalveolar lavage lymphocyte blast transformation studies appear to be reliable ancillary diagnostic tests.[132,160,162–164,171]

Talc and Other Silicate Pneumoconioses

Talc is a silicate compound encountered in several industries, including rubber, plastics, ceramics, paint, paper, and cosmetics. In addition to disease from industrial exposure, examples of talcosis caused by massive inhalation of cosmetic talcum powder have been reported.[117,138] Talc is commonly contaminated with other minerals, such as asbestos, silica, or mica, for example. Histologic reactions, therefore, vary depending on the associated mineral present.[117,136] Hyaline nodules, interstitial fibrosis, or a combination of the two patterns have been described, and foreign body granulomas containing plate-like birefringent

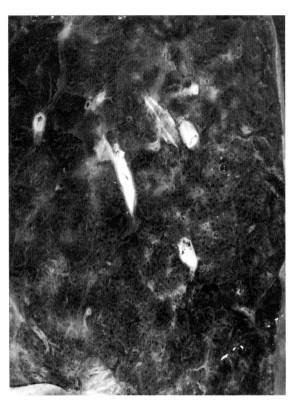

Figure 5–14 Gross appearance of siderosis. Note the brown–orange 'rusty' appearance to the lung. This specimen is from a hematite miner.

particles may be seen. Talc particles can also be found within macrophage cytoplasm or lying free within areas of fibrosis.

The vast majority of inhaled talc particles are smaller than 5 μm in diameter. The presence of larger particles should suggest that there has been intravenous injection of oral medications as the source (see Chapter 13).[110,174] Talc acquired by intravenous injection ranges in size from 14 to 50 μm in greatest dimension. It differs from inhaled talc in that it is located almost exclusively within or around small blood vessels, and it is often admixed with other material, such as methylcellulose.

Other silicates may be encountered in industry or in the environment. Mica, kaolin, bauxite, vermiculite, and fly ash have all been reported to produce pulmonary fibrosis.[116,129,139,151,158,166] These minerals may also be contaminated by silica or asbestos.

Hard Metal Pneumoconiosis

Hard metal is composed of a mixture of tungsten carbide and cobalt, sometimes also with small amounts of other metals, including titanium, tantalum, chromium, or nickel.[112,114,124,176] It exhibits extreme hardness and resistance to high temperatures and therefore is used for grinding, drilling, cutting, or sharpening. Exposure can occur both in the production of hard metal and in industries utilizing this substance, such as in diamond polishing and tool grinding, for example.

Hard metal pneumoconiosis causes a form of diffuse interstitial lung disease, and patients usually present with dyspnea and restrictive pulmonary function tests. Recovery may occur after cessation of exposure, although fatal cases have been described.[121,124,161]

The pathologic findings in most cases of hard metal pneumoconiosis correspond to the form of chronic interstitial pneumonia known as *giant cell interstitial pneumonia* (GIP).[112,121,123,165,169,175] This lesion is characterized by patchy interstitial fibrosis with a scant inflammatory cell infiltrate that is accentuated around bronchioles (Fig. 5–15). The striking feature is the accumulation within adjacent airspaces of alveolar macrophages (a DIP-like reaction, see Chapter 3), many of which are enlarged and multinucleated – hence the name 'giant cell interstitial pneumonia'. A characteristic feature of the multinucleated giant cells is that their cytoplasm often contains one or more engulfed inflammatory cells, either macrophages or neutrophils. Scattered eosinophils may be admixed with the intra-alveolar macrophage infiltrate, and alveolar pneumocytes are usually hyperplastic and may be multinucleated. Microanalytic studies generally identify only tungsten within the tissue, although experimental studies suggest that cobalt, rather than tungsten, is the causative agent in this pneumoconiosis.[112,114,121,161] While the finding of GIP on a biopsy specimen should suggest hard metal pneumoconiosis, rare cases lacking an exposure history or tissue evidence of metal deposition have been reported.[123]

Miscellaneous

Aluminum powder, ore, or dust inhalation most commonly is associated with an asthma-like syndrome and chronic obstructive lung disease.[111] Interstitial fibrosis has been described rarely, but whether this reaction is due to aluminum per se or to a contaminating, more fibrogenic dust such as silica or asbestos, for example, is not clear.[116,125,137,141,142] Sarcoid-like granulomas, DIP (see Chapter 3),[126,140] and pulmonary alveolar proteinosis (see Chapter 15)[156] have been described as unusual manifestations of aluminum-induced lung disease. Granulomas have been associated

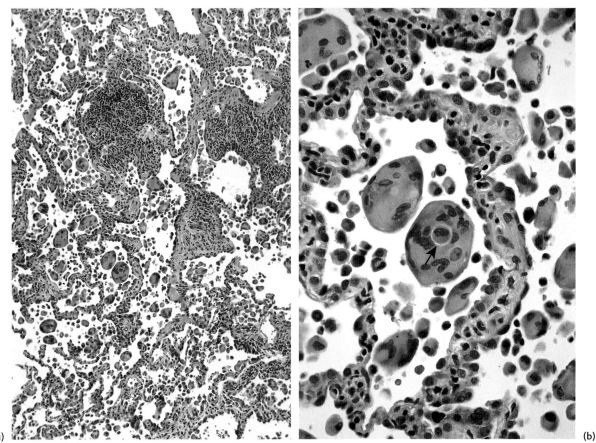

(a)
(b)

Figure 5–15 Hard metal pneumoconiosis (giant cell interstitial pneumonia). (a) Low magnification showing interstitial inflammation and fibrosis associated with increased numbers of alveolar macrophages. Multinucleated giant cells can be appreciated even at low magnification. (b) Higher magnification showing intraalveolar multinucleated giant cells. Note the ingested macrophage (emperipoiesis) within one giant cell (arrow).

rarely with *titanium* exposure,[168] and there is some evidence that titanium may also cause interstitial fibrosis.[157] *Silicon carbide (carborundum)* has been shown to cause a distinctive form of pneumoconiosis characterized by nodular and interstitial fibrosis, intraalveolar pigmented macrophages, and ferruginous bodies.[134,154] Interstitial fibrosis has been described rarely in patients exposed to rare earth elements, especially cerium (*rare earth pneumoconiosis*).[155] Carbon arc lamps have been an important exposure source, and rare elements are also encountered in a variety of industrial settings.

A nodular and granulomatous interstitial pulmonary infiltrate has been described in *vineyard sprayers* exposed to a pesticide composed of copper sulfate and hydrated lime.[177] This lesion may progress to form hyaline scars, and apparently some cases have been misdiagnosed as silicosis. Interstitial fibrosis resembling mixed dust fibrosis has been reported in dentists and dental technicians, so-called *dental technician's pneumoconiosis*, and may be related to inhaled silica, silicates, metal alloys (especially cobalt–chromium–molybdenum), and alginate powder.[14,127,153,159,170,173] Interstitial pneumonia associated with large numbers of foamy macrophages has been attributed to the inhalation of *acrylic resin* in dental laboratory workers.[115]

Although *polyvinyl chloride* (PVC) is not a mineral dust, it warrants discussion. Inhalation of PVC particles produces an interstitial accumulation of macrophages and giant cells, and there may be associated interstitial inflammation and fibrosis. Ultrastructural study demonstrates oval intracytoplasmic particles, apparently representing PVC dust within the macrophages.[120,152] *Fibrous glass* has been suggested as a cause of pneumoconiosis, and particles of this material have been identified by phase microscopy in the lungs of patients with interstitial fibrosis. Most of the patients, however, had other exposure histories, and there is no clear evidence that clinically significant lung fibrosis results from exposure to fibrous glass alone.[131,178] Interstitial fibrosis due to chronic inhalation of *wood smoke* has been described in rare cases.[167,172]

A form of interstitial lung disease has been detected in workers in the flocking industry (*flock worker's lung*).[133,145,146,147] Flocking is a process whereby synthetic fibers (mainly nylon in the reported cases) are cut into short lengths and applied to a fabric to produce a plush finish. Patients present with dyspnea, cough, restrictive ventilatory defects, and interstitial markings on chest radiographs and computed tomography examinations. A lymphocytic bronchiolitis and associated peribronchiolar interstitial pneumonia have been described in about half the cases.[118] Lymphoid hyperplasia is often present as well. Nonspecific interstitial pneumonia and BOOP have been noted less often.[146] The disease is important to recognize, since removal from the workplace is essential. Most patients recover after exposure is terminated.

REFERENCES

General

1. Baxter PJ, Adams PH, Aw T-C, et al, eds: *Hunter's Diseases of Occupations*, 9th ed, London, Hodder Arnold, 2000.
2. Churg A, Green FHY, eds: *Pathology of Occupational Lung Disease*, 2nd ed, Baltimore, Williams & Williams, 1998.
3. Gee JBL, ed: *Occupational Lung Disease*, New York, Churchill Livingstone, 1984.
4. Morgan WKC, Seaton A: *Occupational Lung Diseases*, 3rd ed, Philadelphia, WB. Saunders, 1995.
5. Parkes WR: *Occupational Lung Disorders*, 3rd ed, London, Butterworth-Heinemann, 1994.

Diagnostic Methods for Pneumoconiosis

6. Johnson NF, Haslam PL, Dewar A, et al: Identification of inorganic dust particles in bronchoalveolar lavage macrophages by energy dispersive x-ray microanalysis. Arch Environ Health 41:133, 1986.
7. Leyden DE: Energy dispersive x-ray spectrometry. Spectroscopy 2:28, 1986.
8. Terzakis JA: X-ray microanalysis. Problem solving in surgical pathology. Pathol Annu 20:59, 1985.
9. Vallyathan NV, Green FHY, Craighead JE: Recent advances in the study of mineral pneumoconiosis. Pathol Annu 15:77, 1980.

Silicosis and Mixed Dust Pneumoconiosis

10. Antilla S, Sutinen S, Paakko P, Finell B: Rheumatoid pneumoconiosis in a dolomite worker: A light and electron microscopic, and x-ray microanalytical study. Br J Dis Chest 78:195, 1984.
11. Bailey WC, Brown M, Buechner HA, et al: Silico-mycobacterial disease in sandblasters. Am Rev Respir Dis 110:115, 1974.
12. Benedek TG: Rheumatoid pneumoconiosis. Documentation of onset and pathogenetic considerations. Am J Med 55:515, 1973.
13. Buechner HA, Ansari A: Acute silico-proteinosis. A new pathologic variant of acute silicosis in sandblasters, characterized by histologic features resembling alveolar proteinosis. Dis Chest 55:274, 1969.
14. Centers for Disease Control and Prevention (CDC): Silicosis in dental laboratory technicians – five states 1994–2000. MMWR Morb Mortal Wkly Rep 53:195, 2004.
15. Craighead JE, Emerson RJ, Stanley DE: Slateworker's pneumoconiosis. Hum Pathol 23:1098, 1992.
16. Craighead JE, Kleinerman J, Abraham JL, et al: Diseases associated with exposure to silica and non-fibrous silicate minerals. Arch Pathol Lab Med 112 673, 1988.
17. Craighead JE, Vallyathan NV: Cryptic pulmonary lesions in workers occupationally exposed to dust containing silica. JAMA 244:1939, 1980.
18. Davis GS: Pathogenesis of silicosis: Current concepts and hypotheses. Lung 164:139, 1986.
19. Doll NJ, Stankus RP, Hughes J, et al: Immune complexes and autoantibodies in silicosis. J Allergy Clin Immunol 68:281, 1981.
20. Dumontet C, Biron F, Vitrey D, et al: Acute silicosis due to inhalation of a domestic product. Am Rev Respir Dis 143:880, 1991.
21. Fujimoto K, Müller NL, Kata S, et al: Pneumoconiosis in rush mat workers exposed to clay dye "sendo" dust. Chest 125:737, 2004.
22. Gong H Jr, Tashkin DP: Silicosis due to intentional inhalation of abrasive scouring powder. Case report with long-term survival and vasculitic sequelae. Am J Med 67:358, 1979.
23. Grobbelaar JP, Bateman ED: Hut lung: A domestically acquired pneumoconiosis of mixed aetiology in rural women. Thorax 46:334, 1991.
24. Hamada H, Vallyathan V, Cool CD, et al: Mast cell basic fibroblast growth factor in silicosis. Am J Respir Crit Care Med. 161:2026, 2000.
25. Hoffman EO, Lamberty J, Pizzolato P, et al: The ultrastructure of acute silicosis. Arch Pathol 96:104, 1973.
26. Honma K, Abraham JL, Chiyotani K, et al: Proposed criteria for mixed-dust pneumoconiosis: Definition, descriptions, and guidelines for pathologic diagnosis and clinical correlation. Hum Pathol 35:1515, 2004.
27. Kampalath BN, McMahon JT, Cohen A, et al: Obliterative central bronchitis due to mineral dust in patients with pneumoconiosis. Arch Pathol Lab Med 122:56, 1998.
28. Landrigan PJ: Silicosis. State of the Art Review. Occup Med 2:319, 1987.
29. Leibowitz MC, Goldstein B: Some investigations into the nature and cause of massive fibrosis (MF) in the lungs of South African gold, coal, and asbestos mine workers.

Am J Ind Med 12:129, 1987.

30. McDonald JW, Roggli VL: Detection of silica particles in lung tissue by polarizing light microscopy. Arch Pathol Lab Med 119:242, 1995.

31. Mossman BT, Churg A: Mechanisms in the pathogenesis of asbestosis and silicosis. Am J Respir Crit Care Med 157:1666, 1998.

32. Nugent KM, Dodson RF, Idell S, Devillier JR: The utility of bronchoalveolar lavage and transbronchial lung biopsy combined with energy-dispersive X-ray analysis in the diagnosis of silicosis. Am Rev Respir Dis 140:1438, 1989.

33. Owens MW, Kinasewitz GT, Gonzalez E: Case report: Sandblasters' lung with mycobacterial infection. Am J Med Sci 295:554, 1988.

34. Rom WN, Bitterman PB, Rennard SI, et al: Characterization of the lower respiratory tract inflammation of nonsmoking individuals with interstitial lung disease associated with chronic inhalation of inorganic dusts. Am Rev Respir Dis 136:1429, 1987.

35. Slavin RE, Swedo JL, Brandes D, et al: Extrapulmonary silicosis: A clinical, morphologic, and ultrastructural study. Hum Pathol 16:393, 1985.

36. Snider DE Jr: The relationship between tuberculosis and silicosis. Am Rev Respir Dis 118:455, 1978.

37. Suratt PM, Winn WC, Brody AR, et al: Acute silicosis in tombstone blasters. Am Rev Respir Dis 115:521, 1977.

38. Xipell JM, Ham KN, Price CG, et al: Acute silico-lipoproteinosis. Thorax 32:104, 1977.

39. Ziskind M, Jones RM, Weill H: Silicosis. Am Rev Respir Dis 113:643, 1976.

Asbestos-Related Reactions

40. Aberle DR, Gamsu G, Ray CS: High-resolution CT of benign asbestos-related diseases: Clinical and radiographic correlation. AJR Am J Roentgenol 151:883, 1988.

41. Akira M, Yokoyama K, Yamamoto S, et al: Early asbestosis: Evaluation with high-resolution CT. Radiology 178:409, 1991.

42. Bateman ED, Benatar SR: Asbestos-induced diseases: Clinical perspectives. Q J Med 239:183, 1987.

43. Becklake MR: Fiber burden and asbestos-related lung disease: Determinants of dose–response relationships. Am J Respir Crit Care Med 150:1488, 1994.

44. Bellis D, Andrion A, Delsedime L, Mollo F: Minimal pathologic changes of the lung and asbestos exposure. Hum Pathol 20:102, 1989.

45. Boutin C, Dumortier P, Rey F, et al: Black spots concentrate oncogenic asbestos fibers in the parietal pleura. Thoracoscopic and mineralogic study. Am J Respir Crit Care Med 153:444, 1996.

46. Churg A: Asbestos fibers and pleural plaques in a general autopsy population. Am J Pathol 109:88, 1982.

47. Churg A: Asbestos fiber content of the lungs in patients with and without asbestos airways disease. Am Rev Respir Dis 127:470, 1983.

48. Churg A: Analysis of asbestos fibers from lung tissue: Research and diagnostic uses. Semin Respir Med 7:281, 1986.

49. Churg A: The diagnosis of asbestosis. Hum Pathol 20:97, 1989.

50. Churg A: Asbestos-related disease in the workplace and the environment: Controversial issues. In: Churg A, Katzenstein A, eds: *The Lung: Current Concepts*, Baltimore, Williams & Wilkins, 1993, pp 54–77.

51. Churg A, Stevens B: Enhanced retention of asbestos fibers in the airways of human smokers. Am J Respir Crit Care Med 151:1409, 1995.

52. Churg A, Wright JL, DePaoli L, Wiggs B: Mineralogic correlates of fibrosis in chrysotile miners and millers. Am Rev Respir Dis 139:891, 1989.

53. Churg A, Wright J, Wiggs B, Depaoli L: Mineralogic parameters related to amosite asbestos-induced fibrosis in humans. Am Rev Respir Dis 142:1331, 1990.

54. Craighead JE, Abraham JL, Churg A, et al: The pathology of asbestos-associated diseases of the lungs and pleural cavities: Diagnostic criteria and proposed grading schema. Arch Pathol Lab Med 106:544, 1982.

55. Crouch E, Churg A: Ferruginous bodies and the histologic evaluation of dust exposure. Am J Surg Pathol 8:109, 1984.

56. Cugell DW, Kamp DW: Asbestos and the pleura. Chest 125:1103, 2004.

57. Cullen MR: Controversies in asbestos-related lung cancer. Occup Med 2:259, 1987.

58. De Vuyst P, Dumortier P, Moulin E, et al: Diagnostic value of asbestos bodies in bronchoalveolar lavage fluid. Am Rev Respir Dis 136:1219, 1987.

59. Dodson RF, Greenberg SD, Williams MG Jr, et al: Asbestos content in lungs of occupationally and nonoccupationally exposed individuals. JAMA 252:68, 1984.

60. Dodson RF, Huang J, Williams MG, et al: Lack of asbestos contamination of paraffin. Arch Pathol Lab Med. 122:1103, 1998.

61. Dodson RF, Hurst GA, Williams MG Jr, et al: Comparison of light and electron microscopy for defining occupational asbestos exposure in transbronchial lung biopsies. Chest 94:366, 1988.

62. Dodson RF, O'Sullivan MF, Huang J, et al: Asbestos in extrapulmonary sites: Omentum and mesentery. Chest 117:486, 2000.

63. Dodson RF, Williams MG Jr, Corn CJ, et al: Usefulness of combined light and electron microscopy: Evaluation of sputum samples for asbestos to determine past occupational exposure. Mod Pathol 2:320, 1989.

64. Dodson RF, Williams MG Jr, Corn CJ, et al: Asbestos content of lung tissue, lymph nodes, and pleural plaques from former shipyard workers. Am Rev Respir Dis 142:843, 1990.

65. Dodson RF, Williams MG Jr, O'Sullivan MF, et al: A comparison of the ferruginous body and uncoated fiber content in the lungs of the former asbestos workers. Am Rev Respir Dis 132:143, 1985.

66. Dumortier P, Broucke I, DeVuyst P: Pseudoasbestos bodies and fibers in bronchoalveolar lavage of refractory ceramic fiber users. Am J Respir Crit Care Med 164:499, 2001.

67. Epler GR, Fitz Gerald MX, Gaensler EA, Carrington CB: Asbestos-related disease from household exposure. Respiration 39:229, 1980.

68. Gaensler EA, Jederlinic PJ, Churg A: Idiopathic pulmonary fibrosis in asbestos-exposed workers. Am Rev Respir Dis 144:689, 1991.

69. Ghio AJ, Roggli VL, Richards JH, et al: Oxalate deposition on asbestos bodies. Hum Pathol 34:737, 2003.

70. Guidotti TL, Miller A, Christiani D, et al: Diagnosis and initial management of nonmalignant diseases related to asbestos. Am J Respir Crit Care Med 170:691, 2004.

71. Gylseth B, Skaug V: Relation between pathological grading and lung fibre concentration in a patient with asbestosis. Br J Ind Med 43:754, 1986.

72. Hammar SP, Hallman KO: Localized inflammatory pulmonary disease in subjects occupationally exposed to asbestos. Chest 103:1792, 1993.

73. Hillerdal G: Endemic pleural plaques. Eur J Respir Dis 69:1, 1986.

74. Hillerdal G: Asbestos-related pleural disease. Semin Respir Med 9:65, 1987.

75. Hillerdal G: Rounded atelectasis. Clinical experience with 74 patients. Chest 95:836, 1989.

76. James KR, Bull TB, Fox B: Detection of asbestos fibres by dark ground microscopy. J Clin Pathol 40:1259, 1987.

77. Jones RN: The diagnosis of asbestosis. Am Rev Respir Dis 144:477, 1991.

78. Kane PB, Goldman SL, Pillai BH, et al: Diagnosis of asbestosis by transbronchial biopsy. A method to facilitate demonstration of ferruginous bodies. Am Rev Respir Dis 115:689, 1977.

79. Kuhn C III, Kuo T-T: Cytoplasmic hyalin in asbestosis. A reaction of injured alveolar epithelium. Arch Pathol 95:190, 1973.

80. Lee RJ, Florida RG, Stewart IM: Asbestos contamination in paraffin tissue blocks. Arch Pathol Lab Med 119:528, 1995.

81. Martensson G, Hagberg S, Pettersson K, Thiringer G: Asbestos pleural effusion: A clinical entity. Thorax 42:646, 1987.

82. Roggli VL, Benning TL: Asbestos bodies in pulmonary hilar lymph nodes. Mod Pathol 3:513, 1990.

83. Roggli V, Oury TD, Sporn TA, eds: *Pathology of Asbestos-Associated Diseases*, 2nd ed, New York, Springer, 2005.

84. Rom WN, Travis WD, Brody AR: Cellular and molecular basis of the asbestos-related diseases. Am Rev Respir Dis 143:408, 1991.

85. Rosenstock L, Hudson LD: The pleural manifestations of asbestos exposure. Occup Med 2:383, 1987.

86. Schwartz DA, Galvin JR, Burmeister LF, et al: The clinical utility and reliability of asbestos bodies in bronchoalveolar fluid. Am Rev Respir Dis 144:684, 1991.

87. Sebastien P, Armstrong B, Monchaux G, Bignon J: Asbestos bodies in bronchoalveolar lavage fluid and in lung parenchyma. Am Rev Respir Dis 137:75, 1988.

88. Stephens M, Gibbs AR, Pooley FD, Wagner JC: Asbestos induced diffuse pleural fibrosis: Pathology and mineralogy. Thorax 42:583, 1987.

89. Teschler H, Konietzko N, Schoenfeld B, et al: Distribution of asbestos bodies in the human lung as determined by bronchoalveolar lavage. Am Rev Respir Dis 147:1211, 1993.

90. Tukiainen P, Paskinen E, Korhola O, et al: TruCut needle biopsy in asbestosis and silicosis: Correlation of histological changes with radiographic change and pulmonary function in 41 patients. Br J Ind Med 35:292, 1978.

91. Vathesatogkit P, Harkin TJ, Addrizzo-Harris DJ, et al: Clinical correlation of asbestos bodies in BAL fluid. Chest 126:966, 2004.

92. Vollmer RT, Roggli VL: Asbestos body concentrations in human lung: Predictions from asbestos body counts in tissue sections with a mathematical model. Hum Pathol 16:713, 1985.

93. Wain SL, Roggli VL, Foster WL Jr: Parietal pleural plaques, asbestos bodies and neoplasia. A clinical, pathologic, and roentgenographic correlation of 25 consecutive cases. Chest 86:707, 1984.

94. Williams MG Jr, Dodson RF, Corn C, Hurst GA: A procedure for the isolation of amosite asbestos and ferruginous bodies from lung tissue and sputum. J Toxicol Environ Health 10:627, 1982.

95. Wright JL, Churg A: Morphology of small-airway lesions in patients with asbestos exposure. Hum Pathol 15:68, 1984.

96. Wright JL, Cosio M, Wiggs B, Hogg JC: A morphologic grading scheme for membranous and respiratory bronchioles. Arch Pathol Lab Med 109:163, 1985.

97. Wright RS, Abraham JL, Harber P, et al: Fatal asbestosis 50 years after brief high intensity exposure in a vermiculite expansion plant. Am J Respir Crit Care Med 165:1145, 2002.

98. Yamamoto S: Histopathological features of pulmonary asbestosis with particular emphasis on the comparison with those of usual interstitial pneumonia. Osaka City Med J 43:225, 1997.

99. Zhang P-C, Chung W-B, Chan K-W, Kung ITM: Modified alkali digestion method for pulmonary asbestos fibre counts. Pathology 19:159, 1987.

Coal Workers' Pneumoconiosis

100. Davis JMG, Chapman J, Collins P, et al: Variations in the histological patterns of the lesions of coal workers' pneumoconiosis in Britain and their relationship to lung dust content. Am Rev Respir Dis 128:118, 1983.

101. Fisher ER, Watkins G, Lam NV, et al: Objective pathological diagnosis of coal workers' pneumoconiosis. JAMA 245:1829, 1981.

102. Green FHY, Laquer WA: Coal workers pneumoconiosis. Pathol Annu 15:333, 1980.

103. Hu S-N, Vallyathan V, Green FHY, et al: Pulmonary arteriolar muscularization in coal workers'

pneumoconiosis and its correlation with right ventricular hypertrophy. Arch Pathol Lab Med 114:1063, 1990.

104. Kleinerman J, Green F, Harley RA, et al: Pathology standards for coal worker's pneumoconiosis. Arch Pathol Lab Med 103:375, 1979.

105. Morgan WKC, Lapp NL: Respiratory disease in coal miners. Am Rev Respir Dis 113:531, 1976.

106. Remy-Jardin M, Degreef JM, Beuscart R, et al: Coal worker's pneumoconiosis: CT assessment in exposed workers and correlation with radiographic findings. Radiology 177:363, 1990.

107. Ruckely VA, Gauld SJ, Chapman JS, et al: Emphysema and dust exposure in a group of coal workers. Am Rev Respir Dis 129:528, 1984.

108. Soutar CA: Update on lung diseases in coal miners. Br J Ind Med 44:145, 1987.

109. Vallyathan V, Brower PS, Green FHY, et al: Radiographic and pathologic correlation of coal worker's pneumoconiosis. Am J Respir Crit Care Med 154:741, 1996.

Other Pneumoconioses

110. Abraham JL, Brambilla C: Particle size for differentiation between inhalation and injection pulmonary talcosis. Environ Res 21:94, 1980.

111. Abramson MJ, Wlodarczyle JH, Saunders NA, Hensley MJ: Does aluminum smelting cause lung disease? Am Rev Respir Dis 139:1042, 1989.

112. Antilla S, Sutinen S, Paananen M, et al: Hard metal lung disease: A clinical, histological, ultrastructural and X-ray microanalytical study. Eur J Respir Dis 69:83, 1986.

113. Aronchick JM, Rossman MD, Miller WT: Chronic beryllium disease: Diagnosis, radiographic findings, and correlation with pulmonary function tests. Radiology 163:677, 1987.

114. Auchincloss JH, Abraham JL, Gilbert R, et al: Health hazard of poorly regulated exposure during manufacture of cemented tungsten carbides and cobalt. Br J Ind Med 49:832, 1992.

115. Barrett TE, Pietra GG, Maycock RL, et al: Acrylic resin pneumoconiosis: Report of a case in a dental student. Am Rev Respir Dis 139:841, 1989.

116. Bellott SM, Schade van Westrum JAFM, Wagenvoort CA, Meijer AEFH: Deposition of bauxite dust and pulmonary fibrosis. Pathol Res Pract 179:225, 1984.

117. Berner A, Gylseth B, Levy F: Talc dust pneumoconiosis. A case report. Acta Pathol Microbiol Scand 89:17, 1981.

118. Boag AH, Colby TV, Fraire AE, et al: The pathology of interstitial lung disease in nylon flock workers. Am J Surg Pathol 23:1539, 1999.

119. Butnor KJ, Sporn TA, Ingram P, et al: Beryllium detection in human lung tissue using electron probe x-ray microanalysis. Mod Pathol 16:1171, 2003.

120. Cordasco EM, Demeter SL, Kerkay J, et al: Pulmonary manifestations of vinyl and polyvinyl chloride (interstitial lung disease). Chest 78:828, 1980.

121. Cugell DW, Morgan WKC, Perkins DG, Rubin A: The respiratory effects of cobalt. Arch Intern Med 150:177, 1990.

122. Cullen MR, Cherniack MG, Kominsky JR: Chronic beryllium disease in the United States. Semin Respir Med 7:203, 1986.

123. Daroca PJ, George WJ: Giant cell interstitial pneumonia. South Med J 84:257, 1991.

124. Della Torre F, Cassani M, Segale M, et al: Trace metal lung diseases: A new fatal case of hard metal pneumoconiosis. Respiration 57:248, 1990.

125. De Vuyst P, Dumortier P, Rickaert F, et al: Occupational lung fibrosis in an aluminum polisher. Eur J Respir Dis 68:131, 1986.

126. De Vuyst P, Dumortier P, Schandené L, et al: Sarcoid-like lung granulomatosis induced by aluminum dusts. Am Rev Respir Dis 135:493, 1987.

127. De Vuyst P, Vande Weyer R, De Coster A, et al: Dental technician's pneumoconiosis. A report of two cases. Am Rev Respir Dis 133:316, 1986.

128. Dodson RF, O'Sullivan MF, Corn CJ, et al: Ferruginous body formation on a nonasbestos mineral. Arch Pathol Lab Med 109:849, 1985.

129. Edstrom HW, Rice DMD: "Labrador lung": An unusual mixed dust pneumoconiosis. Can Med Assoc J 126:27, 1982.

130. Eisenbud M, Lisson J: Epidemiological aspects of beryllium-induced nonmalignant lung disease: A 30-year update. J Occup Med 25:196, 1983.

131. Enterline PE, Marsh GM, Esmen NA: Respiratory disease among workers exposed to man-made mineral fibers. Am Rev Respir Dis 128:1, 1983.

132. Epstein PE, Dauber JH, Rossman MD, Daniel RP: Bronchoalveolar lavage in a patient with chronic berylliosis: Evidence for hypersensitivity pneumonitis. Ann Intern Med 97:213, 1987.

133. Eschenbachel WL, Kreiss K, Lougheed D, et al: Nylon flock-associated interstitial lung disease. Am J Respir Crit Care Med 159:2003, 1999.

134. Funahashi A, Schlueter DP, Pintar K, et al: Pneumoconiosis in workers exposed to silicon carbide. Am Rev Respir Dis 129:636, 1984.

135. Funahashi A, Schlueter DP, Pintar K, et al: Welder's pneumoconiosis: Tissue elemental microanalysis by energy-dispersive x-ray analysis. Br J Ind Med 45:14, 1988.

136. Gibbs AE, Pooley FD, Griffiths DM, et al: Talc pneumoconiosis: A pathologic and mineralogic study. Hum Pathol 23:1344, 1992.

137. Gilks B, Churg A: Aluminum-induced pulmonary fibrosis: Do fibers play a role? Am Rev Respir Dis 136:176, 1987.

138. Goldbach PD, Abraham JL, Young WI, et al: Talcum powder pneumoconiosis: Diagnosis by transbronchial biopsy using energy-dispersive X-ray analysis. West J Med 136:439, 1982.

139. Golden EB, Warnock ML, Hulett LD Jr, Churg A: Fly ash lung: A new pneumoconiosis. Am Rev Respir Dis 125:108, 1982.

140. Herbert A, Sterling G, Abraham J, Corrin B: Desquamative interstitial pneumonia in an aluminum welder. Hum Pathol 13:694, 1982.

141. Hull MJ, Abraham JL: Aluminum welding fume-induced pneumoconiosis. Hum Pathol 33:819, 2002.

142. Jederlinic PJ, Abraham JL, Churg A, et al: Pulmonary fibrosis in aluminum oxide workers. Am Rev Respir Dis 142:1179, 1990.

143. Jones Williams W: Beryllium workers sarcoidosis or chronic beryllium disease. Sarcoidosis 6(Suppl 1):34, 1989.

144. Jones Williams WJ, Kelland D: New aid for diagnosing chronic beryllium disease (CBD): Laser ion mass analysis (LIMA). J Clin Pathol 39:900, 1986.

145. Kern DG, Crausman RS, Durand KTH, et al: Flock worker's lung: Chronic interstitial lung disease in the nylon flocking industry. Ann Intern Med 129:261, 1998.

146. Kern DG, Durand KTH, Crausman RS, et al: Chronic interstitial lung disease in nylon flocking industry workers – Rhode Island, 1992–1996. MMWR Morb Mortal Wkly Rep 46:897, 1997.

147. Kern DG, Kuhn C, Ely EW, et al: Flock worker's lung: Broadening the spectrum of clinicopathology, narrowing the spectrum of suspected etiologies. Chest 117:251, 2000.

148. Kotloff RM, Richman PS, Greenacre JK, Rossman MD: Chronic beryllium disease in a dental laboratory technician. Am Rev Respir Dis 147:205, 1993.

149. Kreiss K, Mroz MM, Zhen B, et al: Risks of beryllium disease related to work processes at a metal, alloy, and oxide production plant. Occup Environ Med 54:605, 1997.

150. Kriebel D, Brain JD, Sprince NL, Kazemi H: The pulmonary toxicity of beryllium. Am Rev Respir Dis 137:464, 1988.

151. Landas SK, Schwartz DA: Mica-associated pulmonary interstitial fibrosis. Am Rev Respir Dis 144:718, 1991.

152. Lilis R: Vinyl chloride and polyvinyl chloride exposure and occupational lung disease. Chest 78:826, 1980.

153. Loewen GM, Weiner D, McMahan J: Pneumoconiosis in an elderly dentist. Chest 93:1312, 1988.

154. Masse S, Begin R, Cantin A: Pathology of silicone carbide pneumoconiosis. Mod Pathol 1:104, 1988.

155. McDonald JW, Ghio AJ, Sheehan CE, et al: Rare earth (cerium oxide) pneumoconiosis: Analytical scanning electron microscopy and literature review. Mod Pathol 8:859, 1995.

156. Miller RR, Churg AM, Hutcheon M, Lam S: Pulmonary alveolar proteinosis and aluminum dust exposure. Am Rev Respir Dis 130:312, 1984.

157. Moran CA, Mullick FG, Ishak KG, et al: Identification of titanium in human tissues: Probable role in pathologic processes. Hum Pathol 22:450, 1991.

158. Morgan WKC, Donner A, Higgins ITT, et al: The effects of koalin on the lung. Am Rev Respir Dis 138:813, 1988.

159. Morgenroth K, Kronenberger H, Michalke G, et al: Morphology and pathogenesis of pneumoconiosis in dental technicians. Path Res Pract 179:528, 1985.

160. Mroz MM, Kreiss K, Lezotte DC, et al: Re-examination of the blood lymphocyte transformation test in the diagnosis of chronic beryllium disease. J Allergy Clin Immunol 88:54, 1991.

161. Nemery B, Nagels J, Verbeken E, Dinsdale D, Demedts M: Rapidly fatal progression of cobalt lung in a diamond polisher. Am Rev Respir Dis 141:1373, 1990.

162. Newman LS, Kreiss K: Nonoccupational beryllium disease masquerading as sarcoidosis: Identification by blood lymphocyte proliferative response to beryllium. Am Rev Respir Dis 145:1212, 1992.

163. Newman LS, Kreiss K, King TE Jr, et al: Pathologic and immunologic alterations in early stages of beryllium disease. Reexamination of disease definition and natural history. Am Rev Respir Dis 139:1479, 1989.

164. Newman LS, Mroz MM, Balkissoon R, et al: Beryllium sensitization progresses to chronic beryllium disease: A longitudinal study of disease risk. Am J Respir Crit Care Med 171:54, 2005.

165. Ohori NP, Sciurba FC, Owens GR, et al: Giant-cell interstitial pneumonia and hard-metal pneumoconiosis. A clinicopathologic study of four cases and review of the literature. Am J Surg Pathol 13:581, 1989.

166. Pimental JC, Menezes AP: Pulmonary and hepatic granulomatous disorders due to the inhalation of cement and mica dusts. Thorax 33:219, 1978.

167. Ramage JE, Roggli VL, Bell DY, Piantadosi CA: Interstitial lung disease and domestic wood burning. Am Rev Respir Dis 137:1229, 1988.

168. Redline S, Barna BP, Tomashefski JF, Abraham JL: Granulomatous disease associated with pulmonary deposition of titanium. Br J Ind Med 43:652, 1986.

169. Rolfe MW, Paine R, Davenport RB, Strieter RM: Hard metal pneumoconiosis and the association of tumor necrosis factor-alpha. Am Rev Respir Dis 146:1600, 1992.

170. Rom WN, Lockey JE, Lee JS, et al: Pneumoconiosis and exposures of dental laboratory technicians. Am J Pub Health 74:1252, 1984.

171. Rossman MD, Kern JA, Elias JA, et al: Proliferative response of bronchoalveolar lymphocytes to beryllium. Ann Intern Med 108:687, 1988.

172. Sandoval J, Salas J, Martinez-Guerra ML, et al: Pulmonary arterial hypertension and cor pulmonale associated with chronic domestic woodsmoke inhalation. Chest 103:12, 1993.

173. Seldén A, Sahle W, Johansson L, et al: Three cases of dental technician's pneumoconiosis related to cobalt-chromium-molybdenum dust exposure: Diagnosis and follow-up. Chest 109:837, 1996.

174. Sieniewicz DJ, Nidecker AC: Conglomerate pulmonary disease: A form of talcosis in intravenous and methadone abusers. AJR Am J Roentgenol 135:697, 1980.

175. Sluis-Cremer GK, Glyn Thomas R, Solomon A: Hard-metal lung disease. A report of 4 cases. S Afr Med J 71:598, 1987.

175a. Sood A, Beckett WS, Cullen MR: Variable response to long-term corticosteroid therapy in chronic beryllium disease. Chest 126:2000, 2004.

176. Sprince NL, Oliver C, Eisen EA, et al: Cobalt exposure and lung disease in tungsten carbide production. A cross-sectional study of current workers. Am Rev Respir Dis 138:1220, 1988.

177. Villar TG: Vineyard sprayer's lung. Clinical aspects. Am Rev Respir Dis 110:545, 1974.

178. Weill H, Hughes JN, Hammad YY, et al: Respiratory health in workers exposed to man-made vitreous fibers. Am Rev Respir Dis 128:104, 1983.

6

IMMUNOLOGIC LUNG DISEASE

Although an immunologic pathogenesis is postulated for a large number of lung diseases, this mechanism has been convincingly delineated in only a few, including Goodpasture's syndrome, hypersensitivity pneumonia, and allergic bronchopulmonary aspergillosis. The following sections discuss these entities, as well as related diseases encompassed by the broader categories of alveolar hemorrhage syndrome and pulmonary eosinophilia. Rejection of lung allografts and graft-versus-host disease are additional areas in which immunologic mechanisms are well defined. These and other complications related to transplantation are reviewed in the last section.

HYPERSENSITIVITY PNEUMONIA (EXTRINSIC ALLERGIC ALVEOLITIS)

Hypersensitivity pneumonia, also known as *extrinsic allergic alveolitis*, is a type of immunologic reaction in the lung to inhaled antigens that is thought to involve a combination of immune complex, humoral, and cell-mediated immune reactions.[12,30,37,44] The main etiologic agents include thermophilic bacteria, fungi, and animal proteins (Table 6–1). Other bacteria and bacterial products, as well as insect products, amoebae, and certain chemicals, have been implicated less commonly. The clinical syndromes resulting from reaction to these agents are numerous and are given names reflecting the circumstances of exposure.[7,12,16,37,38] *Farmer's lung, air conditioner lung,* and *humidifier lung* are prototypic examples of reactions to thermophilic actinomycetes, although they tend to have different clinical presentations. A variety of fungi have been implicated in hypersensitivity pneumonia. *Summer-type hypersensitivity pneumonia* is an important form of hypersensitivity pneumonia that occurs in Japan and is thought in most cases to be due to exposure to *Trichosporon cutaneum* in the home.[1] *Cryptococcus albidus* may be etiologic in some cases as well.[75] *Maple bark stripper's disease, malt worker's lung, sequoiosis,* and *suberosis*[26] are all related to fungal

Table 6–1 Major Causes of Hypersensitivity Pneumonia

Antigen	Source	Disease
Thermophilic Bacteria		
Micropolyspora faeni, *Thermoactinomyces vulgaris* }	Moldy hay	Farmer's lung
Thermoactinomyces vulgaris	Moldy compost	Mushroom worker's disease
Thermoactinomyces saccharii	Moldy sugar cane	Bagassosis
Thermoactinomyces vulgaris *Thermoactinomyces candidus* }	Air conditioner ducts, humidifiers	Humidifier lung, air conditioner lung
Fungi		
Cryptostroma corticale	Moldy maple bark	Maple bark stripper's disease
Aspergillus clavatus	Moldy barley	Malt worker's lung
Graphium species, *Pullularia* species	Moldy wood dust	Sequoiosis
Trichosporon cutaneum, Cryptococcus albidus	Home environment	Summer-type hypersensitivity pneumonitis (Japan)
Lyophyllum aggregatum	Indoor mushroom harvesting	Mushroom worker's lung
Penicillium frequentans, Aspergillus fumigatus	Cork dust	Suberosis
Other Bacteria		
Bacillus subtilis	Water	Detergent worker's lung
Bacillus cereus	Water	Humidifier lung
Pseudomonas, acinetobacter, nontuberculous mycobacteria	Metal working fluid	Metal working fluid hypersensitivity pneumonia (machine operator's lung)
Animal Products		
Avian proteins	Bird droppings, feathers	Pigeon breeder's disease, bird fancier's lung
Ox/pig proteins	Pituitary powder	Pituitary snuff-taker's lung
Bacterial Products		
	Cotton	Byssinosis
Amoebae		
	Water	Humidifier lung
Insect Products		
	Grain	Wheat weevil disease
Chemicals		
Trimellitic anhydride (TMA) Methylene diisocyanate (MDI) Toluene diisocyanate (TDI) }	Plastics, rubber manufacturing	Chemical worker's lung
Pyromellitic dianhydride (PMDA)	Epoxy resin	
Naphthylene 1,5 diisocyanate (NDI)	Polyurethane foam production	

exposure. Bacteria other than thermophilic actinomycetes have been implicated in *detergent worker's lung* and some cases of *humidifier lung*. *Metal working fluid hypersensitivity pneumonia* or *machine operator's lung* is an important cause of morbidity in machinists, and a number of bacteria are suspect in its etiology, including pseudomonas, acinetobacter, and nontuberculous mycobacteria.[4,17,20,50] *Pigeon breeder's lung* is a well-known complication of exposure to pigeons, both in persons who raise these birds and in individuals who are passively exposed to wild pigeons.[16] Exposure to pet birds in the home is another important cause of hypersensitivity pneumonia, which is referred to as *bird fancier's lung* or *budgerigar fancier's lung*. In addition to these organic antigens, hypersensitivity pneumonia can rarely be due to inorganic low-molecular-weight chemical exposure, as in plastics or rubber manufacturing, for example.[24] Identification and removal of the etiologic agent of hypersensitivity pneumonia is extremely important, since continued exposure may lead to irreversible lung fibrosis.

Clinical Features

The clinical presentation of hypersensitivity pneumonia may be *acute*, *subacute*, or *chronic*, although overlapping presentations can occur, and patients with chronic or subacute disease can have intermittent acute disease.[12,15,21,22,37,38,41] The acute form follows exposure to large amounts of an offending antigen. It is characterized by severe dyspnea, cough, high fever, and chills developing from 4 to 6 hours following exposure. Centrilobular ground glass and nodular opacities are seen on high-resolution computed tomography (CT) examinations. *Farmer's lung* is a classic example of this form of hypersensitivity pneumonia. Symptoms usually resolve within 12 to 18 hours following cessation of exposure, and the chest infiltrates clear within several days. Reexposure to the antigen results in recrudescence of the illness, and continued intermittent exposure may lead to permanent lung damage related to the development of interstitial fibrosis. Biopsy is generally not necessary to diagnose the acute form of the disease because the temporal relationship of symptoms to exposure is usually obvious, and the diagnosis can therefore be made on clinical grounds. Certain laboratory findings help to confirm the diagnosis, including specific precipitating antibodies in the serum and positive skin tests. Aerosol inhalation challenge can be used in some cases but is not usually advocated for acute cases.

The subacute and chronic forms of hypersensitivity pneumonia present more of a clinical enigma than does the acute form, since the relationship of symptoms to exposure may not be apparent. They result from prolonged exposure to small amounts of antigen. Subacute disease occurs over weeks to months, with symptoms similar to the acute form but less severe. High-resolution CT findings are similar to those for the acute stage, although linear opacities and airtrapping may be seen occasionally. Respiratory disease in mushroom workers often presents with a subacute course.[45] Chronic hypersensitivity pneumonia is a common presentation of *humidifier* or *air conditioner lung* and *budgerigar* or *bird fancier's lung*. Patients with these diseases experience a more insidious onset of dyspnea, often associated with dry cough, fatigue, and malaise.[44]

High-resolution CT shows mid to upper lobe predominant linear interstitial opacities and small nodules, often associated with traction bronchiectasis and honeycomb areas. In longstanding cases, the clinical and radiographic presentation may be difficult to distinguish from idiopathic pulmonary fibrosis (IPF) (see Chapter 3).[15,32] Studies of bronchoalveolar lavage cellular constituents help in diagnosis, since lymphocytosis, often containing predominately CD8 lymphocytes, is prominent.[1,42,43] Lymphocyte proliferation tests utilizing suspected antigens and inhalation provocation tests can also aid in diagnosis.[27,34] Serum precipitating antibodies are often present but are nonspecific, since they can be found in exposed but healthy individuals.[12,37,38,41] Also, they are not present in every case. Skin tests may be helpful, but only avian or fungal antigens can be used, since thermophilic antigens are locally irritating.

Corticosteroids may hasten recovery in the acute stage, and there is some evidence that they may also be useful in the chronic form of the disease.[12,37,38,41] The best treatment, however, is to avoid exposure to the causative antigen. Irreversible lung damage such as interstitial fibrosis or honeycomb lung can develop if exposure to the offending antigen persists.[5,14,15] Therefore, a careful clinical history and thorough investigation of the patient's home and work environment need to be undertaken to identify potential sources of exposure.

Histologic Features

The combination of a cellular chronic interstitial pneumonia that is accentuated in peribronchiolar parenchyma, ill-defined non-necrotizing granulomas, and foci of bronchiolitis obliterans is diagnostic of hypersensitivity pneumonia, although all three components are not always found. Chronic interstitial pneumonia is a constant feature, however, and it can mimic nonspecific interstitial pneumonia (see Chapter 3) (Fig. 6–1).[2,6,7,9,18,19,36,40,48] Early in the course this process is distributed around respiratory bronchioles (Fig. 6–2), and chronic bronchiolitis may be a prominent feature.[31] Lymphoid follicles with germinal centers are occasionally seen, but are usually not prominent. Intervening areas of distal parenchyma may be uninvolved, although later on the process may affect the lung more diffusely. Often, however, even in advanced cases, accentuation of the infiltrate within the interstitium around small bronchioles can be appreciated, and the airway lumens may be narrowed.

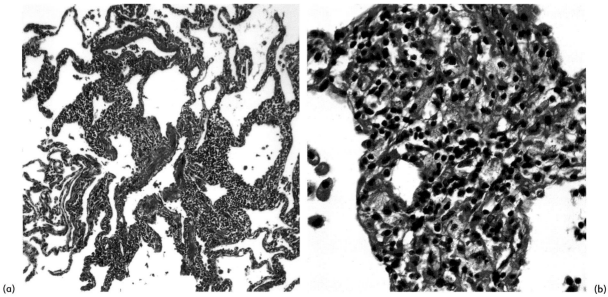

(a)

(b)

Figure 6–1 Hypersensitivity pneumonia. (a) Low magnification view showing a prominent cellular chronic interstitial pneumonia that is accentuated around a respiratory bronchiole. Notice that the lumen of the bronchiole is narrowed by the process. **(b)** Higher magnification showing a mixture of small lymphocytes, plasma cells, and histiocytes within the infiltrate.

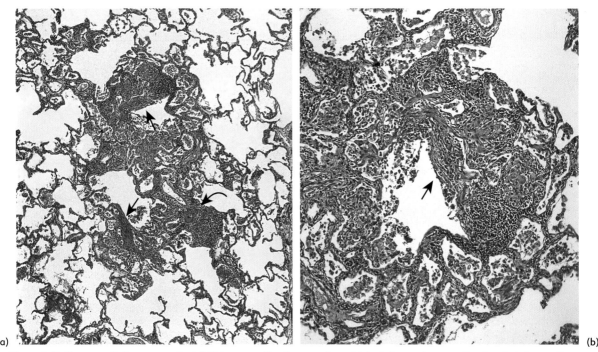

(a)

(b)

Figure 6–2 Hypersensitivity pneumonia. (a) At low magnification a peribronchiolar inflammatory reaction is noted along with a chronic interstitial pneumonia that extends into adjacent alveolar septa. Foci of bronchiolitis obliterans (arrows) and a small ill-defined non-necrotizing granuloma (curved arrow) are seen. **(b)** Higher magnification showing the bronchiolitis obliterans (arrow) as well as the cellular interstitial infiltrate in the wall of the small airway. Note the prominent epithelioid histiocytes.

Lymphocytes comprise the majority of infiltrating cells, with fewer numbers of plasma cells and scattered, plump epithelioid histiocytes that often occur in small clusters around bronchioles.[35] The presence of epithelioid histiocytes is an important clue to the diagnosis (Fig. 6–3). Eosinophils and neutrophils are usually not prominent, and fibrosis is minimal except for advanced chronic cases.[29,47] Small, non-necrotizing granulomas are found in two-thirds of cases and are usually localized to the peribronchiolar interstitium (Fig. 6–4).[19,36] These granulomas contain a mixture of epithelioid histiocytes, multinucleated giant cells, and lymphocytes, and tend to be loosely formed and poorly circumscribed. Foci of bronchiolitis obliterans or bronchiolitis obliterans–organizing pneumonia (BOOP) (see Chapter 2) accompany the other changes in one-half to two-thirds of cases (Fig. 6–5).[6,19] This lesion is characterized by the filling of distal bronchioles and surrounding alveolar ducts and alveolar spaces by plugs of fibroblasts and variable numbers of chronic inflammatory cells within a lightly staining stroma. Foamy macrophages related to bronchiolar obstruction are present within nearby

alveolar spaces in many cases.[19,36] Less commonly, a fibrinous intraalveolar exudate with variable numbers of neutrophils has been described. Vasculitis is not a feature, at least at that stage of disease when a biopsy is usually taken (see later on).

Histologic features that would implicate a specific etiologic agent are usually absent. One exception is *maple bark stripper's disease*,[10] in which 3–5-μm, ovoid, thick-walled, brown spores of the causative organism, *Cryptostroma corticale*, can be identified within the histiocytes or granulomas. Interstitial aggregates of foamy macrophages have been noted in some cases of *pigeon breeder's disease* but likely are nonspecific findings related to bronchiolar obstruction from bronchiolitis obliterans.[16] Staining for specific antigens has been detected in lung tissue by immunofluorescent techniques in a few cases.[12,33,49]

Although the earliest pathologic changes in hypersensitivity pneumonia are not well defined, lung changes have been described in one patient who died several days following his first attack.[3] These changes were characterized by a necrotic, intraalveolar, acute

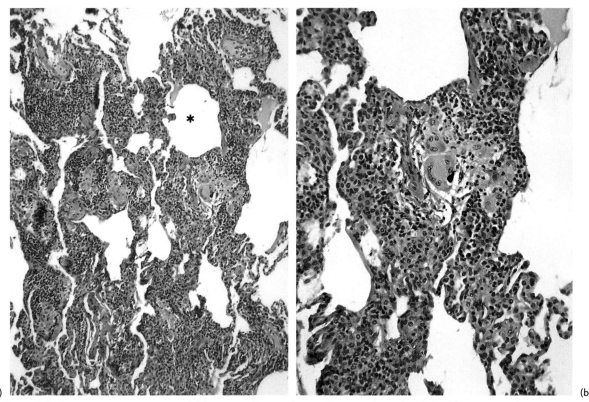

(a)　　　　　　　　　　　　　　　　　　　　　　　　　　　　　　　　　　　　　　(b)

Figure 6–3 Hypersensitivity pneumonia. (a) Low magnification showing large numbers of epithelioid histiocytes and multinucleated giant cells admixed with a chronic inflammatory cell infiltrate in this example. A small bronchiole is at top right (asterisk). (b) Higher magnification showing the mixed cellular infiltrate along with a loosely formed non-necrotizing granuloma.

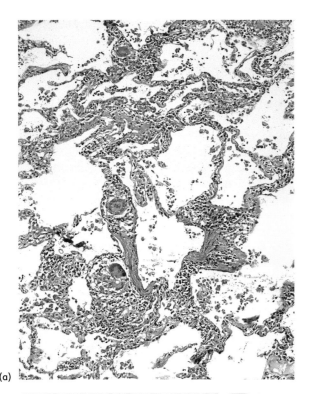

(a)

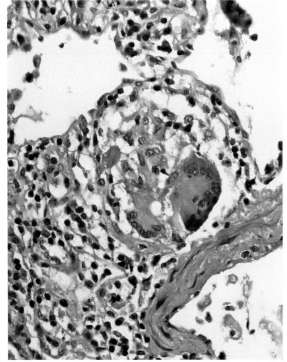

(b)

Figure 6–4 Hypersensitivity pneumonia. (a) Low magnification view showing cellular chronic interstitial pneumonia accentuated around a respiratory bronchiole. **(b)** At higher magnification a loosely formed non-necrotizing granuloma is appreciated in peribronchiolar interstitium.

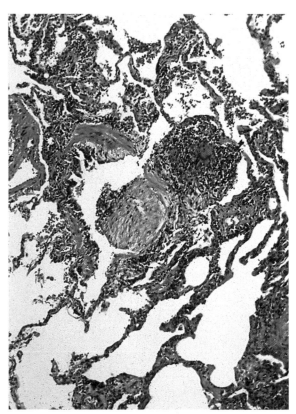

Figure 6–5 Bronchiolitis obliterans in hypersensitivity pneumonia. Note the intraluminal fibrous plug within a small bronchiole. There is a surrounding cellular chronic interstitial pneumonia including an ill-defined non-necrotizing granuloma.

inflammatory cell exudate combined with interstitial pneumonia located predominantly around respiratory bronchioles. Bronchiolitis obliterans was also found, and there was focal acute vasculitis involving alveolar capillaries and small arteries.

Interstitial fibrosis only becomes prominent in advanced disease. Often, the peribronchiolar accentuation is maintained, but the changes can be difficult to distinguish from usual interstitial pneumonia (UIP) at this stage.[5a,18,28,32] The presence of fibrosis, not surprisingly, is associated with a worse prognosis.[47]

Pathologic Diagnosis

The triad of a temporally uniform chronic interstitial pneumonia with peribronchiolar accentuation, non-necrotizing granulomas in peribronchiolar interstitium, and foci of bronchiolitis obliterans is diagnostic, although, as mentioned above, all three components are not always present. The finding of granulomas in a cellular chronic interstitial pneumonia is highly suggestive of the diagnosis, while a cellular chronic interstitial pneumonia with peribronchiolar accentuation should raise the possibility of hypersensitivity pneumonia. Clinical investigation and pertinent laboratory testing should be performed in such cases to confirm or exclude the diagnosis. It should be remembered, however, that even in cases demonstrating the classic diagnostic triad of pathologic findings, an exposure source may not be identifiable.[6] Interestingly, the prognosis seems to be similar whether or not an exposure is identified.

Differential Diagnosis

The main lesions in the histologic differential diagnosis of hypersensitivity pneumonia include other non-infectious interstitial processes and granulomatous infections. UIP, lymphoid interstitial pneumonia (LIP), and sarcoidosis are the main noninfectious interstitial processes, and their differentiating features are listed in Table 6–2 (see also Table 9-2). UIP (see Chapter 3) is distinguished by the characteristic temporal hetero-geneity of the pathologic changes with prominent fibrosis and areas of honeycomb change in most cases. Also, even in areas showing minimal fibrosis, the interstitial pneumonia in UIP contains a less densely cellular infiltrate than that seen in hypersensitivity pneumonia. Epithelioid histiocytes and granulomas do not occur in UIP, and their presence should be a tip-off to the diagnosis. LIP (see Chapter 9) is distinguished from hypersensitivity pneumonia in that its interstitial infiltrate is considerably more cellular, commonly contains prominent germinal centers, and often expands and distorts alveolar septa. It involves the lung diffusely and does not show the peribronchiolar distribution characteristic of hypersensitivity pneumonia. BOOP is usually not seen in LIP, and although epithelioid histiocytes and granulomas can be found, they are usually overshadowed by the lymphocytes and plasma cells. The clinical history may be helpful in some cases, since LIP is commonly associated with Sjögren's syndrome or other autoimmune phenomena, and, of course, an exposure history may be identifiable in patients with hypersensitivity pneumonia. Findings identical to nonspecific interstitial pneumonia (NSIP, see Chapter 3) can be seen in some cases of hypersensitivity pneumonia.[48] The possibility of hypersensitivity pneumonia, therefore, should be excluded clinically before diagnosing NSIP.

Hypersensitivity pneumonia and sarcoidosis may be difficult to distinguish in a few cases, but in general they are readily separable (see Chapter 7). The main histologic differences involve the distribution of the inflammatory reaction, the appearance of the granulomas, and the extent of the interstitial pneumonia. In sarcoidosis, the granulomas are distributed along lymphatic pathways, therefore following interlobular septa and the bronchovascular tree, in contrast to the strictly peribronchiolar distribution in hypersensitivity pneumonia. The granulomas in sarcoidosis are well-circumscribed, tight collections of epithelioid histiocytes, in contrast to the loosely formed histiocyte aggregates in hypersensitivity pneumonia. Partial hyalinization is common in the granulomas of sarcoidosis but is usually not seen in hypersensitivity pneumonia. A

Table 6–2 Differentiating Features of Hypersensitivity Pneumonia and Other Interstitial Inflammatory Disorders

	HP	UIP	LIP	Sarcoidosis
Interstitial pneumonia	Yes	Yes	Yes	No
Appearance	Temporally uniform, cellular	Temporally variegated, scantly cellular	Temporally uniform, densely cellular with alveolar septal distortion	—
Distribution	Peribronchiolar	Random	Diffuse	—
Honeycomb change	Not usually	Usually	No	No
Granulomas	Common	No	Common	Yes
Appearance	Loosely formed	—	Loosely formed	Well formed, well circumscribed
Distribution	Peribronchiolar	—	Random	Lymphangitic
BOOP	Common	No	No	No

Abbreviations: HP = hypersensitivity pneumonia; UIP = usual interstitial pneumonia; LIP = lymphoid interstitial pneumonia; BOOP = bronchiolitis obliterans–organizing pneumonia.

chronic interstitial pneumonia extending beyond the granulomatous foci is a major feature in hypersensitivity pneumonia but does not occur in sarcoidosis. Finally, areas of BOOP are common in hypersensitivity pneumonia but are not seen in sarcoidosis.

Special stains for organisms and cultures should be performed in all cases, to distinguish hypersensitivity pneumonia from granulomatous infections. The one infection that especially may mimic hypersensitivity pneumonia is nontuberculous (*Mycobacterium avium-complex*) mycobacterial infection, caused in most cases by exposure to contaminated hot tubs and known as *hot tub lung* (see Chapter 11). Hot tub lung is commonly associated with a chronic interstitial pneumonia and areas of BOOP in addition to granulomas. The main histologic difference from hypersensitivity pneumonia is that the granulomas tend to be well formed rather than loosely formed, and some contain central necrosis. Also, the chronic interstitial pneumonia is usually confined to the area of granulomatous inflammation rather than affecting the lung more diffusely.

Pulmonary Mycotoxicosis (Organic Dust Syndrome)

Pulmonary mycotoxicosis, or *organic dust syndrome*, is a reaction that follows massive organic dust exposure, and it needs to be distinguished from farmer's lung and other forms of hypersensitivity pneumonia. It is an acute, febrile respiratory illness that classically is associated with unloading silos.[8,11,23,46] Clinically, fever, cough, and respiratory distress develop several hours following exposure. The disease differs from farmer's lung in that most exposed individuals become ill, indicating that it represents a toxic, rather than a hypersensitivity, reaction. Also, most patients do not manifest infiltrates on chest radiographs, precipitating antibodies do not develop, and recurrences do not happen despite continued exposure. The histologic appearance is characterized by an interstitial and intraalveolar neutrophilic and histiocytic infiltrate associated with bronchiolitis. Large numbers of fungal elements can be found within the exudate. Recovery is the rule, and there are no known respiratory tract sequelae.

PULMONARY EOSINOPHILIA

Pulmonary eosinophilia can be defined as a condition in which patchy pulmonary infiltrates occur radiographically, and in which, pathologically, eosinophils are a

Table 6–3 Classification of Pulmonary Eosinophilia
Eosinophilic pneumonia
Simple (Loeffler's syndrome)
Tropical
Chronic
Acute
Mucoid impaction of bronchi
Bronchocentric granulomatosis
Allergic bronchopulmonary aspergillosis
Churg–Strauss syndrome

prominent component of the inflammatory cell infiltrate.[51,93] There is usually, but not always, associated eosinophilia of blood and/or sputum. 'PIE (pulmonary infiltrates with eosinophilia) syndrome' is an older term for pulmonary eosinophilia that is generally no longer used.

There have been several classifications of pulmonary eosinophilia.[51,93] Ours is a modification of an approach by Morrissey et al[79] and is listed in Table 6–3. In the following sections, the pertinent clinical and pathologic features of eosinophilic pneumonia, mucoid impaction of bronchi, bronchocentric granulomatosis, and allergic bronchopulmonary aspergillosis are discussed. Churg–Strauss syndrome is reviewed in Chapter 8.

Eosinophilic Pneumonia

Eosinophilic pneumonia is the most common form of pulmonary eosinophilia.[51,72] It encompasses four clinical syndromes: simple eosinophilic pneumonia (Loeffler's syndrome), tropical eosinophilic pneumonia, chronic (prolonged) eosinophilic pneumonia, and acute eosinophilic pneumonia. Importantly, the histopathologic changes are similar in all four conditions, and the pathologist can only diagnose eosinophilic pneumonia generically from the histologic appearance.

Clinical Syndromes Associated with Eosinophilic Pneumonia

Simple Eosinophilic Pneumonia: Simple eosinophilic pneumonia (Loeffler's syndrome) is a mild, self-limited condition that usually resolves spontaneously in less than 1 month.[79] Patients with this disease generally have fleeting pulmonary infiltrates and peripheral blood eosinophilia, and they may be asymptomatic. Biopsy is generally not necessary, since the clinical symptoms are minimal and the course is short. Tissue changes, reported in only a few cases, are typical of eosinophilic pneumonia.[72]

Tropical Eosinophilic Pneumonia: Biopsy is usually not necessary in tropical eosinophilic pneumonia, which is a well-recognized clinical syndrome in the tropics.[82,85] Patients generally present with high fever, cough, wheezing, fleeting chest infiltrates, and a high blood eosinophil count. Filarial infections have been implicated in the etiology of most cases. Pulmonary lesions are thought to result from an inflammatory reaction to circulating microfilaria. These patients respond to antifilarial drugs.

Chronic Eosinophilic Pneumonia: Chronic eosinophilic pneumonia, in contrast to simple and tropical eosinophilic pneumonia, is likely to require lung biopsy for diagnosis. Clinically, most patients present with a subacute illness characterized by fever, chills, dyspnea, weight loss, and malaise present for several weeks.[57,60,63,67,68,71,75,79] Mild, nonspecific respiratory complaints are less common, and a few individuals are asymptomatic. Women are affected more often than men, and patients frequently have a history of chronic asthma.[74,75] Peripheral blood eosinophilia is usually present, and elevated IgE levels have been reported during the acute phase. Radiographically, patchy, nonsegmental, often-peripheral infiltrates with ill-defined borders are commonly seen. The infiltrates may be transient, and they tend to resolve and reappear in the same location.[67,77] An unusual chest x-ray pattern resembling the 'photographic negative of pulmonary edema' was described by Gaensler and Carrington[61] and is highly suggestive of the diagnosis. It is not specific, however, since other conditions such as BOOP and viral pneumonia can cause the same radiographic appearance.[51] Most patients with chronic eosinophilic pneumonia respond favorably to corticosteroid therapy, although recurrences are common and prolonged therapy may be necessary.[56,57,68,75,76,81]

Many cases of chronic eosinophilic pneumonia are idiopathic, but a number of potential etiologies need to be excluded in all cases (Table 6–4).[51,68,76,79] Probably, the most important one is drug toxicity (see Chapter 4), and the most common drugs associated with this lesion include bleomycin, nitrofurantoin, para-aminosalicylic acid, penicillin, and sulfonamides.[55,62,66,80,88,98,99] Ingestion of L-tryptophan may also produce this lesion.[96] Fungal hypersensitivity, especially to aspergillus (see later on), is an important cause,[58,65,72,77–79,86] and

Table 6–4 Causes of Chronic Eosinophilic Pneumonia
Drug toxicity (ampicillin, bleomycin, cromoglycate, glafenine, hydralazine, naproxen, nitrofurantoin, para-aminosalicylic acid, penicillin, streptomycin, sulfasalazine, sulfonamides, tetracycline)
Other ingestants (L-tryptophan)
Fungal hypersensitivity (*Aspergillus, Curvularia, Drechslera, Helminthosporium, Candida, Torulopsis, Bipolaris, Pseudoallescheria, Fusarium*, etc.)
Parasites (*Ancyclostoma*, ascaris, filaria, *Strongyloides*)
Inhalants (cocaine, nickel carbonyl vapor)
Unknown

parasitic infestation due to various organisms in addition to filaria has been implicated in some cases.[72] Inhalation of substances such as crack cocaine and nickel carbonyl fumes has also been reported to cause eosinophilic pneumonia.[59,72,83] Patients should undergo a comprehensive clinical and laboratory evaluation to identify a cause, including a detailed ingestant (especially drugs) and inhalant history, testing of serum for precipitating antibodies to various organisms, examination of stool for ova and parasites, and sputum cultures for fungi. Although in most patients the illness responds to corticosteroid treatment, it is best if a specific cause can be identified and eliminated in order to prevent recurrence.

The pathogenesis of chronic eosinophilic pneumonia is unknown, but a role has been proposed for the eosinophil-active cytokine interleukin-5 (IL-5).[70]

Acute Eosinophilic Pneumonia: This variant of eosinophilic pneumonia has only been recognized in recent years, although it is likely that cases in the past have been included in the spectrum of chronic eosinophilic pneumonia.[71] Patients present with an acute febrile illness, usually of less than 1 week's duration. Diffuse bilateral infiltrates are present radiographically, and respiratory failure, often requiring mechanical ventilation, develops rapidly.[52–54,87,89] Most patients do not have asthma, and blood eosinophilia is usually not present. The disease responds dramatically to corticosteroid therapy, and recurrences have not been documented. The etiology is unknown in most cases, although parasites (toxocara),[90] drugs (trazodone),[92] toxic inhalants (Scotchguard),[69] heavy dust exposure

(World Trade Center),[91] and cigarette smoking[94,95] have been implicated rarely.

Histologic Features of Eosinophilic Pneumonia

The predominant histologic feature in eosinophilic pneumonia is the filling of alveolar spaces by eosinophils admixed with variable numbers of macrophages (Fig. 6–6).[60,65,68,72,79] The latter cells contain abundant, pale eosinophilic cytoplasm and sometimes are multinucleated. The proportion of eosinophils and macrophages varies; although eosinophils are usually predominant, the macrophages may focally be numerous (Fig. 6–7). Occasionally, eosinophil granules – or even Charcot-Leyden crystals – may be found within the cytoplasm of the macrophages (Fig. 6–8), and evidence of eosinophil degranulation can be demonstrated ultrastructurally as well as by immunofluorescence.[64,65,84] A proteinaceous exudate is often prominent within the alveolar spaces adjacent to areas containing the cellular infiltrate. Necrosis of the intraalveolar cellular infiltrate is common, but parenchymal (interstitial) necrosis does not occur. Eosinophilic abscesses consisting of a central mass of necrotic eosinophils surrounded by palisading histiocytes are occasionally found. Foci of BOOP (see Chapter 2) are frequently associated with the other airspace findings (Fig. 6–9), and changes of diffuse alveolar damage (DAD) have been described in acute eosinophilic pneumonia (Fig. 6–10).[68,72,97]

The airspace exudate in eosinophilic pneumonia is typically accompanied by an interstitial pneumonia characterized by expansion of alveolar septa by a mixture of eosinophils, lymphocytes, and plasma cells with associated alveolar lining cell hyperplasia. Other abnormalities of the interstitial architecture can be seen by electron microscopy, including edema, eosinophil granules – both free and within macrophages – and hydropic changes in macrophages and endothelial cells.[60,64] A mild, non-necrotizing vasculitis involving small arteries and venules is often present as well. It is characterized by a perivascular and sometimes transmural, chronic inflammatory cell infiltrate with numerous eosinophils (Fig. 6–11), and its presence does not indicate a more serious condition such as Churg–Strauss syndrome (see Chapter 8).

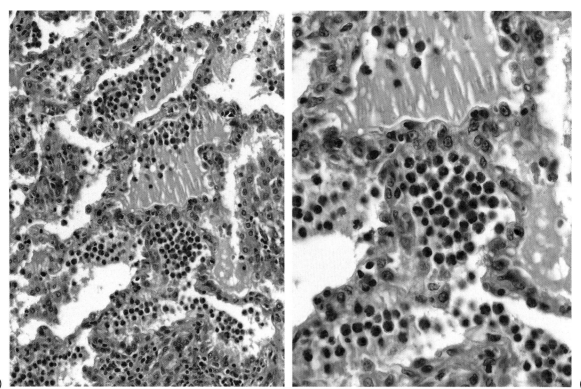

(a) (b)

Figure 6–6 Eosinophilic pneumonia. (a) Low magnification showing the presence of clusters of eosinophils within alveolar spaces associated with a mild chronic interstitial pneumonia. **(b)** Higher magnification showing numerous eosinophils and scattered macrophages filling an alveolar space.

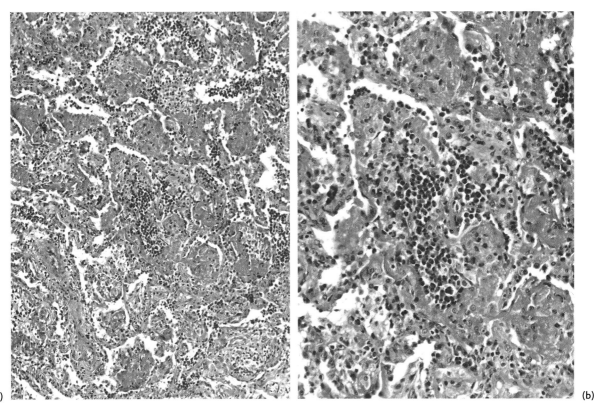

Figure 6–7 Eosinophilic pneumonia. (a) A proteinaceous exudate is prominent in this example within alveolar spaces, in addition to numerous eosinophils and macrophages. There is also a prominent associated chronic interstitial pneumonia. **(b)** Higher magnification of alveolar exudate, showing a mixture of eosinophils, proteinaceous material, and numerous macrophages.

Differential Diagnosis of Eosinophilic Pneumonia

Eosinophilic pneumonia is one pathologic manifestation of *Churg–Strauss syndrome* (see Chapter 8). Sometimes, other features may also be present, including necrotizing granulomatous inflammation and granulomatous vasculitis, and they should suggest the diagnosis. When eosinophilic pneumonia is the sole finding, however, Churg–Strauss syndrome should be considered only if typical clinical features (asthma, high blood eosinophil count, and evidence of vasculitis in two extrapulmonary sites), often accompanied by a positive p-ANCA, are present. It should be remembered that a perivascular eosinophil infiltrate is common in ordinary eosinophilic pneumonia and its presence does not indicate Churg–Strauss syndrome.

Another entity in the differential diagnosis of eosinophilic pneumonia is *eosinophilic granuloma* (see Chapter 15). Although the infiltrate in this condition is also composed of a combination of eosinophils and histiocytes, it differs in that it is predominantly interstitial, rather than intraalveolar, in location. Also, the histiocytes of eosinophilic granuloma (Langerhans cells) have characteristic deeply infolded nuclei, in contrast to the round nuclei of eosinophilic pneumonia. In difficult cases, staining for S-100 antigen or CD1a should help, since only the histiocytes of eosinophilic granuloma, not the macrophages of eosinophilic pneumonia, stain positively.

When macrophages are prominent within the intraalveolar infiltrate of eosinophilic pneumonia, *respiratory bronchiolitis interstitial lung disease/desquamative interstitial pneumonia* (RBILD/DIP) may enter the differential diagnosis (see Chapter 3). Interstitial and perivascular inflammation, necrosis of the intraalveolar exudate, and eosinophilic abscesses are common features of eosinophilic pneumonia that are not seen in RBILD/DIP.

Other conditions may be associated with a prominent eosinophil infiltrate, including various infections (especially coccidioidomycosis, see Chapter 11), dirofilarial nodules (see Chapter 11), and Wegener's granulomatosis

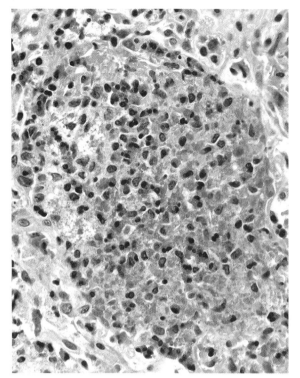

Figure 6–8 Macrophages are prominent in addition to eosinophils in this airspace exudate of eosinophilic pneumonia. Note that many macrophages contain eosinophil granules in their cytoplasm.

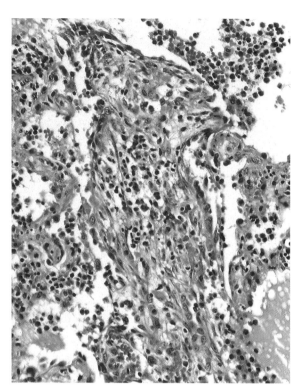

Figure 6–9 BOOP in eosinophilic pneumonia. The characteristic intraluminal fibroblast plug of BOOP is shown. Numerous eosinophils are present along with the fibroblasts and chronic inflammatory cells.

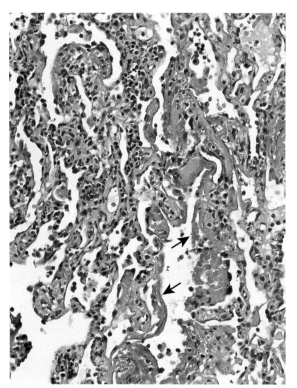

Figure 6–10 Acute eosinophilic pneumonia. Hyaline membranes (arrows) are seen in this example, along with an interstitial and airspace infiltrate of eosinophils.

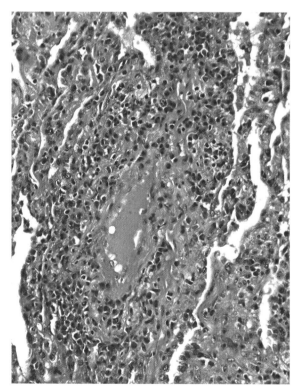

Figure 6–11 Vasculitis in eosinophilic pneumonia. This pulmonary artery is surrounded by a dense eosinophil infiltrate. There is no necrosis of the wall or the infiltrating inflammatory cells.

(eosinophilic variant, see Chapter 8), and a perivascular eosinophil infiltrate has been described in portions of lungs resected from patients with spontaneous pneumothorax.[73] The diagnosis of eosinophilic pneumonia should not be made in cases with unusual pathologic features, especially parenchymal necrosis or necrotizing vasculitis, and caution should be exercised when the clinical and radiographic features do not fit.

Mucoid Impaction of Bronchi

Mucoid impaction of bronchi (MIB) is an uncommon condition affecting segmental and subsegmental bronchi that is characterized by the dilatation and filling of bronchi with characteristic thick mucoid material. The changes are unassociated with proximal bronchial obstruction. MIB differs from the more common postobstructive bronchiectasis with mucous plugging, not only by the lack of bronchial obstruction but also histologically (see further on).

Clinical and Radiographic Features

Most patients with MIB have an underlying lung disease, such as asthma, chronic bronchitis, or cystic fibrosis.[101,104,108,110,120] They may be asymptomatic, or they may manifest signs and symptoms of acute pneumonia occurring distal to the impacted bronchus. Some patients present with symptoms related to an exacerbation of their underlying disease. In many cases, MIB is a manifestation of a fungal hypersensitivity reaction (allergic bronchopulmonary fungal disease – ABPFD, see later on).

The radiographic features of MIB are variable.[101,111] Typically, V- or Y-shaped densities are described that may be associated with distal zones of collapse or areas of consolidation. If there are multiple involved bronchi, the radiographic changes can resemble a cluster of grapes. Frequently, however, the lesions present as isolated, well-circumscribed, rounded densities that are indistinguishable from neoplasms. It is this appearance that usually prompts surgical excision.

Pathologic Features

Grossly, the bronchi in MIB are dilated and filled with firm, rubbery, often laminated, gray to light brown material (Fig. 6–12).[100] Expectorated plugs of such mucoid material may maintain the shape of the parent bronchus (Fig. 6–13). Microscopically, the bronchial walls are thinned and fibrotic with atrophic islands of cartilage, and their lumens are dilated and filled

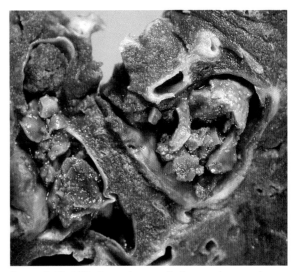

Figure 6–12 **MIB.** Gross photograph showing the typical tan, brown material that fills dilated bronchi. (Photograph courtesy of Dr Michael Mazur, Syracuse, NY.)

with mucinous material (Fig. 6–14). The bronchial epithelium may be compressed and show squamous metaplasia.[100,101,111] A submucosal infiltrate of plasma cells and lymphocytes with variable numbers of eosinophils is present. The impacted intraluminal material usually shows features of so-called *allergic mucin*, characterized by a mixture of mucus, fibrin, eosinophils, Charcot-Leyden crystals, neutrophils, and necrotic cellular debris. Eosinophils usually comprise the majority of cells and frequently appear degenerated. They are tightly clustered and, along with other cellular debris, are arranged in a distinct lamellar configuration (Fig. 6–15).[102,111] Charcot-Leyden crystals, which appear hexagonal in cross-section and bipyramidal in longitudinal section and are related to eosinophil breakdown, may be numerous. In patients with ABPFD (see further on), fungal hyphae can usually be identified within the allergic mucin, and this finding may be the first clue to diagnosis in unsuspected cases (Fig. 6–16). Changes may also be seen in the parenchyma distal to the impaction, including, most commonly, BOOP, eosinophilic pneumonia, and granulomas.[104]

When examining specimens containing MIB, care should be taken to avoid washing the mucoid material out of the bronchi. Multiple microscopic sections of the impacted mucus should be examined using Grocott–Gomori methenamine silver (GMS) stains in addition to hematoxylin and eosin (H and E) to search for fungal hyphae.

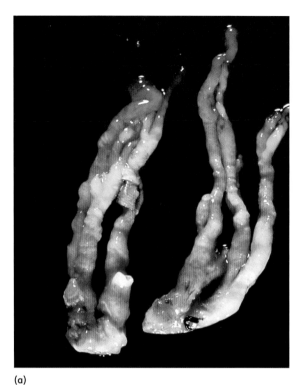

(a)

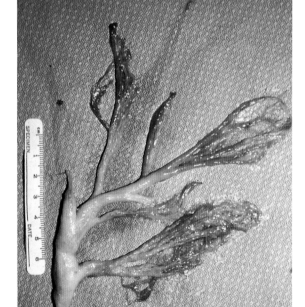

(b)

Figure 6–13 Mucous plugs in MIB. (a) Expectorated plugs have the shape of the branching parent bronchi. **(b)** This plug was removed at bronchoscopy. It shows a delicate distal branching pattern of small bronchi.

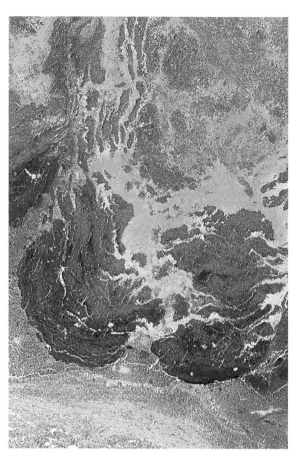

Figure 6–14 MIB. Low magnification showing the characteristic allergic mucin filling a dilated bronchus. The thinned and inflamed bronchial wall is at the bottom.

Differential Diagnosis

MIB must be differentiated from mucous plugging associated with asthma, from postobstructive mucous plugging, and from so-called plastic bronchitis. The mucous plugs in asthma differ in that they lack the distinct lamellated pattern of allergic mucin, although they contain numerous eosinophils and frequently Charcot-Leyden crystals.[102] Postobstructive plugs consist of a mixture of mucus, neutrophils, bronchial epithelial cells, and cell debris, but few eosinophils and no Charcot-Leyden crystals. *Plastic bronchitis (cast bronchitis)* is a rare condition that has been reported in both children and adults, usually in association with infections, bronchiectasis, cystic fibrosis, or cardiac anomalies.[103,106,107,109] It also is commonly encountered in children with the acute chest syndrome of sickle cell disease.[105] The plugs in this lesion are composed of a mixture of neutrophils, cellular debris, and

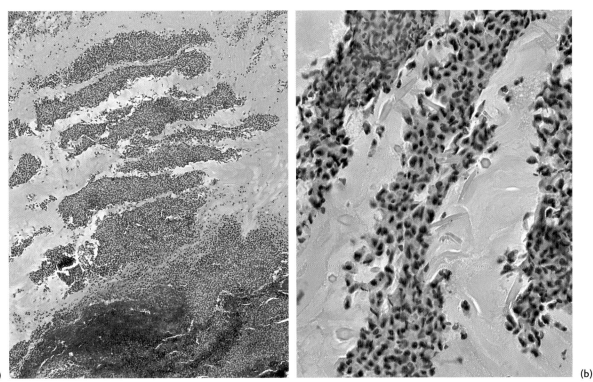

(a)

(b)

Figure 6–15 Allergic mucin. (a) The characteristic lamellar arrangement of necrotic eosinophils and other inflammatory cells within background mucin and proteinaceous exudates is illustrated in this photomicrograph. **(b)** At higher magnification, numerous Charcot-Leyden crystals are seen along with clusters of necrotic eosinophils. The Charcot-Leyden crystals appear hexagonal on cross-section and bipyramidal, needle-shaped on longitudinal section.

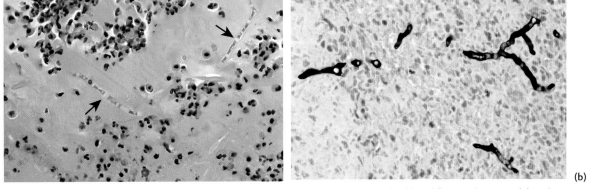

(a)

(b)

Figure 6–16 Fungal hyphae in allergic mucin. Fungal hyphae (arrows) can be visualized in H and E-stained sections **(a)** and are highlighted with GMS **(b)**. Note the irregular fragmented appearance of the organisms.

proteinaceous exudate, but no eosinophils or Charcot-Leyden crystals.

Bronchocentric Granulomatosis

Bronchocentric granulomatosis was first described by Liebow[122] in 1973, and there have been relatively few cases published since then.[113,116,117,120,121,128,130] It is a necrotizing granulomatous process that centers upon and destroys bronchioles. About half the reported cases have occurred in asthmatics with blood and tissue eosinophilia, and they represent a manifestation of ABPFD (see further on).[113,117,120,136] The remaining cases are of uncertain etiology, and many likely represent misdiagnosed or undiagnosed infectious processes.[124] The diagnosis of bronchocentric granulomatosis should be made with caution in patients without asthma or eosinophilia, and the term should not be used for infections or other processes that happen to preferentially affect bronchioles.

Clinical Features

Patients with asthma usually present with fever, cough, or severe wheezing, and peripheral blood eosinophilia is common.[120] Solitary lung infiltrates or regions of atelectasis are the most characteristic radiographic findings. Treatment and prognosis are the same as for ABPFD (see further on).

The nonasthmatic individuals with bronchocentric granulomatosis are clinically more heterogeneous.[120,121] Their presenting manifestations range from absent or minimal symptoms to an acute, febrile respiratory illness. Blood eosinophilia is usually not present. The chest radiographic findings show localized mass lesions or areas of consolidation with atelectasis.[129] Most patients respond to corticosteroids, and some have recovered without therapy.

Histopathologic Features

In the earliest lesion, there is partial replacement of the bronchiolar mucosa by a rim of epithelioid histiocytes that often palisade around the lumen which contains a necrotic inflammatory exudate (Fig. 6–17). Later, both the mucosa and the walls of the bronchioles are totally destroyed by the granulomatous reaction, and the lesion resembles an ordinary necrotizing granuloma except that it is located adjacent to a pulmonary artery in the place normally occupied by a bronchiole (Fig. 6–18). Elastic tissue stains sometimes can help by either outlining the adjacent pulmonary arteries or staining remnants of bronchiolar elastic tissue. Palisading histiocytes usually surround the necrotic

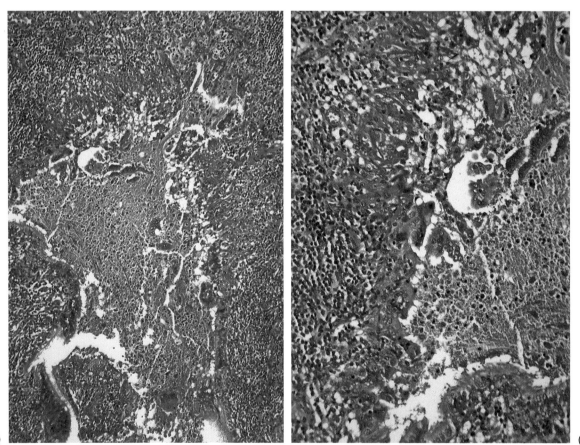

(a)   (b)

Figure 6–17 Bronchocentric granulomatosis. (a) Low magnification of a bronchiole showing partial replacement of the wall by palisading histiocytes. **(b)** Higher magnification showing the palisading histiocytes and fibrinoid necrosis replacing the bronchiolar epithelium. The lumen is filled with necrotic inflammatory debris.

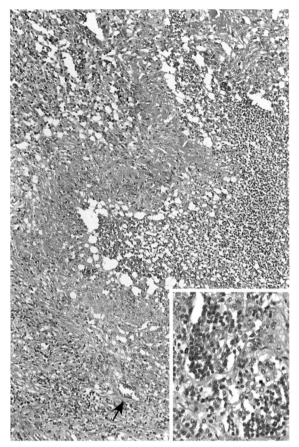

Figure 6–18 Bronchocentric granulomatosis. This necrotizing granuloma has completely replaced a bronchiole. The adjacent pulmonary artery is seen at the bottom (arrow) and is inflamed. Note the inflammatory exudates in the lumen. Eosinophils are prominent in the surrounding parenchyma (inset).

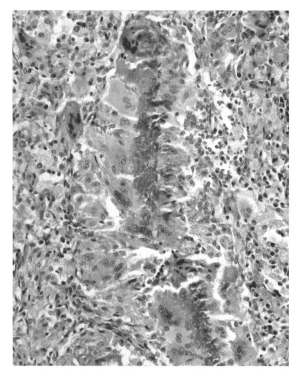

Figure 6–19 Foreign body giant cell reaction in bronchocentric granulomatosis. Coarsely granular to amorphous eosinophilic material is present in this foreign body granuloma. These structures are common in bronchocentric granulomatosis.

zones which are often filled with cellular debris and karyorrhectic nuclei. Remnants of eosinophils may be prominent. Sometimes, fungal hyphae can be identified within the necrosis by means of special stains. The finding of fungal hyphae does not indicate invasive infection, however, since the centers of the granulomas represent bronchiolar lumens, and invasion into adjacent parenchyma is not found. A peculiar foreign body giant cell reaction around clumps of amorphous or coarsely granular orange material, possibly related to necrotic eosinophils, is sometimes seen within the airspace exudate (Fig. 6–19). Eosinophils may be prominent in the surrounding infiltrate, where they are admixed with plasma cells, lymphocytes, histiocytes, and scattered multinucleated giant cells. Inflammation may extend into nearby pulmonary arteries, but a necrotizing vasculitis is not present. Areas of eosinophilic pneumonia are occasionally present in adjacent parenchyma. MIB is a common finding in proximal bronchi, and fungal hyphae are often identified in the impacted mucinous material.

Differential Diagnosis

A variety of conditions can cause bronchocentric necrotizing granulomatous inflammation, including both infectious and noninfectious processes (Fig. 6–20). Bronchocentric granulomas have been reported in 27% of tuberculomas and 8% of histoplasmomas, where they are usually focal findings (see Chapter 11).[128] Examples of tuberculosis, histoplasmosis, and blastomycosis have been described, however, in which the granulomatous inflammation was exclusively bronchocentric, exactly mimicking bronchocentric granulomatosis.[123,125] Similar cases have also been described in echinococcal infection,[114] invasive aspergillosis, and mucormycosis.[126,127] These observations underscore the need to use caution in diagnosing bronchocentric granulomatosis in the absence of asthma, eosinophilia, or MIB.

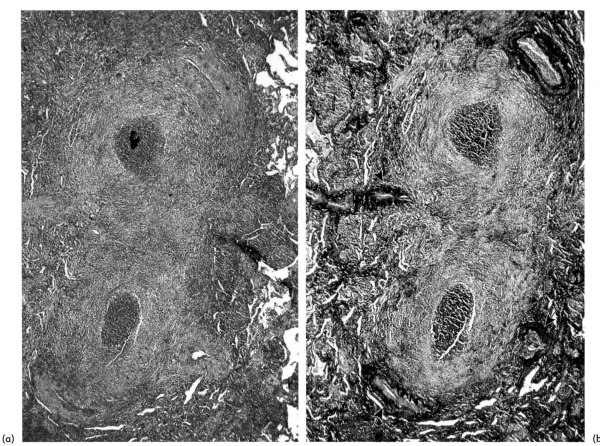

(a)   (b)

Figure 6–20 Bronchocentric granulomas in tuberculosis. Necrotizing granulomas completely replace bronchioles in this example
(a). The bronchocentric location of the granulomas is confirmed by an elastic tissue stain (b) which outlines the adjacent
pulmonary arteries (arrows).

Although the finding of numerous eosinophils
associated with the granulomatous inflammation favors
a noninfectious etiology, some infections, especially
coccidioidomycosis, may be associated with tissue
eosinophilia, and, a bronchocentric distribution to
the granulomas may occur. An infectious etiology,
therefore, should be carefully excluded in all cases, by
both special stains and cultures, before diagnosing
bronchocentric granulomatosis.

A bronchocentric distribution can also be seen in
noninfectious granulomatous processes other than
bronchocentric granulomatosis. Bronchiolar involvement can occur in Wegener's granulomatosis (see
Chapter 8, bronchocentric variant), and likely explains
reports of extrapulmonary disease in some cases of
bronchocentric granulomatosis.[116,118,130] The correct
diagnosis is established by recognizing the necrotizing
vasculitis characteristic of Wegener's. Rheumatoid
nodules can involve bronchioles.[112,122] They are usually

multiple radiographically and occur in patients with
subcutaneous nodules and high rheumatoid titers.
Necrotizing sarcoid granulomatosis can have bronchocentric involvement, but the presence of a granulomatous vasculitis distinguishes it from bronchocentric
granulomatosis.[122] Bronchocentric granulomas have
been reported distal to bronchial obstruction by
tumor.[119]

Allergic Bronchopulmonary Aspergillosis

Allergic bronchopulmonary aspergillosis (ABPA) is a
clinical syndrome occurring predominantly in chronic
asthmatics that is caused by hypersensitivity to
Aspergillus species, usually *A fumigatus*.[30,132,142,147] A
similar reaction has been reported less often to other
fungi, including *Curvularia lunata*,[143,148,152,166] *Drechslera
hawaiiensis*,[152] *Helminthosporium*,[144] *Torulopsis glabrata*,[158]
Candida albicans,[131,150] *Bipolaris*,[148] *Pseudoallescheria*

boydii,[149,156] and *Fusarium vasinfectum*.[134] The term *allergic bronchopulmonary fungal disease* (ABPFD) or *allergic bronchopulmonary mycosis* (ABPM) is a more generic designation that encompasses all potential fungal antigens and is used when the specific organism has not been identified.[135,139,152] The diagnosis of ABPA or the related ABPFD is generally established on the basis of clinical, radiographic, and laboratory findings, and biopsy is usually not undertaken. Tissue may be encountered by the pathologist, however, in clinically unsuspected cases or when irreversibly damaged portions of lung are removed. The pathogenesis is thought to be related to a combination of type I, type III, and possibly type IV, immunologic reactions to fungal antigens.

Clinical Features

The diagnosis of ABPA is based on the presence of asthma, peripheral blood eosinophilia, infiltrates (often transient) on chest radiographs, immediate cutaneous reactivity to aspergillus, elevated total serum IgE, precipitating antibodies to aspergillus, elevated serum levels of IgE and IgG antibodies to aspergillus, and central bronchiectasis.[146,157] The latter two findings are considered pathognomonic of ABPA, although central bronchiectasis is not present in early cases and specific IgE and IgG antibodies may be present in patients without detectable active disease.[141,142] Additional supporting features for ABPA include late cutaneous reactions to aspergillus, a history of expectorating sputum plugs, and culture of aspergillus from sputum.[137,142,151,153] Five stages of disease have been described and their recognition may help in patient management and assessing prognosis.[142,145,146,151,155,157]

Corticosteroids are the treatment of choice for ABPA, although a role for itraconazole has been suggested.[142,159,164] Recurrences are common, however, and, if untreated, may result in irreversible lung damage, including parenchymal fibrosis and bronchiectasis. Patients should be carefully followed with serial chest radiographs, since recurrent infiltrates can occur without associated symptoms. Monitoring serum levels of total IgE and specific IgE and IgG antibodies to aspergillus may also aid in following disease activity. Major surgical resections should be avoided once this diagnosis is established.

Histologic Features

Since tissue examination is generally not necessary for diagnosis, the histopathologic features of ABPA have not been extensively investigated. Several reports have described various combinations of broncho-

centric granulomatosis, eosinophilic pneumonia, and MIB.[120,133,136,140,160,163] Tissue eosinophilia is prominent in most cases. Scattered fungal hyphae usually can be found within the centers of the bronchocentric granulomas and within the intraluminal mucin of MIB. Invasion by fungi into viable tissue or blood vessels is not a feature.

The findings on a lung biopsy specimen of BCG and/or MIB, along with evidence of tissue eosinophilia, is highly suggestive of ABPA (or ABPFD), and if fungal hyphae are also present, these changes are diagnostic. It is especially important for the pathologist to recognize this disease so that appropriate therapy can be instituted. Interestingly, a lesion similar to ABPA or ABPFD may involve the nose and paranasal sinuses and has been termed *allergic aspergillus sinusitis* or *allergic fungal sinusitis*, depending on the organism identified.[138,145,165] It occasionally occurs in association with ABPA or ABPFD.[161,166,173] Histologically, typical allergic mucin with necrotic eosinophils, Charcot-Leyden crystals, and fungal hyphae fills the sinus cavity, an appearance that is identical to MIB.

PULMONARY HEMORRHAGE

For diagnostic purposes, cases of pulmonary hemorrhage can be divided into alveolar hemorrhage syndromes, secondary alveolar hemorrhage, and localized pulmonary hemorrhage (see Table 6–5). The bleeding in the *alveolar hemorrhage syndromes* originates in the alveoli and involves the lungs diffusely. Patients present with hemoptysis, diffuse pulmonary infiltrates, and often anemia, and lung biopsy may be necessary for diagnosis.[168,172,175,190,191,199,212,216,217] *Secondary alveolar hemorrhage* occurs as a complication of another condition which is usually the dominant clinical finding. The diagnosis is generally made clinically and most cases do not require biopsy. *Localized pulmonary hemorrhage* is confined to a lobe or portion of a lobe. It is often treated by lobectomy, and the surgical pathologist may be faced with the difficult task of identifying the source of bleeding.

Careful correlation of clinical, laboratory, and radiographic findings with the pathologic findings is important for diagnosis in all forms of pulmonary hemorrhage. Additionally, the alveolar hemorrhage syndromes are an indication (in fact, the only indication) to perform immunofluorescence studies, and therefore a small aliquot of lung biopsy should be snap-frozen for immunofluorescence in suspected cases.

Table 6–5   Classification of Pulmonary Hemorrhage

I. **Alveolar Hemorrhage Syndromes**
   Goodpasture's syndrome
   Idiopathic pulmonary hemosiderosis
   Capillaritis syndromes (Wegener's granulomatosis,
      microscopic polyangiitis, acute lupus pneumonitis,
      other connective tissue diseases, cryoglobulinemia,
      Henoch-Schönlein purpura, etc.)
   Drug reactions (penicillamine, nitrofurantoin,
      L-tryptophan)
   Inhalant-related (cocaine, trimellitic anhydride,[167]
      pyromellitic dianhydride[185])
   Following hematopoietic stem cell transplantation
   Associated with idiopathic, rapidly progressive
      glomerulonephritis[194,195]

II. **Secondary Alveolar Hemorrhage**
   Infections (necrotizing bacterial pneumonia,
      leptospirosis)
   Renal failure with volume overload
   Thrombocytopenia, other coagulopathies
   Venous congestion (heart failure, mitral valve disease,
      pulmonary venoocclusive disease, fibrosing
      mediastinitis, mediastinal tumors)

III. **Localized Pulmonary Hemorrhage**
   Parenchymal lesions (neoplasm, fungus ball, other
      cavitary masses)
   Airway lesions, (bronchitis/bronchiectasis, neoplasms,
      vascular anomalies, lithiasis)

This section concentrates on Goodpasture's syndrome, idiopathic pulmonary hemosiderosis, secondary alveolar hemorrhage and localized alveolar hemorrhage. The capillaritis syndromes are discussed in Chapter 8, collagen vascular diseases in Chapter 7, drug reactions and cocaine in Chapter 4, and hematopoietic stem cell (bone marrow) transplantation later on in this chapter.

Goodpasture's Syndrome

Goodpasture's syndrome, also known as *anti-glomerular basement membrane (anti-GBM) antibody disease*, is a well-documented example of a type II, or cytotoxic antibody-mediated, immune reaction. Antibodies to glomerular basement membranes, which cross-react with pulmonary basement membranes, have been demonstrated within both the kidney and lung and in the serum. The disease affects men twice as often as women. Most patients are young adults who present with an acute onset of hemoptysis, anemia, azotemia, and diffuse pulmonary infiltrates. The diagnosis can usually be established by performing a kidney biopsy.[206] A proliferative or necrotizing glomerulonephritis that may be focal or diffuse and is often accompanied by crescent formation is the usual finding on light microscopy. Linear staining of the glomerular basement membranes for IgG (or, less commonly, for IgM or IgA) and complement is demonstrable by immunofluorescence. In most cases, circulating anti-GBM antibodies can be identified within the serum. Occasionally, a patient will manifest hemoptysis but minimal or absent renal abnormalities, and, in this case, a lung biopsy is likely to be performed.[173,214] It should be remembered that other types of glomerulonephritis may be accompanied by pulmonary hemorrhage in the absence of antiglomerular basement membrane antibodies.[180,189,194,195] By definition, these examples are not considered to represent Goodpasture's syndrome.

Treatment usually involves a combination of plasmapheresis and immunosuppressive therapy.[184,191] The prognosis seems to be related to the severity of renal disease prior to beginning therapy, with a more favorable outcome in patients having lower serum creatinine and fewer crescents on kidney biopsy specimens. Recurrences may happen, even after prolonged periods of remission.[187,197]

Histopathologic Features

The main histologic abnormality in Goodpasture's syndrome is extensive intraalveolar hemorrhage characterized by the accumulation of fresh blood and hemosiderin within airspaces (Fig. 6–21).[192,206,216] Hemosiderin is a hemoglobin degradation product that requires at least 2 days to form following hemorrhage and is usually cleared from the lungs after 2 to 4 weeks.[209] Its presence indicates a certain chronicity to the process and also verifies that the blood is not iatrogenically related to the lung biopsy procedure. The hemosiderin is usually found within alveolar macrophage cytoplasm but can be deposited extracellularly, and it appears as coarse, brown–yellow refractile granules. Nonspecific thickening of alveolar septa and alveolar pneumocyte hyperplasia commonly accompany the intraalveolar hemorrhage. A neutrophil infiltrate suggestive of capillaritis has been noted within alveolar septa in some cases,[192] and an eosinophil infiltrate has been reported rarely.[188] The presence, however, of extensive inflammation, definite vasculitis involving arteries or veins, or parenchymal necrosis should suggest another diagnosis. By immunofluorescence techniques, linear staining for immunoglobulins (usually

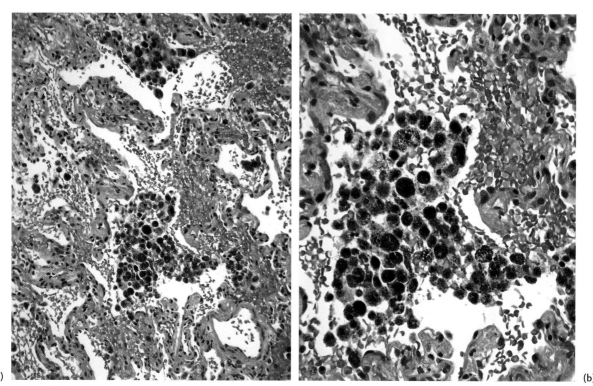

(a)   (b)

Figure 6–21 Goodpasture's syndrome. (a) Blood and hemosiderin fill alveolar spaces in this example. Note that the alveolar septa contain no inflammation. (b) Higher magnification showing hemosiderin-filled macrophages and blood in alveolar space.

IgG and, rarely, IgM or IgA) and complement can be demonstrated along alveolar septa (Fig. 6–22).[171] Ultrastructurally, widened gaps between endothelial cells, fragmentation of the capillary basement membranes, and deposition of ferritin particles along the basement membranes have been noted.[173,178]

Idiopathic Pulmonary Hemosiderosis

Idiopathic pulmonary hemosiderosis (IPH) may have clinical manifestations similar to Goodpasture's syndrome except that renal involvement is absent.[168,186,190,191,198,207] Unlike Goodpasture's syndrome, however, most cases occur in children under 10 years old, with females and males affected equally. A male predominance has been found in the few cases occurring in adults. Familial cases have been described as well.[170,174,198,213] Most patients present with hemoptysis and chest infiltrates and are found to have iron-deficiency anemia. Elevated serum IgA occurs in one-half of patients, but circulating anti-GBM antibodies are absent. An association with celiac disease has been noted in some cases and some children have precipitating antibodies to milk

proteins.[198,203,207,218] Spontaneous remissions and exacerbations are common, and they may recur over many years. Various therapies have been attempted, and corticosteroids, often combined with cytotoxic agents such as azathioprine, seem to have some beneficial effect.[186,198,207] Mortality is significant, but prognosis is difficult to precisely assess because the disease is so uncommon and there are few large series. An 86% 5-year survival was reported recently in a series of 17 children treated with corticosteroids, often combined with azathioprine or hydroxychloroquine.[207] This survival figure, however, is significantly higher than previous reports, and whether or not it represents a valid assessment is unclear.

Histopathologic Features

By light microscopy, IPH is indistinguishable from Goodpasture's syndrome. There is extensive intraalveolar hemorrhage with erythrocytes and hemosiderin. Nonspecific, alveolar septal thickening may be present, but vasculitis, necrosis, and inflammation are absent. Unlike Goodpasture's syndrome, however, no evidence of immunoglobulin or complement deposition is

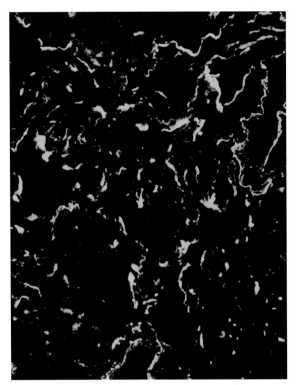

Figure 6–22 Immunofluorescence staining for IgG in Goodpasture's syndrome. Note the linear deposition along alveolar walls.

demonstrable by immunofluorescence techniques.[170] Ultrastructurally, various nonspecific abnormalities of alveolar capillary and epithelial basement membranes have been described, including reduplication, fragmentation, smudging, and thickening.[176,178,181,182,219] Swelling and other abnormalities of capillary endothelial cells that may be associated with luminal narrowing, along with platelet aggregation, have also been described.[176] Evidence of alveolar epithelial injury and repair has been noted in several cases as well.[179,183]

A common finding in IPH is the disruption and encrustation of vascular elastic tissue by iron and calcium deposition (Fig. 6–23). The elastic tissue assumes a thickened, refractile appearance and is often engulfed by foreign body giant cells. This is a nonspecific lesion that is termed *endogenous pneumoconiosis* (see Chapter 13), and it occurs in any condition characterized by chronic bleeding into the lung.[204]

It should be apparent that the histologic findings in IPH are nonspecific. The diagnosis, therefore, is one of exclusion and can be established only after all other causes of alveolar hemorrhage (see Table 6–5) have been eliminated.

Differential Diagnosis of Alveolar Hemorrhage Syndromes

Many of the causes of the alveolar hemorrhage syndrome listed in Table 6–5 can be diagnosed without a lung biopsy, using a combination of clinical history and laboratory studies. Goodpasture's syndrome, Wegener's granulomatosis, microscopic polyangiitis, acute lupus pneumonitis, and IPH are the conditions most likely to be biopsied, and their differentiating features are summarized in Table 6–6.[216] A necrotizing capillaritis occurs in Wegener's granulomatosis[201,215] and systemic lupus erythematosus[200] and is characterized by acute inflammation and necrosis of alveolar septal capillaries with occasional involvement of arterioles (see Chapter 8). Although a similar lesion has been described in some cases of Goodpasture's syndrome as well, it is generally not prominent.[192,216] Immunofluorescent studies are most helpful in interpreting biopsies in which a vasculitis or other histologic findings indicative of a specific disease are absent or subtle. Linear immunofluorescence along alveolar epithelial basement membranes for immunoglobulins and complement is diagnostic of Goodpasture's syndrome, while granular staining along endothelial basement membranes is frequent in systemic lupus erythematosus (see Chapter 7). Electron microscopy complements the immunofluorescent studies and shows dense deposits corresponding to the granular immunofluorescence in cases of systemic lupus erythematosus. Laboratory studies also help in the differential diagnosis. Circulating anti-GBM antibodies are found in Goodpasture's syndrome, antineutrophil cytoplasmic antibodies (ANCA, see Chapter 8) in Wegener's granulomatosis (usually C-ANCA) and in microscopic polyangiitis (usually P-ANCA), and antinuclear and related antibodies are characteristic of lupus. The presence and pattern of extrapulmonary involvement also helps in the differential diagnosis, as IPH is confined to the lung while Goodpasture's syndrome involves lung and kidney only, and other entities commonly involve additional sites such as skin, nervous system, joints and gastrointestinal tract, for example.

Secondary Alveolar Hemorrhage

Secondary causes of diffuse alveolar hemorrhage are listed in Table 6–5. The diagnosis is usually based on clinical and laboratory findings or bronchoalveolar lavage without the need for a biopsy. Infections (mainly necrotizing bacterial pneumonias due to ordinary bacteria, but also uncommon infections such as

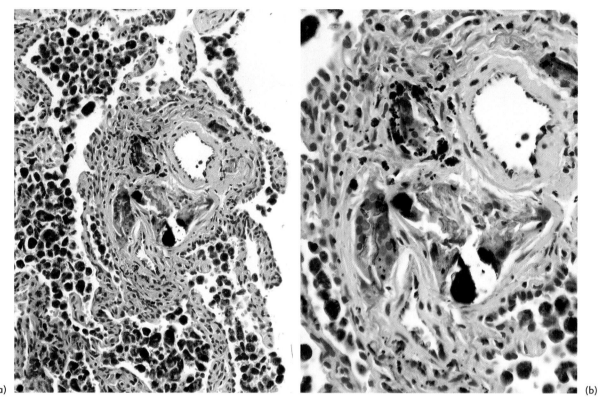

(a)
(b)

Figure 6–23 Endogenous pneumoconiosis in idiopathic pulmonary hemosiderosis. (a) Low magnification showing a foreign body giant cell reaction to altered elastic tissue in perivascular interstitium. Note the large numbers of hemosiderin-filled macrophages in adjacent alveolar spaces. **(b)** Higher magnification better illustrating the foreign body reaction to the altered elastic tissue.

Table 6–6 Differentiating Features of the Major Alveolar Hemorrhage Syndromes

	GPS	WG	MPA	SLE	IPH
Laboratory Findings					
Anti-GBM antibodies	Yes	No	No	No	No
ANCA	No	Usually (mostly C-ANCA)	Usually (mostly P-ANCA)	No	No
ANA	No	No	No	Yes	No
Extrapulmonary Involvement					
Kidney	Usually	Often	Often	Often	No
Other organs	No	Often	Often	Sometimes	No
Pathologic Findings					
Necrotizing capillaritis	Not usually	Yes	Yes	Yes	No
Immunofluorescence	Linear, epithelial bm	Negative	Negative	Granular, endothelial bm	Negative
Electron-dense deposits (EM)	No	No	No	Yes	No

Abbreviations: GPS = Goodpasture's syndrome; WG = Wegener's granulomatosis; MPA = microscopic polyangiitis; SLE = systemic lupus erythematosus; IPH = idiopathic pulmonary hemosiderosis; GBM = glomerular basement membrane; ANCA = antineutrophil cytoplasmic antibodies (C- with cytoplasmic fluorescence, P- with perinuclear fluorescence); ANA = antinuclear antibodies; EM = electron microscopy, bm = basement membrane.

leptospirosis), volume overload in renal failure, and thrombocytopenia or other coagulopathies are the most common causes.[169,177,193,202,205,208,210,217] Rarely, patients with clinically unapparent *mitral stenosis* may undergo lung biopsy, and the features can mimic those of IPH. Other causes of chronic venous congestion can produce a similar picture, including chronic congestive heart failure and obstruction of pulmonary venous outflow in the mediastinum as in fibrosing mediastinitis or slow growing tumors, for example. A similar clinicopathologic picture can also be caused by the rare condition *pulmonary venoocclusive disease* (see Chapter 13). The presence of vascular changes indicating pulmonary hypertension should suggest the correct diagnosis. The findings of occluded venules and small perivenous infarcts are additional helpful features in diagnosing PVOD.

Localized Pulmonary Hemorrhage

Cases in which pulmonary hemorrhage is localized to one portion of lung, usually a lobe, are more common than examples of the alveolar hemorrhage syndrome. Patients present with an acute onset of hemoptysis, which may be massive. Chest radiographs show localized consolidation corresponding to the area of intraalveolar hemorrhage, and bronchoscopy can identify fresh blood emanating from bronchi supplying the affected lobe. Lobectomy is the usual treatment. Some patients with localized bleeding have an obvious mass lesion or cavity that accounts for the hemorrhage, but in many there is no gross abnormality (other than the blood), and these pose a difficult and often frustrating problem for the pathologist. In our experience, the source of bleeding in such cases is almost always the bronchi, and serial sections should be taken from the bronchial tree. Sections of hemorrhagic distal lung are usually not productive. Microscopic foci of granulation tissue, with or without ulceration, broncholithiasis, foci of in situ squamous cell carcinoma, and tiny carcinoid tumors, are examples of abnormalities that may be found in the bronchi to account for the bleeding in some cases.[196,211] In a significant number of cases, however, a source of bleeding cannot be identified despite careful study.

TRANSPLANTATION-RELATED DISORDERS

Lung Transplantation

A number of complications occur following heart–lung or lung transplantation.[221,242,246,248,253] Harvest injury

Table 6–7   Classification of Lung Allograft Rejection

A. Acute (vascular) Rejection (Grade 0–4)
B. Airway Inflammation (Grade 0–4)
C. Chronic Airway Rejection – constrictive bronchiolitis obliterans (a/b – active/inactive)
D. Chronic Vascular Rejection – vascular sclerosis

related to ischemia occurs within a few days after transplantation. It is characterized pathologically by DAD. Hyperacute rejection occurs rarely within minutes to hours of vascular anastomosis.[225] It is thought to result from the presence of preformed antibodies against major allograft antigens. The main pathologic changes include platelet/fibrin thrombi and edema. Acute rejection and infection become important later on, and biopsies are frequently undertaken for diagnosis. After several months, constrictive bronchiolitis obliterans (see Chapter 16), often referred to in this clinical setting as *obliterative bronchiolitis* or *bronchiolitis obliterans syndrome*, can develop. It is thought to be a manifestation of chronic rejection. Arteriosclerotic vascular changes such as intimal fibrosis and medial hypertrophy may be seen in small pulmonary arteries and veins at this stage. The classification of lung allograft rejection is summarized in Table 6–7.[258,259] Other lesions, such as posttransplant lymphoproliferative disorder or recurrence of the original lung disease, may be encountered in long-term survivors.[233a,250,264]

Acute Rejection

Most episodes of acute rejection occur within 3 months following transplantation, although this phenomenon can be seen considerably later. Histologic findings indicative of acute rejection can be encountered in routine surveillance biopsies taken from asymptomatic patients, but they are seen more commonly in the setting of an acute febrile illness.[226,228,233,235–237,240,254,262] The clinical presentation of acute rejection may exactly mimic that of an infection and includes fever, cough, and chest x-ray infiltrates, and a biopsy, usually transbronchial, is taken to differentiate the two entities.[223,240,254]

Histologically, acute rejection is characterized by perivascular and subendothelial mononuclear cell infiltrates, often combined with lymphocytic bronchitis and bronchiolitis (Fig. 6–24).[226,227,235,254,262] It is divided into five grades based on the intensity and extent of the perivascular and interstitial mononuclear cell infiltrates, as listed in Table 6–8.[228,240,258,259] The

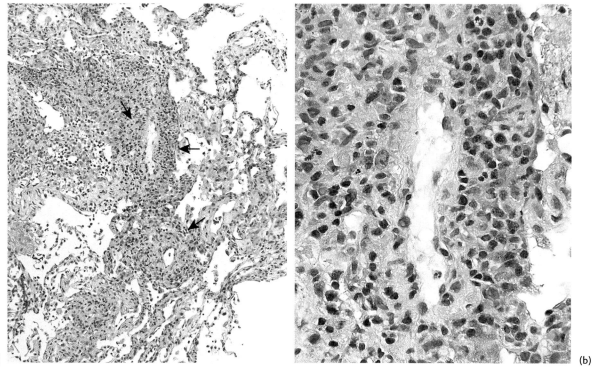

(a)

(b)

Figure 6–24 Acute rejection. (a) At low magnification a dense perivascular mononuclear cell infiltrate is seen (arrows). **(b)** Higher magnification shows numerous reactive lymphocytes and scattered plasma cells in the artery wall and focally extending beneath the endothelium. The changes correspond to grade A2. (Photomicrograph courtesy of Dr Jeffrey L Myers, Ann Arbor, Michigan.)

infiltrate consists of a mixture of small lymphocytes, transformed lymphocytes, and immunoblasts, and the majority are T cells.[234] Eosinophils and neutrophils may be prominent in severe cases and DAD can occur.[231,255] There is some evidence that cases containing proportionately more B cells respond less favorably to antirejection therapy.[262] A low proliferation rate of the cellular infiltrate measured by MIB-1 staining has been reported to be associated with a better response to therapy.[229] Hemosideran deposition within alveolar macrophages commonly accompanies the other changes, and there is some evidence that it is secondary to the acute rejection.[250a]

A lymphocytic bronchitis or bronchiolitis frequently accompanies the perivascular changes of acute rejection, and it can also be graded as listed in Table 6–9.[227,238,249,256,259] Acute inflammation sometimes accompanies the mononuclear cell infiltrate. The presence and/or intensity of airway inflammation does not affect the acute rejection grade, which is based solely on the perivascular and interstitial inflammation. In fact, airway inflammation can occur in the absence of acute rejection, in which case it may be related to

Table 6–8 Grading of Acute Rejection[259]

A0: No significant abnormality

A1: Minimal acute rejection
Occasional perivascular mononuclear cell infiltrates, not visible at low magnification

A2: Mild acute rejection
Frequent perivascular mononuclear cell infiltrates readily apparent at low magnification; subendothelial infiltrates and endothelialitis

A3: Moderate acute rejection
Dense perivascular mononuclear cell infiltrates, usually with endothelialitis, which extend into adjacent alveolar septa and airspaces

A4: Severe acute rejection
Similar to Grade A3, with extensive alveolar septal and airspace involvement and diffuse alveolar damage

Table 6–9 Grading of Airway Inflammation (Lymphocytic Bronchitis/Bronchiolitis)[259]

B0: No airway inflammation

B1: Minimal airway inflammation
Rare scattered mononuclear cells in submucosa

B2: Mild airway inflammation
Circumferential band of mononuclear cells in submucosa along with epithelial cell necrosis and infiltration by lymphocytes; occasional eosinophils present

B3: Moderate airway inflammation
Band-like submucosal mononuclear cell infiltrates with eosinophils, satellitosis, epithelial cell necrosis, and lymphocytic infiltration

B4: Severe airway inflammation
Dense band-like mononuclear cell infiltrate, epithelial necrosis and ulceration with fibrinopurulent exudates

infection. Severe airway inflammation may predict the eventual development of constrictive bronchiolitis obliterans in some cases.[249,256]

In all cases, special stains for organisms should be carefully examined and a search made for other indicators of infection, especially viral inclusions. The presence of prominent alveolar exudates should raise the suspicion of infection.[227] Perivascular lymphoid infiltrates are not specific for rejection and can also be seen in infections, especially cytomegalovirus (CMV).[230,248] Rejection should not be diagnosed in the presence of an identifiable infection.

Chronic Rejection

Constrictive bronchiolitis obliterans (see Chapter 16) occurs in up to 50% of long-term survivors of lung or heart–lung transplantation after a mean interval of 10 months and is considered a manifestation of chronic rejection.[220,222,223,232,241,245,260,263] The terms *bronchiolitis obliterans*, *obliterative bronchiolitis*, and *cicatricial bronchiolitis obliterans* have been used interchangeably for this lesion, and *bronchiolitis obliterans syndrome* is used in reference to the clinical manifestations.[234,245,294]

Clinically, patients with constrictive bronchiolitis obliterans usually present with progressive dyspnea, and pulmonary function tests show severe obstructive and mild restrictive defects. Only minimal and non-specific changes are seen on chest radiographs, although lower lobe bronchial dilatation may be found

on high-resolution CT scans.[243] The course is often rapidly progressive, although some cases respond to enhanced immunosuppressive therapy.[232,241,245]

The main pathologic finding is the presence of fibrosis occurring in the submucosa of terminal and respiratory bronchioles, causing luminal narrowing and/or obstruction (see Chapter 16, Figs 16–18 to 16–21). There may be an associated mononuclear cell infiltrate with ongoing epithelial injury in 'active' cases. Both T and B lymphocytes are identified, and alterations in bronchiolar basement membranes have been described.[234,252] Mast cells and dendritic cells may be prominent.[244,257] 'Inactive' lesions are characterized by dense scarring with minimal inflammation that replaces bronchioles. In this late stage, the histologic changes are often subtle, characterized only by small scars present adjacent to pulmonary arteries. Sometimes, remnants of bronchiolar smooth muscle are seen within and around the scars. An increase in collagen III has been noted by immunohistochemistry in the fibrous areas.[265]

The combination of acute inflammation in airways and histologic evidence of acute rejection elsewhere appears to predispose to the development of this lesion, and patients with lymphocytic bronchiolitis even without acute rejection also are at increased risk.[239] Late acute rejection and lymphocytic bronchiolitis are associated with an even higher risk of constrictive bronchiolitis obliterans.[239]

It should be remembered that although constrictive bronchiolitis obliterans is an important airway lesion in transplant recipients, examples of BOOP (see Chapter 2) may also occur.[220,224,247,251,261] They usually present sooner following transplantation, and are associated with infection, aspiration, or other demonstrable injury, including often acute rejection.

Hematopoietic Stem Cell Transplantation (Bone Marrow Transplantation)

Bone marrow transplantation is a potentially curative mode of therapy for some patients with otherwise fatal leukemias, aplastic anemia, lymphoma, and other malignancies and rare metabolic defects. 'Hematopoietic stem cell transplantation' is the preferred terminology since donor cells may be provided from fetal cord blood and peripheral blood in addition to bone marrow. The procedure consists of suppression of the patient's own bone marrow by various regimens that usually include both chemotherapy and total body irradiation, followed by intravenous infusion of donor stem cells. The stem cell source can be either from another person (allogeneic) or from the patient's own stored marrow (autologous). Pulmonary complications occur in approximately one-half of patients and are associated with high mortality.[242,276,279,286a,287]

Infectious pneumonias are the most common pulmonary complication of hematopoietic stem cell transplantation, and CMV is the most frequently identified organism.[272,273,280,287,291] Bacteria, including both Gram-negative and Gram-positive organisms, are also important pathogens, with herpes and other viruses, fungi, and pneumocystis occurring less frequently.

An idiopathic *interstitial pneumonia* accounts for a large proportion of pulmonary abnormalities following allogenic hematopoietic stem cell transplantation (so-called *idiopathic pneumonia syndrome*).[273,278,280,286a,287,290,291] This lesion usually occurs within 3 months following transplantation and is associated with a high mortality rate. Histologically, some examples resemble DAD (see Chapter 2) with hyaline membranes, alveolar pneumocyte hyperplasia, and fibroblast proliferation, while others are more suggestive of nonspecific interstitial pneumonia (see Chapter 3). The etiology of this lesion is unknown but may be related to previous irradiation and/or chemotherapy, to an undiagnosed viral (such as CMV or herpesvirus 6) infection,[271] or to graft-versus-host disease.

Diffuse alveolar hemorrhage has been described in a significant proportion of hematopoietic stem cell transplant patients.[266–268,277,286a,292] It usually occurs within 2 weeks of transplantation and is associated with high mortality rates. The cause is unknown, but other pulmonary complications, especially DAD and infections, are common accompanying features.[177,267]

Constrictive bronchiolitis obliterans (obliterative bronchiolitis) occurs in approximately 10% of long-term survivors of hematopoietic stem cell transplantation and is identical to the lesion complicating lung transplantation, as discussed in the previous section and in Chapter 16.[270,273,278,281,282,285,288,293,294] Most patients present with dyspnea and evidence of airflow obstruction, and chest radiographs usually show hyperinflation without parenchymal infiltrates. In approximately one-half of cases, an infectious etiology can be identified, and these cases tend to occur sooner following transplantation (median, 90 days) than the noninfectious variety (median, 180 days).[270,288] Most evidence suggests that noninfectious constrictive bronchiolitis obliterans is related to graft-versus-host disease, either as a primary cause or because these patients receive increased immunosuppression that predisposes them to viral or other infections.[281,285,288,293] This is not the entire explanation, however, since the disease has also been reported in patients receiving autologous transplants.[283] Other lesions may occur in long-term survivors, including a nonclassifiable type of interstitial pneumonia, BOOP, DAD, and LIP (see Chapter 9).[282,284] A form of *lymphocytic bronchitis* has been described in some patients dying after bone marrow transplantation and has also been attributed to graft-versus-host disease.[269,294] As with solid organ transplantation, post-transplant lymphoproliferative disorder can also occur.[233a]

A vasculopathy involving small arteries and arterioles in lung and gastrointestinal tract has been reported rarely in children following hematopoietic stem cell transplantation.[286] The affected vessels show luminal narrowing or occlusion by intimal fibrosis, often with a peculiar myxoid appearance. Foamy change is frequently found in the intima as well. This lesion is thought to be multifactorial in etiology, related both to prior chemotherapy and radiation and to graft-versus-host disease. Cases of *pulmonary venoocclusive disease* (see Chapter 13) have been reported rarely.[289] Peculiar vascular occlusion by cellular debris within a basophilic exudate associated with hemorrhagic infarcts (so-called *pulmonary cytolytic thrombi*) has been described rarely. Affected patients have nodular lesions radiographically.[274,275] The etiology of this lesion is unknown, but prognosis is excellent.

REFERENCES

Hypersensitivity Pneumonia

1. Ando M, Konishi K, Yoneda R, Tamura M: Difference in the phenotypes of bronchoalveolar lavage lymphocytes in patients with summer-type hypersensitivity pneumonitis, farmer's lung, ventilation pneumonitis and bird fancier's lung: Report of a nationwide epidemiologic study in Japan. J Allergy Clin Immunol 87:1002, 1991.
2. Barrios R, Fortoul TL, Lupi-Herrera E: Pigeon breeder's disease: Immunofluorescence and ultrastructural observations. Lung 164:55, 1986.
3. Barrowcliff DF, Arblaster PG: Farmer's lung: A study of an early acute fatal case. Thorax 23:490, 1968.
4. Bernstein DI, Lummus ZL, Santilli G, et al: Machine operator's lung: A hypersensitivity pneumonitis disorder associated with exposure to metalworking fluid aerosols. Chest 108:636, 1995.
5. Bourke SJ, Banham SW, Carter R, et al: Longitudinal course of extrinsic allergic alveolitis in pigeon breeders. Thorax 44:415, 1989.

5a. Churg A, Muller NL, Flint J, Wright JL: Chronic hypersensitivity pneumonitis. Am J Surg Pathol 30:201, 2006.

6. Coleman A, Colby TV: Histologic diagnosis of extrinsic allergic alveolitis. Am J Surg Pathol 12:514, 1988.

7. Dickie H, Rankin J: Farmer's lung. An acute granulomatous interstitial pneumonitis occurring in agricultural workers. JAMA 167:1069, 1958.

8. Emanuel DA, Marx JJ Jr, Ault B, et al: Organic dust toxic syndrome (pulmonary mycotoxicosis) – a review of the experience in central Wisconsin. In: Dosman JA, Cockroft DW, eds: *Principles of Health and Safety in Agriculture*, Boca Raton, Florida, CRC Press, 1989, pp 72–75.

9. Emanuel DA, Wenzel FJ, Bowerman CI, Lawton BR: Farmer's lung. Clinical, pathologic, and immunologic study of twenty-four patients. Am J Med 37:392, 1964.

10. Emanuel DA, Wenzel FJ, Lawton BR: Pneumonitis due to *Cryptostroma corticale* (Maple-bark disease). N Engl J Med 274:1413, 1966.

11. Emanuel DA, Wenzel FJ, Lawton BR: Pulmonary mycotoxicosis. Chest 67:293, 1975.

12. Fink J: Hypersensitivity pneumonitis. J Allergy Clin Immunol 74:1, 1984.

13. Ghose T, Landrigan P, Killeen R, Dill J: Immunopathological studies in patients with Farmer's lung. Clin Allergy 4:119, 1974.

14. Greenberger PA, Pien LC, Patterson R, et al: End-stage lung and ultimately fatal disease in a bird fancier. Am J Med 86:119, 1989.

15. Hayakawa H, Shiral M, Sato A, et al: Clinicopathological features of chronic hypersensitivity pneumonitis. Respirology 7:359, 2002.

16. Hensley G, Garancis J, Cherayil G, Fink J: Lung biopsies of pigeon breeder's disease. Arch Pathol 87:572, 1969.

17. Hodgson MJ, Bracker A, Yang C, et al: Hypersensitivity pneumonitis in a metal-working environment. Am J Ind Med 39:616, 2001.

18. Jacobs RL, Andrews CP, Coalson J: Organic antigen-induced interstitial lung disease: Diagnosis and management. Ann Allergy Asthma Immunol 88:30, 2002.

19. Kawanami O, Basset F, Barrios R, et al: Hypersensitivity pneumonitis in man. Light- and electron-microscopic studies of 18 lung biopsies. Am J Pathol 110:275, 1983.

20. Kreiss K, Cox-Ganser J: Metalworking fluid-associated hypersensitivity pneumonitis: A workshop summary. Am J Ind Med 32:423, 1997.

21. Lacasse Y, Selman M, Costabel U, et al: Clinical diagnosis of hypersensitivity pneumonitis. Am J Respir Crit Care Med 168:952, 2003.

22. Matar LD, McAdams HP, Sporn TA: Hypersensitivity pneumonitis. AJR Am J Roentgenol 174:1061, 2000.

23. May JJ, Stallones L, Darrow D, Pratt DS: Organic dust toxicity (pulmonary mycotoxicosis) associated with silo unloading. Thorax 41:919, 1986.

24. Merget R, Marczynski B, Chen Z, et al: Haemorrhagic hypersensitivity pneumonitis due to naphthylene 1,5-diisocyanate. Eur Respir J 19:377, 2002.

25. Miyagawa T, Hamagami S, Tanigawa N: *Cryptococcus albidus*-induced summer-type hypersensitivity pneumonitis. Am J Respir Crit Care Med 161:961, 2000.

26. Morell F, Roger A, Cruz MJ, et al: Suberosis: Clinical study and new etiologic agents in a series of eight patients. Chest 124:1145, 2003.

27. Ohtani Y, Kojima K, Sumi Y, et al: Inhalation provocation tests in chronic bird fancier's lung. Chest 118:1382, 2000.

28. Ohtani Y, Saiki S, Kitaichi M, et al: Chronic bird fancier's lung: Histopathological and clinical correlation. An application of the 2002 ATS/ERS consensus classification of the idiopathic interstitial pneumonias. Thorax 60:665, 2005.

29. Pardo A, Barrios R, Gaxiola M, et al: Increase of lung neutrophils in hypersensitivity pneumonitis is associated with lung fibrosis. Am J Respir Crit Care Med 161:1698, 2000.

30. Pepys J, Simon G: Asthma, pulmonary eosinophilia, and allergic alveolitis. Med Clin North Am 57:573, 1973.

31. Pérez-Padilla R, Gaxiola M, Salas J, et al: Bronchiolitis in chronic pigeon breeder's disease: Morphologic evidence of a spectrum of small airway lesions in hypersensitivity pneumonitis induced by avian antigens. Chest 110:371, 1996.

32. Pérez-Padilla R, Salas J, Chapela R, et al: Mortality in Mexican patients with chronic pigeon breeder's lung compared with those with usual interstitial pneumonia. Am Rev Respir Dis 148:49, 1993.

33. Popp W, Braun W, Zwick H, et al: Detection of antigen-specific antibodies on lung tissue in a patient with hypersensitivity pneumonitis. Virchows Arch [A Pathol Anat] 413:223, 1988.

34. Ramírez-Venegas A, Sansores RH, Pérez-Padilla R, et al: Utility of a provocation test for diagnosis of chronic pigeon breeder's disease. Am J Respir Crit Care Med 158:862, 1998.

35. Reijula K, Sutinen S: Ultrastructure of extrinsic allergic bronchiolo-alveolitis. Pathol Res Pract 181:418, 1986.

36. Reyes CN, Wenzel FJ, Lawton BR, Emanuel DA: The pulmonary pathology of farmer's lung disease. Chest 81:142, 1982.

37. Reynolds H: Hypersensitivity pneumonitis: Correlation of cellular and immunologic changes with clinical phases of disease. Lung 166:189, 1988.

38. Rose C, King TE Jr: Controversies in hypersensitivity pneumonitis. Am Rev Respir Dis 145:1, 1992.

39. Salvaggio JE, DeShazo RD: Pathogenesis of hypersensitivity pneumonitis. Chest 89:190S, 1986.

40. Seal R, Hapke E, Thomas G: The pathology of acute and chronic stages of farmer's lung. Thorax 23:469, 1968.

41. Selman M, Chapela R, Raghu G: Hypersensitivity pneumonitis: Clinical manifestations, pathogenesis, diagnosis, and therapeutic strategies. Sem Respir Med 14:353, 1993.

42. Semenzato G, Chilosi M, Ossi E, et al: Bronchoalveolar lavage and lung histology. Comparative analysis of inflammatory and immunocompetent cells in patients

with sarcoidosis and hypersensitivity pneumonitis. Am Rev Respir Dis 132:400, 1985.

43. Soler P, Nioche S, Valeyre D, et al: Role of mast cells in the pathogenesis of hypersensitivity pneumonitis. Thorax 42:565, 1987.

44. Suda T, Sato A, Ida M, et al: Hypersensitivity pneumonitis associated with home ultrasonic humidifiers. Chest 107:711, 1995.

45. Tsushima K, Fujimoto K, Yamazaki Y, et al: Hypersensitivity pneumonia induced by spores of lyophyllum aggregatum. Chest 120:1085, 2001.

46. Von Essen S, Robbins RA, Thompson AB, Rennard SI: Organic dust syndrome: An acute febrile reaction to organic dust exposure distinct from hypersensitivity pneumonitis. J Toxicol 28:389, 1990.

47. Vourlekis JS, Schwarz MI, Cherniak RM, et al: The effect of pulmonary fibrosis on survival in patients with hypersensitivity pneumonitis. Am J Med 116:662, 2004.

48. Vourlekis JS, Schwarz MI, Cool CD, et al: Nonspecific interstitial pneumonitis as the sole histologic expression of hypersensitivity pneumonitis. Am J Med 112:490, 2002.

49. Wenzel F, Emanuel D, Gray R: Immunofluorescent studies in patients with farmer's lung. J Allergy Clin Immunol 48:224, 1971.

50. Zacharisen MC, Kadambi AR, Schlueter DP, et al: The spectrum of respiratory disease associated with exposure to metal working fluids. J Occup Environ Med 40:1, 1998.

Eosinophilic Pneumonia

51. Allen JN, Davis WB: Eosinophilic lung diseases. Am J Respir Crit Care Med 150:1423, 1994.

52. Allen JN, Pacht ER, Gadek JE, Davis WB: Acute eosinophilic pneumonia as a reversible cause of noninfectious respiratory failure. N Engl J Med 321:569, 1989.

53. Badesch DB, King TE Jr, Schwarz MI: Acute eosinophilic pneumonia: A hypersensitivity phenomenon? Am Rev Respir Dis 139:249, 1989.

54. Buchheit J, Eid N, Rodgers G Jr, Feger T, Yakoub O: Acute eosinophilic pneumonia with respiratory failure: A new syndrome. Am Rev Respir Dis 145:716, 1992.

55. Buscaglia AJ, Cowden FE, Brill H: Pulmonary infiltrates associated with naproxen. JAMA 251:65, 1984.

56. Capewell S, Chapman BJ, Alexander F, et al: Corticosteroid treatment and prognosis in pulmonary eosinophilia. Thorax 44:925, 1989.

57. Carrington CB, Addington WW, Goff AM, et al: Chronic eosinophilic pneumonia. N Engl J Med 280:787, 1969.

58. Chapman BJ, Capewell S, Gibson R, et al: Pulmonary eosinophilia with and without allergic bronchopulmonary aspergillosis. Thorax 44:919, 1989.

59. Forrester JM, Steele AW, Waldron JA, Parsons PE: Crack lung: An acute pulmonary syndrome with a spectrum of clinical and histopathologic findings. Am Rev Respir Dis 142:462, 1990.

60. Fox B, Seed W: Chronic eosinophilic pneumonia. Thorax 35:570, 1980.

61. Gaensler EA, Carrington CB: Peripheral opacities in chronic eosinophilic pneumonia: The photographic negative of pulmonary edema. AJR Am J Roentgenol 128:1, 1977.

62. Gheysens B, Van Mieghem W: Pulmonary infiltrates with eosinophilia due to glafenine. Eur J Respir Dis 65:456, 1984.

63. Gonzalez EB, Haynes D, Weeder VW: Chronic eosinophilic pneumonia (Carrington's) with increased serum IgE levels. A distinct subset? Arch Intern Med 148:2622, 1988.

64. Gonzalez EB, Swedo JL, Rajaraman S, et al: Ultrastructural and immunohistochemical evidence for release of eosinophilic granules in vivo: Cytotoxic potential in chronic eosinophilic pneumonia. J Allergy Clin Immunol 79:755, 1987.

65. Grantham J, Meadows J III, Gleich G: Chronic eosinophilic pneumonia: Evidence for eosinophil degranulation and release of major basic protein. Am J Med 80:89, 1986.

66. Ho D, Tashkin DP, Bein ME, Sharma O: Pulmonary infiltrates with eosinophilia associated with tetracycline. Chest 76:33, 1979.

67. Hayakawa H, Sata A, Toyoshima M, et al: A clinical study of idiopathic eosinophilic pneumonia. Chest 105:1482, 1994.

68. Jederlinic PJ, Sicilian L, Gaensler EA: Chronic eosinophilic pneumonia. A report of 19 cases and a review of the literature. Medicine (Baltimore) 67:154, 1988.

69. Kelly KJ, Ruffing R: Acute eosinophilic pneumonia following intentional inhalation of Scotchguard. Ann Allergy 71:358, 1993.

70. Kita H, Sur S, Hunt LW, et al: Cytokine production at the site of disease in chronic eosinophilic pneumonitis. Am J Respir Crit Care Med 153:1437, 1996.

71. Libby D, Murphy T, Edwards A, et al: Chronic eosinophilic pneumonia: An unusual cause of acute respiratory failure. Am Rev Resp Dis 122:497, 1980.

72. Liebow A, Carrington CB: The eosinophilic pneumonias. Medicine (Baltimore) 48:251, 1969.

73. Luna E, Tomashefski JF Jr, Brown D, et al: Reactive eosinophilic pulmonary vascular infiltration in patients with spontaneous pneumothorax. Am J Surg Pathol 18:195, 1994.

74. Marchand E, Etienne-Mastroianni B, Chanez P, et al: Idiopathic chronic eosinophilic pneumonia and asthma: How do they influence each other? Eur Respir J 22:8, 2003.

75. Marchand E, Reynaud-Gaubert M, Lauque D, et al: Idiopathic chronic eosinophilic pneumonia: A clinical and follow-up study of 62 cases. Medicine (Baltimore) 77:299, 1998.

76. McCarthy DS, Pepys J: Cryptogenic pulmonary eosinophilias. Clin Allergy 3:339, 1973.

77. Miyagawa Y, Nagata N, Shigematsu N: Clinicopathological study of migratory lung infiltrates. Thorax 46:233, 1991.

78. Miyazaki E, Sugisaki K, Shigenaga T, et al: A case of acute eosinophilic pneumonia caused by inhalation of *Trichosporon terrestre*. Am J Respir Crit Care Med 151:541, 1995.

79. Morrissey WL, Gaensler EA, Carrington CB, Turner HB: Chronic eosinophilic pneumonia. Respiration 32:453, 1975.

80. Nader DA, Schillaci RF: Pulmonary infiltrates with eosinophilia due to naproxen. Chest 83:280, 1983.

81. Naughton M, Fahy J, FitzGerald MX: Chronic eosinophilic pneumonia. A long-term follow-up of 12 patients. Chest 103:162, 1993.

82. Neva FA, Kaplan AP, Pacheco G, Gray L, Danaraj TJ: Tropical eosinophilia. J Allergy Clin Immunol 55:422, 1975.

83. Oh PI, Balter MS: Cocaine induced eosinophilic lung disease. Thorax 47:478, 1992.

84. Olopade CO, Crotty TB, Douglas WW, et al: Chronic eosinophilic pneumonia and idiopathic bronchiolitis obliterans organizing pneumonia: Comparison of eosinophil number and degranulation by immunofluorescence staining for eosinophil-derived major basic protein. Mayo Clin Proc 70:137, 1995.

85. Ottesen EA, Nutman TB: Tropical pulmonary eosinophilia. Annu Rev Med 43:417, 1992.

86. Pacheco A, Cuevas M, Carbelo B, et al: Eosinophilic lung disease associated with *Candida albicans*. Eur Respir J 12:502, 1998.

87. Philit F, Etienne-Mastroianni B, Parrot A, et al: Idiopathic acute eosinophilic pneumonia: A study of 22 patients. Am J Respir Crit Care Med 166:1235, 2002.

88. Poe R, Condemi J, Weinstein S, Schuster R: Adult respiratory distress syndrome related to ampicillin sensitivity. Chest 77:449, 1980.

89. Pope-Harman A, Davis WB, Allen ED, et al: Acute eosinophilic pneumonia: A summary of 15 cases and review of the literature. Medicine (Baltimore) 75:334, 1996.

90. Roig J, Romeu J, Riera C, et al: Acute eosinophilic pneumonia due to Toxocariasis with bronchoalveolar lavage findings. Chest 102:294, 1992.

91. Rom WN, Weiden M, Garcia R, et al: Acute eosinophilic pneumonia in a New York City firefighter exposed to World Trade Center dust. Am J Respir Crit Care Med 166:797, 2002.

92. Salerno SM, Strong JS, Roth BJ, Sakata V: Eosinophilic pneumonia and respiratory failure associated with a trazodone overdose. Am J Respir Crit Care Med 152:2170, 1995.

93. Shannon JJ, Lynch JP III: Eosinophilic pulmonary syndromes. Clin Pulm Med 2:19, 1995.

94. Shintani H, Fujimura, Masaki M, Ishiura Y, Noto M: A case of cigarette smoking-induced acute eosinophilic pneumonia showing tolerance. Chest 117:227, 2000.

95. Shiota Y, Kawai T, Matsumoto H, et al: Acute eosinophilic pneumonia following cigarette smoking. Intern Med 39:830, 2000.

96. Strumpf IJ, Drucker RD, Anders KH, Cohen S, Fajolu O: Acute eosinophilic pulmonary disease associated with the ingestion of L-tryptophan-containing products. Chest 99:8, 1991.

97. Tazelaar HD, Linz LJ, Colby TV, et al: Acute eosinophilic pneumonia: Histopathologic findings in nine patients. Am J Respir Crit Care Med 155:296, 1997.

98. Wang KK, Bowyer BA, Fleming CR, Schroeder KW: Pulmonary infiltrates and eosinophilia associated with sulfasalazine. Mayo Clin Proc 59:343, 1984.

99. Yousem SA, Lifson JD, Colby TV: Chemotherapy-induced eosinophilic pneumonia. Relation to bleomycin. Chest 88:103, 1985.

Mucoid Impaction of Bronchi

100. Hutcheson J, Shaw R, Paulson D, Kee J Jr: Mucoid impaction of the bronchi. Am J Clin Pathol 33:427, 1960.

101. Irwin R, Thomas H III: Mucoid impaction of the bronchus. Am Rev Respir Dis 108:955, 1973.

102. Jelihovsky T: The structure of bronchial plugs in mucoid impaction, bronchocentric granulomatosis and asthma. Histopathology 7:153, 1983.

103. Jett JR, Tazelaar HD, Keim LW, Ingrassia TS III: Plastic bronchitis: An old disease revisited. Mayo Clin Proc 66:305, 1991.

104. Morgan A, Bogomoletz W: Mucoid impaction of the bronchi in relation to asthma and plastic bronchitis. Thorax 23:356, 1968.

105. Moser C, Nussbaum E, Cooper DM: Plastic bronchitis and the role of bronchoscopy in the acute chest syndrome of sickle cell disease. Chest 120:608, 2001.

106. Muller W, von der Hardt H, Rieger C: Idiopathic and symptomatic plastic bronchitis in childhood. A report of three cases and review of the literature. Respiration 52:214, 1987.

107. Pérez-Soler A: Cast bronchitis in infants and children. Am J Dis Child 143:1024, 1989.

108. Sanerkin N, Seal R, Leopold J: Plastic bronchitis, mucoid impaction of the bronchi, and allergic bronchopulmonary aspergillosis and their relationship to bronchial asthma. Ann Allergy 24:586, 1966.

109. Seear M, Hui H, Magee F, et al: Bronchial casts in children: A proposed classification based on nine cases and a review of the literature. Am J Respir Crit Care Med. 155:364, 1997.

110. Spotnitz M, Overholt E: Mucoid impaction of the bronchi associated with aspergillus. Dis Chest 52:92, 1967.

111. Urschel H Jr, Paulson D, Shaw R: Mucoid impaction of the bronchi. Ann Thorac Surg 2:1, 1966.

Bronchocentric Granulomatosis

112. Bonafede RP, Benatar SR: Bronchocentric granulomatosis and rheumatoid arthritis. Br J Dis Chest 81:197, 1987.

113. Clee MD, Lamb D, Clark RA: Bronchocentric

granulomatosis: A review and thoughts on pathogenesis. Br J Dis Chest 77:227, 1983.

114. Den Hertog RW, Wagenaar SS, Westermann CJJ: Bronchocentric granulomatosis and pulmonary echinococcosis. Am Rev Respir Dis 126:344, 1982.

115. Fannin SW, Hagley MT, Seibert JD, Koenig TJ: Bronchocentric granulomatosis, acute renal failure, and high titer antineutrophil cytoplasmic antibodies: Possible variants of Wegener's granulomatosis. J Rheumatol 20:507, 1993.

116. Goodman D, Sacca J: Pulmonary cavitation, allergic aspergillosis, and bronchocentric granulomatosis. Chest 72:368, 1977.

117. Hanson G, Flod N, Wells I, Novey H, Galant S: Bronchocentric granulomatosis: A complication of allergic bronchopulmonary aspergillosis. J Allergy Clin Immunol 59:83, 1977.

118. Hellems SO, Kanner RE, Renzetti AD Jr: Bronchocentric granulomatosis associated with rheumatoid arthritis. Chest 83:831, 1983.

119. Houser SL, Mark EJ: Bronchocentric granulomatosis with mucus impaction due to bronchogenic carcinoma: An association with clinical relevance. Arch Pathol Lab Med 124:1168, 2000.

120. Katzenstein A, Liebow A, Friedman P: Bronchocentric granulomatosis, mucoid impaction, and hypersensitivity reactions to fungi. Am Rev Respir Dis 111:497, 1975.

121. Koss M, Robinson R, Hochholzer L: Bronchocentric granulomatosis. Hum Pathol 12:632, 1981.

122. Liebow AA: Pulmonary angiitis and granulomatosis. Am Rev Respir Dis 108:1,1973.

123. Maguire GP, Lee M, Rosen Y, Lyons HA: Pulmonary tuberculosis and bronchocentric granulomatosis. Chest 89:606, 1986.

124. Myers JL: Bronchocentric granulomatosis. Disease or diagnosis? Chest 96:3, 1989.

125. Myers JL, Katzenstein AA: Granulomatous infection mimicking bronchocentric granulomatosis. Am J Surg Pathol 10:317, 1986.

126. Tazelaar HD, Baird AM, Mill M, et al: Bronchocentric mycosis occurring in transplant recipients. Chest 96:92, 1989.

127. Tron V, Churg A: Chronic necrotizing pulmonary aspergillosis mimicking bronchocentric granulomatosis. Pathol Res Pract 181:621, 1986.

128. Ulbright T, Katzenstein A-LA: Solitary necrotizing granulomas of the lung: Differentiating features and etiology. Am J Surg Pathol 4:13, 1980.

129. Ward S, Heyneman LE, Flint JDA, et al: Bronchocentric granulomatosis: Computed tomographic findings in five patients. Clin Radiol 55:296, 2000.

130. Wiedemann HP, Bensinger RE, Hudson LD: Bronchocentric granulomatosis with eye involvement. Am Rev Respir Dis 126:347, 1982.

Allergic Bronchopulmonary Aspergillosis

131. Akiyama K, Mathison DA, Riker JB, et al: Allergic bronchopulmonary candidiasis. Chest 85:699, 1984.

132. Akiyama K, Takizawa H, Suzuki M, et al: Allergic bronchopulmonary aspergillosis due to *Aspergillus oryzae*. Chest 91:285, 1987.

133. Aubrey M-C, Fraser R: The role of bronchial biopsy and washing in the diagnosis of allergic bronchopulmonary aspergillosis. Mod Pathol 11:607, 1998.

134. Backman KS, Roberts M, Patterson R: Allergic bronchopulmonary mycosis caused by *Fusarium vasinfectum*. Am J Respir Crit Care Med 152:1379, 1995.

135. Benatar S, Allan B, Hewitson R, Don P: Allergic bronchopulmonary stemphyliosis. Thorax 35:515, 1980.

136. Bosken C, Myers J, Greenberger P, Katzenstein A: Pathologic features of allergic bronchopulmonary aspergillosis. Am J Surg Pathol 12:216, 1988.

137. Breslin ABX, Jenkins CR: Experience with allergic bronchopulmonary aspergillosis: Some unusual features. Clin Allergy 14:21, 1984.

138. Cody DT II, Neel HB III, Ferreiro JA, Roberts GD: Allergic fungal sinusitis. The Mayo Clinic experience. Laryngoscope 104:1074, 1994.

139. Glancy J, Elder J, McAleer R: Allergic bronchopulmonary fungal disease without clinical asthma. Thorax 36:345, 1981.

140. Golbert T, Patterson R: Pulmonary allergic aspergillosis. Ann Intern Med 72:395, 1970.

141. Greenberger PA, Miller TP, Roberts M, Smith LL: Allergic bronchopulmonary aspergillosis in patients with and without evidence of bronchiectasis. Ann Allergy 70:333, 1993.

142. Greenberger PA, Patterson R: Allergic bronchopulmonary aspergillosis and the evaluation of the patient with asthma. J Allergy Clin Immunol 81:646, 1988.

143. Halwig JM, Brueske DA, Greenberger PA, et al: Allergic bronchopulmonary curvariosis. Am Rev Respir Dis 132:186, 1985.

144. Hendrick DJ, Ellithorpe DB, Lyon F, et al: Allergic bronchopulmonary helminthosporiosis. Am Rev Respir Dis 126:935, 1982.

145. Katzenstein A, Sale S, Greenberger P: Pathologic findings in allergic aspergillus sinusitis, a newly recognized form of sinusitis. Am J Surg Pathol 7:439, 1983.

146. Kumar R: Mild, moderate, and severe forms of allergic bronchopulmonary aspergillosis: A clinical and serologic evaluation. Chest 124:890, 2003.

147. Laham MN, Carpenter JL: *Aspergillus terreus*, a pathogen capable of causing infective endocarditis, pulmonary mycetoma, and allergic bronchopulmonary aspergillosis. Am Rev Respir Dis 125:769, 1982.

148. Lake FR, Froudist JH, McAleer R, et al: Allergic bronchopulmonary fungal disease caused by Bipolaris and Curvularia. Aust N Z J Med 21:871, 1991.

149. Lake FR, Tribe AE, McAleer R, Froudist J, Thompson PJ: Mixed allergic bronchopulmonary fungal disease due to *Pseudallescheria boydii* and *Aspergillus*. Thorax 45:489, 1990.

150. Lee TM, Greenberger PA, Oh S, et al: Allergic bronchopulmonary candidiasis: Case report and

suggested diagnostic criteria. J Allergy Clin Immunol 80:816, 1987.

151. Lee TM, Greenberger PA, Patterson R, et al: Stage V (fibrotic) allergic bronchopulmonary aspergillosis. Arch Intern Med 147:319, 1987.

152. McAleer R, Kroenert D, Elder J, Froudist J: Allergic bronchopulmonary disease caused by *Curvularia lunata* and *Drechslera hawaiiensis*. Thorax 36:338, 1981.

153. McCarthy D, Pepys J: Allergic bronchopulmonary aspergillosis. Clinical immunology: (1) Clinical features. Clin Allergy 1:261, 1971.

154. McCarthy D, Simon G, Hargreave F: The radiological appearances in allergic bronchopulmonary aspergillosis. Clin Radiol 21:366, 1970.

155. Mendelson EB, Fisher MR, Mintzer RA, et al: Roentgenographic and clinical staging of allergic bronchopulmonary aspergillosis. Chest 87:334, 1985.

156. Miller MA, Greenberger PA, Amerian R, et al: Allergic bronchopulmonary mycosis caused by *Pseudoallescheria boydii*. Am Rev Respir Dis 148:810, 1993.

157. Patterson R, Greenberger PA, Radin RC, Roberts M: Allergic bronchopulmonary aspergillosis: Staging as an aid to management. Ann Intern Med 96:286, 1982.

158. Patterson R, Samuels BS, Phair JJ, Roberts M: Bronchopulmonary torulopsosis. Int Arch Allergy Appl Immunol 69:30, 1982.

159. Safirstein B, D'Souza M, Simon G, Tai E, Pepys J: Five-year follow-up of allergic bronchopulmonary aspergillosis. Am Rev Respir Dis 108:450, 1973.

160. Scadding J: The bronchi in allergic aspergillosis. Scand J Respir Dis 48:372, 1967.

161. Shah A, Khan ZU, Chaturvedi S, Malik GB, Randhawa HS: Concomitant allergic *Aspergillus* sinusitis and allergic bronchopulmonary aspergillosis associated with familial occurrence of allergic bronchopulmonary aspergillosis. Ann Allergy 64:507, 1990.

162. Sher TH, Schwartz HJ: Allergic *Aspergillus* sinusitis with concurrent allergic bronchopulmonary *Aspergillus*: Report of a case. J Allergy Clin Immunol 81:844, 1988.

163. Slavin RG, Bedrossian CW, Hutcheson PS, et al: A pathologic study of allergic bronchopulmonary aspergillosis. J Allergy Clin Immunol 81:718, 1988.

164. Stevens DA, Schwartz HJ, Lee JY, et al: A randomized trial of itraconazole in allergic bronchopulmonary aspergillosis. N Engl J Med 342:756, 2000.

165. Torres C, Jae YR, El-Naggar AK, et al: Allergic fungal sinusitis: A clinicopathologic study of 16 cases. Hum Pathol 27:795, 1996.

166. Travis WD, Kwon-Chung KJ, Kleiner DE, et al: Unusual aspects of allergic bronchopulmonary fungal disease: Report of two cases due to *Curvularia* organisms associated with allergic fungal sinusitis. Hum Pathol 22:1240, 1991.

Alveolar Hemorrhage Syndromes

167. Ahmad D, Patterson R, Morgan WKC, et al: Pulmonary haemorrhage and haemolytic anaemia due to trimellitic anhydride. Lancet 1:328, 1979.

168. Albelda SM, Gefter WB, Epstein DM, Miller WT: Diffuse pulmonary hemorrhage: A review and classification. Radiology 154:289, 1985.

169. Barnett VT, Bergmann F, Humphrey H, Chediak J: Diffuse alveolar hemorrhage secondary to superwarfarin ingestion. Chest 102:1301, 1992.

170. Beckerman R, Taussig L, Pinnas J: Familial idiopathic pulmonary hemosiderosis. Am J Dis Child 133:609, 1979.

171. Beechler C, Enquist R, Hunt K, et al: Immunofluorescence of transbronchial biopsies in Goodpasture's syndrome. Am Rev Respir Dis 121:869, 1980.

172. Bonsib SM, Walker WP: Pulmonary-renal syndrome: Clinical similarity amidst etiologic diversity. Mod Pathol 2:129, 1989.

173. Brambilla CG, Brambilla EM, Stoebner P, Dechelette E: Idiopathic pulmonary hemorrhage. Ultrastructural and mineralogic study. Chest 81:120, 1982.

174. Breckenridge RL Jr, Ross JS: Idiopathic pulmonary hemosiderosis. A report of familial occurrence. Chest 75:636, 1979.

175. Collard HR, Schwarz MI: Diffuse alveolar hemorrhage. Clin Chest Med 25:583, 2004.

176. Corrin B, Jagusch M, Dewar A, et al: Fine structural changes in idiopathic pulmonary haemosiderosis. J Pathol 153:249, 1987.

177. DeLassence A, Fleury-Feith J, Escudier E, et al: Alveolar hemorrhage. Diagnostic criteria and results in 194 immunocompromised hosts. Am J Respir Crit Care Med 151:157, 1995.

178. Donald K, Edwards R, McEvoy J: Alveolar capillary basement membrane lesions in Goodpasture's syndrome and idiopathic pulmonary hemosiderosis. Am J Med 59:642, 1975.

179. Donlan C, Srodes C, Duffy F: Idiopathic pulmonary hemosiderosis. Electron microscopic immunofluorescent and iron kinetic studies. Chest 68:577, 1975.

180. Goldstein J, Weil J, Liel Y: Intrapulmonary hemorrhages and immune complex glomerulonephritis masquerading as Goodpasture's syndrome. Hum Pathol 17:754, 1986.

181. Gonzalez-Crussi F, Hull M, Grosfeld J: Idiopathic pulmonary hemosiderosis: Evidence of capillary basement membrane abnormality. Am Rev Respir Dis 114:689, 1976.

182. Hyatt R, Adelstein E, Halazun J, Lukens J: Ultrastructure of the lung in idiopathic pulmonary hemosiderosis. Am J Med 52:822, 1972.

183. Irwin R, Cottrell T, Hsu K, et al: Idiopathic pulmonary hemosiderosis: An electron microscopic and immunofluorescent study. Chest 65:41, 1974.

184. Johnson J, Moore J Jr, Austin H III, et al: Therapy of anti-glomerular basement membrane antibody disease. Analysis of prognostic significance of clinical, pathologic and treatment factors. Medicine (Baltimore) 64:219, 1985.

185. Kaplan V, Baur X, Czuppon A, Ruegger M, Russi E, Speich R: Pulmonary hemorrhage due to inhalation of

vapor containing pyromellitic dianhydride. Chest 104:644, 1993.

186. Kiper N, Gocmen A, Ozcelik U, et al: Long-term clinical course of patients with idiopathic pulmonary hemosiderosis (1979–1994): Prolonged survival with low-dose corticosteroid therapy. Pediatr Pulmonol 27:180, 1999.

187. Klasa RJ, Abboud RT, Ballon HS, Grossman L: Goodpasture's syndrome: Recurrence after a five-year remission. Case report and review of the literature. Am J Med 84:751, 1988.

188. Komadina KH, Houk RW, Vicks SL, et al: Goodpasture's syndrome associated with pulmonary eosinophilic vasculitis. J Rheumatol 15:1298, 1988.

189. Kradin RL, Kiprov D, Dickersin GR, et al: Immune complex disease with fatal pulmonary hemorrhage. Arch Pathol Lab Med 105:582, 1981.

190. Leatherman JW: Immune alveolar hemorrhage. Chest 91:891, 1987.

191. Leatherman JW, Davies SF, Hoidal JR: Alveolar hemorrhage syndromes: Diffuse microvascular lung hemorrhage in immune and idiopathic disorders. Medicine (Baltimore) 63:343, 1984.

192. Lombard CM, Colby TV, Elliott CG: Surgical pathology of the lung in anti-basement membrane antibody-associated Goodpasture's syndrome. Hum Pathol 20:445, 1989.

193. Luks AM, Lakshminarayanan S, Hirschmann JV: Leptospirosis presenting as diffuse alveolar hemorrhage: A case report and literature review. Chest 123:639, 2003.

194. Mac-Moune Lai F, Li EKM, Suen MWM, Lui SF, Li PKT, Lai KN: Pulmonary hemorrhage: A fatal manifestation in IgA nephropathy. Arch Pathol Lab Med 118:542, 1994.

195. Masson RG, Rennke HG, Gottlieb MN: Pulmonary hemorrhage in a patient with fibrillary glomerulonephritis. N Engl J Med 326:36, 1992.

196. McLean TR, Beall AC Jr, Jones JW: Massive hemoptysis due to bronchiolithiasis. Ann Thorac Surg 52:1173, 1991.

197. Mehler PS, Brunvand MW, Hutt MP, Anderson RJ: Chronic recurrent Goodpasture's syndrome. Am J Med 82:833, 1987.

198. Milman N, Pedersen FM: Idiopathic pulmonary haemosiderosis. Epidemiology, pathogenic aspects and diagnosis. Respir Med 92:902, 1998.

199. Morgan P, Turner-Warwick M: Pulmonary haemosiderosis and pulmonary haemorrhage. Br J Dis Chest 75:225, 1981.

200. Myers JL, Katzenstein A-LA: Microangiitis in lupus-induced pulmonary hemorrhage. Am J Clin Pathol 85:552, 1986.

201. Myers JL, Katzenstein A-LA: Wegener's granulomatosis presenting with massive pulmonary hemorrhage and capillaritis. Am J Surg Pathol 11:895, 1987.

202. Nathan PE, Torres AV, Smith AJ, Gagliardi AJ, Rapeport KB: Spontaneous pulmonary hemorrhage following coronary thrombolysis. Chest 101:1150, 1992.

203. Pacheco A, Casanova C, Fogue L, Sueiro A: Long-term clinical follow-up of adult idiopathic pulmonary hemosiderosis and celiac disease. Chest 99:1525, 1991.

204. Pai U, McMahon J, Tomashefski JF Jr: Mineralizing pulmonary elastosis in chronic cardiac failure: "Endogenous pneumoconiosis" revisited. Am J Clin Pathol 101:22, 1994.

205. Pea L, Roda L, Boussaud V, Lonjon B: Desmopressin therapy for massive hemoptysis associated with severe leptospirosis. Am J Respir Crit Care Med 167:726, 2003.

206. Proskey A, Weatherbee L, Easterling R, et al: Goodpasture's syndrome: A report of five cases and review of the literature. Am J Med 48:162, 1970.

207. Saeed MM, Woo MS, MacLaughlin EF, et al: Prognosis in pediatric idiopathic pulmonary hemosiderosis. Chest 116:721, 1999.

208. Santalo M, Domingo P, Fontcuberta J, et al: Diffuse pulmonary hemorrhage associated with anticoagulant therapy. Eur J Respir Dis 69:114, 1986.

209. Sherman JM, Winnie G, Thomassen MJ, et al: Time course of hemosiderin production and clearance by human pulmonary macrophages. Chest 86:409, 1984.

210. Smith L, Katzenstein A: Pathogenesis of massive pulmonary hemorrhage in acute leukemia. Arch Intern Med 142:2149, 1982.

211. Spark RP, Sobonya RE, Armbruster RJ, Marco JD, Rotkis TC: Pathologic bronchial vasculature in a case of massive hemoptysis due to chronic bronchitis. Chest 99:504, 1991.

212. Specks U: Diffuse alveolar hemorrhage syndromes. Curr Opin Rheumatol 13:12, 2001.

213. Thaell JF, Greipp PR, Stubbs SE, Siegal GP: Idiopathic pulmonary hemosiderosis. Two cases in a family. Mayo Clin Proc 53:113, 1978.

214. Tobler A, Schurch E, Altermatt HJ, Im Hof V: Anti-basement membrane antibody disease with severe pulmonary haemorrhage and normal renal function. Thorax 46:68, 1991.

215. Travis WD, Carpenter HA: Diffuse pulmonary hemorrhage. An uncommon manifestation of Wegener's granulomatosis. Am J Surg Pathol 11:702, 1987.

216. Travis WD, Colby TV, Lombard C, Carpenter HA: A clinicopathologic study of 34 cases of diffuse pulmonary hemorrhage with lung biopsy confirmation. Am J Surg Pathol 14:1112, 1990.

217. vonVigier RO, Trummler SA, Laux-End R, et al: Pulmonary renal syndrome in childhood: A report of twenty-one cases and a review of the literature. Pediatr Pulmonol 29:282, 2000.

218. Wright PH, Menzies IS, Pounder RE, Keeling PWN: Adult idiopathic pulmonary haemosiderosis and coeliac disease. Q J Med 50:95, 1981.

219. Yeager H, Powell D, Weinberg R, et al: Idiopathic pulmonary hemosiderosis. Ultrastructural studies and response to azathioprine. Arch Intern Med 136:1145, 1976.

Transplantation-Related Disorders

Lung Transplantation

220. Abernathy EC, Hruban RH, Baumgartner WA, Reitz BA, Hutchins GM: The two forms of bronchiolitis obliterans in heart-lung transplant recipients. Hum Pathol 22:1102, 1991.

221. Burke CM, Baldwin JC, Morris AJ, et al: Twenty-eight cases of human heart-lung transplantation. Lancet 1:517, 1986.

222. Burke CM, Theodore J, Dawkins KD, et al: Post-transplant obliterative bronchiolitis and other late lung sequelae in human heart-lung transplantation. Chest 86:824, 1984.

223. Cagle PT, Brown RW, Frost A, et al: Diagnosis of chronic lung transplant rejection by transbronchial biopsy. Mod Pathol 8:137, 1995.

224. Chaparro C, Chamberlain D, Maurer J, et al: Bronchiolitis obliterans organizing pneumonia (BOOP) in lung transplant recipients. Chest 110:1150, 1996.

225. Choi JK, Kearns J, Palevsky HI, et al: Hyperacute rejection of a pulmonary allograft: Immediate clinical and pathologic findings. Am J Respir Crit Care Med 160:1015, 1999.

226. Clelland CA, Higenbottam TW, Stewart S, Scott JP, Wallwork J: The histological changes in transbronchial biopsy after treatment of acute lung rejection in heart-lung transplants. J Pathol 161:105, 1990.

227. Colombat M, Groussard O, Lautrette A, et al: Analysis of the different histologic lesions observed in transbronchial biopsy for the diagnosis of acute rejection. Clinicopathologic correlations during the first 6 months after lung transplantation. Hum Pathol 36:387, 2005.

228. De Hoyos A, Chamberlain D, Schvartzman R, et al: Prospective assessment of a standardized pathologic grading system for acute rejection in lung transplantation. Chest 103:1813, 1993.

229. Fasano M, Yousem S, Jagirdar J: MIB-1 as a predictor of response in lung allografts with moderate acute cellular rejection. Am J Surg Pathol 22:749, 1998.

230. Fend F, Prior C, Margreiter R, Mikuz G: Cytomegalovirus pneumonitis in heart-lung transplant recipients: Histopathology and clinicopathologic considerations. Hum Pathol 21:918, 1990.

231. Gerhardt SG, Tuder RM, Girgis RE, et al: Pulmonary eosinophilia following lung transplantation for sarcoidosis in two patients. Chest 123:629, 2003.

232. Glanville AR, Baldwin JC, Burke CM, et al: Obliterative bronchiolitis after heart-lung transplantation: Apparent arrest by augmented immunosuppression. Ann Intern Med 107:300, 1987.

233. Guilinger RA, Paradis IL, Dauber JH, et al: The importance of bronchoscopy with transbronchial biopsy and bronchoalveolar lavage in the management of lung transplant recipients. Am J Respir Crit Care Med 152:2037, 1995.

233a. Halkos ME, Miller JI, Mann KP, et al: Thoracic presentations of post-transplant lymphoproliferative disorders. Chest 126:2013, 2004.

234. Hasegawa S, Ockner DM, Ritter JH, et al: Expression of class II major histocompatibility complex antigens (HLA-DR) and lymphocyte subset immunotyping in chronic pulmonary transplant rejection. Arch Pathol Lab Med 119:432, 1995.

235. Higenbottam T, Stewart S, Penketh A, Wallwork J: Transbronchial lung biopsy for the diagnosis of rejection in heart-lung transplant patients. Transplantation 46:532, 1988.

236. Hopkins PM, Aboyoun CL Chhajed PN, et al: Prospective analysis of 1,235 transbronchial lung biopsies in lung transplant recipients. J Heart Lung Transpl 21:1062, 2002.

237. Hruban RH, Beschorner WE, Baumgartner WA, et al: Depletion of bronchus-associated lymphoid tissue associated with lung allograft rejection. Am J Pathol 132:6, 1988.

238. Hruban RH, Beschorner WE, Baumgartner WA, et al: Diagnosis of lung allograft rejection by bronchial intraepithelial Leu-7 positive lymphocytes. J Thorac Cardiovasc Surg 96:939, 1988.

239. Husain AN, Siddiqui MT, Holmes EW, et al: Analysis of risk factors for the development of bronchiolitis obliterans syndrome. Am J Respir Crit Care Med 159:829, 1999.

240. Husain AN, Siddiqui MT, Montoya A, et al: Post-lung transplant biopsies: An 8-year Loyola experience. Mod Pathol 9:126, 1996.

241. Keller CA, Cagle PT, Brown RW, et al: Bronchiolitis obliterans in recipients of single, double, and heart-lung transplantation. Chest 107:973, 1995.

242. Kotloff RM, Ahya VN, Crawford SW: Pulmonary complications of solid organ and hematopoietic stem cell transplantation. Am J Respir Crit Care Med 170:22, 2004.

243. Lentz D, Bergin CJ, Berry GJ, Stoehr C, Theodore J: Diagnosis of bronchiolitis obliterans in heart-lung transplantation patients: Importance of bronchial dilatation on CT. AJR Am J Roentgenol 159:463, 1992.

244. Leonard CT, Soccal PM, Singer L, et al: Dendritic cells and macrophages in lung allografts: A role in chronic rejection. Am J Respir Crit Care Med 161:1349, 2000.

245. Levine SM, Bryan CL: Bronchiolitis obliterans in lung transplant recipients. The "thorn in the side" of lung transplantation. Chest 107:894, 1995.

246. Marchevsky A, Hartman G, Walts A, Ross D, Koerner S, Waters P: Lung transplantation: The pathologic diagnosis of pulmonary complications. Mod Pathol 4:133, 1991.

247. Miyagawa-Hayashino A, Wain JC, Mark EJ: Lung transplantation biopsy specimens with bronchiolitis obliterans or bronchiolitis obliterans organizing pneumonia due to aspiration. Arch Pathol Lab Med 129:223, 2005.

248. Nakhleh RE, Bolman RM III, Henke CA, Hertz MI: Lung transplant pathology: A comparative study of pulmonary acute rejection and cytomegaloviral infection. Am J Surg Pathol 15:1197, 1991.

249. Ohori NP, Iacono AT, Grgurich WF, Yousem SA: Significance of acute bronchitis/bronchiolitis in the

lung transplant recipient. Am J Surg Pathol 18:1192, 1994.

250. Rosendale B, Yousem SA: Discrimination of Epstein-Barr virus-related posttransplant lymphoproliferations from acute rejection in lung allograft recipients. Arch Pathol Lab Med 119:418, 1995.

250a. Sandmeier P, Speich R, Grebski E, et al: Iron accumulation in lung allografts is associated with acute rejection but not with adverse outcome. Chest 128:1379, 2005.

251. Siddiqui MT, Garrity ER, Husain AN: Bronchiolitis obliterans organizing pneumonia-like reactions: A nonspecific response or an atypical form of rejection or infection in lung allograft recipients? Hum Pathol 27:714, 1996.

252. Siddiqui MT, Garrity ER, Martinez R, Husain AN: Bronchiolar basement membrane changes and bronchiolitis obliterans in lung allografts study. Mod Pathol 9:320, 1996.

253. Tazelaar H, Yousem S: The pathology of combined heart-lung transplantation: An autopsy study. Hum Pathol 19:1403, 1988.

254. Trulock EP, Ettinger NA, Brunt EM, Pasque MK, Kaiser LR, Cooper JD: The role of transbronchial lung biopsy in the treatment of lung transplant recipients: An analysis of 200 consecutive procedures. Chest 102:1049, 1992.

255. Yousem SA: Graft eosinophilia in lung transplantation. Hum Pathol 23:1172, 1992.

256. Yousem SA: Lymphocytic bronchitis/bronchiolitis in lung allograft recipients. Am J Surg Pathol 17:491, 1993.

257. Yousem SA: The potential role of mast cells in lung allograft rejection. Hum Pathol 28:179, 1997.

258. Yousem SA, Berry GJ, Brunt EM, et al: A working formulation for the standardization of nomenclature in the diagnosis of heart and lung rejection: Lung Rejection Study Group. J Heart Transplant 9:593, 1990.

259. Yousem SA, Berry GJ, Cagle PT, et al: Revision of the 1990 working formulation for the classification of pulmonary allograft rejection: Lung Rejection Study Group. J Heart Lung Transpl 15:1, 1996.

260. Yousem SA, Burke CM, Billingham ME: Pathologic pulmonary alterations in long-term human heart-lung transplantation. Hum Pathol 16:911, 1985.

261. Yousem SA, Duncan SR, Griffith BP: Interstitial and airspace granulation tissue reactions in lung transplant recipients. Am J Surg Pathol 16:877, 1992.

262. Yousem SA, Martin T, Paradis IL, Keenan R, Griffith BP: Can immunohistological analysis of transbronchial biopsy specimens predict responder status in early acute rejection of lung allografts? Hum Pathol 25:525, 1994.

263. Yousem SA, Paradis I, Griffith BP: Can transbronchial biopsy aid in the diagnosis of bronchiolitis obliterans in lung transplant recipients? Transplantation 57:151, 1994.

264. Yousem SA, Randhawa P, Locker J, et al: Posttransplant lymphoproliferative disorders in heart-lung transplant recipients: Primary presentation in the allograft. Hum Pathol 20:361, 1989.

265. Zhang L, Ward C, Snell GI, et al: Scar collagen deposition in the airways of allografts of lung transplant recipients. Am J Respir Crit Care Med 155:2072, 1997.

Bone Marrow Transplantation

266. Afessa, B, Tefferi A, Litzow MR, et al: Diffuse alveolar hemorrhage in hematopoietic stem cell transplant recipients. Am J Respir Crit Care Med 166:641, 2002.

267. Agusti C, Ramirez J, Picado C, et al: Diffuse alveolar hemorrhage in allogenic bone marrow transplantation. A postmortem study. Am J Respir Crit Care Med 151:1006, 1995.

268. Ben-Abraham R, Paret G, Cohen R, et al: Diffuse alveolar hemorrhage following allogeneic bone marrow transplantation in children. Chest 124:660, 2003.

269. Beschorner WE, Saral R, Hutchins GM, et al: Lymphocytic bronchitis associated with graft-vs-host disease in recipients of bone marrow transplants. N Engl J Med 299:1030, 1978.

270. Chan CK, Hyland RH, Hutcheon MA, et al: Small-airways disease in recipients of allogeneic bone marrow transplants. An analysis of 11 cases and a review of the literature. Medicine (Baltimore) 66:327, 1987.

271. Cone RW, Hackman RC, Huang M-L, et al: Human herpesvirus 6 in lung tissue from patients with pneumonitis after bone marrow transplantation. N Engl J Med 329:156, 1993.

272. Cordonnier C, Bernaudin J, Bierling P, et al: Pulmonary complications occurring after allogeneic bone marrow transplantation. A study of 130 consecutive transplanted patients. Cancer 58:1047, 1986.

273. Griese M, Rampf U, Hofmann D, et al: Pulmonary complications after bone marrow transplantation in children: Twenty-four years of experience in a single pediatric center. Pediatr Pulmonol 30:393, 2000.

274. Gulbahce HE, Manivel JC, Jessurun J: Pulmonary cytolytic thrombi: A previously unrecognized complication of bone marrow transplantation. Am J Surg Pathol 24:1147, 2000.

275. Gulbahce HE, Pambuccian SE, Jessurun J, et al: Pulmonary nodular lesions in bone marrow transplant recipients: Impact of histologic diagnosis on patient management and prognosis. Am J Clin Pathol 121:205, 2004.

276. Hamilton PJ, Pearson ADJ: Bone marrow transplantation and the lung. Thorax 41:497, 1986.

277. Jules-Elysee K, Stover DE, Yahalom J, White DA, Gulati SC: Pulmonary complications in lymphoma patients treated with high-dose therapy and autologous bone marrow transplantation. Am Rev Respir Dis 146:485, 1992.

278. Khurshid I, Anderson LC: Non-infectious pulmonary complications after bone barrow transplantation. Postgrad Med J 78:257, 2002.

279. Krowka MJ, Rosenow EC III, Hoaglund HC: Pulmonary complications of bone marrow transplantation. Chest 87:237, 1985.

280. Meyers JD, Flournoy N, Thomas E: Nonbacterial pneumonia after allogeneic marrow transplantation: A

review of ten years' experience. Rev Infect Dis 4:1119, 1982.

281. Ostrow D, Buskard N, Hill R, et al: Bronchiolitis obliterans complicating bone marrow transplantation. Chest 87:828, 1985.

282. Palmas A, Tefferi A, Myers JL, et al: Late-onset noninfectious pulmonary complications after allogeneic bone marrow transplantation. Br J Haematol 100:680, 1998.

283. Paz HL, Crilley P, Patchefsky A, Schiffman RL, Brodsky I: Bronchiolitis obliterans after autologous bone marrow transplantation. Chest 101:775, 1992.

284. Perreault C, Cousineau S, D'Angelo G, et al: Lymphoid interstitial pneumonia after allogeneic bone marrow transplantation. A possible manifestation of chronic graft-versus-host disease. Cancer 55:1, 1985.

285. Ralph D, Springmeyer S, Sullivan K, et al: Rapidly progressive air-flow obstruction in marrow transplant recipients. Possible association between obliterative bronchiolitis and chronic graft-vs-host disease. Am Rev Respir Dis 129:641, 1984.

286. Selby DM, Rudzki JR, Bayever ES, et al: Vasculopathy of small muscular arteries in pediatric patients after bone marrow transplantation. Hum Pathol 30:734, 1999.

286a. Sharma S, Nadrous HF, Peters SG, et al: Pulmonary complications in adult blood and marrow transplant recipients. Autopsy findings. Chest 128:1385, 2005.

287. Sloane JP, Depledge MH, Powles RL, et al: Histopathology of the lung after bone marrow transplantation. J Clin Pathol 36:546, 1983.

288. Urbanski S, Kossakowska A, Curtis J, et al: Idiopathic small airways pathology in patients with graft-versus-host disease following allogeneic bone marrow transplantation. Am J Surg Pathol 11:965, 1987.

289. Williams LM, Fussell S, Veith RW, et al: Pulmonary veno-occlusive disease in an adult following bone marrow transplantation: Case report and review of the literature. Chest 109:1388, 1996.

290. Wingard JR, Mellits ED, Sostrin MB, et al: Interstitial pneumonitis after allogeneic bone marrow transplantation. Nine-year experience at a single institution. Medicine (Baltimore) 67:175, 1988.

291. Wise RH Jr, Shin MS, Gockerman JP, et al: Pneumonia in bone marrow transplant patients. AJR Am J Roentgenol 143:707, 1984.

292. Witte RJ, Gurney JW, Robbins RA, et al: Diffuse pulmonary alveolar hemorrhage after bone marrow transplantation: Radiographic findings in 39 patients. AJR Am J Roentgenol 157:461, 1991.

293. Wyatt SE, Nunn P, Hows JM, et al: Airways obstruction associated with graft versus host disease after bone marrow transplantation. Thorax 39:887, 1984.

294. Yousem SA: The histological spectrum of pulmonary graft-versus-host disease in bone marrow transplant recipients. Hum Pathol 26:668, 1995.

7

SYSTEMIC DISEASES INVOLVING THE LUNG

This chapter discusses the most common systemic diseases in which lung involvement may be prominent and a lung biopsy may be useful for diagnosis. No attempt has been made to include all systemic illnesses in which pulmonary lesions have been described. A list of the less common diseases that can have pulmonary involvement is provided at the end of the chapter (Table 7–4).

COLLAGEN VASCULAR DISEASES

Pulmonary involvement is a significant complication of many collagen vascular diseases, and it sometimes precedes the onset of the disease.[1,3,6] Interstitial lung disease is the most common manifestation, but a variety of other lesions can occur as well. The following sections review the pulmonary manifestations of the major collagen vascular diseases.

Rheumatoid Arthritis

Pulmonary changes related to rheumatoid arthritis may involve both the pleura and the parenchyma and are summarized in Table 7–1.[10,11,23]

Pleural Lesions

Pleurisy, often associated with pleural effusion, is the most common clinical manifestation of lung involvement. A characteristic granular appearance to the parietal pleura can be seen by thoracoscopic examination.[12] A pleural biopsy may be done in patients with effusions to exclude an infectious etiology. Occasionally, decortication is necessary to treat recurrent symptomatic effusions that are unresponsive to medical therapy. Histologic findings are usually nonspecific and include chronic inflammation, mesothelial hyperplasia, and fibrinoid deposits. Multinucleated giant cells have also been reported. Rarely, necrobiotic nodules that are identical to those in the subcutaneous tissues may be found.

Table 7–1 Lung Involvement in Rheumatoid Arthritis

Pleural Lesions
   Nonspecific pleuritis
   Necrobiotic nodules

Parenchymal Lesions
   Interstitial pneumonia and fibrosis
      UIP
      NSIP
   BOOP
   Airway lesions
      Constrictive bronchiolitis obliterans (obliterative
        bronchiolitis)
      Follicular bronchiolitis
   Others
      Necrobiotic nodules
      Caplan's syndrome
      Vasculitis
      Pulmonary hypertension
      Secondary amyloidosis

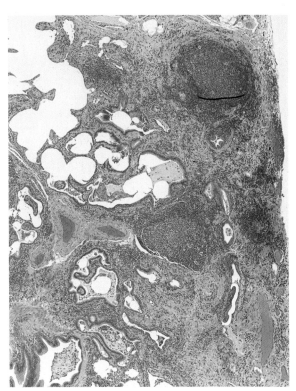

Figure 7–1 Rheumatoid lung. This patient had typical findings of UIP. In this area of honeycomb change there are two prominent lymphoid follicles containing reactive germinal centers. Although reactive lymphoid hyperplasia in UIP is not specific for rheumatoid lung, its presence should suggest the possibility of that diagnosis.

Parenchymal Lesions

A variety of pathologic processes occur in the lungs in rheumatoid arthritis. Interstitial pneumonia and fibrosis are common, and include both usual interstitial pneumonia (UIP) and nonspecific interstitial pneumonia (NSIP) (see Chapter 3).[1,4,5,6,7,18,23] UIP is a temporally and spatially variegated interstitial pneumonia characterized by areas of mild interstitial inflammation alternating with collagen-type fibrosis, honeycomb areas, small areas of active fibrosis (fibroblast foci), and normal lung. NSIP is a more uniform process characterized by a mixture of interstitial chronic inflammation and fibrosis with minimal architectural distortion. Traditionally, UIP was considered the most common interstitial pneumonia in rheumatoid arthritis, but more recent studies indicate a higher incidence of NSIP.[5,7] The prognosis of UIP associated with rheumatoid arthritis (and other collagen vascular diseases) appears to be better than UIP alone.[5] Sometimes, lymphoid aggregates with germinal centers are prominent in the background of UIP or NSIP (Fig. 7–1).[7,23] Although this finding is not specific for rheumatoid arthritis, its presence in UIP or NSIP should raise the possibility of underlying rheumatoid arthritis in cases lacking a pertinent history. Immunofluorescent studies have demonstrated deposits of IgM, presumably representing rheumatoid factor, and IgG within the alveolar septa and capillary walls.[11]

Bronchiolitis obliterans–organizing pneumonia (BOOP, see Chapter 2) is another finding in patients with rheumatoid arthritis.[1,2,6,18,21] It is characterized by plugs of fibroblasts and chronic inflammatory cells within distal bronchioles, alveolar ducts, and peribronchiolar alveolar spaces. This lesion may mimic the interstitial pneumonias radiographically. Its prognosis is not as good as BOOP occurring without an associated disease.[2]

Less often, constrictive bronchiolitis obliterans (obliterative bronchiolitis, see Chapter 16) occurs in rheumatoid arthrititis.[14–16] This lesion is characterized histologically by destruction of bronchioles and replacement by scar tissue. It differs from BOOP in that the reaction is confined to bronchioles, and their lumens are narrowed (constricted) by circumferential, mural fibrous tissue rather than being filled by intraluminal fibrous tissue plugs. Individuals with obliterative bronchiolitis present with an acute onset of dyspnea associated with hyperinflation of the lungs, and they usually pursue a progressive downhill course, with high mortality rates. Some of the reported patients had received penicillamine, and the role of this or other drugs in the etiology is uncertain.

Follicular bronchiolitis is another bronchiolar lesion that occurs occasionally (see Chapters 9 and 16).[7,10,13,22] It usually is encountered in the background of an interstitial pneumonia, but occasionally is the only abnormality.[7,15] It is characterized by lymphoid aggregates, often with reactive germinal centers that are present in the walls of bronchioles and may compress their lumens. Lymphoid aggregates may also occur along interlobular septa and in subpleural areas. This process can occur in other collagen vascular diseases (especially Sjögren's syndrome), as well as in patients with certain immunodeficiency states, and in hypersensitivity reactions.

Necrobiotic nodules identical to subcutaneous rheumatoid nodules have been reported in the lung but are rare.[1,17,24] They are usually subpleural and may be multiple or solitary. High serum titers of rheumatoid factor and subcutaneous nodules are frequent accompanying features. Histologically, they consist of a necrotic center bound by palisading histiocytes and surrounded by plasma cells and lymphocytes (Fig. 7–2). A moderate vasculitis, which is usually not necrotizing, is commonly present in the adjacent parenchyma. Such lesions must be differentiated from other necrotizing granulomas, especially the more common infectious granulomas and certain noninfectious granulomatous vasculitides. The results of cultures and special stains for organisms should exclude infection. The differentiation between rheumatoid nodules and Wegener's granulomatosis may be more difficult, especially when vasculitis is prominent. Finding numerous multinucleated giant cells, neutrophils, and eosinophils within the infiltrate favors Wegener's granulomatosis, whereas extension of the lesion through the visceral pleura is characteristic of rheumatoid nodules but less common in Wegener's (Fig. 7–3). Of course, a necrotizing vasculitis is characteristic of Wegener's (see Chapter 8), while the vasculitis in rheumatoid nodules is not necrotizing. In histologically difficult cases, the clinical and laboratory findings should help to clarify the diagnosis.

Caplan's syndrome (see Chapter 5) was first described in coal miners with rheumatoid arthritis, and it may occur in association with a variety of pneumoconioses. It is characterized by the presence of multiple necrobiotic nodules that are similar to those described previously, except that there is accompanying deposition of dust particles.[1]

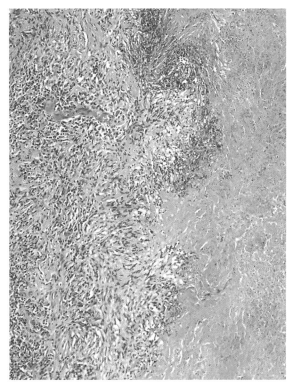

Figure 7–2 Rheumatoid nodule. An irregularly shaped necrotizing granuloma is seen that replaces lung parenchyma. It is characterized by a rim of palisading histiocytes around central necrosis, and there is a surrounding chronic inflammatory cell infiltrate. Nuclear debris is focally prominent in the necrotic zone (top).

Rarely, a vasculitis that involves predominantly small pulmonary arteries and venules has been described in patients with rheumatoid arthritis, although it more commonly involves extrapulmonary organs.[8] The deposition of immunoglobulins and complement has been demonstrated within vascular walls by immunofluorescence. Some examples of acute capillaritis (see Chapter 8), characterized by necrotizing acute inflammation of the alveolar capillary walls, occur in rheumatoid arthritis.[18] Pulmonary hypertension has been reported in rare cases.[9,20] Secondary amyloidosis, which may complicate rheumatoid arthritis, can involve the lung as well (see later on).

Systemic Lupus Erythematosus

A variety of pleural and parenchymal changes may be seen in systemic lupus erythematosus (SLE) (Table 7–2). Pleuritis and pleural effusion are common clinical manifestations, and pleural fibrosis and an acute

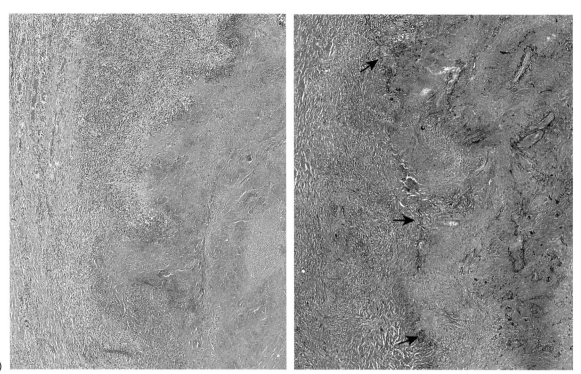

(a)   (b)

Figure 7–3 Rheumatoid nodule. (a) Extension of the necrotizing granulomatous inflammation into the pleura (left). **(b)** An elastic tissue stain shows partial destruction of the pleural elastic tissue (arrows) by the necrotizing process.

Table 7–2 Lung Involvement in Systemic Lupus Erythematosus	
Pleural Lesions	**Parenchymal Lesions**
Fibrinous pleuritis	NSIP
(pleural effusion)	UIP
Fibrosis of pleura	BOOP
	DAD*
	Intraalveolar hemorrhage*
	Vascular lesions
	Intimal, medial thickening
	Vasculitis
	Pulmonary hypertension

*The clinical syndrome manifested by patients with this finding is known as acute lupus pneumonitis (see text).

fibrinous pleuritis are often found at autopsy.[30,40] A variety of parenchymal lesions also occur.[1,6,30] Interstitial pneumonia is encountered occasionally, and most cases are NSIP.[5,30] UIP is uncommon.[2,7] A more cellular interstitial infiltrate of lymphocytes with lymphoid nodules,

suggestive of lymphoid interstitial pneumonia (LIP) (see Chapter 9), has been described occasionally.[36,43] It is not clear, however, whether the reported cases represent LIP or cellular NSIP. Some examples of BOOP have occurred in the setting of SLE.[1,2,28,32,36,38] Hematoxylin bodies can be observed rarely in the lung.[30]

Acute lupus pneumonitis is an uncommon, but dramatic, manifestation of SLE that is characterized clinically by fever, tachypnea, severe hypoxemia, and diffuse infiltrates.[36,40,41,43,45] Some cases occur in patients with antiphospholipid antibodies, and the resulting clinical syndrome is referred to as 'catastrophic antiphospholipid syndrome'.[25] A lung biopsy is usually required to establish the diagnosis. The most frequently observed pathologic abnormality in this condition is diffuse alveolar damage (DAD) (see Chapter 2) characterized by interstitial and intraalveolar edema and hyaline membrane formation.[6,36] Less commonly, the pathologic changes consist of massive intraalveolar hemorrhage with erythrocytes and hemosiderin-laden macrophages filling airspaces (Fig. 7–4).[27,31,35,36,41,48] Clinically, this form of the disease may mimic other alveolar hemorrhage syndromes (see Chapter 6), especially Goodpasture's syndrome, since patients may

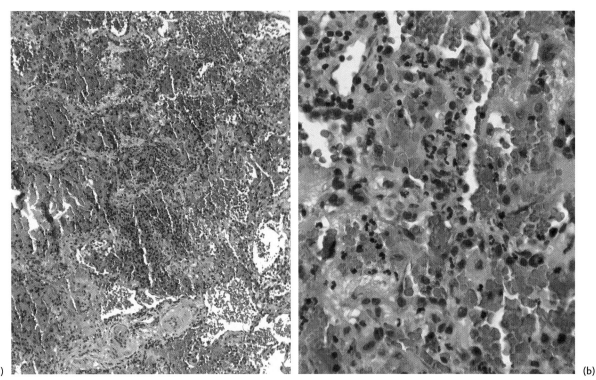

(a)   (b)

Figure 7–4 Acute lupus pneumonitis. (a) Low magnification view showing extensive intraalveolar hemorrhage. There is also a patchy acute inflammatory cell infiltrate present within alveolar septa that causes disruption in places. **(b)** Higher magnification showing acute inflammation in an alveolar septum that is indicative of a necrotizing capillaritis.

present with hemoptysis, respiratory distress, and renal failure. Laboratory tests should distinguish these two diseases, but sometimes biopsy is performed before the results of laboratory tests are known. The distinction of these diseases can often be made from routine histologic sections because evidence of acute necrotizing capillaritis (see Chapter 8) is usually present in cases of SLE-induced hemorrhage (Fig. 7–4b).[19,41,48] This lesion is characterized by expansion and destruction of alveolar septa by necrotic neutrophils, and it may be accompanied by a necrotizing arteriolitis.[19,41] Ultrastructural and immunofluorescent studies are also useful in the differential diagnosis. Granular staining of capillary basement membranes for immunoglobulins and complement is common in SLE (Fig. 7–5a), and elution techniques have demonstrated that the immunoglobulin deposits in this disease possess activity against DNA.[26,30,40] This appearance contrasts with the linear immunofluorescent staining of the alveolar basement membranes for immunoglobulins and complement that is characteristic of Goodpasture's syndrome. Granular staining of alveolar lining cell and mesothelial cell nuclei for immunoglobulins and complement has also

been demonstrated in SLE (Fig. 7–5b).[42] This intranuclear staining is ascribable to bound antinuclear antibody, a form of an in situ antinuclear antibody (ANA) test. Ultrastructurally, electron-dense deposits, corresponding to the granular immune complex deposits demonstrated by immunofluorescence, can often be found within alveolar capillary basement membranes in cases of SLE (Fig. 7–5c).[27,41] They may have an internal structure composed of concentric rings similar to the fingerprint pattern of deposits seen in glomerular basement membranes.[27] Tubuloreticular inclusions have also been noted in endothelial cell cytoplasm but are not specific for SLE.[34]

A variety of pulmonary vascular changes have been reported in SLE. Intimal thickening, medial hypertrophy, and periadventitial fibrosis are common findings at autopsy.[30] Acute changes of fibrinoid necrosis and vasculitis are found less often, usually in the setting of pulmonary hemorrhage (see earlier section).[41] Pulmonary hypertension has been attributed to SLE occasionally and in some cases may be related to anticardiolipin antibodies.[26,29,30,39,43,44,46,47] Pulmonary venoocclusive disease has been reported rarely.[33]

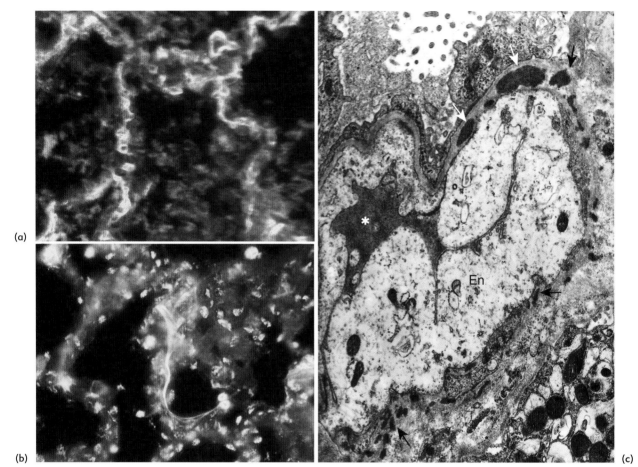

(a)

(b)

(c)

Figure 7–5 Acute lupus pneumonitis. Immunofluorescence showing granular staining of alveolar capillary basement membranes **(a)** and alveolar pneumocyte nuclei (from another case) **(b)** for IgG. Staining for complement was also present.
(c) Electron micrograph of a capillary showing numerous electron-dense deposits along the endothelial basement membrane (arrows). The capillary lumen is marked by an asterisk, and the endothelial cell cytoplasm labeled En. (Photo (c) courtesy of the late Dr Charles 'Chick' Kuhn.)

Progressive Systemic Sclerosis (Scleroderma)

Interstitial fibrosis, usually involving the lower lobes, develops in most patients with scleroderma and is a prominent finding at autopsy.[1,52,57,59,61] It is generally a manifestation of widespread systemic disease, although rarely it may antecede other manifestations of scleroderma. Both UIP and NSIP have been found at biopsy[4,5,6] and some studies report a predominance of NSIP.[49–51,54] There is some evidence that occult, recurrent aspiration of gastric contents due to gastro-esophageal reflux may contribute to interstitial fibrosis in some cases.[53] Pleural fibrosis and adhesions are common accompanying findings at autopsy, although pleural effusion is infrequent during life.[59] DAD has been reported rarely.[56]

Pulmonary vascular changes also occur in scleroderma and may be associated with clinically evident pulmonary hypertension.[58,60,61] They appear to be more frequent in patients with the CREST variant of scleroderma.[58,61] The severity of the vascular abnormalities does not correlate with the extent of interstitial fibrosis. Thickening of the intima and media of the pulmonary arteries is the most common finding (Fig. 7–6). Concentric fibrous proliferation may be seen within the intima, and there may be mucinous foci that stain with periodic acid–Schiff (PAS) and Alcian blue. Focal mucinous degeneration may be found within the media as well, where it is associated with disruption of elastic fibers. These arterial lesions are thought to be analogous to the renal vascular changes seen in the malignant systemic hypertension of scleroderma. Staining of

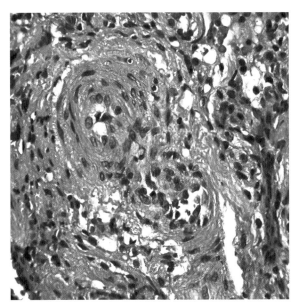

Figure 7–6 Pulmonary hypertension in scleroderma. There is prominent medial and intimal hypertrophy in this small artery. This change was not related to interstitial fibrosis.

endothelium for immunoglobulins and complement has been reported in one study.[55]

Polymyositis and Dermatomyositis

Interstitial pneumonia and interstitial fibrosis also occur in dermatomyositis and polymyositis but less frequently than in the other collagen vascular diseases.[1,64,65,68,70,71] Most cases resemble NSIP, although UIP occurs occasionally as does DAD.[4,5,7,62,64–67] LIP was noted in one case.[64] BOOP has been described in association with interstitial pneumonia in several cases, and it may be the predominant finding.[2,64,65,68,70,71] Vasculitis occurs rarely,[68] and primary pulmonary hypertension has been reported in one case.[63] Pulmonary hemorrhage and capillaritis have been reported in two cases, although the pathologic description is not convincing.[69] Another important cause of lung infiltrates in polymyositis or dermatomyositis is acute bronchopneumonia, related either to aspiration or to a depressed cough reflex secondary to underlying respiratory muscle weakness.[3] Pulmonary abnormalities may precede or initially overshadow the more common manifestations of the disease.[1,64]

Mixed Connective Tissue Disease

Patients who manifest overlapping clinical features of SLE, progressive systemic sclerosis, and polymyositis are considered to have mixed connective tissue disease.[72] High titers of circulating antibody to nuclear ribonuclear protein (RNP) can be identified in most. Not surprisingly, pleuropulmonary manifestations are common in these patients, since they are also common in the individual connective tissue diseases comprising the syndrome. Radiographic and functional evidence of interstitial fibrosis is frequent, but has not been well characterized pathologically.[1,72,74,76,77] NSIP has been reported in some cases.[5] Vascular changes identical to those seen in primary pulmonary hypertension have also been described, including plexiform lesions, fibrinoid necrosis, and arteritis.[73] Massive pulmonary hemorrhage has been described rarely.[75]

Sjögren's Syndrome

In Sjögren's syndrome, there is lymphocytic infiltration and atrophy of the salivary glands with resulting dryness of the mouth and other mucous membranes. Various collagen vascular diseases, most often rheumatoid arthritis, may be associated with Sjögren's syndrome. Lung involvement is common and is characterized both by manifestations of the associated rheumatic disease and by lesions related more specifically to Sjögren's syndrome itself (see Table 7–3). The former category includes nonspecific pleuritis, UIP, and NSIP.[4,5,7,78,79,81,85,91] In fact, NSIP is reported to be the most common biopsy finding in Sjögren's disease patients with lung involvement.[85] Lymphocytic infiltration and atrophy of the tracheobronchial mucous glands, similar to that seen in the major salivary glands, is a finding more specific to Sjögren's syndrome.

Table 7–3   Lung Involvement in Sjögren's Syndrome
Related to associated rheumatic disease
Pleuritis
Interstitial pneumonia and fibrosis (UIP, NSIP)
Specific to Sjögren's syndrome
Lymphocytic infiltration and atrophy of tracheobronchial mucous glands
Peribronchiolar lymphocytic infiltration with obstructive lung disease
Plexogenic pulmonary hypertension
Lymphoproliferative disorders
Follicular bronchiolitis
LIP
Lymphomatoid granulomatosis
Malignant lymphoma
Amyloidosis

Increased numbers of CD4-positive T lymphocytes have been noted in the infiltrate.[89] This process may lead to pulmonary infection because of the loss of normal mucus production with impairment of bronchociliary clearance mechanisms. Narrowing of the small airways and obstructive lung disease, as well as multiple bullae, have been described and are thought to be related to peribronchiolar lymphocytic infiltration.[84,86] Plexogenic pulmonary hypertension occurs rarely.[83,90]

A variety of lymphoproliferative diseases may involve the lung in Sjögren's syndrome, including follicular bronchiolitis, LIP, lymphomatoid granulomatosis, and malignant lymphoma (usually low-grade B-cell lymphoma, less often large B-cell).[78,80,82,85,87,88,91,92] These conditions are discussed in detail in Chapter 9. Clinically, the presence of hilar lymph node enlargement with multiple pulmonary nodules is highly suggestive of the development of lymphoma.[91] Amyloidosis (see text following) has been reported in several cases of Sjögren's syndrome, and it may be accompanied by LIP.[86,88,91,96]

AMYLOIDOSIS

Amyloidosis may involve the lung parenchyma either diffusely or in a nodular form, or it may be confined to the tracheobronchial tree.[94,95,101,102,112,115] As in other sites, amyloid in the lung appears as an amorphous eosinophilic material in the hematoxylin and eosin (H and E) stain.[100] It is metachromatic with crystal violet stain, and appears apple-green when stained with Congo red and examined under polarized light. Electron microscopy reveals a haphazard array of fine, non-branching, beaded fibrils ranging from 7.5 to 10 nm in width. Most, but not all, examples of pulmonary amyloidosis have been shown by means of potassium permanganate oxidation and immunohistochemical techniques to be immunoglobulin-derived (AL amyloid).[94,96,102,107,109,110,114]

Diffuse Alveolar Septal Amyloidosis

Diffuse alveolar septal amyloidosis is a frequent finding at autopsy in patients with disseminated primary amyloidosis or amyloidosis associated with multiple myeloma.[112] Secondary amyloidosis, in which there is an associated condition predisposing to amyloid deposition, involves the lung less often. Significant pulmonary impairment during life in any type of amyloidosis is uncommon and is probably more often related to cardiac failure from amyloid involvement of the heart than to deposition of amyloid within the lungs.[110,112]

Rarely, primary lung involvement with alveolar septal amyloidosis occurs in the absence of extrapulmonary involvement.[95,101,102,112] Patients with this condition present with progressive dyspnea, and fine reticulonodular interstitial infiltrates are found on chest radiographs. Lung biopsy is necessary for diagnosis. By light microscopy, amyloid deposits are seen along the alveolar septa and within the media of blood vessels (Figs 7–7 and 7–8). In some cases they are focal, involving occasional vessels and scattered portions of alveolar septa, but they may be extensive, involving large areas of interstitium. The deposits impart a homogeneous pink appearance to the media of the involved vessels and thicken the alveolar septa by the accumulation of amorphous eosinophilic material that may bulge into the alveolar spaces. By electron microscopy, the characteristic fibrils can be seen within the interstitial space and alveolar capillary basement membranes.[99,109] Pleural involvement occurs rarely and may be associated with pleural effusion.[93,103,106] Some cases are associated with benign lymphoid infiltrates such as LIP, and there may be an associated collagen vascular disease, especially Sjögren's syndrome.[97]

Diffuse alveolar septal amyloidosis needs to be distinguished from diffuse interstitial fibrosis with extensive collagen deposition. The presence of glassy-appearing globular deposits that affect blood vessels in addition to alveolar septa is a tip-off to the diagnosis. The lack of other features usually associated with interstitial fibrosis (inflammation, fibroblast foci, honeycomb areas) should also suggest the diagnosis. Of course, the use of special stains, such as Congo red or crystal violet, immunohistochemical stains for amyloid proteins, or electron microscopy should confirm the diagnosis.

Nodular Pulmonary Amyloidosis

This form of amyloidosis is usually not associated with amyloid deposition in other organs.[95,96,101,102,107,111,113] Patients are generally asymptomatic or have mild chest complaints. Chest radiographs show solitary or multiple, well-circumscribed masses that are often peripherally located; cavitation, and even hilar lymphadenopathy, can occur. The clinical differential diagnosis usually includes metastatic tumor and tuberculosis or other granulomatous disease. Open lung biopsy is generally performed for diagnosis, although transthoracic needle biopsy may be adequate in some cases.[108]

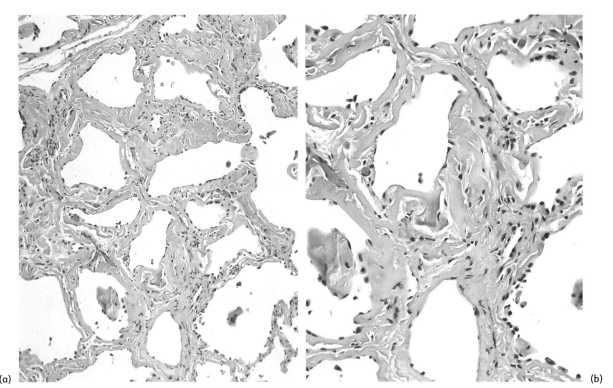

(a)   (b)

Figure 7–7 Alveolar septal amyloidosis. (a) Low magnification view showing thickening of alveolar septa by amorphous-appearing eosinophilic material. (b) Higher magnification emphasizing the amorphous appearance of the amyloid within alveolar septa.

Grossly, the lesions are discrete, tumor-like nodules that appear gray–tan and waxy. They average from 1 to 3 cm in diameter, although masses as large as 15 cm have been described. Histologically, they are composed of dense accumulations of typical amorphous eosinophilic material that is sharply demarcated from the surrounding lung (Fig. 7–9). A Congo red stain typically shows apple-green birefringence in polarized light, and immunohistochemical stains for amyloid P and A proteins may be positive. Aggregates of plasma cells and lymphocytes may be found within the nodules, and foreign body giant cells are frequently seen engulfing the amyloid (Fig. 7–10). Foci of calcification and bone and cartilage formation are common, and occasionally zones of necrosis are present.

Sometimes, conventional staining techniques are negative for amyloid in cases that otherwise are histologically typical. Some of these cases occur in patients with *light chain deposition disease* and have been shown by immunohistochemistry and electron microscopy to contain immunoglobulin light chain deposits rather than true amyloid.[105] In difficult cases or when ancillary special techniques are not available, the clinical findings should help in the differential diagnosis, since renal involvement is prominent in light chain deposition disease, and most affected patients also have evidence of plasma cell myeloma. A few cases, however, have been reported in patients lacking evidence of light chain deposition disease elsewhere, and are of uncertain histogenesis.[104] For practical purposes, those lesions that histologically resemble an amyloid nodule but lack the typical staining characteristics can be termed 'amyloid-like nodules'.[104]

The main lesion in the differential diagnosis of nodular amyloidosis or amyloid-like nodules is pulmonary hyalinizing granuloma (see Chapter 15).[98,116] Radiographically, this entity also manifests solitary or multiple pulmonary masses, and patients usually have few symptoms. Histologically, unlike the lesions of nodular amyloidosis, pulmonary hyalinizing granulomas are composed of thick, acellular collagen bundles that are arranged in a distinct lamellar configuration; ossification, cartilage formation, and foreign body granulomas are not found.

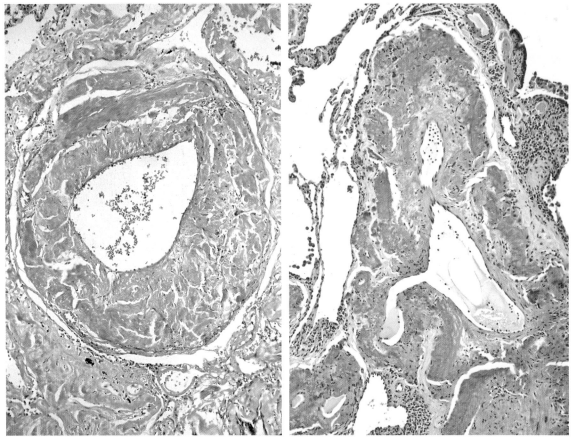

(a)   (b)

Figure 7–8 Vascular involvement in alveolar septal amyloidosis. (a) Abundant amorphous globules of amyloid replace most of this artery wall. Note the amyloid in the surrounding parenchyma as well. (b) A Congo red stain highlights amyloid deposition in another artery.

Tracheobronchial Amyloidosis

Tracheobronchial amyloidosis, in which deposits of amyloid are confined to the tracheobronchial tree, constitutes a rare form of pulmonary amyloidosis.[95,96,102,114] These deposits may be solitary or multiple. As solitary deposits, they often mimic carcinoma, either because they form a mass or because they produce distal pneumonia or collapse related to bronchial occlusion. Multiple deposits may involve extensive portions of the conducting airways. Major presenting manifestations include wheezing, stridor, recurrent chest infections, and hemoptysis. The diagnosis can usually be made by bronchial biopsy, and bronchoscopy may also be therapeutic by removing the bulk of the obstructing tissue. Histologically, the amorphous eosinophilic material typical of amyloid is present within the submucosa of bronchi (Fig. 7–11). It surrounds mucous glands and cartilage, which may become atrophied.

Foreign body giant cells, calcification, and ossification are common associated features.

SARCOIDOSIS

Sarcoidosis is a multisystem granulomatous disease of unknown cause, and it is probably the most common interstitial lung disease encountered by the surgical pathologist. Lung involvement is present in most patients, and pulmonary lesions may be the sole manifestation of the disease. The diagnosis is based on a characteristic spectrum of clinical, radiographic, and laboratory findings combined with compatible histologic features, and lung biopsy is frequently undertaken for diagnosis.[119,128,146] Endobronchial and transbronchial biopsy techniques are especially useful, because they are relatively noninvasive and will show granulomas in over 60% of cases, even in the absence of radiographically

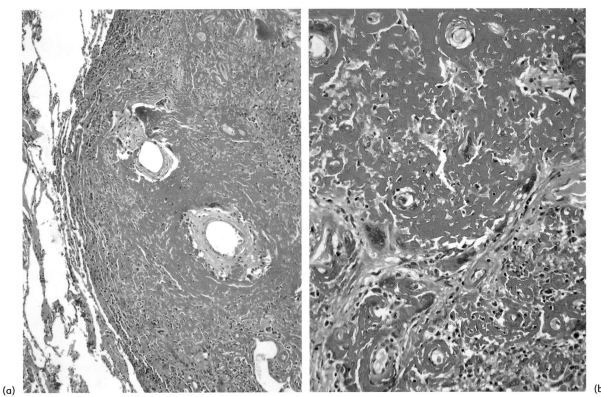

Figure 7–9 Nodular amyloidosis. (a) Low magnification view showing a well-circumscribed nodule of amorphous eosinophilic material replacing a portion of parenchyma. **(b)** Higher magnification showing foreign body giant cells engulfing the amyloid in places.

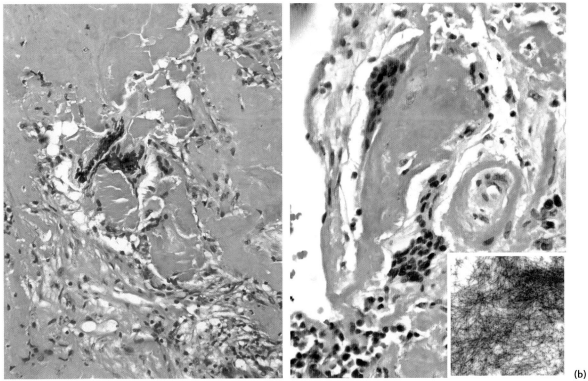

Figure 7–10 Nodular amyloidosis. (a) Higher magnification view of the foreign body giant cell reaction to the amyloid material (center). **(b)** A Congo red stain highlights the foreign body giant cell reaction. Inset is an electron micrograph showing the typical haphazardly arranged thin fibrils characteristic of amyloid (×25,000, courtesy of the late Dr Charles 'Chick' Kuhn).

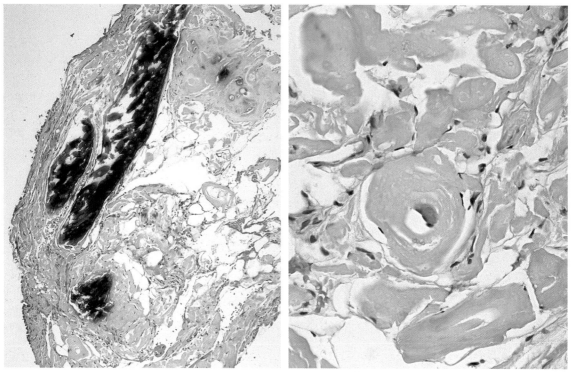

(a) (b)

Figure 7-11 Tracheobronchial amyloidosis. (a) Bronchial biopsy shows extensive amyloid deposition in the bronchial wall. The bronchial epithelium is on the left. Calcification is prominent and the cartilage (top) is atrophic. **(b)** Higher magnification showing the amorphous amyloid deposits.

apparent lung infiltrates (see Chapter 17).[153,159,164] Transbronchial needle aspiration of enlarged hilar and mediastinal lymph nodes combined with transbronchial biopsy is also useful.[172]

Clinical and Radiographic Findings

Sarcoidosis most frequently affects young to middle-aged adults, usually less than 40 years old, although there is a wide age range including even the elderly.[123a] Blacks and women appear to be at higher risk than other groups. The disease has been reported in patients with HIV infection, usually in individuals with CD4 lymphocyte counts greater than 200 cells/μL, many of whom have also been receiving highly active antiretroviral therapy (HAART).[145,147,149,171] Some cases have also been reported in patients receiving interferon-α for hepatitis C.[163,168] Patients usually present with mild, nonspecific chest complaints such as dyspnea and cough, although many are asymptomatic.[128,146] Restrictive defects on pulmonary function testing and low diffusing capacity are common in symptomatic patients. Radiographically, bilateral interstitial opacities are usually found, and there may be associated hilar lymph node enlargement.[148] Other radiographic abnormalities occur less frequently, including solitary or multiple nodular densities, localized areas of consolidation, and peripheral opacities.[134,151,158,161] Pleural effusion occurs rarely.[120,178] On computed tomography (CT), thickened bronchovascular bundles constitute the most common finding.[150] A radiographic staging system has been devised that appears to correlate with prognosis: stage I – hilar adenopathy alone without parenchymal infiltrates (best prognosis); stage II – hilar adenopathy and parenchymal infiltrates; stage III – parenchymal infiltrates alone (poorest prognosis). Corticosteroids are used to treat progressive symptomatic disease.[119] Therapy with antifibrotic agents such as colchicine and pirfenidone has been tried in progressive disease, but the results have not been beneficial. Therapy with substances that block tumor necrosis factor alpha (TNFα), such as pentoxifylline, thalidomide, etanercept, or infliximab, is another promising approach.[119]

Histologic Features

Classic Sarcoidosis

Involvement of the lung in sarcoidosis is manifested by non-necrotizing granulomatous inflammation

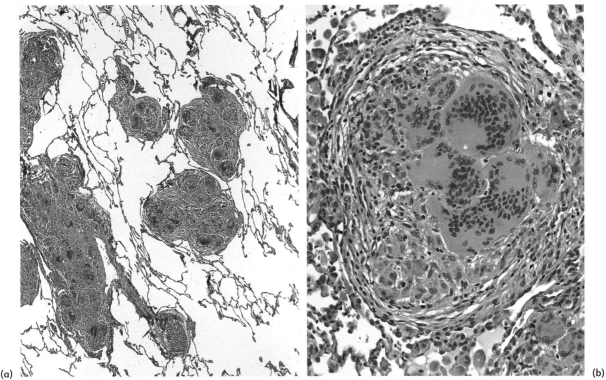

(a) (b)

Figure 7–12 Sarcoidosis. (a) Low magnification view showing characteristic well-circumscribed, non-necrotizing granulomas within the interstitium. Note the lack of inflammation in adjacent alveolar septa. **(b)** Higher magnification of a typical granuloma, showing the tightly packed central epithelioid histiocytes and multinucleated giant cells that are surrounding by a thin rim of fibroblasts.

similar to that occurring in extrapulmonary organs.[117,123,126,138,146,173] The granulomas characteristically are composed of tightly clustered epithelioid histiocytes and, occasionally, multinucleated giant cells with few intervening lymphocytes or other inflammatory cells (Fig. 7–12). Their borders are usually well circumscribed and often surrounded by a thin rim of concentrically arranged fibroblasts with scattered chronic inflammatory cells. Hyalinized fibrous tissue may replace portions of granulomas or even entire granulomas and it may be extensive (Fig. 7–13). Small foci of central necrosis can be found in the granulomas occasionally and may raise the suspicion of infection.[137] Although reticulin stains are said to demonstrate a preserved reticulin network in such cases but not in infections,[146] this technique is not useful in our experience.

The granulomas involve predominantly the interstitium rather than airspaces. They may be scattered individually with little distortion of the underlying lung architecture (Fig. 7–14), or they can form confluent masses that replace portions of lung parenchyma (Fig. 7–15). In either situation, a characteristic distribution along lymphatic pathways can usually be observed. This pattern is most easily recognized in partially involved areas of parenchyma, where the granulomas can be seen coursing along bronchovascular bundles, interlobular septa, and the pleura (Fig. 7–16). Although a narrow rim of chronic inflammatory cells commonly surrounds the granulomas, significant interstitial pneumonia extending into adjacent lung tissue is usually not seen.

A number of nonspecific cytoplasmic inclusions may be present within the granulomas and their component histiocytes, including asteroid, Schaumann, and conchoid bodies (Fig. 7–17).[141] Large, polarizable crystalline structures are also common and should not be confused with inhaled exogenous material (Fig. 7–18).[157,175] They are composed mainly of calcium oxalate and smaller amounts of calcium carbonate, and are thought to represent degradation products of cell metabolism. Irregularly shaped dense bodies and tadpole-shaped structures have been noted within the histiocytes by electron microscopy.[127,129,177] Although some

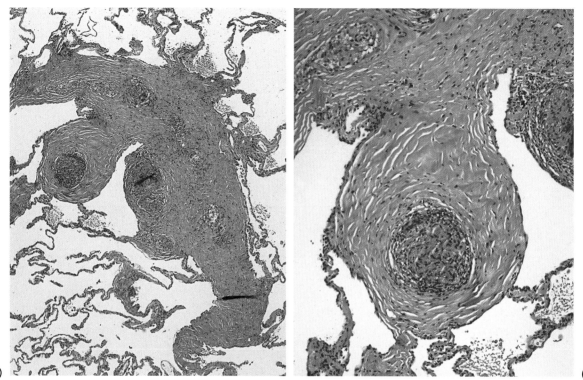

(a)   (b)

Figure 7–13 Hyalinized fibrosis in sarcoidosis. (a) Low magnification shows extensive hyalinized fibrosis that replaces areas of granulomatous inflammation. **(b)** Higher magnification shows small residual granuloma surrounded by hyalinized fibrosis.

investigators have postulated that these cytoplasmic inclusions represent microorganisms,[177] it seems more likely that they are related to lysosomes.

A granulomatous vasculitis frequently accompanies the other changes in sarcoidosis, especially in cases with extensive parenchymal involvement by granulomas (Fig. 7–19).[162,170] It is characterized by non-necrotizing granulomas within the intima and media of blood vessels that often compress the lumens but do not cause necrosis of the blood vessel walls. Rarely, pulmonary hypertension may occur secondary to granulomatous occlusion of vessels.[136,166]

Necrotizing Sarcoid Granulomatosis

Necrotizing sarcoid granulomatosis was first described by Liebow[144] in 1973, and there have been only a few subsequent reports.[125,133,142,143,154,160,164,167] The clinical presentation is similar to that of classic sarcoidosis, and there is a female predominance. The radiographic findings differ, however, in that nodular opacities are the most common finding, and they are usually multiple and bilateral. Hilar lymphadenopathy is frequently present as well, and pleural effusions are common. Extrathoracic involvement does not usually occur,

although ocular, neurologic, cardiac, hepatic, and splenic involvement has been reported rarely.[75,76,143,154] The clinical course is generally benign, and most patients respond to corticosteroid therapy.

Necrotizing sarcoid granulomatosis differs histologically from classic sarcoidosis by the presence of large areas of parenchymal necrosis in a background of confluent, non-necrotizing, 'sarcoid-like' granulomas (Fig. 7–20).[125,142,144,167] Additionally, there is an associated prominent vasculitis that is more widespread than can be explained by extension from parenchymal granulomatous inflammation (Fig. 7–21).[125,144] The vasculitis may be granulomatous or it may be characterized by transmural chronic inflammation. Multinucleated giant cells are prominent in some cases, but significant necrosis is usually not a feature.

In the past there was considerable debate whether necrotizing sarcoid granulomatosis was a variant of sarcoidosis or represented a distinct entity. Current evidence suggests that it is best considered a variant of sarcoidosis, probably corresponding to so-called nodular sarcoid.[151,154,161] A more important issue, because of the combination of granulomatous inflammation and necrosis with vasculitis, is the distinction from

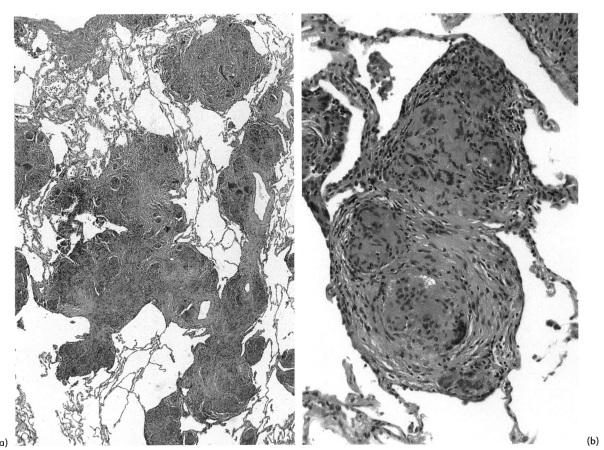

Figure 7–14 Interstitial involvement in sarcoidosis. (a) At low magnification the granulomas are seen to infiltrate and expand alveolar septa. They also course along an interlobular septum (right). The airspaces contain scattered histiocytes but are otherwise not involved. **(b)** Higher magnification illustrating the interstitial location of the granuloma. Note also the typical well-circumscribed appearance.

Wegener's granulomatosis. This distinction is usually not difficult, because non-necrotizing granulomas are not features of Wegener's. Also, the vasculitis of Wegener's is characteristically more necrotizing and often suppurative.

Special Stains and Additional Studies

Special stains for acid-fast bacilli and fungi, of course, need to be carefully examined, and all cases should be cultured.[137] More sophisticated techniques for identifying an infectious etiology, such as the polymerase chain reaction (PCR), have also been utilized, with varying results.[131] Some studies found evidence of mycobacterial DNA (either *M. tuberculosis* or nontuberculous organisms), but usually only in a minority of cases, while others were entirely negative.[121,132,155,156,176] The findings raise the possibility that cell wall-defective

mycobacteria or persistent intracellular mycobacterial DNA might be important in pathogenesis. Other investigators have identified propionibacterium by both PCR and culture, although the role, if any, of this indigenous skin anaerobic bacterium in producing sarcoidosis is not clear.[139] The current view is that an infectious agent may act as a trigger for inflammation in genetically susceptible individuals rather than causing a true infection.[131]

Angiotensin-converting enzyme (ACE) has been demonstrated within epithelioid cells of sarcoid granulomas by means of immunohistologic and autoradiographic techniques.[118,152] Staining of epithelioid histiocytes has been demonstrated with a monoclonal anti-Kveim antibody, although this staining is not specific for sarcoidosis.[140] The associated lymphoid cells have been shown by immunohistochemistry to consist mainly of helper (CD4) T cells with the capacity to proliferate.[122,124,174] Immunohistochemical staining

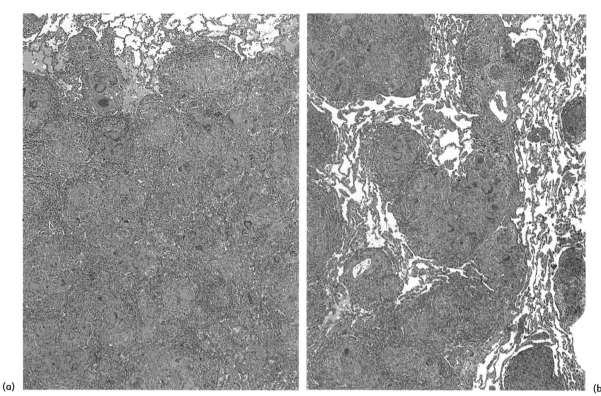

(a)

(b)

Figure 7–15 Confluent granulomas in sarcoidosis. (a) In this example, confluent granulomas have replaced a portion of lung parenchyma in a nodular fashion. (b) The interstitial location of the granulomas can still be appreciated at the periphery of the nodule.

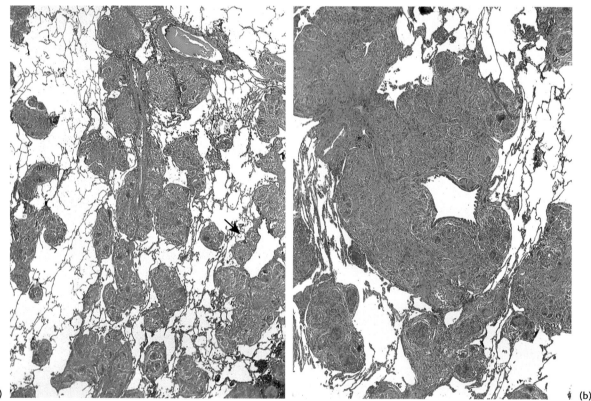

(a)

(b)

Figure 7–16 Lymphangitic distribution of the granulomas in sarcoidosis. (a) Low magnification view showing granulomas along an interlobular septa with central vein (center) and around a small bronchiole (right, arrow). (b) Higher magnification of peribronchiolar granulomas from same case as in (a). Note the narrowing of the bronchiolar lumen.

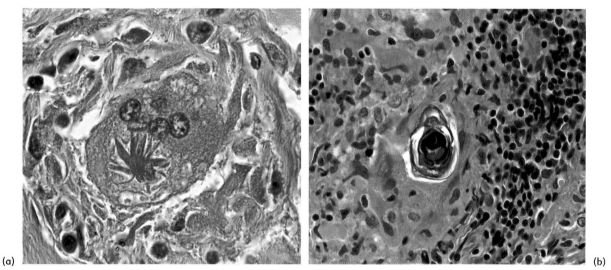

(a)   (b)

Figure 7–17 Cytoplasmic inclusions in sarcoidosis. (a) Asteroid body. **(b)** Schaumann body.

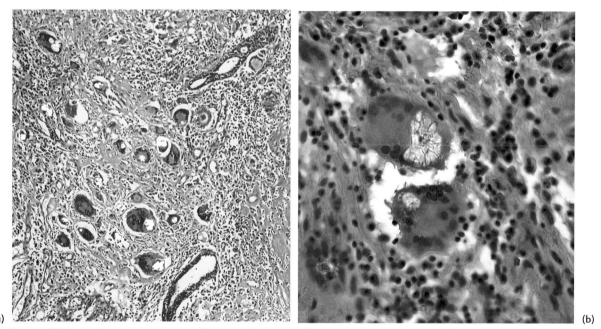

(a)   (b)

Figure 7–18 Crystalline inclusions in sarcoidosis. (a) At low magnification under partially polarized light, large crystalline structures are seen within multinucleated giant cells. **(b)** Higher magnification view of H and E-stained section, showing large sheet-like refractile yellow crystals.

for various matrix metalloproteinases has been demonstrated in sarcoid granulomas.[135]

Differential Diagnosis

The major conditions in the differential diagnosis of sarcoidosis include infection, berylliosis and other occupational lung diseases, talc granulomatosis (intravenous drug abuser's lung), and hypersensitivity pneumonia. Additionally, Wegener's granulomatosis enters the differential diagnosis of necrotizing sarcoid granulomatosis. As noted earlier, special stains for acid-fast bacteria and fungi must be carefully examined in each case to exclude an infection, and all specimens

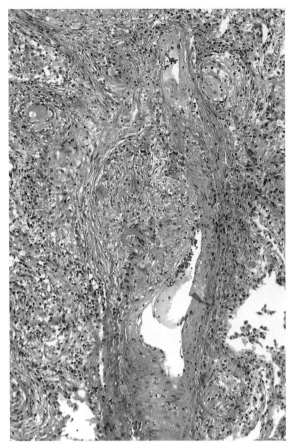

Figure 7–19 Vascular involvement in sarcoidosis. Non-necrotizing granulomas are seen partially replacing the wall of this pulmonary artery. The artery is present adjacent to an area of granulomatous inflammation (top and left). There is no necrosis of the vessel wall.

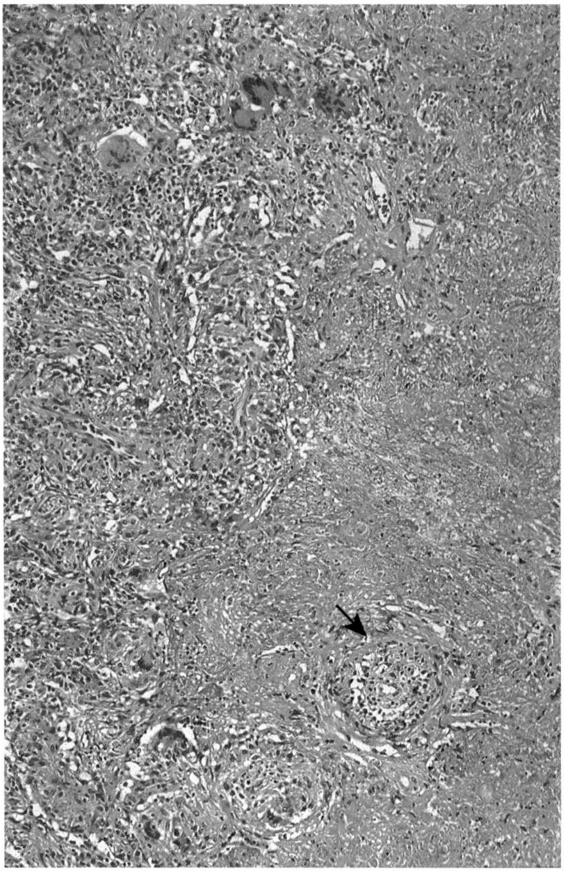

Figure 7–20 Necrotizing sarcoid granulomatosis. Low magnification view showing large area of parenchymal necrosis surrounded by confluent non-necrotizing granulomas. Vascular inflammation is also present (arrow).

should be cultured. In necrotizing sarcoid granulomatosis, the presence of vasculitis occurring away from the areas of necrosis helps distinguish the changes from tuberculosis and fungal infections before the results of cultures are known. It should be remembered, however, that vasculitis can be seen in infectious granulomas, where it occurs in or directly adjacent to the granulomatous inflammation (see Chapter 11), and, therefore, necrotizing sarcoid granulomatosis should be considered only if the vasculitis is severe and occurs at some distance away from the inflamed areas. Although it is uncommon for most infections to cause non-necrotizing, sarcoid-like granulomas that may be confused with ordinary sarcoidosis, this tissue reaction is common in both cryptococcal and *Mycobacterium avium-intracellulare* complex (MAC, see Chapter 11) infections. Cryptococci are easily visible in H and

E-stained sections as well as in Gomori's methenamine silver (GMS) stains, however, while diagnosis of MAC infection usually requires culture, although the organisms occasionally are visible in acid-fast stains. An important clue to infection rather than sarcoidosis is the presence of airspace in addition to interstitial granulomas along with intraluminal organization (BOOP). Many cases of MAC infection occur in patients exposed to hot tubs (so-called *hot tub lung*, see Chapter 11), and, therefore, clinical history may help in diagnosis.

Berylliosis is very rare, and there are no specific histologic or radiologic findings that distinguish it from sarcoidosis, although focal necrosis and vasculitis are said to be more common in sarcoidosis.[123,146] The diagnosis of berylliosis must be based on the clinical history of exposure and on analysis of tissue (see Chapter 5).

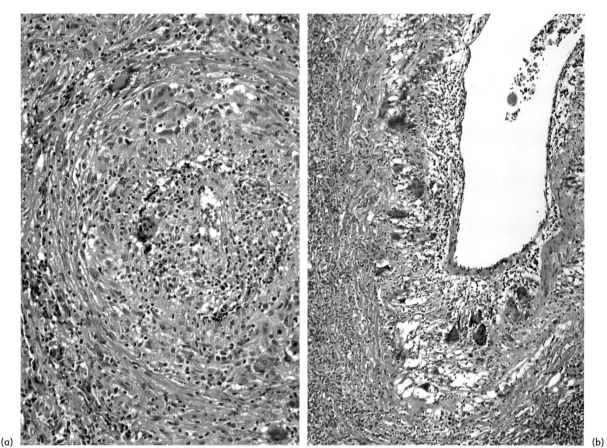

Figure 7–21 Vasculitis in necrotizing sarcoid granulomatosis. (a) This artery is infiltrated by epithelioid histiocytes and chronic inflammatory cells and the lumen is narrowed. Necrosis is not seen. (b) Multinucleated giant cells are prominent in this example.

Lymphocyte stimulation tests using cells obtained at bronchoalveolar lavage may also help in diagnosis.

The presence of crystalline structures in sarcoid granulomas may initially suggest an occupational lung disease such as *talc pneumoconiosis*. The characteristic lymphangitic distribution of the granulomas excludes most inhalational diseases, however, and, of course, a thorough clinical history usually clarifies the situation. In questionable cases, tissue analysis will establish the correct diagnosis. The possibility of *talc granulomatosis* as occurs in intravenous drug abusers (drug abuser's lung, see Chapter 13) may also be considered because of the crystals. Histologically, talc granulomatosis differs from sarcoidosis in that the granulomas are usually of the foreign body type rather than sarcoid-like and they are confined to small blood vessels and the surrounding interstitium. Also, larger inclusions of methylcellulose and other exogenous substances are usually present in addition to talc.

Hypersensitivity pneumonia (see Chapter 6) sometimes enters the differential diagnosis of sarcoidosis, although the differentiation is not difficult in most cases. Pathologic features that should suggest hypersensitivity pneumonia include ill-defined or poorly circumscribed granulomas, a prominent interstitial pneumonia extending away from the granulomas, and areas of bronchiolitis obliterans. Additionally, the inflammatory reaction in hypersensitivity pneumonia is localized to, or at least accentuated around, bronchioles rather than following the lymphangitic distribution characteristic of sarcoidosis.

The Surgical Pathology Report in Sarcoidosis

The diagnosis of sarcoidosis is based on a combination of clinical, laboratory, radiographic, and pathologic findings, and, therefore, it is not possible for the

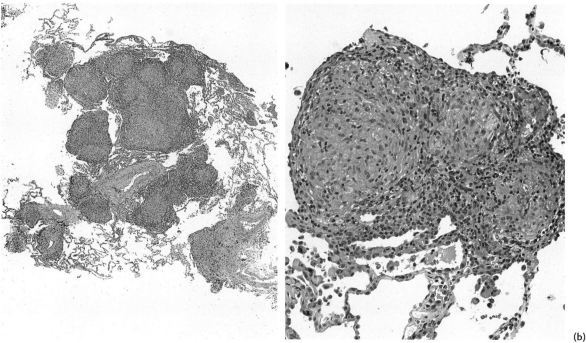

(a)

(b)

Figure 7–22 Transbronchial biopsy in sarcoidosis. (a) Numerous typical, well-demarcated, non-necrotizing granulomas are seen in this example. **(b)** Higher magnification shows the tight, well-circumscribed appearance of a granuloma. Note the lack of inflammation in the adjacent alveolar septa.

pathologist to specifically diagnose 'sarcoidosis' based on the histologic findings alone. Rather, the pathologist can provide only a descriptive diagnosis of 'non-necrotizing granulomas', which can be further interpreted by the clinicians in the appropriate context. In cases that show the typical morphology and distribution of sarcoid granulomas, however, it is justified, and frequently very helpful to clinicians, to diagnose 'noncaseating granulomas consistent with sarcoidosis'. Conversely, if the granulomas are not typical of sarcoidosis, this observation should be communicated to the clinicians so that other diseases in the differential diagnosis will be seriously considered.

Transbronchial Biopsy in Sarcoidosis

Transbronchial lung biopsy (TBB) is the usual mode of sampling lung tissue in cases of suspected sarcoidosis (see Chapter 17), while open lung biopsy is generally utilized only in cases when TBB is nonproductive or when the diagnosis is unsuspected clinically.[137,157,159,170] Although abundant, typical, non-necrotizing granulomatous inflammation may be sampled (Fig. 7–22), the findings are often more subtle. Scattered, small,

compressed or distorted granulomas within the bronchial walls or adjacent alveolar septa may be the only finding (Fig. 7–23). The granulomas may consist only of a few multinucleated histiocytes, and the typical lymphangitic distribution may not be appreciable. It is important in such cases to carefully examine multiple levels from each block so that even subtle granulomatous inflammation is not missed.[169] Simply identifying even a single tiny granuloma may be sufficient to confirm the clinical impression on a TBB.

MISCELLANEOUS DISEASES

There are a large number of other diseases that occasionally have associated lung involvement, and they are listed in Table 7–4. Systemic vasculitides involving lung, including Behçet's disease and polyarteritis, are discussed in Chapter 8. It should be noted that BOOP (see Chapter 2) has been reported in association with many and varied conditions. Since BOOP is a relatively common pathologic finding, we do not consider it a specific manifestation of another disease unless it is noted in more than a few isolated case reports.

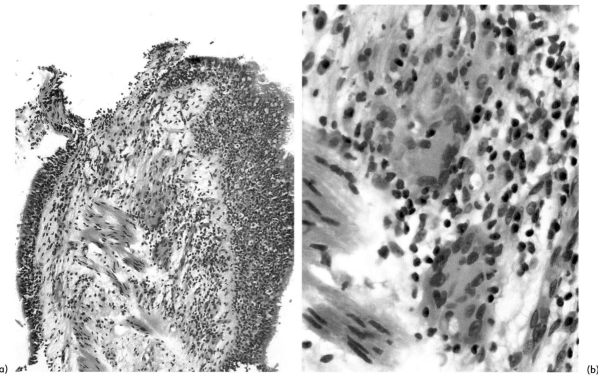

(a) (b)

Figure 7–23 Bronchial biopsy in sarcoidosis. In this example, only a small, ill-defined granuloma is present in the bronchial wall (a). At higher magnification (b), the loose cluster of epithelioid histiocytes and multinucleated giant cells is better appreciated.

Table 7–4 Other Diseases Occasionally Associated with Lung Involvement	
Disease	**Lung Involvement**
Storage Diseases	
Gaucher's disease[179,226,229]	Pulmonary hypertension, interstitial, intraalveolar, and intracapillary Gaucher cells
Hermansky–Pudlak syndrome[193,214a,225,236]	Interstitial fibrosis, vacuolated alveolar pneumocytes
Fabry's disease[228]	Vacuolization of vascular media and intima
Niemann–Pick Type B disease[216]	Endogenous lipoid pneumonia
Histiocytic Disorders	
Malacoplakia[181,185,187,199]	Nodular infiltrates of histiocytes, Michaelis-Gutman bodies, often due to *Rhodacoccus equi* in AIDS
Whipple's disease[201,238]	Peribronchiolar and perivascular infiltrate of PAS-positive histiocytes
Erdheim Chester disease[191,224]	Lymphangitic interstitial infiltrates of CD68+, S-100–, and CD1a– histiocytes with abundant eosinophilic or foamy cytoplasm and fibrosis
Gastrointestinal Diseases	
Ulcerative colitis, Crohn's disease[180,182,184,188,189,197,212,232,237]	Bronchitis, bronchiectasis, acute/chronic bronchiolitis, granulomatous bronchiolitis, necrotic nodules, acute bronchopneumonia, BOOP, interstitial pneumonia/fibrosis
Celiac disease[190,217,230]	Bronchitis, peribronchial fibrosis, abscess cavities, idiopathic pulmonary hemosiderosis

Continued

Table 7–4 Other Diseases Occasionally Associated with Lung Involvement—*cont'd*

Disease	Lung Involvement
Dermatologic Disorders	
Pyoderma gangrenosum[206,209,235]	Steroid-responsive acute bronchopneumonia, abscesses
Sweet's syndrome (acute febrile neutrophilic dermatosis)[231]	Steroid-responsive acute bronchopneumonia
Pseudoxanthoma elasticum[200]	Disruption and calcification of elastic fibers
Stevens–Johnson syndrome/toxic epidermal necrolysis[204,207]	Constrictive bronchiolitis obliterans
Birt-Hogg-Dubé syndrome[180a,193a]	Cysts, pneumothorax
Metabolic Disorders	
Ehlers–Danlos syndrome[186,240]	Cysts, fibrous pseudotumors, arteriovenous anastomoses, pneumothorax, pulmonary hemorrhage
Cutis laxa[186]	Emphysema, pulmonary artery stenosis
Marfan's syndrome[239]	Bullae, pneumothorax
Diabetes mellitus[194,221]	Perivascular xanthogranulomatosis; infections, especially zygomycosis
Hematological Disorders	
Sickle cell anemia[195,196,213,219,233,234]	Infarcts due to intravascular sickling, bronchopneumonia, fat emboli, pulmonary hypertension, plastic bronchitis
Chronic granulomatous disease[214]	Suppurative granulomas; microabscesses, often containing fungi or bacteria; eosinophilia; pigmented macrophages
Cryofibrinogenemia[215]	Fibrin thrombi in small blood vessels
Chronic Liver Disease[205,210,220,222,241]	
(cirrhosis, nodular regenerative hyperplasia)	Vasodilatation, arteriovenous shunts, pulmonary hypertension
Miscellaneous Diseases	
Ankylosing spondylitis[198,203,208,223]	Upper lobe fibrobullous lesions, aspergillus mycetomas, mycobacterial infections
Myasthenia gravis[211]	Chronic interstitial pneumonia
Juvenile arthritis[218]	Follicular bronchiolitis, lymphoid interstitial pneumonia, pulmonary hypertension
Endometriosis[183,192,202,227]	Pneumothorax, hemothorax, pulmonary nodules

REFERENCES

Collagen Vascular Diseases

General

1. Lamblin C, Bergoin C, Saelens T, Wallaert B: Interstitial lung diseases in collagen vascular diseases. Eur Respir J 18:69s, 2001.
2. Lohr RH, Boland BJ, Douglas WW, et al: Organizing pneumonia. Features and prognosis of cryptogenic, secondary, and focal variants. Arch Intern Med 157:1323, 1997.
3. Lynch JP III, Hunninghake GW: Pulmonary complications of collagen vascular disease. Annu Rev Med 43:17, 1992.
4. Nagao T, Nagai S, Kitaichi M, et al: Usual interstitial pneumonia: Idiopathic pulmonary fibrosis versus collagen vascular diseases. Respiration 68:151, 2001.
5. Nakamura Y, Chida K, Suda T, et al: Nonspecific interstitial pneumonia in collagen vascular diseases: Comparison of the clinical characteristics and prognostic significance with usual interstitial pneumonia. Sarcoidosis Vasc Diffuse Lung Dis 20:235, 2003.
6. Tanaka, N, Newell JD, Brown KK, et al: Collagen vascular disease-related lung disease. High-resolution computed tomography findings based on the pathologic classification. J Comput Assist Tomogr 28:351, 2004.
7. Tansey D, Wells, AU, Colby TV, et al: Variations in histological patterns of interstitial pneumonia between connective tissue disorders and their relationship to prognosis. Histopathology 44:585, 2004.

Rheumatoid Arthritis

8. Armstrong JG, Steele RH: Localised pulmonary arteritis in rheumatoid disease. Thorax 37:313, 1982.
9. Asherson RA, Morgan SH, Hackett D, et al: Rheumatoid

arthritis and pulmonary hypertension. A report of three cases. J Rheumatol 12:154, 1985.

10. Athreya B, Doughty R, Bookspan M, et al: Pulmonary manifestations of juvenile rheumatoid arthritis. A report of eight cases and review. Clin Chest Med 1:361, 1980.

11. Cervantes-Perez P, Toro-Perez A, Rodriguez-Jurado P: Pulmonary involvement in rheumatoid arthritis. JAMA 243:1715, 1980.

12. Faurschou P, Francis D, Faarup P: Thoracoscopic, histological, and clinical findings in nine cases of rheumatoid pleural effusion. Thorax 40:371, 1985.

13. Fortoul TI, Cano-Valle F, Oliva E, Barrios R: Follicular bronchiolitis in association with connective tissue diseases. Lung 163:305, 1985.

14. Hakala M, Paakko P, Sutinen S, et al: Association of bronchiolitis with connective tissue disorders. Ann Rheum Dis 45:656, 1986.

15. Hayakawa H, Sato A, Imokawa S, et al: Bronchiolar disease in rheumatoid arthritis. Am J Respir Crit Care Med 154:1531, 1996.

16. Herzog C, Miller R, Hoidal J: Bronchiolitis and rheumatoid arthritis. Am Rev Respir Dis 124:636, 1981.

17. Jolles H, Mosely PL, Peterson MW: Nodular pulmonary opacities in patients with rheumatoid arthritis. A diagnostic dilemma. Chest 96:1022, 1989.

18. Lee H-K, Kim DS, Yoo B, et al: Histopathologic pattern and clinical features of rheumatoid arthritis-associated interstitial lung disease. Chest 127:2019, 2005.

19. Mark E, Ramirez J: Pulmonary capillaritis and hemorrhage in patients with systemic vasculitis. Arch Pathol Lab Med 109:413, 1985.

20. Morikawa J, Kitamura K, Habuchi Y, et al: Pulmonary hypertension in a patient with rheumatoid arthritis. Chest 93:876, 1988.

21. Rees JH, Woodhead MA, Sheppard N, DuBois R: Rheumatoid arthritis and cryptogenic organizing pneumonitis. Respir Med 85:243, 1991.

22. Yousem SA, Colby TV, Carrington CB: Follicular bronchitis/bronchiolitis. Hum Pathol 16:700, 1985.

23. Yousem SA, Colby TV, Carrington CB: Lung biopsy in rheumatoid arthritis. Am Rev Respir Dis 131:770, 1985.

24. Yue CC, Park CH, Kushner I: Apical fibrocavitary lesions of the lung in rheumatoid arthritis. Report of two cases and review of the literature. Am J Med 81:741, 1986.

Systemic Lupus Erythematosus

25. Asherson R, Cervera R, Piette J-C, et al: Catastrophic antiphospholipid syndrome: Clinical and laboratory features of 50 patients. Medicine (Baltimore) 77:195, 1998.

26. Asherson RA, Higenbottam TW, Dinh Xuan AT, et al: Pulmonary hypertension in a lupus clinic: Experience with twenty-four patients. J Rheumatol 17:1292, 1990.

27. Churg A, Franklin W, Chan K, et al: Pulmonary hemorrhage and immune-complex deposition in the lung. Complications in a patient with systemic lupus erythematosus. Arch Pathol Lab Med 104:388, 1980.

28. Gammon RB, Bridges TA, Al-Nezir H, Alexander CB, Kennedy JI Jr: Bronchiolitis obliterans organizing pneumonia associated with systemic lupus erythematosus. Chest 102:1171, 1992.

29. Gladman DD, Sternberg L: Pulmonary hypertension in systemic lupus erythematosus. J Rheumatol 12:365, 1985.

30. Haupt HM, Moore GW, Hutchins GM: The lung in systemic lupus erythematosus. Analysis of the pathologic changes in 120 patients. Am J Med 71:791, 1981.

31. Hughson MD, He Z, Henegar J, McMurray R: Alveolar hemorrhage and renal microangiopathy in systemic lupus erythermatosus. Immune complex small vascular injury with apoptosis. Arch Pathol Lab Med 125:475, 2001.

32. Katzenstein A, Myers J, Prophet W, et al: Bronchiolitis obliterans and usual interstitial pneumonia. A comparative clinicopathologic study. Am J Surg Pathol 10:373, 1986.

33. Kishida Y, Kanai Y, Kuramochi S, Hosoda Y: Pulmonary venoocclusive disease in a patient with systemic lupus erythematosus. J Rheumatol 20:2161, 1993.

34. Lyon MG, Bewtra C, Kenik JG, Hurley JA: Tubuloreticular inclusions in systemic lupus pneumonitis. Report of a case and review of the literature. Arch Pathol Lab Med 108:599, 1984.

35. Marino C, Pertschuk L: Pulmonary hemorrhage in systemic lupus erythematosus. Arch Intern Med 141:201, 1981.

36. Matthay R, Schwarz M, Petty T, et al: Pulmonary manifestations of systemic lupus erythematosus: Review of twelve cases of acute lupus pneumonitis. Medicine (Baltimore) 54:397, 1974.

37. Miller LR, Greenberg SD, McLarty JW: Lupus lung. Chest 88:265, 1985.

38. Min JK, Hong YS, Park SH, et al: Bronchiolitis obliterans organizing pneumonia as an initial manifestation in patients with systemic lupus erythematosus. J Rheumatol 24:2254, 1997.

39. Miyata M, Suzuki K, Sakuma F, et al: Anticardiolipin antibodies are associated with pulmonary hypertension in patients with mixed connective tissue disease or systemic lupus erythematosus. Int Arch Allergy Immunol 100:351, 1993.

40. Murin S, Wiedemann HP, Matthay RA: Pulmonary manifestations of systemic lupus erythematosus. Clin Chest Med 19:641, 1998.

41. Myers JM, Katzenstein AA: Microangiitis in lupus-induced pulmonary hemorrhage. Am J Clin Pathol 85:552, 1986.

42. Pertschuk L, Moccia L, Rosen Y, et al: Acute pulmonary complications in systemic lupus erythematosus. Immunofluorescence and light microscopic study. Am J Clin Pathol 68:553, 1977.

43. Pines A, Kaplinsky N, Olchovsky D, et al: Pleuropulmonary manifestations of systemic lupus erythematosus: Clinical features of its subgroups.

Prognostic and therapeutic implications. Chest 88:129, 1985.

44. Roncoroni AJ, Alvarez C, Molinas F: Plexogenic arteriopathy associated with pulmonary vasculitis in systemic lupus erythematosus. Respiration 59:52, 1992.

45. Santos-Ocampo AS, Mandell BF, Fessler BJ: Alveolar hemorrhage in systemic lupus erythematosus. Presentation and management. Chest 118:1083, 2000.

46. Schwartzberg M, Lieberman DH, Getzoff B, Ehrlich GE: Systemic lupus erythematosus and pulmonary vascular hypertension. Arch Intern Med 144:605, 1984.

47. Wilson L, Tomita T, Braniecki M: Fatal pulmonary hypertension in identical twins with systemic lupus erythematosus. Hum Pathol 22:295, 1991.

48. Zamora MR, Warner ML, Tuder R, Schwarz MI: Diffuse alveolar hemorrhage and systemic lupus erythematosus: Clinical presentation, histology, survival and outcome. Medicine (Baltimore) 76:192, 1997.

Progressive Systemic Sclerosis (Scleroderma)

49. Bouros D, Wells AU, Nicholson AG, et al: Histopathologic subsets of fibrosing alveolitis in patients with systemic sclerosis and their relationship to outcome. Am J Respir Crit Care Med 165:1581, 2002.

50. Desai SR, Veeraraghavan S, Hansell DM, et al: CT features of lung disease in patients with systemic sclerosis: Comparison with idiopathic pulmonary fibrosis and nonspecific interstitial pneumonia. Radiology 232:560, 2004.

51. Fujita J, Yoshinouchi T, Ohtsuki Y, et al: Non-specific interstitial pneumonia as pulmonary involvement of systemic sclerosis. Ann Rheum Dis 60:281, 2001.

52. Harrison NK, Myers AR, Corrin B, et al: Structural features of interstitial lung disease in systemic sclerosis. Am Rev Respir Dis 144:706, 1991.

53. Johnson DA, Drane WE, Curran J, et al: Pulmonary disease in progressive sclerosis. A complication of gastroesophageal reflux and occult aspiration? Arch Intern Med 149:589, 1989.

54. Kim D-S, Yoo B, Lee, J-S, et al: The major histopathologic pattern of pulmonary fibrosis in scleroderma is nonspecific interstitial pneumonia. Sarcoid Vasc Diffuse Lung Dis 19:121, 2002.

55. Magro CM, Morrison C, Pope-Harman A, et al: Direct and indirect immunofluorescence as a diagnostic adjunct in the interpretation of nonneoplastic medical lung disease. Am J Clin Pathol 119:279, 2003.

56. Muir TE, Tazelaar HD, Colby TV, Myers JL: Organizing diffuse alveolar damage associated with progressive systemic sclerosis. Mayo Clin Proc 72:639, 1997.

57. Rossi GA, Bitterman PB, Rennard SI, et al: Evidence for chronic inflammation as a component of the interstitial lung disease associated with progressive systemic sclerosis. Am Rev Respir Dis 131:612, 1985.

58. Stupi AM, Steen VD, Owens GR, et al: Pulmonary hypertension in the CREST syndrome variant of systemic sclerosis. Arthritis Rheum 29:515, 1986.

59. Weaver A, Divertie M, Titus J: Pulmonary scleroderma. Dis Chest 54:490, 1980.

60. Young R, Mark G: Pulmonary vascular changes in scleroderma. Am J Med 64:998, 1978.

61. Yousem SA: The pulmonary pathologic manifestations of the CREST syndrome. Hum Pathol 21:467, 1990.

Polymyositis–Dermatomyositis

62. Arakawa H, Yamada H, Kurihara Y, et al: Nonspecific interstitial pneumonia associated with polymyositis and dermatomyositis. Serial high-resolution CT findings and functional correlation. Chest 123:1096, 2003.

63. Bunch T, Tancredi R, Lie J: Pulmonary hypertension in polymyositis. Chest 79:105, 1981.

64. Cottin V, Thivolet-Béjui F, Reynaud-Gaubert M, et al: Interstitial lung disease in amyopathic dermatomyositis, dermatomyositis and polymyositis. Eur Respir J 22:245, 2003.

65. Douglas WW, Tazelaar HD, Hartman TE, et al: Polymyositis-dermatomyositis-associated interstitial lung disease. Am J Respir Crit Care Med 164:1182, 2001.

66. Fujisawa T, Suda T, Nakamura Y, et al: Differences in clinical features and prognosis of interstitial lung diseases between polymyositis and dermatomyositis. J Rheumatol 32:58, 2005.

67. Kang EH, Lee EB, Shin KC, et al: Interstitial lung disease in patients with polymyositis, dermatomyositis, and amyopathic dermatomyositis. Rheumatology (Oxford) 44:1282, 2005.

68. Lakhanpal S, Lie JT, Conn DL, Martin WJ: Pulmonary disease in polymyositis/dermatomyositis: A clinicopathological analysis of 65 autopsy cases. Ann Rheum Dis 46:23, 1987.

69. Schwarz MI, Sutarik JM, Nick JA, et al: Pulmonary capillaritis and diffuse alveolar hemorrhage. A primary manifestation of polymyositis. Am J Respir Crit Care Med 151:2037, 1995.

70. Takizawa H, Shiga J, Moroi Y, et al: Interstitial lung disease in dermatomyositis: Clinicopathological study. J Rheumatol 14:102, 1987.

71. Tazelaar HD, Viggiano RW, Pickersgill J, et al: Interstitial lung disease in polymyositis and dermatomyositis: Clinical features and prognosis as correlated with histologic findings. Am Rev Respir Dis 141:427, 1990.

Mixed Connective Tissue Disease

72. Bennett R, O'Connell D: Mixed connective tissue disease: A clinicopathologic study of 20 cases. Semin Arthritis Rheum 10:25, 1980.

73. Hosoda Y, Suzuki Y, Takano M, et al: Mixed connective tissue disease with pulmonary hypertension: A clinical and pathological study. J Rheumatol 14:826, 1987.

74. Prakash UBS, Luthra HS, Divertie MB: Intrathoracic manifestations in mixed connective tissue disease. Mayo Clin Proc 60:813, 1985.

75. Sanchez-Guerrero J, Cesarman G, Alarcón-Segovia D: Massive pulmonary hemorrhage in mixed connective tissue disease. J Rheumatol 16:1132, 1989.

76. Sullivan WD, Hurst DJ, Harmon CE, et al: A prospective evaluation emphasizing pulmonary involvement in patients with mixed connective tissue disease. Medicine (Baltimore) 63:92, 1984.

77. Wiener-Kronish J, Solinger A, Warnock M, et al: Severe pulmonary involvement in mixed connective tissue disease. Am Rev Respir Dis 124:499, 1981.

Sjögren's Syndrome

78. Asherson R, Muncey F, Pambakian H, et al: Sjögren's syndrome and fibrosing alveolitis complicated by pulmonary lymphoma. Ann Rheum Dis 46:701, 1987.

79. Constantopoulos SH, Papadimitriou CS, Moutsopoulos HM: Respiratory manifestations in primary Sjögren's syndrome. A clinical, functional, and histologic study. Chest 88:226, 1985.

80. Deheinzelin D, Capelozzi VL, Kairalla RA, et al: Interstitial lung disease in primary Sjögren's syndrome. Am J Respir Crit Care Med 154:794, 1996.

81. Fairfax AJ, Haslam PL, Pavia D, et al: Pulmonary disorders associated with Sjögren's syndrome. Q J Med 199:279, 1981.

82. Ferreiro J, Robalino B, Saldana M: Primary Sjögren's syndrome with diffuse cerebral vasculitis and lymphocytic interstitial pneumonitis. Am J Med 82:1227, 1987.

83. Hedgpeth M, Boulware D: Pulmonary hypertension in primary Sjögren's syndrome. Ann Rheum Dis 47:251, 1988.

84. Inase N, Usui Y, Tachi H, et al: Sjögren's syndrome with bronchial gland involvement and multiple bullae. Respiration 57:286, 1990.

85. Ito I, Nagai S, Kitaichi M, et al: Pulmonary manifestations of primary Sjögren's syndrome. Am J Respir Crit Care Med 171:632, 2005.

86. Kobayashi H, Matsuoka R, Kitamura S, et al: Sjögren's syndrome with multiple bullae and pulmonary nodular amyloidosis. Chest 94:438, 1988.

87. Koss M, Hochholzer L, Langloss J, et al: Lymphoid interstitial pneumonia: Clinicopathologic and immunopathological findings in 18 cases. Pathology 19:178, 1987.

88. Liebow A, Carrington C: Diffuse pulmonary lymphoreticular infiltrations associated with dysproteinemia. Med Clin North Am 57:809, 1973.

89. Papiris SA, Saetta M, Turato G, et al: CD-4 positive T-lymphocytes infiltrate the bronchial mucosa of patients with Sjögren's syndrome. Am J Respir Crit Care Med 156:637, 1997.

90. Sato T, Matsubara O, Tanaka Y, Kasuga T: Association of Sjögren's syndrome with pulmonary hypertension: Report of two cases and review of the literature. Hum Pathol 24:199, 1993.

91. Strimlan C, Rosenow E III, Divertie M, Harrison E: Pulmonary manifestations of Sjogren's syndrome. Chest 70:354, 1976.

92. Weisbrot I: Lymphomatoid granulomatosis of the lung, associated with a long history of benign lymphoepithelial lesions of the salivary glands and lymphoid interstitial pneumonia. Am J Clin Pathol 66:792, 1976.

Amyloidosis

93. Berk JL, Keane J, Seldin DC, et al: Persistent pleural effusions in primary systemic amyloidosis. Chest 124:969, 2003.

94. Berk JL, O'Regan A, Skinner M: Pulmonary and tracheobronchial amyloidosis. Semin Respir Med 23:155, 2002.

95. Cordier JF, Loire R, Brune J: Amyloidosis of the lower respiratory tract. Clinical and pathologic features in a series of 21 patients. Chest 90:827, 1986.

96. DaCosta P, Corrin B: Amyloidosis localized to the lower respiratory tract: Probable immunoamyloid nature of the tracheobronchial and nodular pulmonary forms. Histopathology 9:703, 1985.

97. DeSai SR, Nicholson AG, Stewart S, et al: Benign pulmonary lymphocytic infiltration and amyloidosis: Computed tomographic and pathologic features in three cases. J Thoracic Imag 12:215, 1997.

98. Engleman P, Liebow A, Gmelich J, Friedman P: Pulmonary hyalinizing granuloma. Am Rev Respir Dis 115:997, 1977.

99. Eshun-Wilson K, Frandsen N, Christensen H: Pulmonary alveolar septal amyloidosis. A scanning and transmission electron microscopy study. Virchows Arch (Pathol Anat) 371:89, 1976.

100. Falk RH, Comenzo RL, Skinner M: The systemic amyloidoses. N Engl J Med 337:898, 1997.

101. Howard ME, Ireton J, Daniels F, et al: Pulmonary presentation of amyloidosis. Respirology 6:61, 2000.

102. Hui AN, Koss MN, Hochholzer L, Wehunt WD: Amyloidosis presenting in the lower respiratory tract. Clinicopathologic, radiologic, immunohistochemical, and histochemical studies on 48 cases. Arch Pathol Lab Med 110:212, 1986.

103. Kavuru MD, Adamo JP, Ahmad M, et al: Amyloidosis and pleural disease. Chest 98:20, 1990.

104. Khoor A, Myers JL, Tazelaar HD, Kurtin PJ: Amyloid-like pulmonary nodules, including localized light-chain deposition. Clinicopathologic analysis of three cases. Am J Clin Pathol 121:200, 2004.

105. Kijner CH, Yousem SA: Systemic light chain deposition disease presenting as multiple pulmonary nodules. A case report and review of the literature. Am J Surg Pathol 12:405, 1988.

106. Knapp M, Roggli V, Kim J, et al: Pleural amyloidosis. Arch Pathol Lab Med 112:57, 1988.

107. Laden SA, Cohen ML, Harley RA: Nodular pulmonary amyloidosis with extrapulmonary involvement. Hum Pathol 15:594, 1984.

108. Möllers MJ, van Schaik JPJ, van der Putte SCJ: Pulmonary amyloidoma. Histologic proof yielded by transthoracic coaxial fine needle biopsy. Chest 102:1597, 1992.

109. Monreal FA: Pulmonary amyloidosis: Ultrastructural

study of early alveolar septal deposits. Hum Pathol 15:388, 1984.

110. Planes C, Kleinknecht D, Brauner M, et al: Diffuse interstitial lung disease due to AA amyloidosis. Thorax 47:323, 1992.

111. Schoen FJ, Alexander RW, Hood I, Dunn LJ: Nodular pulmonary amyloidosis. Description of a case with ultrastructure. Arch Pathol Lab Med 104:66, 1980.

112. Smith R, Hutchins G, Moore G, Humphrey R: Type and distribution of pulmonary parenchymal and vascular amyloid. Am J Med 66:96, 1979.

113. Stokes MB, Jagirdar J, Burchstin O, et al: Nodular pulmonary immunoglobulin light chain deposits with coexistent amyloid and nonamyloid features in an HIV-infected patient. Mod Pathol 10:1059, 1997.

114. Toyoda M, Ebihara Y, Kato H, Kita S: Tracheobronchial AL amyloidosis: Histologic, immunohistochemical, ultrastructural, and immunoelectron microscopic observations. Hum Pathol 24:970, 1993.

115. Utz JP, Swensen SJ, Gertz MA: Pulmonary amyloidosis. The Mayo Clinic experience from 1980 to 1993. Ann Intern Med 124:407, 1996.

116. Yousem SA, Hochholzer L: Pulmonary hyalinizing granuloma. Am J Clin Pathol 87:1, 1987.

Sarcoidosis

117. Abe S, Munakata M, Nishimura M, et al: Gallium-67 scintigraphy, bronchoalveolar lavage, and pathologic changes in patients with pulmonary sarcoidosis. Chest 85:650, 1984.

118. Allen RKA, Chai SY, Dunbar MS, Mendelsohn FAO: In vitro autoradiographic localization of angiotensin-converting enzyme in sarcoid lymph nodes. Chest 90:315, 1986.

119. Baughman RP, Lower EE, duBois RM: Sarcoidosis. Lancet 361:1111, 2003.

120. Beekman J, Zimmet S, Chun B, Miranda A, Katz S: Spectrum of pleural involvement in sarcoidosis. Arch Intern Med 136:323, 1976.

121. Bocart D, Lecossier D, De Lassence A, Valeyre D, Battesti J-P, Hance AJ: A search for mycobacterial DNA in granulomatous tissues from patients with sarcoidosis using the polymerase chain reaction. Am Rev Respir Dis 145:1142, 1992.

122. Campbell DA, Poulter LW, DuBois RM: Immunocompetent cells in bronchoalveolar lavage reflect the cell populations in transbronchial biopsies in pulmonary sarcoidosis. Am Rev Respir Dis 132:1300, 1985.

123. Carrington C, Gaensler E, Mikus J, Schacter A, Burke G, Goff A: Structure and function in sarcoidosis. Ann N Y Acad Sci 278:265, 1976.

123a. Chevalet P, Clément R, Rodat O, et al: Sarcoidosis diagnosed in elderly subjects. Retrospective study of 30 cases. Chest 126:1423, 2004.

124. Chilosi M, Menestrina F, Capelli P, et al: Immunohistochemical analysis of sarcoid granulomas. Evaluation of Ki67 + and interleukin-1 + cells. Am J Pathol 131:191, 1988.

125. Churg A, Carrington C, Gupta R: Necrotizing sarcoid granulomatosis. Chest 76:406, 1979.

126. Crystal R, Roberts W, Hunninghake G, et al: Pulmonary sarcoidosis: A disease characterized and perpetuated by activated lung T-lymphocytes. Ann Intern Med 94:73, 1981.

127. Danel C, Dewar A, Corrin B, et al: Ultrastructural changes in bronchoalveolar lavage cells in sarcoidosis and comparison with the tissue granuloma. Am J Pathol 112:7, 1983.

128. DeRemee RA. Sarcoidosis. Mayo Clin Proc 70:177, 1995.

129. Dewar A, Corrin B, Turner-Warwick M: Tadpole shaped structures in a further patient with granulomatous lung disease. Thorax 39:466, 1984.

130. Drake WP, Pei Z, Pride DT, et al: Molecular analysis of sarcoidosis tissues for mycobacterium species DNA. Emerg Infect Dis 8:1334, 2002.

131. DuBois RM, Goh N, McGrath D, Cullinan P: Is there a role for microorganisms in the pathogenesis of sarcoidosis? J Intern Med 253:4, 2003.

132. Ghossein RA, Ross DG, Salomon RN, Rabson AR: A search for mycobacterial DNA in sarcoidosis using the polymerase chain reaction. Am J Clin Pathol 101:733, 1994.

133. Gibbs AR, Williams WJ, Kelland D: Necrotizing sarcoidal granulomatosis: A problem of identity. A study of seven cases. Sarcoidosis 4:94, 1987.

134. Glazer HS, Levitt RG, Shackelford GD: Peripheral pulmonary infiltrates in sarcoidosis. Chest 86:741, 1984.

135. Gonzaléz AA, Segura AM, Horiba K, et al: Matrix metalloproteinases and their tissue inhibitors in the lesions of cardiac and pulmonary sarcoidosis: An immunohistochemical study. Hum Pathol 33:1158, 2002.

136. Hoffstein V, Ranganathan N, Mullen JBM: Sarcoidosis simulating pulmonary veno-occlusive disease. Am Rev Respir Dis 134:809, 1986.

137. Hsu RM, Connors AF Jr, Tomashefski JF Jr: Histologic, microbiologic, and clinical correlates of the diagnosis of sarcoidosis by transbronchial biopsy. Arch Pathol Lab Med 120:364, 1996.

138. Huang C, Heurich A, Rosen Y, et al: Pulmonary sarcoidosis. Roentgenographic, functional, and pathologic correlations. Respiration 37:337, 1979.

139. Ishige I, Usui Y, Takemura T, Yoshinobu E: Quantitative PCR of mycobacterial and propionibacterial DNA in lymph nodes of Japanese patients with sarcoidosis. Lancet 354:120, 1999.

140. Ishioka S, Fujihara M, Takaishi M, et al: Anti-Kveim monoclonal antibody. New monoclonal antibody reacting to epithelioid cells in sarcoid granulomas. Chest 98:1255, 1990.

141. Kirkpatrick CJ, Curry A, Bisset DL: Light and electron-microscopic studies on multinucleated giant cells in sarcoid granuloma: New aspects of asteroid and Schaumann bodies. Ultrastruct Pathol 12:581, 1988.

142. Koss M, Hochholzer L, Feigin D, et al: Necrotizing sarcoid-like granulomatosis. Clinical, pathologic, and immunopathologic findings. Hum Pathol 11(Suppl):510, 1981.

143. LeGall F, Loeuillet L, Delaval Ph, et al: Necrotizing sarcoid granulomatosis with and without extrapulmonary involvement. Path Res Pract 192:306, 1996.

144. Liebow A: Pulmonary angiitis and granulomatosis. Am Rev Respir Dis 108:1, 1973.

145. Lowery WS, Whitlock WL, Dietrich RA, Fine JM: Sarcoidosis complicated by HIV infection: Three case reports and a review of the literature. Am Rev Respir Dis 142:887, 1990.

146. Mitchell D, Scadding J, Heard B, Hinson K: Sarcoidosis: Histopathological definition and clinical diagnosis. J Clin Pathol 30:395, 1977.

147. Morris DG, Jasmer RM, Huang L, et al: Sarcoidosis following HIV infection. Evidence for CD4$^+$ lymphocyte dependence. Chest 124:929, 2003.

148. Muller NL, Mawson JB, Mathieson JR, et al: Sarcoidosis: Correlation of extent of disease at CT with clinical, functional, and radiographic findings. Radiology 171:613, 1989.

149. Naccache J-M, Antoine M, Wislez M, et al: Sarcoid-like pulmonary disorder in human immunodeficiency virus-infected patients receiving antiretroviral therapy. Am J Respir Crit Care Med 159:2009, 1999.

150. Nishimura K, Itoh H, Kitaichi M, et al: Pulmonary sarcoidosis: Correlation of CT and histopathologic findings. Radiology 189:105, 1993.

151. Onal E, Lopata M, Lourenco R: Nodular pulmonary sarcoidosis. Clinical, roentgenographic, and physiologic course in five patients. Chest 72:296, 1977.

152. Pertschuk LP, Silverstein E, Friedland J: Immunohistologic diagnosis of sarcoidosis. Detection of angiotensin-converting enzyme in sarcoid granulomas. Am J Clin Pathol 75:350, 1981.

153. Poe R, Israel R, Utell M, Hall W: Probability of a positive transbronchial lung biopsy result in sarcoidosis. Arch Intern Med 139:761, 1979.

154. Popper HH, Klemen H, Colby TV, Churg A: Necrotizing sarcoid granulomatosis – is it different from nodular sarcoidosis? Pneumologie 57:268, 2003.

155. Popper HH, Klemen H, Hoefler G, Winter E: Presence of mycobacterial DNA in sarcoidosis. Hum Pathol 28:796, 1997.

156. Popper HH, Winter E, Hofler G: DNA of Mycobacterium tuberculosis in formalin-fixed, paraffin-embedded tissue in tuberculosis and sarcoidosis detected by polymerase chain reaction. Am J Clin Pathol 101:738, 1994.

157. Reid JD, Andersen ME: Calcium oxalate in sarcoid granulomas with particular reference to the small ovoid body and a note on the finding of dolomite. Am J Clin Pathol 90:545, 1988.

158. Rockoff SD, Rohatgi PK: Unusual manifestations of thoracic sarcoidosis. AJ Am J Roentgenol 144:513, 1985.

159. Roethe R, Fuller P, Byrd R, Hafermann D: Transbronchoscopic lung biopsy in sarcoidosis. Optimal number and sites for diagnosis. Chest 77:400, 1980.

160. Rolfes DB, Weiss MA, Sanders MA: Necrotizing sarcoid granulomatosis with suppurative features. Am J Clin Pathol 82:602, 1984.

161. Romer F: Sarcoidosis with large nodular lesions simulating pulmonary metastases. An analysis of 126 cases of intrathoracic sarcoidosis. Scand J Respir Dis 58:11, 1977.

162. Rosen Y, Moon S, Huang C, et al: Granulomatous pulmonary angiitis in sarcoidosis. Arch Pathol Lab Med 101:170, 1977.

163. Rubinowitz AN, Naidich DP, Alinsonorin C: Interferon-induced sarcoidosis. J Comput Assist Tomogr 27:279, 2003.

164. Shorr AF, Torrington KG, Hnatiuk OW: Endobronchial biopsy for sarcoidosis. A prospective study. Chest 120:109, 2001.

165. Singh N, Cole S, Krause P, et al: Necrotizing sarcoid granulomatosis with extrapulmonary involvement. Am Rev Respir Dis 124:189, 1981.

166. Smith L, Lawrence J, Katzenstein A: Vascular sarcoidosis: A rare cause of pulmonary hypertension. Am J Med Sci 38:44, 1983.

167. Stephen J, Braimbridge M, Corrin B, et al: Necrotizing "sarcoidal" angiitis and granulomatosis of the lungs. Thorax 31:356, 1976.

168. Tahan V, Ozseker F, Guneylioglu D, et al: Sarcoidosis after use of interferon for chronic hepatitis C. Report of a case and review of the literature. Dig Dis Sci 48:169, 2003.

169. Takemura T, Matsui Y, Oritsu M, et al: Pulmonary vascular involvement in sarcoidosis: Granulomatous angiitis and microangiopathy in transbronchial lung biopsies. Virchows Arch A Pathol Anat Histopathol 418:361, 1991.

170. Takemura T, Matsui Y, Shigeki S, Mikami R: Pulmonary vascular involvement in sarcoidosis: A report of 40 autopsy cases. Hum Pathol 23:1216, 1992.

171. Trevenzoli M, Cattelan AM, Marino F, et al: Sarcoidosis and HIV infection: A case report and a review of the literature. Postgrad Med J 79:535, 2003.

172. Trisolini R, Lazzari L, Cancellieri A, et al: The value of flexible transbronchial needle aspiration in the diagnosis of stage I sarcoidosis. Chest 124:2126, 2003.

173. Tukiainen P, Taskinen E, Korhola O, et al: Trucut needle biopsy in sarcoidosis. Relationship between histology of the biopsy specimens and radiographic features and pulmonary function. Br J Dis Chest 77:243, 1983.

174. van Maarsseven AC, Mullink H, Alons CL, Stam J: Distribution of T-lymphocyte subsets in different portions of sarcoid granulomas: Immunohistologic analysis with monoclonal antibodies. Hum Pathol 17:493, 1986.

175. Visscher D, Churg A, Katzenstein A-LA: Significance of crystalline inclusions in lung granulomas. Mod Pathol 1:415, 1988.

176. Vokurka M, Lecossier D, duBois RM, et al: Absence of DNA from mycobacteria of the *M. tuberculosis* complex

in sarcoidosis. Am J Respir Crit Care Med 156:1000, 1997.

177. Wang N-S, Schraufnagel DE, Sampson MG: The tadpole-shaped structures in human non-necrotizing granulomas. Am Rev Respir Dis 123:560, 1981.

178. Wilen S, Rabinowitz J, Ulreich S, Lyons H: Pleural involvement in sarcoidosis. Am J Med 57:200, 1974.

Other Systemic Diseases

179. Amir G, Ron N: Pulmonary pathology in Gaucher's disease. Hum Pathol 30:666, 1999.

180. Butland R, Cole P, Citron K, Turner-Warwick M: Chronic bronchial suppuration and inflammatory bowel disease. Q J Med 197:63, 1981.

180a Butnor KJ, Guinee DG Jr: Pleuropulmonary pathology of Birt-Hogg-Dubé syndrome. Am J Surg Pathol 30:395, 2006.

181. Byard RW, Bourne AJ, Thorner PS: Malacoplakia of the lung – a review. Surg Pathol 4:301, 1991.

182. Camus P, Piard F, Ashcroft T, et al: The lung in inflammatory bowel disease. Medicine (Baltimore) 72:151, 1993.

183. Carter EJ, Ettensohn DB: Catamenial pneumothorax. Chest 98:713, 1990.

184. Casey MB, Tazelaar HD, Myers JL, et al: Noninfectious lung pathology in patients with Crohn's disease. Am J Surg Pathol 27:213, 2003.

185. Colby T, Hunt S, Pelzmann K, Carrington C: Malakoplakia of the lung: A report of two cases. Respiration 39:295, 1980.

186. Corrin B, Simpson CGB, Fisher C: Fibrous pseudotumours and cyst formation in the lungs in Ehlers-Danlos syndrome. Histopathology 17:478, 1990.

187. Crouch E, Wright J, White V, Churg A: Malakoplakia mimicking carcinoma metastatic to lung. Am J Surg Pathol 8:151, 1984.

188. Dawson A, Gibbs AR, Anderson G: An unusual perilobular pattern of pulmonary interstitial fibrosis associated with Crohn's disease. Histopathology 23:553, 1993.

189. Desai SJ, Gephardt GN, Stoller JK: Diffuse panbronchiolitis preceding ulcerative colitis. Chest 45:1342, 1989.

190. Edwards C, Williams A, Asquith P: Bronchopulmonary disease in coeliac patients. J Clin Pathol 38:361, 1985.

191. Egan AJM, Boardman LA, Tazelaar HD, et al: Erdheim-Chester disease. Clinical, radiologic, and histopathologic findings in five patients with interstitial lung disease. Am J Surg Pathol 23:17, 1999.

192. Flieder DB, Moran CA, Travis WD, et al: Pleuro-pulmonary endometriosis and pulmonary ectopic deciduosis: A clinicopathologic and immunohistochemical study of 10 cases with emphasis on diagnostic pitfalls. Hum Pathol 29:1495, 1998.

193. Garay S, Gardella J, Fazzini E, Goldring R: Hermansky-Pudlak syndrome. Pulmonary manifestations of a ceroid storage disorder. Am J Med 66:737, 1979.

193a.Graham RB, Nolasco M, Peterlin B, Garcia CK: Nonsense mutations in folliculin presenting as isolated familial

194. Hansen LA, Prakash UBS, Colby TV: Pulmonary complications in diabetes mellitus. Mayo Clin Proc 64:791, 1989.

195. Haque AA, Gokhale S, Rampy BA, et al: Pulmonary hypertension in sickle cell hemoglobinopathy: A clinicopathologic study of 20 cases. Hum Pathol 33:1037, 2002.

196. Haupt H, Moore G, Bauer T, Hutchins G: The lung in sickle cell disease. Chest 81:332, 1982.

197. Higenbottam T, Cochrane G, Clark T, et al: Bronchial disease in ulcerative colitis. Thorax 35:581, 1980.

198. Hillerdal G: Ankylosing spondylitis lung disease – an underdiagnosed entity? Eur J Respir Dis 64:437, 1983.

199. Hodder RV, St George-Hyslop P, Chalvardjian A, et al: Pulmonary malakoplakia. Thorax 39:70, 1984.

200. Jackson A, Loh C: Pulmonary calcification and elastic tissue damage in pseudoxanthoma elasticum. Histopathology 4:607, 1980.

201. James TN, Healy Bulkley B: Whipple bacilli within the tunica media of pulmonary arteries. Chest 86:454, 1984.

202. Karpel JP, Appel D, Merav A: Pulmonary endometriosis. Lung 163:151, 1985.

203. Kchir MM, Mtimet S, Kochbati S, et al: Bronchoalveolar lavage and transbronchial biopsy in spondyloarthropathies. J Rheumatol 19:913, 1992.

204. Kim MJ, Lee KY: Bronchiolitis obliterans in children with Stevens-Johnson syndrome: Follow-up with high resolution CT. Pediatr Radiol 26:22, 1996.

205. Krowka M, Cortese D: Pulmonary aspects of chronic liver disease and liver transplantation. Mayo Clin Proc 60:407, 1985.

206. Kruger S, Piroth W, Takyi BA, et al: Multiple aseptic pulmonary nodules with central necrosis in association with pyoderma gangrenosum. Chest 119:977, 2001.

207. Lebargy F, Wolkenstein P, Gisselbrecht M, et al: Pulmonary complications in toxic epidermal necrolysis: A prospective clinical study. Intensive Care Med 23:1237, 1997.

208. Levy H, Hurwitz MD, Strimling M, Zwi S: Ankylosing spondylitis lung disease and *Mycobacterium scrofulaceum*. Br J Dis Chest 82:84, 1988.

209. McCulloch AJ, McEvoy A, Jackson JD, Jarvis EH: Severe steroid responsive pneumonitis associated with pyoderma gangrenosum and ulcerative colitis. Thorax 40:314, 1985.

210. McDonnell PJ, Toye PA, Hutchins GM: Primary pulmonary hypertension and cirrhosis: Are they related? Am Rev Respir Dis 127:437, 1983.

211. McFadden RG, Craig ID, Paterson NAM: Interstitial pneumonitis in myasthenia gravis. Br J Dis Chest 78:187, 1984.

212. Moles K, Varghese G, Hayes J: Pulmonary involvement in ulcerative colitis. Br J Dis Chest 82:79, 1988.

213. Moser C, Nussbaum E, Cooper DM: Plastic bronchitis and the role of bronchoscopy in the acute chest syndrome of sickle cell disease. Chest 120:608, 2001.

spontaneous pneumothorax in adults. Am J Respir Crit Care Med 172:39, 2005.

214. Moskaluk CA, Pogrebniak HW, Pass HI, et al: Surgical pathology of the lung in chronic granulomatous disease. Am J Clin Pathol 102:684, 1994.

214a. Nakatani Y, Nakamura N, Sano J, et al: Interstitial pneumonia in Hermansky–Pudlak syndrome: significance of foamy swelling/degeneration of type-2 pneumocytes. Virch Arch 437:304, 2000.

215. Nash JW, Ross P, Crowson AN, et al: The histopathologic spectrum of cryofibrinogenemia in four anatomic sites. Skin, lung, muscle, and kidney. Am J Clin Pathol 119:114, 2003.

216. Nicholson AG, Wells AU, Hooper J, et al: Successful treatment of endogenous lipoid pneumonia due to Niemann-Pick type B disease with whole-lung lavage. Am J Respir Crit Care Med 165:128, 2002.

217. Pacheco A, Casanova C, Fogue L, Sueiro A: Long-term clinical follow-up of adult idiopathic pulmonary hemosiderosis and celiac disease. Chest 99:1525, 1991.

218. Padeh S, Laxer RM, Silver MM, Silverman ED: Primary pulmonary hypertension in a patient with systemic-onset juvenile arthritis. Arthritis Rheum 34:1575, 1991.

219. Powars D, Weidman JA, Odom-Maryon T, et al: Sickle cell chronic lung disease: Prior morbidity and the risk of pulmonary failure. Medicine (Baltimore) 67:66, 1988.

220. Raffy O, Sleiman C, Vachiery F, et al: Refractory hypoxemia during liver cirrhosis. Hepatopulmonary syndrome or "primary" pulmonary hypertension? Am J Respir Crit Care Med 153:1169, 1996.

221. Reinila A: Perivascular xanthogranulomatosis in the lungs of diabetic patients. Arch Pathol Lab Med 100:542, 1976.

222. Rodriguez-Roisin R, Agusti AGN, Roca J: The hepatopulmonary syndrome: New name, old complexities. Thorax 47:897, 1992.

223. Rosenow E III, Strimlan C, Muhm J, Ferguson R: Pleuropulmonary manifestations of ankylosing spondylitis. Mayo Clin Proc 52:641, 1977.

224. Rush WL, Andriko AW, Galateau-Salle F, et al: Pulmonary pathology of Erdheim-Chester disease. Mod Pathol 13:747, 2000.

225. Schinella RA, Greco MA, Garay SM, et al: Hermansky-Pudlak syndrome: A clinicopathologic study. Hum Pathol 16:366, 1985.

226. Schneider E, Epstein C, Kaback M, Brandes D: Severe pulmonary involvement in adult Gaucher's disease. Report of three cases and review of the literature. Am J Med 63:475, 1977.

227. Slasky BS, Siewers RD, Lecky JW, et al: Catamenial pneumothorax: The roles of diaphragmatic defects and endometriosis. AJR Am J Roentgenol 138:639, 1982.

228. Smith P, Heath D, Rodgers B, Helliwell T: Pulmonary vasculature in Fabry's disease. Histopathology 19:567, 1991.

229. Smith R, Hutchins G, Sack G Jr, Ridolfi R: Unusual cardiac, renal, and pulmonary involvement in Gaucher's disease. Am J Med 65:352, 1978.

230. Stevens FM, Connolly CE, Murray JP, McCarthy CF: Lung cavities in patients with coeliac disease. Digestion 46:72, 1990.

231. Takimoto CH, Warnock M, Golden JA: Sweet's syndrome with lung involvement. Am Rev Respir Dis 143:177, 1991.

232. Vandenplas O, Casel S, Delos M, et al: Granulomatous bronchiolitis associated with Crohn's disease. Am J Respir Crit Care Med 158:1676, 1998.

233. Vichinsky EP, Neumayr LD, Earles AN, et al: Causes and outcomes of the acute chest syndrome in sickle cell disease. N Engl J Med 342:1855, 2000.

234. Vichinsky E, Williams R, Das M, et al: Pulmonary fat embolism: A distinct cause of severe acute chest syndrome in sickle cell anemia. Blood 83:3107, 1994.

235. Vignon-Pennamen MD, Zelinsky-Gurung A, Janssen F, et al: Pyoderma gangrenosum with pulmonary involvement. Arch Dermatol 125:1239, 1989.

236. White DA, Smith GJW, Cooper JAD Jr, et al: Hermansky-Pudlak syndrome and interstitial lung disease: Report of a case with lavage findings. Am Rev Respir Dis 130:138, 1984.

237. Wilcox P, Miller R, Miller G, et al: Airway involvement in ulcerative colitis. Chest 92:18, 1987.

238. Winberg C, Rose M, Rappaport H: Whipple's disease of the lung. Am J Med 65:873, 1978.

239. Wood JR, Bellamy D, Child AH, Citron KM: Pulmonary disease in patients with Marfan syndrome. Thorax 39:780, 1984.

240. Yost BA, Vogelsang JP, Lie JT: Fatal hemoptysis in Ehlers-Danlos syndrome: Old malady with a new curse. Chest 107:1465, 1995.

241. Yutani C, Imakita M, Ishibashi-Ueda H, et al: Nodular regenerative hyperplasia of the liver associated with primary pulmonary hypertension. Hum Pathol 19:726, 1988.

PULMONARY VASCULITIS

This chapter reviews the main vasculitides affecting the lung – Wegener's granulomatosis, Churg–Strauss syndrome, and microscopic polyangiitis. These three entities are often referred to as antineutrophil cytoplasmic antibody (ANCA, see later on) associated vasculitides, since serum ANCA are usually present.[3,4] Other less common capillaritis syndromes and vasculitides that rarely involve the lung are also briefly discussed.

In the past, Wegener's granulomatosis and Churg–Strauss syndrome were encompassed under the category of *pulmonary angiitis and granulomatosis.*[2] Although now outdated, this term was useful because it included several entities that were characterized by parenchymal necrosis and vascular infiltration, and thus all were considered in the same histologic differential diagnosis. Also included under this term were bronchocentric granulomatosis, necrotizing sarcoid granulomatosis, and lymphomatoid granulomatosis. Bronchocentric granulomatosis is a manifestation of allergic bronchopulmonary fungal disease in most cases and is discussed in Chapter 6. Necrotizing sarcoid granulomatosis is more likely a variant of sarcoidosis rather than a true vasculitis, and it is discussed with sarcoidosis in Chapter 6. Lymphomatoid granulomatosis is a form of lymphoma and is reviewed in Chapter 9.

WEGENER'S GRANULOMATOSIS

Clinical Features

Wegener's granulomatosis is a systemic necrotizing vasculitis that involves the lung in most cases.[5,10,17,35,76] Middle-aged adults are usually affected, with a mean age ranging from 40 to 55 years, although there is a wide age range, with cases reported both in children and in the elderly.[33,39,47,60,74] The gender ratio is about equal in most series. The classic, generalized form of the disease is manifested by a triad of upper respiratory tract and lung involvement along with glomerulonephritis. Tracheobronchial involvement may be a prominent component,[18] and other organs are frequently affected as well, including, especially, skin, joints, middle ear, eye, and nervous system.[64] Sometimes only one or two sites of the classic triad are involved, however, and when lung lesions are the sole manifestation, the disease has been referred to as *limited* or *localized* Wegener's granulomatosis.[13,14,21,25,26] More recently, the term 'limited' (as opposed to 'severe') has been used for cases in which the manifestations pose no threat to either the patient's life or the functioning of a vital organ.[67] Nodular pulmonary involvement without associated respiratory impairment falls under this category, while diffuse pulmonary hemorrhage would be considered severe. Limited Wegener's granulomatosis isolated to the lungs can be especially difficult to diagnose, since it is often unsuspected clinically.

The most common presenting complaints in Wegener's granulomatosis include fever, malaise, weight loss, cough, chest pain, and hemoptysis.[5,17,35] There may also be signs and symptoms related to extrapulmonary involvement, such as rhinorrhea, nasal ulceration, or sinus pain, for example. Some patients present with hematuria or renal failure, while otitis media, skin lesions, arthralgias, myalgias, arthritis, neurologic abnormalities, or eye lesions may be present in others. Serum ANCA (see text following) are usually present. Radiographically, multiple, often cavitary, nodular densities are the most frequent findings, although localized areas of consolidation, and even solitary nodules, may occur.[17,35,37,41,55,59] A lung biopsy is usually required for diagnosis, although biopsy of other sites such as skin or upper respiratory tract, for example, may occasionally be productive, especially in combination with ANCA testing.[7,20,23,32] Transbronchial lung biopsy is diagnostic in a few cases.[58]

Antineutrophil Cytoplasmic Antibodies (ANCA)

ANCA are autoantibodies to components of neutrophil and monocyte granules.[27,28,36,53,56,57,61] They can be detected both by indirect immunofluorescence and by enzyme-linked immunosorbent assay (ELISA) techniques.[36,77] Two types are identified: C-ANCA, characterized by a diffuse granular cytoplasmic immunofluorescent staining pattern, and P-ANCA, characterized by a perinuclear staining pattern. C-ANCA are directed primarily against a 29-kd neutral serine protease, proteinase-3, a component of neutrophil azurophilic granules, and are also referred to as PR3-ANCA. Most P-ANCA are directed against myeloperoxidase and are

known as MPO-ANCA. A variety of other substrates have been identified less commonly for some P-ANCA, including enolase, catalase, cathepsin G, elastase, lactoferrin, and lysozyme, for example. In such cases, the immunofluorescent pattern is often 'atypical'.[4,73] Currently, the use of both immunofluorescence and ELISA techniques is advocated for diagnosis.[42,56,57]

C-ANCA are highly specific for Wegener's granulomatosis, although false-positives have been reported in various settings, including infections, connective tissue diseases, fibrotic lung diseases, chronic hypersensitivity pneumonia, pulmonary embolus, malignancy, and inflammatory bowel disease.[15,19,24,29,38,48] C-ANCA are found in over 90% of generalized Wegener's cases and in about 60% of localized cases. P-ANCA are less specific and are more commonly encountered in other diseases, especially crescentic glomerulonephritis, microscopic polyangiitis and Churg-Strauss syndrome. They are found, however, in 5–10% of cases of Wegener's granulomatosis.[30,40] ANCA can be utilized to follow disease activity as well as aid in diagnosis, and they may have a role in pathogenesis.[11,12,38,46,62]

Treatment and Prognosis

Without treatment, generalized Wegener's granulomatosis usually follows a fulminant and almost uniformly fatal course, although more indolent variants have been described.[43] The treatment of choice is cyclophosphamide, usually in combination with corticosteroids, and dramatic responses are obtained in most cases.[5,6,10,17,35,37,51] About 75–80% of patients achieve complete remission with this regimen, and there is a greater than 80% 5-year survival.[1,3,35,40,54] Recurrences are common, however. Treatment with a less toxic regimen using methotrexate instead of cyclophosphamide and corticosteroids has been advocated for patients with limited disease.[1,40,54,67] Beneficial results with trimethoprim–sulfamethoxazole has been noted in some cases of indolent Wegener's, and there is some evidence that treatment with this drug following cyclophosphamide and corticosteroids reduces the incidence of relapses.[22,63,65,75]

Pathologic Features

The histologic diagnosis of Wegener's granulomatosis requires evidence of a necrotizing vasculitis that is usually associated with necrotizing granulomatous inflammation.[13,16,31,37,44,45,70,78] The histologic findings may vary, however, and the changes are best approached

Table 8–1 Histologic Variants of Wegener's Granulomatosis

Classic Wegener's
Necrotizing granulomatous inflammation with
  prominent parenchymal necrosis
    May be bronchocentric (*bronchocentric variant*)
    Eosinophils may be prominent (*eosinophilic variant*)
Necrotizing vasculitis

BOOP-like variant
Extensive intraluminal organization (BOOP) lacking
  large areas of necrosis
Small necrotic foci, microabscesses, suppurative
  granulomas
Necrotizing vasculitis

Alveolar hemorrhage and capillaritis
Fresh blood and hemosiderin in alveolar spaces
Acute inflammation and necrosis of alveolar septa
  (necrotizing capillaritis)

by dividing them into three histologic categories as summarized in Table 8–1. The purpose of this histologic classification is primarily for the pathologist to facilitate diagnosis. The categories generally have little clinical significance, although the hemorrhage and capillaritis variant may be associated with a more fulminant course.

Classic Wegener's Granulomatosis

The *classic variant* is the most common form of Wegener's, and is characterized by large areas of parenchymal necrosis which typically are irregularly, haphazardly or 'geographically' shaped (Fig. 8–1).[13,31,37,70,78] The necrotic zones have jagged, infiltrating borders with inclusion of small islands of residual, viable lung at their periphery. They usually appear deeply basophilic or 'dirty' and contain remnants of nuclear debris. They are bounded by epithelioid histiocytes, often arranged in a palisading configuration, and distinct multinucleated giant cells containing darkly staining nuclei and dense

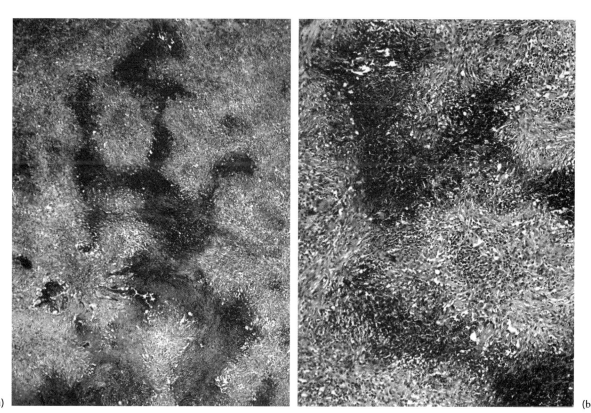

(a)　　　　　　　　　　　　　　　　　　　　　　　　　　　　　　　(b)

Figure 8–1 Wegener's granulomatosis. (a) Low magnification showing the characteristic, darkly staining, haphazard or geographic shaped necrotizing granulomatous inflammation. **(b)** Higher magnification showing the nuclear debris within the necrotic zones that accounts for the basophilic, 'dirty' appearance. Note the surrounding rim of epithelioid histiocytes and chronic inflammatory cells.

eosinophilic cytoplasm may be numerous (Fig. 8–2). Smaller microscopic foci of microabscess-like necrosis with a round or irregular configuration are generally also present. They contain a central suppurative exudate rimmed by variable numbers of lymphocytes, plasma cells, histiocytes, and fibroblasts. Smaller suppurative granulomas are also common and are characterized by palisading histiocytes that are arranged with their long axes perpendicular to the necrotic center (Fig. 8–2b). Sometimes, necrotic collagen that assumes a deeply eosinophilic glassy appearance is present within the suppurative granulomas (Fig. 8–3). Background fibrosis and nonspecific chronic inflammation are typically present, and neutrophils are usually a prominent component of the inflammatory process. Eosinophils are often present, but are usually not numerous.

Necrotizing vasculitis is usually not difficult to identify in classic Wegener's. In florid cases, vessel walls are partly to completely replaced by an inflammatory infiltrate that contains varying proportions of neutrophils, chronic inflammatory cells, eosinophils, and epithelioid histiocytes (Fig. 8–4). Neutrophils are a fairly constant component, however, and fibrinoid necrosis

may be prominent. Often the vessels are partially involved, with only a portion of their circumference containing the inflammatory cell infiltrate and necrosis (Fig. 8–5). In the most subtle cases, scattered karyorrhectic neutrophils are present in vessel walls. Regardless of the extent of the vasculitis, it is important that necrosis be present either in the vessel walls or in the infiltrating inflammatory cells in order to diagnose the prerequisite necrotizing vasculitis. Both arteries and veins are usually affected by the vasculitis, and an elastic tissue stain can demonstrate their differentiation (Fig. 8–6). We do not recommend using this stain routinely for diagnostic purposes, however, since it emphasizes inflamed and occluded vessels without discriminating a necrotizing vasculitis, and thus it may lead to overdiagnosis. It is important that the vasculitis be found in viable parenchyma, since vessels within any necrotic foci regardless of etiology, will contain necrotic cellular debris in their walls that can be mistaken for vasculitis.

A small vessel vasculitis that affects mainly alveolar septal capillaries (capillaritis, see later on) and occasionally small arterioles (arteriolitis) and venules is also

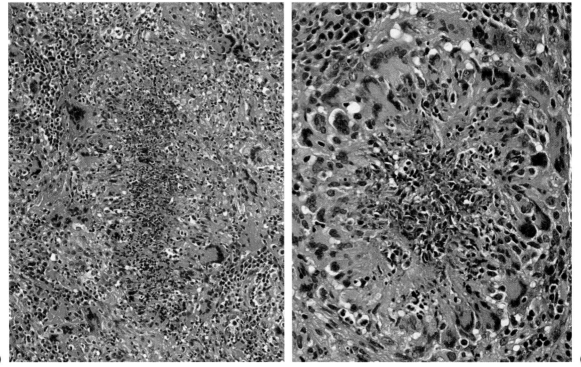

(a)   (b)

Figure 8–2 Suppurative granulomas in Wegener's. (a) Numerous densely staining multinucleated giant cells are present around this small necrotizing granuloma. Necrotic neutrophils are present within the central necrosis. **(b)** Palisading histiocytes surround central suppuration in this necrotizing granuloma.

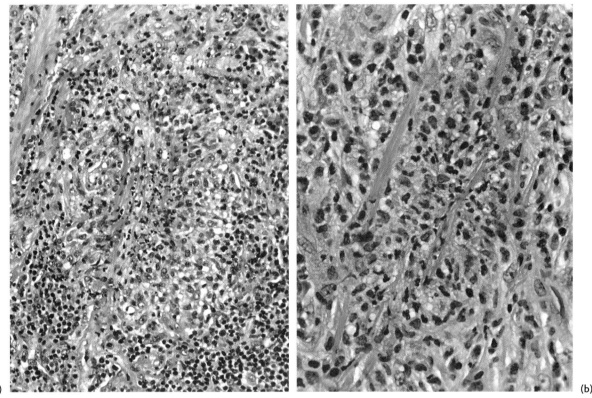

(a) (b)

Figure 8–3 Collagen fibers in granulomas of Wegener's. (a) Collagen bundles are encompassed by this suppurative granuloma. **(b)** Higher magnification showing glassy-appearing collagen bundles surrounded by neutrophils and epithelioid histiocytes.

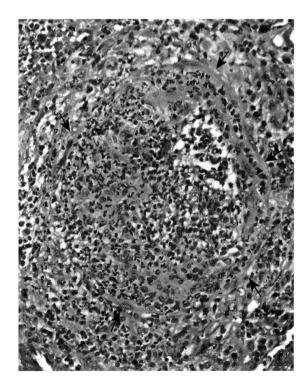

Figure 8–4 Necrotizing vasculitis in Wegener's. The wall of this artery (arrows) is almost completely replaced and destroyed by neutrophils and histiocytes. Only a small part of the media (top right) remains viable.

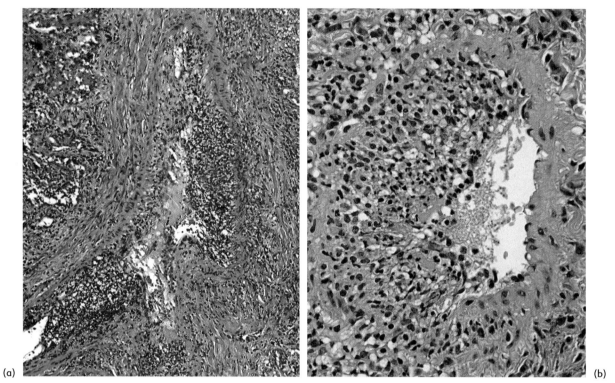

Figure 8–5 Patchy involvement of blood vessel walls by necrotizing vasculitis in Wegener's. (a) Low magnification shows two separate foci of necrotizing vasculitis in a medium-sized artery. **(b)** Higher magnification of another artery showing characteristic eccentric involvement of the wall. Note the focus of fibrinoid necrosis in this example.

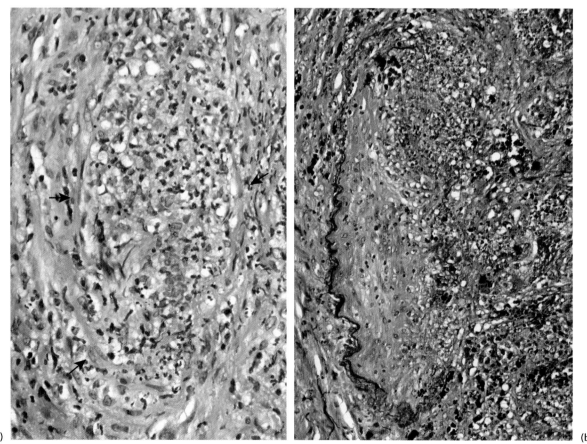

Figure 8–6 Necrotizing vasculitis involving a vein in Wegener's. (a) In hematoxylin–eosin, the vein is infiltrated by neutrophils and histiocytes, causing nearly total obliteration. Note residual media (arrows). **(b)** Elastic tissue stain shows partial destruction of the vascular elastic layer. The presence of a single elastic lamina identifies the vessel as a vein.

common in Wegener's granulomatosis.[49,68,70,78] It is usually found in parenchyma peripheral to areas of more typical granulomatous inflammation, although in rare cases it constitutes the major histologic finding (see capillaritis and hemorrhage variant, later on). Capillaritis is identified by the presence of acute inflammation that expands and dissolves alveolar septa (Fig. 8–7). Sometimes histiocytes and eosinophils are admixed with the neutrophils. Since capillaries are composed only of endothelium and basement membrane, it is not possible by light microscopy to appreciate involvement by inflammation. Rather, capillaritis can only be inferred from the alveolar septal location of the inflammation.

Occasionally, the necrotizing granulomatous inflammation in classic Wegener's centers upon and destroys bronchioles, and, when prominent, this finding constitutes the so-called *bronchocentric variant* (Fig. 8–8).[79] In rare cases, eosinophils are present in large numbers in the infiltrate surrounding the necrotizing granulomas and such cases have been termed the *eosinophil variant*.[80] Blood eosinophilia is usually not present in eosinophilic Wegener's, although it has been reported in some cases.[52] Both histologic variants occur in a background of otherwise classic Wegener's and the clinical manifestations are no different. They need to be recognized only to insure that they are not confused with other entities, such as bronchocentric granulomatosis (see Chapter 6) and Churg–Strauss syndrome (see later on).

BOOP-Like Wegener's Granulomatosis

The *BOOP-like variant* of Wegener's is characterized by extensive intraluminal organization that superficially resembles bronchiolitis obliterans–organizing pneumonia (BOOP, see Chapter 2) (Fig. 8–9).[72] Distinct multinucleated giant cells are often visible within the intraalveolar fibrosis at low magnification and are important clues to the diagnosis. Hemosiderin deposition is often prominent within the fibrosis as well. Although large areas of necrotizing granulomatous inflammation typical of classic Wegener's are not present, tiny foci of 'dirty' necrosis are seen, as are small suppurative granulomas and microabscesses (Fig. 8–10). Acute

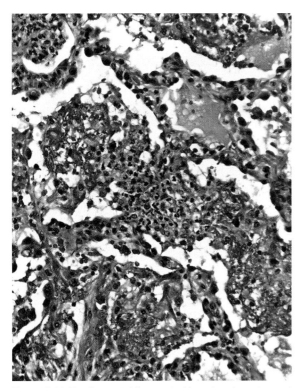

Figure 8–7 Capillaritis in Wegener's. Note the expansion and disruption of an alveolar septum (center) by acute inflammation and histiocytes. Proteinaceous exudates are seen in the adjacent alveolar spaces.

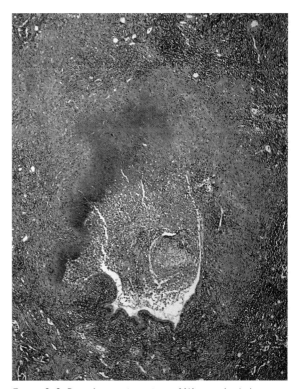

Figure 8–8 Bronchocentric variant of Wegener's. At low magnification, the bronchiole wall is seen to be partially replaced by necrotizing granulomatous inflammation (top). The typical vasculitis was seen elsewhere in this example.

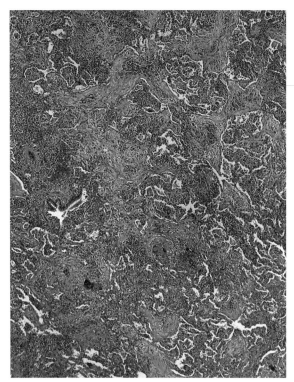

Figure 8–9 BOOP-like Wegener's. Low magnification view showing lightly staining plugs of fibroblasts within alveolar ducts and alveoli that are typical of BOOP. Darkly staining multinucleated giant cells can be appreciated even at this low magnification, and they are a clue to the diagnosis.

inflammatory cells are usually numerous in the background inflammatory cell infiltrate, and necrotizing vasculitis is a prominent feature (Fig. 8–11).

Alveolar Hemorrhage and Capillaritis Variant of Wegener's

The *alveolar hemorrhage and capillaritis* variant can be dramatic clinically and is often difficult to diagnose pathologically.[8–10,34,49,66,68,69] Patients with this form of the disease present with hemoptysis and diffuse pulmonary infiltrates. Their course is often fulminant, mortality is high, and the diagnosis needs to be established quickly so that therapy can be instituted promptly.

Histologically, alveolar hemorrhage is the most prominent abnormality, with a mixture of blood and hemosiderin filling alveolar spaces. Additionally, there is a variable inflammatory cell infiltrate in alveolar septa that contains a prominent component of neutrophils (Fig. 8–12). Capillaritis is identified by patchy expansion

of alveolar septa by neutrophils that frequently show individual cell necrosis. Disruption and necrosis of the involved septa often accompany the cellular infiltrate, and there may be a focal, associated histiocyte infiltrate along with scattered eosinophils (Fig. 8–13). In difficult cases, serially sectioning the blocks can often facilitate the demonstration of small vessel vasculitis. Granulomatous inflammation is not a feature of this form of Wegener's. Although the diagnosis of hemorrhage and capillaritis can be made in such cases, the diagnosis of Wegener's granulomatosis requires clinical input, such as a history of documented Wegener's previously, typical granulomatous inflammation in other sites,[50] or a positive C-ANCA, to distinguish the findings from other capillaritis syndromes (see later on).

Differential Diagnosis

The main lesions in the differential diagnosis of Wegener's granulomatosis include granulomatous infections and other noninfectious granulomatous and vasculitic lung lesions. Because Wegener's granulomatosis shares several histologic features with granulomatous infections, cultures should be taken, and a careful search of special stains for organisms should be performed in all cases before making the diagnosis of Wegener's. It should be remembered that vasculitis commonly accompanies infectious granulomas, but this vasculitis is not necrotizing. Since organisms may not be identifiable by special stains in all infectious necrotizing granulomas (presumably because they have been removed by the inflammatory reaction),[71] the pathologist must maintain strict criteria for the necrotizing vasculitis that is necessary for diagnosing Wegener's.

The differentiating features of the ANCA-associated vasculitides are summarized in Table 8–2. Necrotizing sarcoid granulomatosis (see Chapter 7) enters the differential diagnosis because of extensive necrotizing granulomatous inflammation and vasculitis. Nonnecrotizing granulomas, the hallmark of this disease, are not features of Wegener's. Also, the suppuration characteristic of Wegener's is not seen in necrotizing sarcoid granulomatosis. Lymphomatoid granulomatosis (see Chapter 9) enters the differential diagnosis because of parenchymal necrosis and prominent vascular infiltration. That disease, however, is characterized by a lymphoid infiltrate that is usually atypical, and neither true granulomatous inflammation nor a necrotizing vasculitis is present.

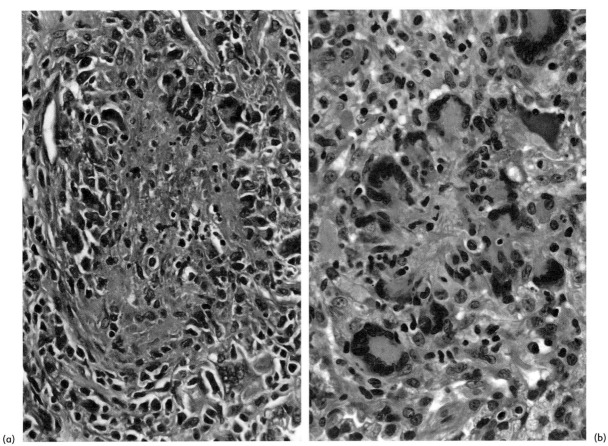

(a)

(b)

Figure 8–10 BOOP-like Wegener's. (a) Higher magnification of a small necrotizing granuloma. Note the dirty necrosis surrounded by epithelioid histiocytes. **(b)** A small suppurative, palisading granuloma is present in this case.

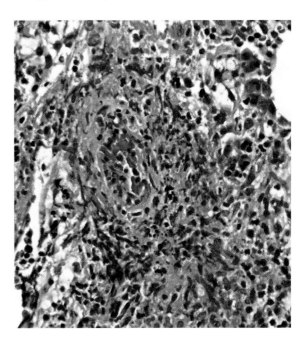

Figure 8–11 Typical necrotizing vasculitis from a case of BOOP-like Wegener's. Vasculitis is not difficult to find in this variant of Wegener's.

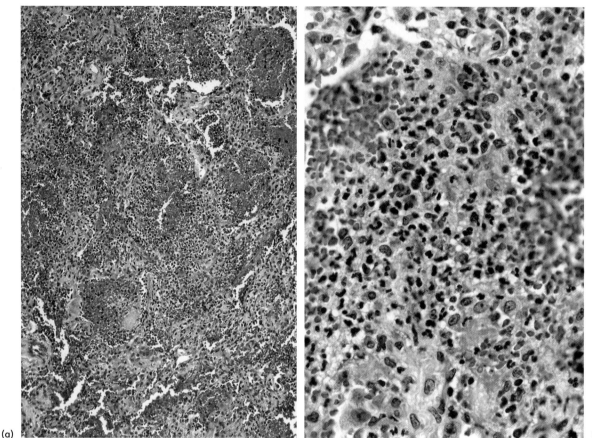

(a)   (b)

Figure 8–12 Hemorrhage and capillaritis variant of Wegener's. (a) Low magnification showing extensive intraalveolar hemorrhage along with a cellular infiltrate thickening many alveolar septa. **(b)** Higher magnification showing marked expansion and destruction of an alveolar septum by acute inflammatory cells and histiocytes, changes indicative of necrotizing capillaritis.

CHURG–STRAUSS SYNDROME

Churg–Strauss syndrome, also known as allergic angiitis and granulomatosis, is an uncommon systemic vasculitis that frequently involves the lung. Clinical criteria for diagnosis include the combination of asthma, high blood eosinophil count (greater than 1500/μL), and evidence of vasculitis involving two or more extrapulmonary sites.[90] The diagnosis is most often made by biopsying extrapulmonary tissues, usually skin, nerve, or muscle, and thus there have been only a few detailed descriptions of the pathologic findings in the lung.[83,84,88,89,90]

Clinical Features

Churg–Strauss syndrome occurs exclusively in patients with chronic asthma, and blood eosinophilia is a prominent associated finding.[82,86,88,91] The mean age is 38 years, although there is a wide age range, including children and the elderly. Extrapulmonary involvement is most commonly manifested by skin lesions, peripheral neuropathy, or heart failure; mild segmental glomerulonephritis is seen in some cases, but renal failure is usually not a feature, and destructive lesions of the upper respiratory tract and nasal sinuses are not found, although allergic nasal polyps are common.[83,86,89,90] A P-ANCA is present in about 70% of patients.[85,88,91] Some cases occur following use of the leukotriene receptor antagonists montelukast and zafirlukast.[87,92] The latter drugs decrease the need for steroids in the treatment of asthma, and the decreased steroid dose is thought to unmask an underlying vasculitis. The radiographic changes are characterized most commonly by patchy, often transient, alveolar opacities, in contrast to the more discrete, mass-like densities typical of

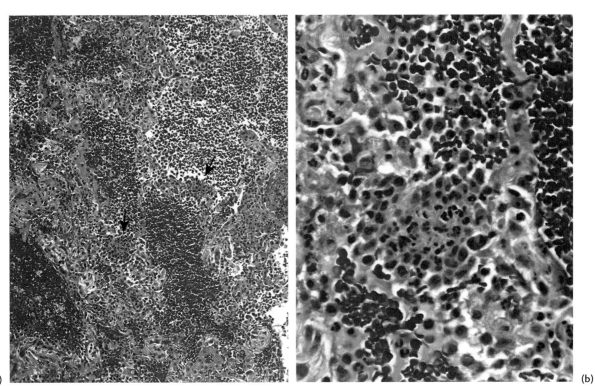

(a) (b)

Figure 8–13 Hemorrhage and capillaritis variant of Wegener's. (a) In this example, the capillaritis is more focal, characterized by small areas of inflammation (arrows). **(b)** Higher magnification of one of the areas of capillaritis shows focal expansion and replacement of alveolar septum by neutrophils and histiocytes. Note the prominent associated intraalveolar hemorrhage.

Table 8–2 Contrasting Features of Pulmonary ANCA-Associated Vasculitides

	WG	CSS	MPA
Asthma	No	Yes	No
Eosinophilia	Usually not	Yes, high	No
ANCA	60–95%, usually C-ANCA	50–70%, usually P-ANCA	70–80%, usually P-ANCA
Radiographic findings	Multiple, often bilateral, nodules, may cavitate	Patchy airspace opacities, often transient	Bilateral diffuse airspace opacities
Glomerulonephritis	Frequent	Occasional, mild	Usual
Necrotizing URT lesions	Common	No	No
Necrotizing granulomatous inflammation	Yes (except hemorrhage and capillaritis variant)	In classic cases only, often absent	No
Necrotizing vasculitis	Yes	Yes	Yes (capillaritis only)
Tissue eosinophilia	Rare	Yes (eosinophilic pneumonia)	No

Abbreviations: WG = Wegener's granulomatosis; CSS = Churg–Strauss syndrome; MPA = microscopic polyangiitis; URT = upper respiratory tract.

Wegener's granulomatosis.[81,82] The disease usually responds to corticosteroids, although in some patients cytotoxic agents are necessary.[83,85,88,90] In fatal cases, death is most often caused by heart failure or intracranial hemorrhage.

Histologic Features

There is a spectrum of histologic changes in the lung. A combination of eosinophilic pneumonia, granulomatous inflammation and necrotizing vasculitis is considered pathognomonic, but is present only infrequently.[88,89] The areas of eosinophilic pneumonia are composed of a mixture of eosinophils and macrophages filling alveolar spaces, usually accompanied by an interstitial chronic inflammatory cell infiltrate containing eosinophils (Fig. 8–14). Eosinophil abscesses may occur, and parenchymal necrosis is often prominent. The granulomatous inflammation is usually necrotizing and often characterized by small palisading histiocytes arranged around central necrosis (so-called palisaded granulomas) (Fig. 8–15). The vasculitis affects arteries and veins and

is characterized by either granulomatous inflammation or less organized chronic inflammatory cells with numerous eosinophils in vessel walls (Fig. 8–16). Multinucleated giant cells may be prominent, and fibrinoid necrosis is often present. Changes of asthma often accompany the other findings. They include goblet cell hyperplasia, thickened basement membrane, hypertrophied smooth muscle, and eosinophils in bronchial walls, along with intraluminal mucinous exudates containing eosinophils.

More commonly, eosinophilic pneumonia occurs either by itself or along with a necrotizing vasculitis, but without granulomatous inflammation. The presence of accompanying parenchymal necrosis should suggest the diagnosis, but clinical correlation is required in such cases to confirm the diagnosis.

Differential Diagnosis

Uncomplicated *eosinophilic pneumonia* (see Chapter 6) is the most important lesion to distinguish from Churg–Strauss syndrome, since it is more common and usually

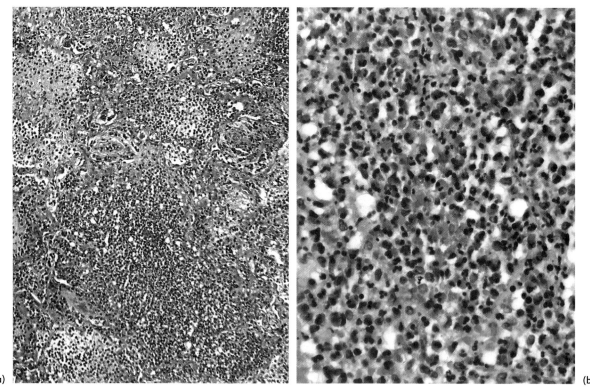

(a)   (b)

Figure 8–14 Eosinophilic pneumonia in Churg–Strauss syndrome. (a) Low magnification showing filling of alveoli by eosinophils (top) along with parenchymal necrosis (bottom). **(b)** Higher magnification illustrating the numerous eosinophils in the cellular infiltrate.

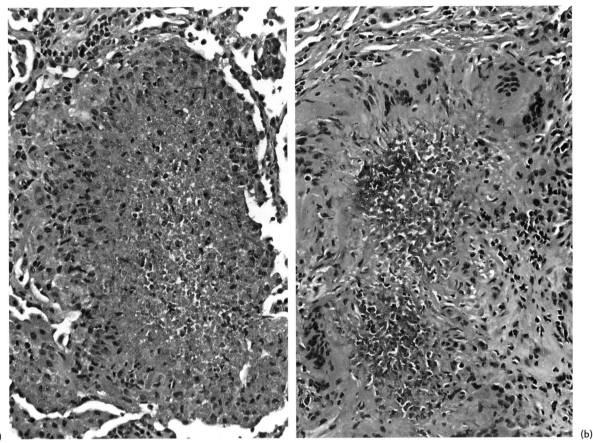

(a)   (b)

Figure 8–15 Necrotizing granulomas in Churg–Strauss syndrome. (a) Numerous necrotic eosinophils fill the center of this granuloma, and palisading histiocytes are seen on the periphery. (b) Remnants of eosinophils are seen in the center of this granuloma, and eosinophils are also seen in the surrounding viable parenchyma.

less severe. It does not have associated parenchymal necrosis, and a necrotizing vasculitis is not a feature, although infiltration of blood vessel walls by chronic inflammation and eosinophils is common. Eosinophilic pneumonia can occur as a manifestation of Churg–Strauss syndrome, as noted earlier, but other supporting clinical and laboratory findings are necessary for diagnosis in such cases.

The eosinophilic variant of *Wegener's granulomatosis* also enters the differential diagnosis (see Table 8–2). It usually has more extensive parenchymal necrosis. Although eosinophils are striking in the inflammatory cell infiltrate, areas of eosinophilic pneumonia do not occur. Of course, clinical findings help, since asthma and eosinophilia are characteristic of Churg–Strauss syndrome and usually not present in Wegener's.

Bronchocentric granulomatosis (see Chapter 6) needs to be distinguished from Churg–Strauss syndrome. Although eosinophilic pneumonia may be found in this condition, the granulomatous process is confined to bronchioles and peribronchiolar parenchyma. A necrotizing vasculitis is absent, and there is often associated mucoid impaction of bronchi.

CAPILLARITIS SYNDROMES

A variety of diseases are associated with a necrotizing capillaritis in the lungs, including, most commonly, microscopic polyangiitis, Wegener's granulomatosis, and lupus (Table 8–3), and most are associated with alveolar hemorrhage.[69,108,114] Older terms that have been used for necrotizing capillaritis include *microangiitis*,[109] *hypersensitivity angiitis*, and *microscopic polyarteritis*.[113] A knowledge of laboratory and clinical features is usually required to distinguish the diseases associated with capillaritis, since the histologic changes are identical.

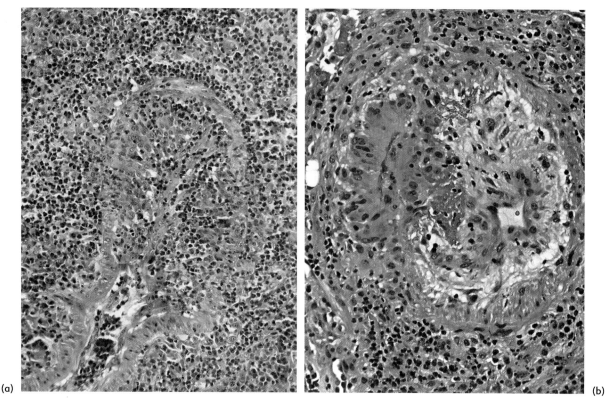

(a)   (b)

Figure 8–16 Vasculitis in Churg–Strauss syndrome. (a) A striking eosinophil infiltrate permeates this artery and the surrounding parenchyma. (b) This artery is partially involved by granulomatous inflammation, and there is focal fibrinoid necrosis. Note the eosinophils in the adjacent parenchyma (bottom).

Table 8–3   Capillaritis Syndromes
Microscopic polyangiitis
Wegener's granulomatosis
Acute lupus pneumonitis
Miscellaneous
Rheumatoid arthritis
Polymyositis
Henoch–Schönlein purpura
Cryoglobulinemia
Drug reactions (sulfonamides, diphenylhydantoin, propylthiouracil, etc)
Behçets's disease
Isolated ANCA-negative hemorrhage and capillaritis

Histologic Features of Capillaritis

Recognition of necrotizing capillaritis on biopsy specimens can be difficult, since capillaries lack a media and intima, and it is not possible to directly visualize inflammation and necrosis of their walls. Rather, only the end result of the inflammatory process is visible, and it is manifest by a neutrophil infiltrate in alveolar septa (Fig. 8–17).[49,94,108,109] Usually, nuclear dust is prominent in the infiltrate, and there may also be admixed eosinophils and histiocytes. The affected alveolar septa are expanded, disrupted, and replaced by the acute inflammatory infiltrate, and a proteinaceous exudate containing nuclear debris and acute inflammatory cells accumulates in adjacent alveolar spaces. Alveolar hemorrhage consisting of both hemosiderin and fresh blood and often admixed with karyorrhectic cell debris almost always accompanies the capillaritis. Sometimes an arteriolitis or venulitis is present as well, although it is uncommon.

Acute capillaritis needs to be distinguished from an early acute bacterial bronchopneumonia. Finding nuclear dust in alveolar septa is important, as is associated alveolar hemorrhage. Caution should be exercised if acute inflammation is more prominent within alveolar spaces than in alveolar septa, and if hemorrhage is absent.

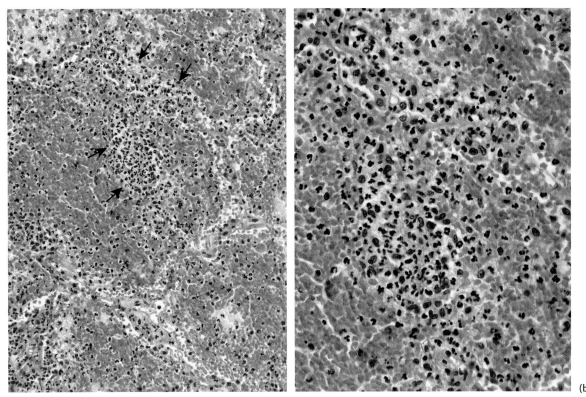

(a) (b)

Figure 8–17 Microscopic polyangiitis. (a) Low magnification view showing prominent alveolar hemorrhage and capillaritis (arrows). **(b)** Higher magnification of necrotizing capillaritis showing the typical expansion and disruption of alveolar septum by neutrophils.

Microscopic Polyangiitis

Microscopic polyangiitis is a systemic vasculitis involving the kidney in over 90% of cases and the lung in up to 50%.[1,91,103,106] It is the most common cause of the pulmonary renal syndrome.[1] Most patients are adults, with a mean age of 50 to 55 years, and a slight male predominance is reported in most series.[91,101,106,107] Pulmonary involvement is usually manifested by alveolar hemorrhage, and dyspnea, cough, and hemoptysis are common presenting complaints. Rare cases have occurred in a background of idiopathic pulmonary fibrosis,[98,102,110] and hyperinflation with obstructive lung disease has also been reported.[95] Evidence of glomerulonephritis with hematuria and renal failure is usually present, and most patients are anemic. Involvement of the musculoskeletal system, gastrointestinal tract, and skin is common, but upper respiratory tract lesions do not occur. ANCA are present in 70–80%, and are of the P-ANCA (anti-MPO) variety. Radiographically, bilateral airspace opacities are characteristic. Treatment is the same as for Wegener's granulomatosis,

consisting of cyclophosphamide and corticosteroids.[1,106,107,114] Mortality is high, approaching 30% in the first 6 months in some series, and relapses are common. Diffuse alveolar damage is a common finding at autopsy.[93]

Other Diseases Associated With Capillaritis

Capillaritis is present focally in many otherwise typical cases of Wegener's granulomatosis (see Fig. 8–7), but it is overshadowed by the vasculitis involving small and medium-sized arteries and veins, and thus largely goes unnoticed. Occasional cases of *Wegener's granulomatosis*, however, as previously noted, are characterized by alveolar hemorrhage and capillaritis, and the diagnosis in such cases requires the presence of C-ANCA or evidence of Wegener's elsewhere.[30,49,68]

One of the main pathologic findings in *acute lupus pneumonitis* (see Chapter 7) is alveolar hemorrhage and capillaritis, and similar changes have also been reported in patients with *rheumatoid arthritis, polymyositis,* and *mixed connective tissue disease.*[108,109,115–117,121] Immune complex deposition has been noted in the lung in some cases.[109,116]

Alveolar hemorrhage presumably due to capillaritis is a rare complication of *Henoch–Schönlein purpura*, and occurs more often in adults with this condition than in children.[111] *Cryoglobulinemia* causes a small vessel vasculitis, and alveolar hemorrhage and capillaritis have been reported as rare reactions to drugs such as *sulfonamides, diphenylhydantoin,* and *propylthiouracil.*[96,99,120]

Behçet's disease is a systemic vasculitis characterized by the triad of uveitis and oral and genital ulceration. Pulmonary involvement is uncommon and usually manifests clinically as hemoptysis. Small vessel vasculitis with capillaritis is seen in such cases, and immune complex deposition may be detected in the affected vessels.[100] Vasculitis involving large pulmonary arteries is a more common finding, however, and the subsequent development of arterial aneurysms is an important complication.[97,105,112,118,119]

Examples of isolated alveolar hemorrhage and capillaritis have been described that are unassociated with extrapulmonary disease or the presence of ANCA.[104] Whether these cases represent limited forms of Wegener's granulomatosis or microscopic polyangiitis or whether they represent a separate disease is uncertain. Seven of eight reported cases recovered, however, and none developed signs of systemic disease.

MISCELLANEOUS VASCULITIDES

Polyarteritis Nodosa

Polyarteritis nodosa (PAN) is a systemic arteritis that involves medium-sized arteries, most often in the kidney, gastrointestinal tract, heart, and liver. Pulmonary involvement is common at autopsy and is characterized by arteritis confined to bronchial arteries and identical to that occurring in other organs.[129] Clinically significant lung involvement during life, however, is rare.[130] ANCA are present in only 15–20% of cases.[3]

Giant Cell Arteritis

Rarely, pulmonary arteries are involved by granulomatous inflammation with giant cells identical to that occurring in the temporal arteries in temporal arteritis.[122,123,125,127,131,133] Some patients may also have associated temporal arteritis.

Takayasu's Arteritis

Takayasu's arteritis is a rare form of vasculitis that involves the large arteries, especially the aorta and its branches, and, less often, the pulmonary arteries.[126] It primarily affects young women. Patients may present with signs of pulmonary artery obstruction or pulmonary hypertension.[124,128] Pathologically, the lesion resembles giant cell arteritis with a transmural chronic inflammatory cell infiltrate containing multinucleated histiocytes. Later on, the inflammatory cell infiltrate may be replaced by fibrosis. Changes resembling plexiform arteriopathy have been reported in a few cases.[128]

REFERENCES

General

1. Jennette JC, Falk RJ: Small-vessel vasculitis. N Engl J Med 337:1511, 1997.
2. Liebow A: The J. Burns Amberson Lecture: Pulmonary angiitis and granulomatosis. Am Rev Respir Dis 108:1, 1973.
3. Savage COS, Harper L, Adu D: Primary systemic vasculitis. Lancet 349:553, 1997.
4. Seo P, Stone JH: The antineutrophil cytoplasmic antibody-associated vasculitis. Am J Med 117:39, 2004.

Wegener's Granulomatosis

5. Anderson G, Coles ET, Crane M, et al: Wegener's granuloma. A series of 265 British cases seen between 1975 and 1985. A report by a sub-committee of the British Thoracic Society Research Committee. Q J Med 83:427, 1992.
6. Andrassy K, Erb A, Koderisch J, et al: Wegener's granulomatosis with renal involvement: Patient survival and correlations between initial renal function, renal histology, therapy and renal outcome. Clin Nephrol 35:139, 1991.
7. Barksdale SK, Hallahan CW, Kerr GS, et al. Cutaneous pathology in Wegener's granulomatosis. A clinicopathologic study of 75 biopsies in 46 patients. Am J Surg Pathol 19:161, 1995.
8. Bax J, Gooszen H, Hoorntje S: Acute fulminating alveolar hemorrhage as presenting symptom in Wegener's granulomatosis. Anticytoplasmic antibodies as a diagnostic tool. Eur J Respir Dis 71:202, 1987.
9. Bosch X, Lopez-Soto A, Mirapeix E, et al: Antineutrophil cytoplasmic antibody-associated alveolar capillaritis in patients presenting with pulmonary hemorrhage. Arch Pathol Lab Med 118:517, 1994.
10. Brandwein S, Esdaile J, Danoff D, Tannenbaum H: Wegener's granulomatosis. Clinical features and outcome in 13 patients. Arch Intern Med 143:476, 1983.

11. Braun MG, Csernok E, Gross WL, Muller-Hermelik HK: Proteinase 3, the target antigen of anticytoplasmic antibodies circulating in Wegener's granulomatosis: Immunolocalization in normal and pathologic tissues. Am J Pathol 139:831, 1991.

12. Brockmann H, Schwarting A, Kriegsmann J, et al: Proteinase-3 as the major autoantigen of c-ANCA is strongly expressed in lung tissue of patients with Wegener's granulomatosis. Arthritis Res 4:220, 2002.

13. Carrington C, Liebow A: Limited forms of angiitis and granulomatosis of Wegener's type. Am J Med 41:497, 1966.

14. Cassan S, Coles D, Harrison E Jr: The concept of limited forms of Wegener's granulomatosis. Am J Med 49:366, 1970.

15. Cho C, Asuncion A, Tatum AH: False-positive antineutrophil cytoplasmic antibody in aspergillosis with oxalosis. Arch Pathol Lab Med 119:558, 1995.

16. Coulomb L'Hermine A, Capron F, Zou W, et al: Expression of the chemokine RANTES in pulmonary Wegener's granulomatosis. Hum Pathol 32:320, 2001.

17. Cordier J-F, Valeyre D, Guillevin L, Loire R, Brechot J-M: Pulmonary Wegener's granulomatosis: A clinical and imaging study of 77 cases. Chest 97:906, 1990.

18. Daum TE, Specks U, Colby TV, et al: Tracheobronchial involvement in Wegener's granulomatosis. Am J Respir Crit Care Med 151:522, 1995.

19. Davenport A, Lock RJ, Wallington TB: Clinical relevance of testing for antineutrophil cytoplasm antibodies (ANCA) with a standard indirect immunofluorescence ANCA test in patients with upper or lower respiratory tract symptoms. Thorax 49:213, 1994.

20. Del Buona EA, Flint A: Diagnostic usefulness of nasal biopsy in Wegener's granulomatosis. Hum Pathol 22:107, 1991.

21. DeRemee R, McDonald T, Harrison E Jr, Coles D: Wegener's granulomatosis. Anatomic correlates, a proposed classification. Mayo Clin Proc 51:777, 1976.

22. DeRemee RA, McDonald TJ, Weiland LH: Wegener's granulomatosis: Observations on treatment with antimicrobial agents. Mayo Clin Proc 60:27, 1985.

23. Devaney KO, Travis WD, Hoffman G, Leavitt R, Lebovics R, Fauci AS: Interpretation of head and neck biopsies in Wegener's granulomatosis: A pathologic study of 126 biopsies in 70 patients. Am J Surg Pathol 14:555, 1990.

24. Edgar JDM, McMillan SA, Bruce IN, Conlan SK: An audit of ANCA in routine clinical practice. Postgrad Med J 71:605, 1995.

25. Fauci AS, Haynes BF, Katz P, Wolff SM: Wegener's granulomatosis: Prospective clinical and therapeutic experience with 85 patients for 21 years. Ann Intern Med 98:76, 1983.

26. Fauci A, Wolff S: Wegener's granulomatosis: Studies in eighteen patients and a review of the literature. Medicine (Baltimore) 52:535, 1973.

27. Fienberg R, Mark EJ, Goodman M, et al: Correlation of antineutrophil cytoplasmic antibodies with the extrarenal histopathology of Wegener's (pathergic) granulomatosis and related forms of vasculitis. Hum Pathol 24:160, 1993.

28. Gal AA, Salinas FF, Staton GW Jr: The clinical and pathological spectrum of antineutrophil cytoplasmic autoantibody-related pulmonary disease. A comparison between perinuclear and cytoplasmic antineutrophil cytoplasmic autoantibodies. Arch Pathol Lab Med 118:1209, 1994.

29. Gal AA, Velasquez A: Antineutrophil cytoplasmic autoantibody in the absence of Wegener's granulomatosis or microscopic polyangiitis: Implications for the surgical pathologist. Mod Pathol 15:197, 2002.

30. Gaudin PB, Askin FB, Falk RJ, Jennette JC: The pathologic spectrum of pulmonary lesions in patients with anti-neutrophil cytoplasmic autoantibodies specific for anti-proteinase 3 and anti-myeloperoxidase. Am J Clin Pathol 104:7, 1995.

31. Gephardt GN, Shah LF, Tubbs RR, Ahmad M: Wegener's granulomatosis: Immunomicroscopic and ultrastructural study of four cases. Arch Pathol Lab Med 114:961, 1990.

32. Goulart RA, Mark EJ, Rosen S: Tumefactions as an extravascular manifestation of Wegener's granulomatosis. Am J Surg Pathol 19:145, 1995.

33. Hall SL, Miller LC, Duggan E, et al: Wegener granulomatosis in pediatric patients. J Pediatr 106:739, 1985.

34. Haworth SJ, Savage CO, Carr D, et al: Pulmonary haemorrhage complicating Wegener's granulomatosis and microscopic polyarteritis. Br Med J 290:1775, 1985.

35. Hoffman GS, Kerr GS, Leavitt RY, et al: Wegener granulomatosis: An analysis of 158 patients. Ann Intern Med 116:488, 1992.

36. Hoffman GS, Specks U: Antineutrophil cytoplasmic antibodies. Arthritis Rheum 41:1521, 1998.

37. Katzenstein A-LA, Locke WK: Solitary lesions in Wegener's granulomatosis. A clinicopathologic study of 25 cases. Am J Surg Pathol 19:545, 1995.

38. Kerr GS, Fleisher TA, Hallahan CW, et al: Limited prognostic value of changes in antineutrophil cytoplasmic antibody titer in patients with Wegener's granulomatosis. Arthritis Rheum 36:365, 1993.

39. Krafcik SS, Covin RB, Lynch JPIII, Sitrin RG: Wegener's granulomatosis in the elderly. Chest 109:430, 1996.

40. Langford CA, Hoffman GS: Wegener's granulomatosis. Thorax 54:629, 1999.

41. Lee KS, Kim TS, Fujimoto K, et al: Thoracic manifestation of Wegener's granulomatosis: CT findings in 30 patients. Eur Radiol 13:43, 2003.

42. Lim LCL, Taylor JG, Schmitz JL, et al: Diagnostic usefulness of antineutrophil cytoplasmic autoantibody serology. Am J Clin Pathol 111:363, 1999.

43. MacFarlane DG, Bourne JT, Dieppe PA, Easty DD: Indolent Wegener's granulomatosis. Ann Rheum Dis 42:398, 1983.

44. Mark EJ, Flieder DB, Matsubara O: Treated Wegener's granulomatosis: Distinctive pathological findings in the lungs of 20 patients and what they tell us about the natural history of the disease. Hum Pathol 28:450, 1997.

45. Mark EJ, Matsubara O, Tarr-Liu NS, Fienberg R: The pulmonary biopsy in the early diagnosis of Wegener's (pathergic) granulomatosis: A study based on 35 open lung biopsies. Hum Pathol 19:1065, 1988.

46. Markey BA, Warren JS: Use of anti-neutrophil cytoplasmic antibody assay to distinguish between vasculitic disease activity and complications of cytotoxic therapy. Am J Clin Pathol 102:589, 1994.

47. McHugh K, Manson D, Eberhard BA, et al: Wegener's granulomatosis in childhood. Pediatr Radiol 21:552, 1991.

48. Merkel PA, Polisson RP, Chang Y, et al: Prevalence of antineutrophil cytoplasmic antibodies in a large inception cohort of patients with connective tissue disease. Ann Intern Med 126:866, 1997.

49. Myers JL, Katzenstein AA: Wegener's granulomatosis presenting with massive pulmonary hemorrhage and capillaritis. Am J Surg Pathol 11:895, 1987.

50. Odeh M, Best L-A, Kerner H, et al: Localized Wegener's granulomatosis relapsing as diffuse massive intra-alveolar hemorrhage. Chest 104:955, 1993.

51. Pinching AJ, Lockwood CM, Pussell BA, et al: Wegener's granulomatosis: Observations on 18 patients with severe renal disease. Q J Med 52:435, 1983.

52. Potter MB, Fincher RK, Finger DR: Eosinophilia in Wegener's granulomatosis. Chest 116:1480, 1999.

53. Rao JK, Weinberger M, Oddone EZ, et al: The role of antineutrophil cytoplasmic antibody (C-ANCA) testing in the diagnosis of Wegener granulomatosis. A literature review and meta-analysis. Ann Intern Med 123:925, 1995.

54. Reinhold-Keller E, Beuge N, Ute L, et al: An interdisciplinary approach to the care of patients with Wegener's granulomatosis. Arthritis Rheum 43:1021, 2000.

55. Reuter M, Schnabel A, Wesner F, et al: Pulmonary Wegener's granulomatosis: Correlation between high-resolution CT findings and clinical scoring of disease activity. Chest 114:500, 1998.

56. Savige J, Dimech W, Fritzler M, et al: Addendum to the international consensus statement on testing and reporting of antineutrophiol cytoplasmic antibodies: Quality control guidelines, comments, and recommendations for testing in other autoimmune diseases. Am J Clin Pathol 120:312, 2003.

57. Savige J, Gillis D, Benson E, et al: International consensus statement on testing and reporting antineutrophil cytoplasmic antibodies (ANCA). Am J Clin Pathol 111:507, 1999.

58. Schnabel A, Hull-Ulrich K, Falloff K, Reuter M, Gross WL: Efficacy of transbronchial biopsy in pulmonary vaculitides. Eur Respir J 10:2738, 1997.

59. Shin MS, Young KR, Ho KJ: Wegener's granulomatosis. Upper respiratory tract and pulmonary radiographic manifestations in 30 cases with pathogenic consideration. Clin Imag 22:99, 1998.

60. Singer J, Sachet I, Howitzer T: Paediatric Wegener's granulomatosis: Two case histories and a review of the literature. Clin Radiol 42:50, 1990.

61. Specks U, Homburger HA: Anti-neutrophil cytoplasmic antibodies. Mayo Clin Proc 69:1197, 1994.

62. Specks U, Wheatley CL, McDonald TJ, et al: Anticytoplasmic autoantibodies in the diagnosis and follow-up of Wegener's granulomatosis. Mayo Clin Proc 64:28, 1989.

63. Spiera H, Lawson W, Weinrauch H: Wegener's granulomatosis treated with sulfamethoxazole-trimethoprim. Report of a case. Arch Intern Med 148:2065, 1988.

64. Stavrou P, Deutsch J, Rene C, Laws DE, Luqmani RA, Murray PI: Ocular manifestations of classical and limited Wegener's granulomatosis. Q J Med 86:719, 1993.

65. Stegeman CA, Tervaert JWC, de Jong PE, Kallenberg CGM: Trimethoprim-sulfamethoxazole (co-trimoxazole) for the prevention of relapse of Wegener's granulomatosis. N Engl J Med 335:16, 1996.

66. Stokes TC, McCann BG, Rees RT, et al: Acute fulminating intrapulmonary haemorrhage in Wegener's granulomatosis. Thorax 37:315, 1982.

67. Stone JH; Wegener's Granulomatosis Etanercept Trial Research Group: Limited versus severe Wegener's granulomatosis: Baseline data on patients in the Wegener's granulomatosis etanercept trial. Arthritis Rheum 48:2299, 2003.

68. Travis WD, Carpenter HA, Lie JT: Diffuse pulmonary hemorrhage. An uncommon manifestation of Wegener's granulomatosis. Am J Surg Pathol 11:702, 1987.

69. Travis WD, Colby TV, Lombard C, Carpenter HA: A clinicopathologic study of 34 cases of diffuse pulmonary hemorrhage with lung biopsy confirmation. Am J Surg Pathol 14:1112, 1990.

70. Travis WD, Hoffman GS, Leavitt RY, et al: Surgical pathology of the lung in Wegener's granulomatosis. Review of 87 open lung biopsies from 67 patients. Am J Surg Pathol 15:315, 1991.

71. Ulbright T, Katzenstein A: Solitary necrotizing granulomas of the lung: Differentiating features and etiology. Am J Surg Pathol 4:13, 1980.

72. Uner AH, Rozum-Slota B, Katzenstein A-LA: BOOP-like variant of Wegener's granulomatosis. A clinicopathologic study of 16 cases. Am J Surg Pathol 20:794, 1996.

73. Vassilopoulos D, Niles JL, Villa-Forte A, et al: Prevalence of antineutrophil cytoplasmic antibodies in patients with various pulmonary diseases or multiorgan dysfunction. Arthritis Rheum 49:151, 2003.

74. Wadsworth DT, Siegel MJ, Day DL: Wegener's granulomatosis in children: Chest radiographic manifestations. AJR Am J Roentgenol 163:901, 1994.

75. West BC, Todd JR, King JW: Wegener granulomatosis and trimethoprim-sulfamethoxazole. Complete remission after a twenty-year course. Ann Intern Med 106:840, 1987.

76. Wolff S, Fauci A, Horn R, Dale D: Wegener's granulomatosis. Ann Intern Med 81:513, 1974.

77. Wong RCW, Silvestrini RA, Savige JA, et al: Diagnostic value of classical and atypical antineutrophil cytoplasmic antibody (ANCA) immunofluorescence patterns. J Clin Pathol 52:124, 1999.

78. Yoshikawa Y, Watanabe T: Pulmonary lesions in Wegener's granulomatosis: A clinicopathologic study of 22 autopsy cases. Hum Pathol 17:401, 1986.

79. Yousem SA: Bronchocentric injury in Wegener's granulomatosis: A report of five cases. Hum Pathol 22:535, 1991.

80. Yousem S, Lombard C: Eosinophilic variant of Wegener's granulomatosis. Hum Pathol 19:682, 1988.

Churg–Strauss Syndrome

81. Buschman DL, Waldron JA, King TE: Churg-Strauss pulmonary vasculitis: High-resolution computed tomography scanning and pathologic findings. Am Rev Respir Dis 142:458, 1990.

82. Choi YH, Im J-G, Han BK, et al: Thoracic manifestation of Churg-Strauss syndrome: Radiologic and clinical findings. Chest 117:117, 2000.

83. Chumbley L, Harrison E Jr, DeRemee R: Allergic granulomatosis and angiitis (Churg-Strauss syndrome). Report and analysis of 30 cases. Mayo Clin Proc 52:477, 1977.

84. Finan MC, Winkelmann RK: The cutaneous extravascular necrotizing granuloma (Churg-Strauss granuloma) and systemic disease: A review of 27 cases. Medicine (Baltimore) 62:142, 1983.

85. Gross WL: Churg-Strauss syndrome: Update on recent developments. Curr Opin Rheumatol 14:11, 2002.

86. Guillevin L, Cohen P, Gayraud M, et al: Churg-Strauss syndrome: Clinical study and long-term follow-up of 96 patients. Medicine (Baltimore) 78:26, 1999.

87. Jamaleddine G, Diab K, Tabbarah Z, et al: Leukotriene antagonists and the Churg-Strauss syndrome. Semin Arthritis Rheum 31:211, 2002.

88. Katzenstein A-LA: Diagnostic features and differential diagnosis of Churg-Strauss syndrome in the lung. Am J Clin Pathol 114:767, 2000.

89. Koss M, Antonovych T, Hochholzer L: Allergic granulomatosis (Churg-Strauss syndrome). Pulmonary and renal morphologic findings. Am J Surg Pathol 5:21, 1981.

90. Lanham JG, Elkon KB, Pusey CD, Hughes GR: Systemic vasculitis with asthma and eosinophilia: A clinical approach to the Churg-Strauss syndrome. Medicine (Baltimore) 63:65, 1984.

91. Lhote F, Guillevin L: Polyarteritis nodosa, microscopic polyangiitis, and Churg-Strauss syndrome: Clinical aspects and treatment. Rheum Dis North Am 21:911, 1995.

92. Wechsler ME, Finn D, Gunawardena D: Churg-Strauss syndrome in patients receiving montelukast as treatment for asthma. Chest 117:708, 2000.

Capillaritis Syndrome

93. Akikusa B, Kondo Y, Irabu N, et al: Six cases of microscopic polyarteritis exhibiting acute interstitial pneumonia. Pathol Int 45:580, 1995.

94. Akikusa B, Sata T, Ogawa M, et al: Necrotizing alveolar capillaritis in autopsy cases of microscopic polyangiitis. Arch Pathol Lab Med 121:144, 1997.

95. Brugiere O, Raffy O, Sleiman O, et al: Progressive obstructive lung disease associated with microscopic polyangiitis. Am J Respir Crit Care Med 155:739, 1997.

96. Dhillon SS, Singh D, Doe N, et al: Diffuse alveolar hemorrhage and pulmonary capillaritis due to propylthiouracil. Chest 116:1485, 1999.

97. Erkan F, Cavdar T: Pulmonary vasculitis in Behçet's disease. Am Rev Respir Dis 146:232, 1992.

98. Eschun GM, Mink SN, Sharma S: Pulmonary interstitial fibrosis as a presenting manifestation in perinuclear antineutrophilic cytoplasmic antibody microscopic polyangiitis. Chest 123:297, 2003.

99. Gaffey C, Chun B, Harvey J, Manz H: Phenytoin-induced systemic granulomatous vasculitis. Arch Pathol Lab Med 110:131, 1986.

100. Gamble CN, Wiesner KB, Shapiro RF, Boyer WJ: The immune complex pathogenesis of glomerulonephritis and pulmonary vasculitis in Behçet's disease. Am J Med 66:1031, 1979.

101. Guillevin L, Durand-Gasselin B, Cevallos R, et al: Microscopic polyangiitis. Clinical and laboratory findings in eighty-five patients. Arthritis Rheum 42:421, 1999.

102. Homma S, Matsushita H, Nakata K: Pulmonary fibrosis in myeloperoxidase antineutrophil cytoplasmic antibody-associated vasculitides. Respirology 9:190, 2004.

103. Jennette JC, Thomas DB, Falk RJ: Microscopic polyangiitis (microscopic polyarteritis). Semin Diagn Pathol 18:3, 2001.

104. Jennings CA, King TE, Tuder R, et al: Diffuse alveolar hemorrhage with underlying isolated pauciimmune pulmonary capillaritis. Am J Respir Crit Care Med 155:1101, 1997.

105. Lakhanpal S, Tani K, Lie JT, et al: Pathologic features of Behçet's syndrome: A review of Japanese autopsy registry data. Hum Pathol 16:790, 1985.

106. Lhote F, Cohen P, Genereau T, et al: Microscopic polyangiitis: Clinical aspects and treatment. Ann Med Interne (Paris) 147:165, 1996.

107. Lauque D, Cadranel J, Lazor R, et al: Microscopic polyangiitis with alveolar hemorrhage: A study of 29 cases and review of the literature. Medicine (Baltimore) 79:222, 2000.

108. Mark EJ, Ramirez JF: Pulmonary capillaritis and hemorrhage in patients with systemic vasculitis. Arch Pathol Lab Med 109:413, 1985.

109. Myers JL, Katzenstein AA: Microangiitis in lupus-induced pulmonary hemorrhage. Am J Clin Pathol 85:552, 1986.

110. Nada AK, Torres VE, Ryu JH, Lie JT, Holley KE: Pulmonary fibrosis as an unusual clinical manifestation of a pulmonary-renal vasculitis in elderly patients. Mayo Clin Proc 65:847, 1990.

111. Nadrous HF, Yu AC, Specks U, Ryu JH: Pulmonary involvement in Henoch-Schönlein purpura. Mayo Clin Proc 79:1151, 2004.

112. Raz I, Okon E, Chajek-Shaul T: Pulmonary manifestations in Behçet's syndrome. Chest 95:585, 1989.

113. Savage COS, Winearls CG, Evans DJ, et al: Microscopic polyarteritis: Presentation, pathology and prognosis. Q J Med 56:467, 1985.

114. Schwarz MI, Brown KK: Small vessel vasculitis of the lung. Thorax 55:502, 2000.

115. Schwarz MI, Sutarik JM, Nick JA, et al: Pulmonary capillaritis and diffuse alveolar hemorrhage. A primary manifestation of polymyositis. Am J Respir Crit Care Med 151:2037, 1995.

116. Schwarz MI, Zamora MR, Hodges TN, et al: Isolated pulmonary capillaritis and diffuse alveolar hemorrhage in rheumatoid arthritis and mixed connective tissue disease. Chest 113:1609, 1998.

117. Scott D, Bacon P, Tribe C: Systemic rheumatoid vasculitis: A clinical and laboratory study of 50 cases. Medicine (Baltimore) 60:288, 1981.

118. Slavin R, deGroot W: Pathology of the lung in Behçet's disease. Case report and review of the literature. Am J Surg Pathol 5:779, 1981.

119. Stricker H, Malinverni R: Multiple, large aneurysms of pulmonary arteries in Behçet's disease. Clinical remission and radiologic resolution after corticosteroid therapy. Arch Intern Med 149:925, 1989.

120. Yermakov V, Hitti I, Sutton A: Necrotizing vasculitis associated with diphenylhydantoin: Two fatal cases. Hum Pathol 13:182, 1983.

121. Zamora MR, Warner ML, Tuder R, et al: Diffuse alveolar hemorrhage and systemic lupus erythematosus: Clinical presentation, histology, survival, and outcome. Medicine (Baltimore) 76:192, 1997.

Miscellaneous Pulmonary Angiitides

122. Bradley JD, Pinals RS, Blumenfeld HB, Poston WM: Giant cell arteritis with pulmonary nodules. Am J Med 77:135, 1984.

123. Doyle L, McWilliam L, Hasleton P: Giant cell arteritis with pulmonary involvement. Br J Dis Chest 82:88, 1988.

124. Elsasser S, Solèr M, Bolliger CT, et al: Takayasu disease with predominant pulmonary involvement. Respiration 67:213, 2000.

125. Glover MU, Muniz J, Bessone L, et al: Pulmonary artery obstruction due to giant cell arteritis. Chest 91:924, 1987.

126. Kerr KM, Auger WR, Fedullo PF, et al: Large vessel pulmonary arteritis mimicking chronic thromboembolic disease. Am J Respir Crit Care Med 152:367, 1995.

127. Ladanyi M, Fraser R: Pulmonary involvement in giant cell arteritis. Arch Pathol Lab Med 111:1178, 1987.

128. Lie JT: Isolated pulmonary Takayasu arteritis: Clinicopathologic characteristics. Mod Pathol 9:469, 1996.

129. Matsumoto T, Homma S, Okada M, et al: The lung in polyarteritis nodosa: A pathologic study of 10 cases. Hum Pathol 24:717, 1993.

130. Nick J, Tuder R, May R, Fisher J: Polyarteritis nodosa with pulmonary vasculitis. Am J Respir Crit Care Med 153:450, 1996.

131. Okubo S, Kunieda T, Ando M, et al: Idiopathic isolated pulmonary arteritis with chronic cor pulmonale. Chest 94:665, 1988.

132. Wagenaar SS, van den Bosch JMM, Westermann CJJ, et al: Isolated granulomatous giant cell vasculitis of the pulmonary elastic arteries. Arch Pathol Lab Med 110:962, 1986.

133. Wagenaar SS, Westermann CJJ, Corrin B: Giant cell arteritis limited to large elastic pulmonary arteries. Thorax 36:876, 1981.

PRIMARY LYMPHOID LUNG LESIONS

Infiltrative lung diseases in which lymphocytes are the main cellular component include a divergent group of disorders spanning a spectrum from inflammatory reactions to malignant neoplasms. Our understanding of these disorders has paralleled the exponential growth of knowledge in the general field of hematopathology over the last two decades. New concepts have evolved and terminology has changed for pulmonary lymphoid lesions just as they have for extrapulmonary lymphoproliferative diseases. This chapter reviews the main lymphoid lesions originating in the lung (Table 9–1). In doing so, it departs somewhat from the implicit objective of the monograph (surgical pathology of *non-neoplastic* lung disease) because it includes selected neoplastic lymphoid lesions. The fact that many of these lesions enter the differential diagnosis of the non-neoplastic conditions, we believe, justifies this transgression.

SMALL LYMPHOCYTIC PROLIFERATIONS

The small lymphocytic proliferations in the lung consist of entities in which mature, small lymphocytes comprise the main cellular components. Most are thought to be derived from bronchus-associated lymphoid tissue (BALT; see later on) and include both reactive and neoplastic conditions (see Table 9–1).

Bronchus-Associated Lymphoid Tissue (BALT) and Reactive Lymphoid Hyperplasia

Aggregates of lymphoid tissue that normally are inconspicuous occur along the bronchial tree, especially at branch points, and are known as *bronchus-associated lymphoid tissue* (BALT).[17,23] Together with analogous tissue in the gastrointestinal tract (*gut-associated lymphoid tissue* [GALT]), they comprise the so-called *mucosal-associated lymphoid tissue* (MALT). They are thought to participate in immunological reactions to airborne antigens, and they can be the source of various

Table 9–1   Primary Lymphoid Lung Lesions
Small lymphocytic proliferations
Reactive lymphoid hyperplasia
Follicular bronchiolitis
Lymphoid interstitial pneumonia
Nodular lymphoid hyperplasia
Low-grade B-cell lymphoma of MALT
Lymphomatoid granulomatosis (LYG)
Miscellaneous (posttransplant lymphoproliferative disorders, non-Hodgkin's lymphomas, Hodgkin's disease, intravascular lymphomatosis)

pathologic lesions, ranging from hyperplasias to malignant neoplasms.

Sometimes, lymphoid follicles with reactive germinal centers are seen in the interstitium, not only around bronchioles, but also along the interlobular septa in biopsies containing other processes (Fig. 9–1). This reactive lymphoid hyperplasia is most often seen in chronic interstitial pneumonias, especially those associated with rheumatoid lung, chronic hypersensitivity pneumonia, and, occasionally, nonspecific interstitial pneumonia. It also occurs in chronic pneumonic processes such as postobstructive pneumonia and organizing infectious pneumonias. It should not be confused with follicular bronchiolitis or lymphoid interstitial pneumonia (see later on), because it is a focal change that is overshadowed by the associated chronic inflammatory process.

Follicular Bronchiolitis

Follicular bronchiolitis, also referred to as follicular hyperplasia of BALT, is an uncommon disorder characterized by the presence of hyperplastic lymphoid follicles containing reactive germinal centers that are present in the walls of bronchioles (Fig. 9–2).[11,15,28] The bronchioles are usually narrowed by the process, and sometimes an intraluminal acute inflammatory cell exudate is present. In a few cases, overlapping features of follicular bronchiolitis and lymphoid interstitial

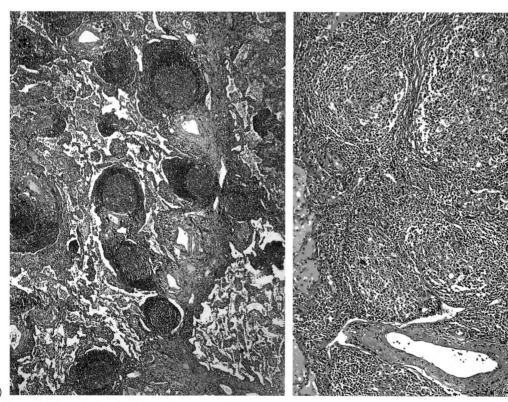

(a)   (b)

Figure 9–1   **Reactive lymphoid hyperplasia in postobstructive pneumonia.** (a) Low magnification showing lymphoid follicles containing reactive germinal centers that are arranged along an interlobular septum. (b) Higher magnification of the lymphoid follicles, highlighting the reactive germinal centers.

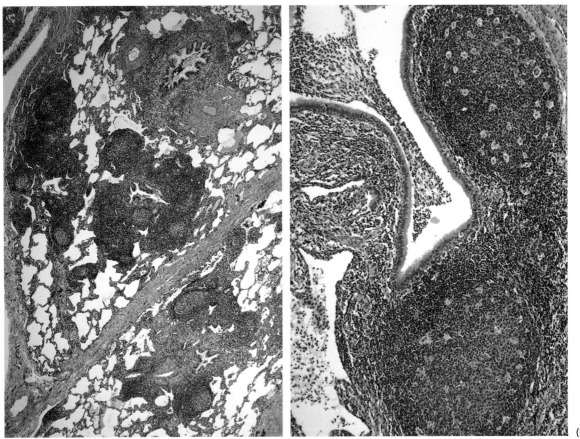

(a)

(b)

Figure 9–2 Follicular bronchiolitis. (a) Low magnification view showing lymphoid follicles with germinal centers that surround and narrow small bronchioles. (b) A higher magnification illustrates the reactive germinal centers around a narrowed bronchiole. Note the acute inflammatory cell exudate in the bronchiole lumen.

pneumonia (see later on) can be found. The diagnosis of follicular bronchiolitis should be restricted, however, to cases in which the lymphoid infiltrate is confined to bronchioles and the immediate peribronchiolar interstitium, without significant extension into more distal parenchyma.

Clinically, follicular bronchiolitis affects persons over a wide age range, from young children to adults. It can occur in association with collagen vascular diseases, especially Sjögren's syndrome or rheumatoid arthritis, and it can be seen in patients with congenital or acquired immunodeficiency, including AIDS.[7,11,15,28] Patients usually present with dyspnea or cough, and bilateral reticular or reticulonodular infiltrates are seen on chest radiographs. Centrilobular nodules often associated with peribronchial nodules and ground glass opacities are characteristically seen on chest CT scans.[7] Peripheral eosinophilia has been reported in some patients in whom it was thought to be a manifestation of a

hypersensitivity reaction, and hypergammaglobulinemia occurs occasionally.[28]

Lymphoid Interstitial Pneumonia

Lymphoid interstitial pneumonia (LIP), also known as diffuse lymphoid hyperplasia of BALT, is a diffuse pulmonary disorder characterized by an interstitial infiltrate of mature lymphocytes and a variable admixture of plasma cells and other mononuclear cells.[8,10,13,22] It is commonly associated with other conditions, including human immunodeficiency virus (HIV) infections, especially in children, Sjögren's syndrome, chronic active hepatitis, and other autoimmune disorders.[3–5,10,13,21,22,25–27] The pathogenesis is unknown, although HIV RNA has been demonstrated in some cases by in situ hybridization,[26] and Epstein-Barr virus (EBV) DNA in others by both in situ hybridization and the polymerase chain reaction (PCR) technique.[2,14]

Clinical Features

Clinically, patients with LIP usually present with progressive dyspnea or cough.[10,13,15,22,24] Some may have symptoms that are suggestive of recurrent infection. Most of the reported cases have been in adults, with a mean age in the mid 50s, and there is a female preponderance. The disease also occurs in children, often in association with HIV infection, and it is considered diagnostic of AIDS in this population.[4,12,18,25] The chest radiograph shows a spectrum of changes that range from bibasilar streaky densities to coarse, reticulonodular shadows.[8,10,13] Soft, fluffy alveolar densities are present less commonly. Thickened bronchovascular bundles, varying-sized nodules, ground glass opacities, and small cysts are common on computed tomography (CT) scans.[24] Pleural effusion may occasionally be seen, but hilar lymph node enlargement does not occur. Pulmonary function studies show a restrictive defect and decreased diffusing capacity. Dysproteinemias, especially hypergammaglobulinemia, are common, and patients with associated Sjögren's syndrome may

also have rheumatoid factor or antinuclear antibodies in their serum.

The clinical course of LIP is variable. In some cases the lesion remains stable, but in others there is progressive deterioration of lung function with eventual end-stage interstitial fibrosis and honeycomb lung.[10,13,22,24] Steroid therapy has been helpful in a number of patients, and cyclophosphamide and chlorambucil have been used in a few.[13,22,27] The development of malignant lymphoma occasionally is a complication.[1,6,10,12,13,20]

Histologic Features

Microscopically, the lung in LIP shows a predominantly interstitial cellular infiltrate that diffusely involves the distal parenchyma (Fig. 9–3).[10,13,15,22] The alveolar septa are usually markedly expanded and often distorted by the process, and small airways and blood vessels may be infiltrated (Fig. 9–4). A mixture of small lymphocytes, plasma cells, and histiocytes comprise the infiltrating cells. Small aggregates of epithelioid histiocytes and loosely formed non-necrotizing granulomas, often

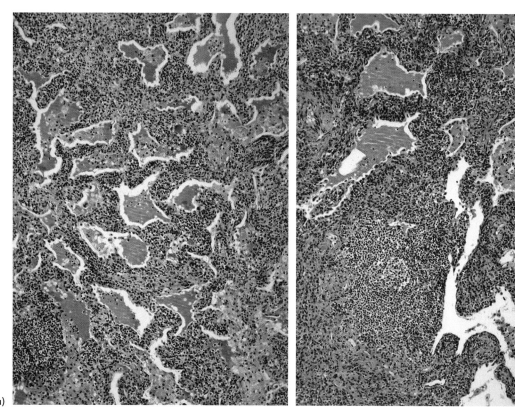

(a)   (b)

Figure 9–3 LIP. Low magnification views showing uniform-appearing alveolar septal thickening (a) as well as some architectural distortion (b). Note the proteinaceous exudate present in alveolar spaces in both figures, and a small lymphoid aggregate with germinal center in B.

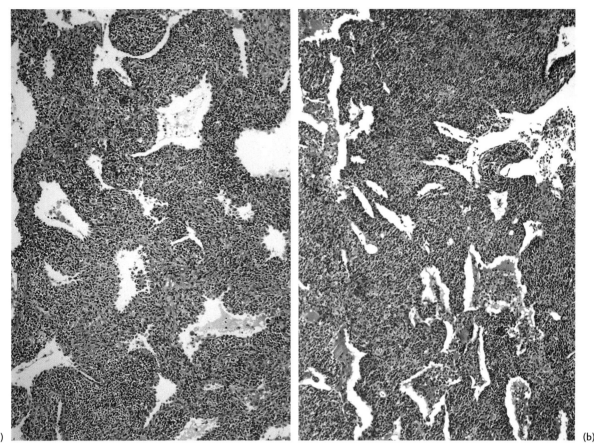

(a)   (b)

Figure 9–4 LIP. (a) This photomicrograph shows the typical densely cellular appearance of widened alveolar septa. Note that some alveolar spaces appear compressed. **(b)** The alveolar septal thickening is irregular in this example. Scattered lightly staining histiocytes can be appreciated in the infiltrate even at this low magnification.

containing multinucleated giant cells, are frequently present (Fig. 9–5). Nodular lymphoid aggregates containing reactive germinal centers are common, and lymphoepithelial lesions are occasionally present.[15,38] By immunohistochemical staining, the interstitial lymphoid cells generally mark as T cells, except in the germinal centers, where they stain with CD20 as B cells.[2,26] Staining for immunoglobulin light chains consistently shows polyclonality in the plasma cells, and heavy chain gene rearrangements are absent.[1,8,10,15] Fibrosis is usually minimal, although type 2 pneumocyte hyperplasia may be prominent. Necrosis is absent. Sometimes the cellular infiltrate spills into alveolar spaces, and small numbers of lymphocytes and histiocytes may accumulate in these areas. An eosinophilic, proteinaceous exudate often fills alveolar spaces adjacent to the cellular interstitial infiltrate. In cases with dysproteinemia, plasma cells may be especially prominent, and Russell bodies and deposits of hyaline

'para-amyloid' may be seen.[13] Nodular amyloidosis (see Chapter 7) has been found along with LIP in several patients with Sjögren's syndrome.[3]

Differential Diagnosis

There may be overlap in some reported cases of LIP and *follicular bronchiolitis*, since the point at which peribronchiolar lymphoid hyperplasia is sufficiently extensive to warrant a diagnosis of LIP is not well defined. Our approach is to diagnose LIP only when there is *diffuse* involvement of alveolar septa extending well beyond the peribronchiolar interstitium. All other cases are classified as follicular bronchiolitis. It may be, however, that follicular bronchiolitis and LIP represent different ends of a spectrum of the same disease.[15]

Other conditions characterized by an interstitial chronic inflammatory cell infiltrate also enter the differential diagnosis, including *nodular lymphoid hyperplasia*, *hypersensitivity pneumonia*, and *nonspecific interstitial*

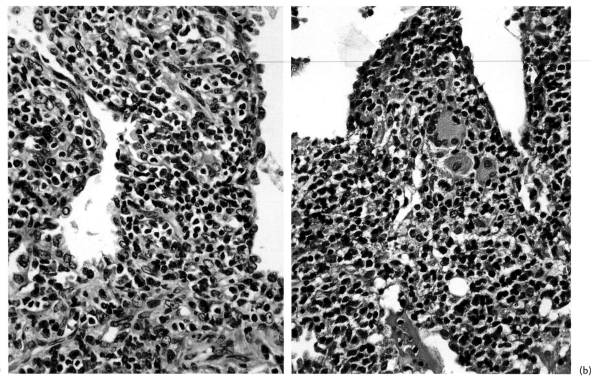

(a) (b)

Figure 9–5 Higher magnification of the cellular infiltrate in LIP showing the characteristic mixture of small lymphocytes and plasma cells **(a)**. Epithelioid histiocytes and multinucleated giant cells are seen in addition to the lymphocytes and plasma cells in another case **(b)**.

pneumonia (NSIP), and their differentiating features are summarized in Tables 9–2 and 9–3. Nodular lymphoid hyperplasia is discussed in detail later on in this chapter. Hypersensitivity pneumonia (see Chapter 6) enters the differential diagnosis especially when granulomas are prominent. The density and distribution of the infiltrate are the most important features in differentiating these two entities. In LIP, the alveolar septa are distorted by a dense lymphoplasmacytic infiltrate, while alveolar septa are only mildly thickened by chronic inflammation in hypersensitivity pneumonia. Furthermore, the interstitial infiltrate is patchy with peribronchiolar accentuation in hypersensitivity pneumonia, compared to diffuse in LIP. The finding of bronchiolitis obliterans also favors hypersensitivity pneumonia, since it does not occur in LIP, but it is not always present. Of course, the clinical history and appropriate laboratory data should help in difficult cases. The degree of cellularity is the most helpful feature in distinguishing LIP and NSIP (see Chapter 3). In LIP, the infiltrate is usually so intense that alveolar spaces, at least focally, are narrowed or compressed, whereas this type of architectural distortion is not seen in NSIP. Also, germinal centers are

usually prominent in LIP but are only focal findings, if present at all, in NSIP. Fibrosis may be extensive in NSIP but is not a prominent feature of LIP.

A number of lymphoproliferative disorders enter the differential diagnosis of LIP, and immunohistochemistry for lymphoid markers along with flow cytometry and T- and B-cell gene rearrangement studies in selected cases can facilitate diagnosis. *Low-grade B-cell lymphoma of MALT* (*extranodal marginal zone B-cell lymphoma*) is probably the most difficult to distinguish from LIP. It is discussed later on in this chapter, and the main differentiating features are summarized in Table 9–3. Briefly, the finding of a monomorphous lymphoid infiltrate (even if only focally present in an otherwise mixed cellular background) containing mainly CD20-positive B lymphocytes along with a lymphangitic distribution to the infiltrate indicate lymphoma.[38] Demonstration of monoclonality by immunohisto-chemical techniques can help in difficult cases, as can demonstration of immunoglobulin heavy chain gene rearrangements.[1,6,8,10,45,50] *Chronic lymphocytic leukemia* is characterized by a uniform infiltrate of small lymphocytes that stain for CD20 and usually also

Table 9–2 Contrasting Features of Lymphoid Interstitial Pneumonia, Hypersensitivity Pneumonia, and Nonspecific Interstitial Pneumonia

	LIP	HP	NSIP
Distortion of alveolar septa by dense interstitial infiltrate	Usual	No	No
Peribronchiolar accentuation of the interstitial infiltrate	No	Usual	Common
Foci of BOOP	No	Common	Common
Histiocytes/non-necrotizing granulomas	Common	Common	No
Germinal centers	Usual	Uncommon	Uncommon

Abbreviations: LIP = lymphoid interstitial pneumonia; HP = hypersensitivity pneumonia; NSIP = nonspecific interstitial pneumonia; BOOP = bronchiolitis obliterans–organizing pneumonia.

Table 9–3 Contrasting Features of Primary Lymphoid Lung Lesions

	LIP	Nodular Lymphoid Hyperplasia	Low-Grade Lymphoma of MALT	LYG
Radiographic Features	Bilateral reticular or reticulonodular infiltrates	Nodular, usually solitary, opacities	Solitary/multiple nodules, localized infiltrates	Nodular opacities, usually multiple and bilateral
Histologic Features				
Infiltrate	Polymorphous small lymphocytes and plasma cells	Polymorphous small lymphocytes and plasma cells, central scar	Usually monomorphous (small lymphocytes)	Usually polymorphous, variable numbers of large atypical lymphoid cells
Distribution	Random, diffuse	Random	Lymphangitic	Random
Germinal centers	Common	Usually prominent	Occasional	No
Necrosis	Absent	Absent	Absent	Usually present
Immunohistochemistry				
Lymphocytes	CD3 (CD20 in germinal centers)	CD3 (CD20 in germinal centers)	CD20, often CD43	CD20 (large, lymphoid cells), CD3 (small lymphoid cells), often EBV+ (large cells)
Plasma cells	Polyclonal	Polyclonal	Sometimes monoclonal	Polyclonal

CD23.[19] The infiltrate may demonstrate a striking peribronchiolar localization.[16] *Plasma cell myeloma* enters the differential diagnosis when plasma cells are prominent in the infiltrate. It differs in that the plasma cells are usually immature or otherwise abnormal, monoclonality is demonstrated by immunohistochemical techniques, and lymphoid cells are not numerous.[9] *Lymphomatoid granulomatosis* (LYG) is discussed later on in this chapter. It differs from LIP in that there is prominent vascular involvement, parenchymal

necrosis, and atypical large lymphoid cells. Also, LYG destroys the lung in a 'cross-country' fashion rather than being confined to the interstitium.

Nodular Lymphoid Hyperplasia

Nodular lymphoid hyperplasia of the lung is histologically similar to LIP but differs radiographically and grossly in that it causes localized mass-like densities rather than diffuse infiltrates.[29] The term 'pseudolymphoma' has been used historically for this lesion,[35] but is no longer accepted because of the potential confusion with lymphoma. 'Inflammatory pseudotumor'[34] is another term that can be used since it does not raise the specter of malignancy, and it more correctly describes the nature of the process. Inflammatory pseudotumor, however, has been used indiscriminately and incorrectly in the past for various other lung lesions, and, thus, for diagnostic purposes it is best used parenthetically with nodular lymphoid hyperplasia.

Clinical Features

Most patients with nodular lymphoid hyperplasia are middle-aged adults, averaging 50 to 60 years old.[29,31,35,41,43] The lesion occurs at a slightly earlier age than lymphoma, and it may occur in young adults as well. The majority of patients are asymptomatic. Cough and fever are common in symptomatic individuals.

Associated conditions such as Sjögren's syndrome or systemic lupus erythematosus have been reported in some patients but are not common. Solitary nodules or infiltrates are the usual radiographic findings, although multiple lesions occur rarely.[29] Pleural effusion is seen occasionally, but hilar lymph node enlargement is not a feature.

Pathologic Features

Nodular lymphoid hyperplasia can be considered to represent the residuum of a healing inflammatory or infectious process, and, therefore, histologic changes indicative of inflammation and scarring are necessary for diagnosis. At low magnification, a nodular mass can be appreciated that replaces a portion of lung parenchyma and is sharply demarcated from surrounding normal structures (Fig. 9–6). Lung architecture is usually at least partly obliterated by this process.

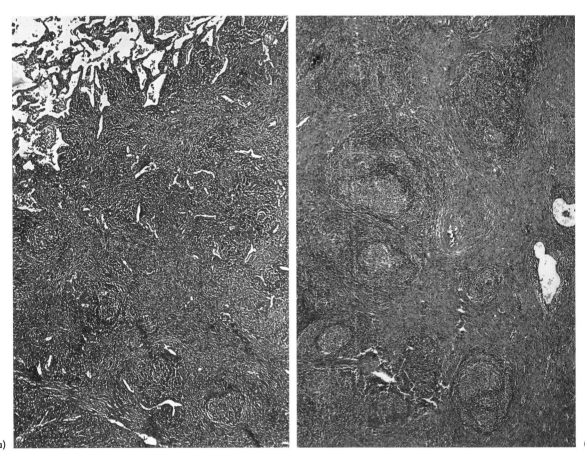

(a)   (b)

Figure 9–6 Nodular lymphoid hyperplasia. (a) Low magnification view showing a sharply demarcated nodule composed of lymphoid aggregates with germinal centers that are present in a background of fibrosis and chronic inflammatory cells. **(b)** Higher magnification from the center of the lesion showing numerous reactive germinal centers within dense fibrosis. Scattered entrapped alveoli with hyperplastic lining cells are also present (right).

Evidence of the interstitial nature of the lesion, however, can be found both at its center, where residual alveolar spaces lined by hyperplastic pneumocytes are often identified, and peripherally, where alveolar septa are infiltrated for a short distance. Scarring is most prominent at the center and is characterized by densely packed collagen bundles admixed with scattered fibroblasts and chronic inflammatory cells (Fig. 9–7). Necrosis is absent. The associated inflammatory cell infiltrate is polymorphous, containing numerous reactive-appearing germinal centers in addition to lymphocytes, plasma cells, and, sometimes, epithelioid histiocytes (Fig. 9–8). Neutrophils and eosinophils may also be present, and foci of organizing pneumonia are common in the surrounding parenchyma.

By immunohistochemical techniques, reactivity for both T- and B-cell antigens is found in the lymphoid infiltrate.[29] The germinal center cells stain for CD20, while the interfollicular lymphoid cells stain for CD3, CD43, and CD5. Both kappa and lambda light chains are seen in the plasma cells and no immunoglobulin heavy chain rearrangements are identified.

Differential Diagnosis

Nodular lymphoid hyperplasia needs to be differentiated from low-grade lymphoma of MALT.[31,33,35] This lesion is discussed in the next section, and the differentiating features of these entities are summarized in Table 9–3. LIP also enters the differential diagnosis, since the polymorphous infiltrate is similar for both conditions. They differ, however, in that nodular lymphoid hyperplasia is a discrete mass lesion that is usually solitary, while LIP is a diffuse interstitial process. Fibrosis is a prominent component of nodular lymphoid hyperplasia but not in LIP. Another lymphoid lesion that is occasionally encountered in lung biopsy specimens and may enter the differential diagnosis is an *intrapulmonary lymph node*.[32] These structures are generally located in the subpleural parenchyma, and they may be multiple. They are identical to ordinary lymph nodes, with a peripheral capsule and subcapsular and medullary sinuses (Fig. 9–9). Anthracosis is often prominent within them, and hyalinized nodules or germinal centers may be seen as well.

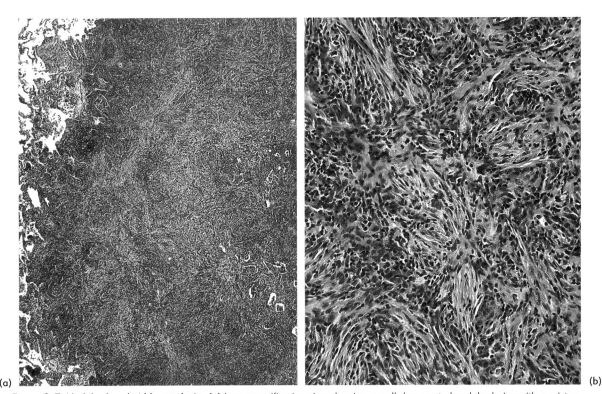

(a) (b)

Figure 9–7 Nodular lymphoid hyperplasia. (a) Low magnification view showing a well-demarcated nodular lesion with a mixture of inflammatory cells and fibrosis in the center. (b) A dense lymphoid and plasma cell infiltrate within background fibrosis is seen at higher magnification. Germinal centers were not prominent in this example.

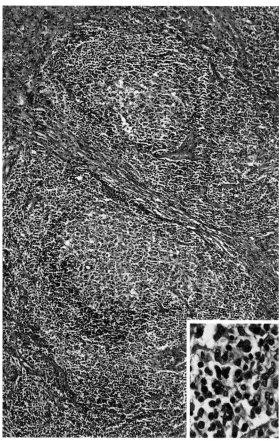

Figure 9–8 Nodular lymphoid hyperplasia. Higher magnification view showing prominent lymphoid follicles with reactive germinal centers in one area. Large numbers of plasma cells were seen elsewhere (inset).

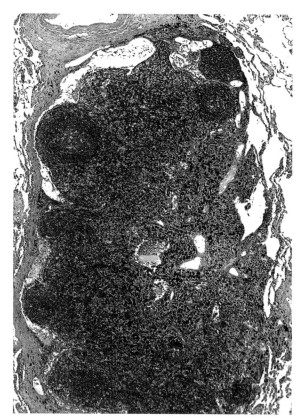

Figure 9–9 Intrapulmonary lymph node. Note the well-formed capsule (left), the subcapsular sinus, and scattered germinal centers. Adjacent lung parenchyma is seen on the left and the right.

Low-Grade B-Cell Lymphoma of MALT (Extranodal Marginal Zone B-Cell Lymphoma)

Clinical Features

Low-grade lymphoma of MALT is the most common primary lymphoma of the lung. It affects predominantly middle-aged and older adults, usually in the sixth or seventh decade, although there is a wide age range.[31,37,39,40,43,45,47,51] Patients are usually asymptomatic or have only mild respiratory complaints. Many patients have associated autoimmune diseases, most often Sjögren's syndrome, and monoclonal gammopathy is a common accompanying finding. Solitary nodules or localized infiltrates are the most common radiographic findings, while multiple opacities occur in about 25%. Diffuse interstitial infiltrates are uncommon. Hilar

lymphadenopathy is usually absent. The prognosis is excellent, with less than 10% of patients in most series dying from lymphoma. Even in patients with multifocal disease, the lesions may remain stable or only slowly progress over many years. In a few patients, however, the process may eventuate in a high-grade malignant lymphoma.[43] Concurrent large cell lymphoma has been reported in some patients, and, surprisingly, its presence seems to have no adverse effect on prognosis.[45]

Pathologic Features

MALT lymphomas are densely cellular, predominantly interstitial lesions that tend to form mass-like lesions, although occasionally they diffusely infiltrate the interstitium (Fig. 9–10). The proclivity for interstitial involvement can usually be appreciated at the periphery of solid nodules, where alveolar septa are widened by the cellular infiltrate (Fig. 9–11). Elsewhere there is confluent nodular expansion of the interstitium, and even in the most densely cellular central portions of the

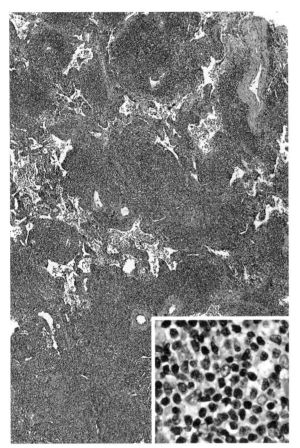

Figure 9–10 Low-grade B-cell lymphoma of MALT. Low magnification view showing expansion of the interstitium by a densely cellular infiltrate that appears most prominent around small arteries. Inset is a higher magnification showing the predominance of small lymphoid cells.

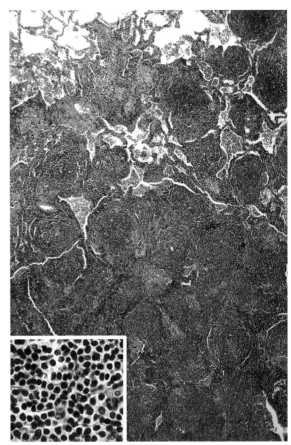

Figure 9–11 Low-grade B-cell lymphoma of MALT. In this example at low magnification, there is nodular replacement of lung parenchyma (bottom). The cellular infiltrate extends into the alveolar septa at the periphery of the nodule (top), thus indicating interstitial involvement. The inset is a higher magnification showing predominantly small lymphoid cells in the infiltrate.

lesion, slit-like remnants of alveolar spaces can often be identified (Fig. 9–12). Most typically, the cellular infiltrate is composed of a monomorphous collection of small lymphoid cells that are closely spaced with little intervening stroma or fibrosis.[31,36,47,51] Variable numbers of other cells, including plasma cells, immunoblasts, and histiocytes, can be found in focal areas as well. Occasionally, small, often atrophic-appearing, germinal centers are seen, and non-necrotizing granulomas may be present, especially near the periphery (Fig. 9–12b).[31,33,36,43,48,51] Vascular permeation by the lymphoid cells is common, but necrosis does not occur. Lymphoepithelial lesions characterized by infiltration of bronchiolar epithelium by the neoplastic lymphocytes can be found in most cases (Fig. 9–13).[37,38,45] Amyloid deposits are occasionally found as well.[37,45]

A helpful feature in diagnosing lymphoma is identification of a lymphangitic distribution to the cellular infiltrate. This feature can be appreciated best at low magnification examination, where the cellular infiltrate is seen to follow along the bronchovascular tree and the interlobular septa, often with extension into the pleura (Fig. 9–14). It is most readily apparent in diffusely infiltrating lesions, but it can often be observed in the parenchyma peripheral to mass lesions as well. Involvement of peribronchial or hilar lymph nodes, of course, confirms the diagnosis, but is very uncommon. Likewise, involvement of the parietal pleura is also considered diagnostic of lymphoma, but is equally uncommon.[31] Infiltration of the visceral pleura and ulceration of

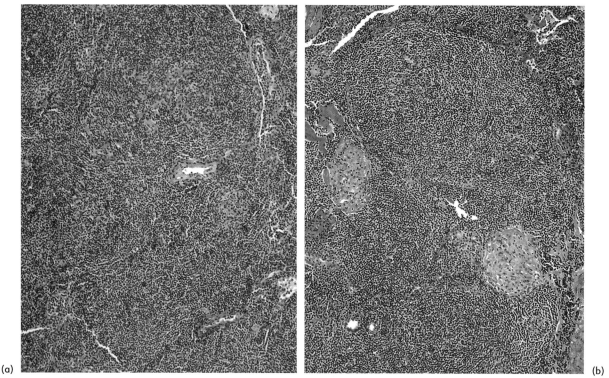

(a)   (b)

Figure 9–12 Low-grade B-cell lymphoma of MALT. (a) Nodular expansion of perivascular interstitium by the cellular infiltrate.
Scattered histiocytes and abortive germinal centers are seen in this example. **(b)** Well-formed non-necrotizing granulomas are
seen in another case.

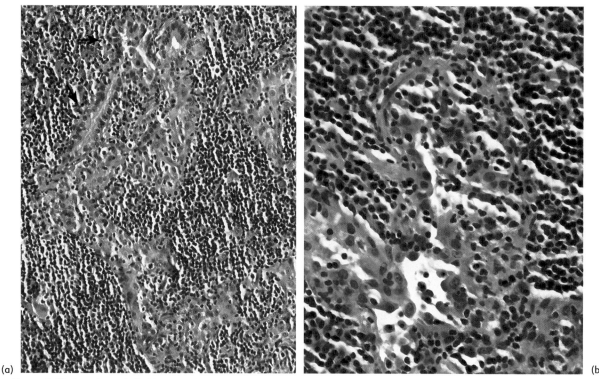

(a)   (b)

Figure 9–13 Lymphoepithelial lesion in low-grade B-cell lymphoma of MALT. (a) Low magnification showing infiltration of
bronchiolar epithelium by the lymphoid cells. A small portion of residual uninvolved bronchiolar epithelium is seen at top left
(arrows). **(b)** Higher magnification showing the typical eosinophilic appearance of the epithelium and the numerous intraepithelial
lymphoid cells.

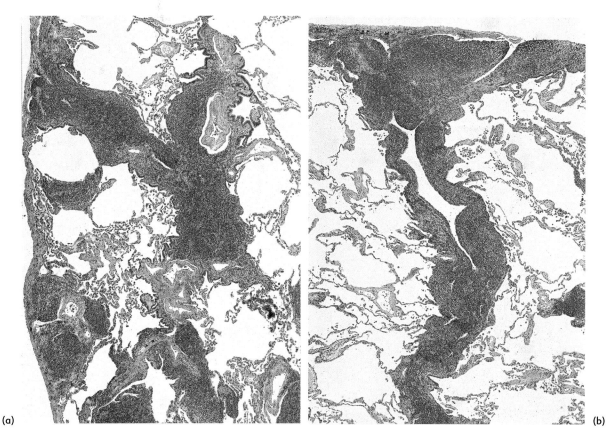

(a)   (b)

Figure 9–14 Lymphangitic distribution in low-grade B-cell lymphoma of MALT. (a) The cellular infiltrate is present around the bronchovascular bundle (top) and extends into the pleura (left). **(b)** The infiltrate in this area courses along an interlobular septum and onto the pleura (top).

bronchi occur frequently in lymphoma, but may be seen in inflammatory conditions as well.[13,35]

Immunohistochemical techniques demonstrate that most of the lymphoid cells stain for CD20 and often also for CD43 (Fig. 9–15). Staining for CD3 and CD45RO (UCHL-1) is seen in only a minority of cells, while staining is negative for CD5 and CD10. The finding of coexpression of CD20 and CD43 in the lymphocytes of lymphoepithelial lesions helps to differentiate lymphoma from reactive lesions, in which the lymphocytes are either CD3- and CD43-positive or CD20-positive and CD43-negative.[38] Immunoglobulin light chain restriction is common,[30,31,36,40–43,46–48,51,52] and clonal immunoglobulin gene rearrangements can be identified by PCR techniques.[37,44,49,50,53]

LYMPHOMATOID GRANULOMATOSIS

It has been over 30 years since the first cases of lymphomatoid granulomatosis (LYG) were reported by

Liebow et al[72] in a classic article in 1972. The authors noted unique clinicopathologic characteristics with overlapping features of Wegener's granulomatosis and malignant lymphoma – hence the name. While the clinical and radiographic manifestations closely resembled Wegener's granulomatosis, the pathologic findings suggested lymphoma. The fact that lymph nodes, bone marrow, and spleen were usually not involved, however, even when the disease had spread beyond the lung, argued against a lymphomatous origin. Now, more than 30 years after its description, and despite the development of sophisticated laboratory techniques and enormous strides in knowledge of hematopathology, controversy remains about the nature of LYG, whether neoplastic or reactive, although a relationship to Wegener's granulomatosis has been unequivocally negated.

Clinical Features

LYG affects men twice as often as women, and the mean age of onset is 48 years, with a wide age range. Most

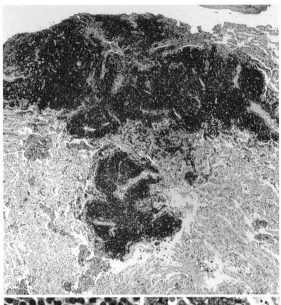

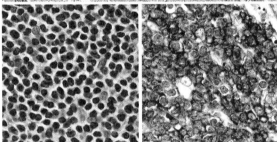

Figure 9–15 Immunohistochemical staining in low-grade B-cell lymphoma of MALT. Low magnification view showing staining for CD20 along interlobular septum and onto the pleura (top). At higher magnification (left inset) the predominantly small lymphoid cell population is better appreciated, and almost all the cells are seen to stain for CD20 (right inset).

patients have symptoms related to lung involvement, such as cough, chest pain, or hemoptysis, or they present with various systemic complaints, including fever, weight loss, and malaise.[69,71,72,83,85] Extrapulmonary manifestations, especially skin lesions or neurologic signs, are common and occasionally precede the onset of lung lesions.[55,57,67,74] Glomerulonephritis does not occur, although clinically silent, infiltrative kidney lesions are common autopsy findings. Involvement of the upper respiratory tract is rare. The usual chest radiographic findings are bilateral, discrete, rounded masses that often suggest metastatic tumor. Hilar lymph node enlargement is usually not present.

LYG may occur in individuals with impaired cellular immunity, including AIDS.[54,62,63,77,86] It has also been reported in renal transplant patients,[69,72] but these cases would now be diagnosed as posttransplant lymphoproliferative disorder (see later on). The development of malignant lymphoma involving lymph nodes has been reported in approximately 10% of patients.[59,69,72]

The prognosis for LYG is poor, with reported mortality rates ranging from 30% to 70%.[59,69,71] Combination chemotherapy appears to be the appropriate therapy, as discussed later on. Remission may be more difficult to achieve in patients who relapse following more conservative therapy.[64,73] Response to interferon-α2b has been reported in a few patients.[55,89] Remission has also been reported in one patient treated with the monoclonal anti-CD20 antibody rituximab.[68] That case was unusual, however, in that the patient had only a mediastinal mass without lung or other organ involvement. Radiation therapy may aid in localized lesions.[80]

Pathologic Features

The classic histologic findings in LYG include a mixed mononuclear cell infiltrate, prominent vascular infiltration by the mononuclear cells, and variable necrosis.[69,71,72,85] Typically there are well-demarcated cellular nodules containing central necrosis that efface both interstitial and airspace architecture (Fig. 9–16). Necrosis may be scant to absent in a minority of cases, and often in such cases a fibrinoid or proteinaceous exudate is seen within adjacent airspaces. Vascular infiltration by the cells is a prominent finding, and both arteries and veins are involved. Characteristically, there is a marked expansion of the intima by the infiltrating cells, and the lumen may be narrowed or obliterated (Fig. 9–17). The media is also infiltrated and expanded, but, in contrast to inflammatory vasculitides, the vessel walls usually remain intact without significant necrosis (Fig. 9–18).

The cellular infiltrate is composed of a mixture of small lymphocytes, histiocytes, plasma cells, and large lymphoid cells with varying degrees of atypia. Multinucleated histiocytes and neutrophils are not features, however, and well-formed granulomas are not present. Eosinophils are usually not numerous, although they are occasionally seen. The large lymphoid cells include immunoblast-like cells with vesicular nuclei containing prominent nucleoli, cells with folded or angulated darkly staining nuclei, and occasionally bizarre and sometimes multinucleated cells.

A spectrum of atypia is seen, ranging from a bland-appearing infiltrate containing mostly small lymphocytes

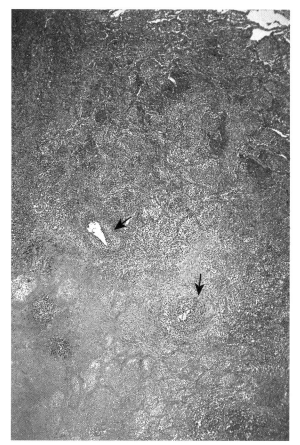

Figure 9–16 LYG. Low magnification view showing central necrosis surrounded by a thick rim of darkly staining cells. Note the vascular infiltration that can be appreciated even at low magnification (arrows).

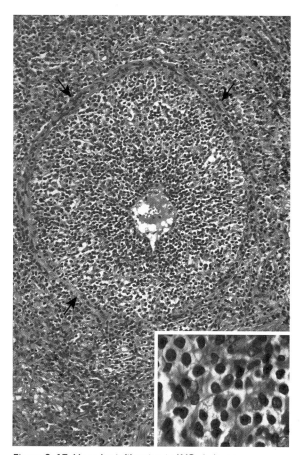

Figure 9–17 Vascular infiltration in LYG. A dense mononuclear cell infiltrate thickens the intima of this artery and narrows the lumen. Note that the media (arrows) remains intact. The inset is a higher magnification of the infiltrate, showing a mixture of mononuclear cells, mainly small lymphoid cells with minimal atypia.

and histiocytes with only rare atypical lymphoid cells (see Figs 9–17 and 9–18) to an obviously malignant infiltrate containing mainly large lymphoid cells (Fig. 9–19) (see Grading, later on). Often there is a mixture of large atypical cells with small lymphocytes and other benign inflammatory cells (Fig. 9–20). In most cases, scattered areas of recognizable lymphoma characterized by small nests or clusters of large, atypical lymphoid cells can be found after careful search, even when most of the infiltrate appears bland (Figs 9–21 and 9–22). The atypical cells tend to be most numerous in blood vessel walls, especially in or near areas of necrosis.

Immunophenotype and Relation to Epstein-Barr Virus

Early immunophenotyping studies indicated that the majority of lymphoid cells in LYG were T cells.[56,64,76,81]

Although T-cell gene rearrangements were identified in only a few cases (none from the lung),[64,76] LYG was generally considered a form of T-cell lymphoma. More recent studies, however, have provided evidence that most cases rather represent a form of B-cell lymphoma in which reactive T cells comprise the majority of cells (so-called T-cell-rich B-cell lymphoma).[61,62,74,78,79,82] Using immunohistochemistry, several studies have demonstrated that while the small lymphoid cells stain with CD3 and CD45RO as T cells, the large atypical lymphoid cells usually mark with CD20 as B cells. Furthermore, light chain restriction has been demonstrated in the B cells by immunohistochemistry, and immunoglobulin heavy chain gene rearrangements can be identified in most.[61,74,79,82] Myers et al[79] and Morice et al[78] additionally demonstrated that the large

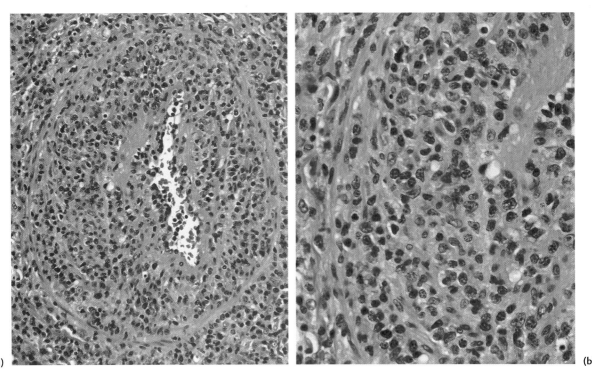

(a)   (b)

Figure 9–18 Vascular infiltration in LYG. (a) In this pulmonary artery, both intima and media are infiltrated and expanded by a mixed mononuclear cell infiltrate. Note that the wall is otherwise intact and there is no necrosis. **(b)** Higher magnification showing the permeation of the muscle layers by a mixture of mononuclear cells with minimal atypia.

lymphoid cells in a few cases stain for T-cell antigens but not CD20, thus indicating that some cases are T-cell lymphomas.

A relationship between LYG and Epstein-Barr virus (EBV) infection was postulated by Liebow in his initial description of the disease and has been subsequently confirmed.[60,70,75,77,79,82,84,87–89] Using the PCR technique, Katzenstein and Peiper[70] identified EBV genomes in 72% of cases. Others have confirmed this finding by means of in situ hybridization, and have shown that labeling for EBV is confined to the large B lymphocytes, which are also the proliferating cells.[61,62,79,88] LYG cases of apparent T-cell origin, however, do not contain evidence of EBV infection.[79]

Grading

Early studies provided evidence that increased numbers of large, atypical lymphoid cells were associated with a worse prognosis.[69] Subsequently, some investigators have graded the proportion of atypical cells from 1 to 3, with Grade 1 containing mainly small lymphocytes and histiocytes with only rare atypical cells, Grade 2 containing increased numbers of atypical cells in a mixed cellular background, and Grade 3 containing monomorphous sheets of atypical cells equivalent to lymphoma.[64,73] Currently, some groups utilize the number of EBV-infected cells in determining grade, with Grade 1 containing none to few, Grade 2 containing moderate numbers, and Grade 3 containing large numbers.[65,66] There is no agreement, however, even among the same investigators, about the precise numbers of EBV-infected cells required for each grade. Also, there is no evidence supporting the utility of this method of grading, and it may not be completely relevant since evidence of EBV infection is not present in every case.

Treatment

It is widely accepted that Grade 3 LYG is a variant of diffuse large B-cell lymphoma in most cases and should be treated as such. The diagnosis in such cases is best expressed as 'diffuse large B-cell lymphoma, lymphomatoid granulomatosis type' so that clinicians clearly understand the treatment options. There is considerable controversy, however, on the nature and treatment of Grades 1 and 2. In our opinion, the fact that areas recognizable as lymphoma are present at

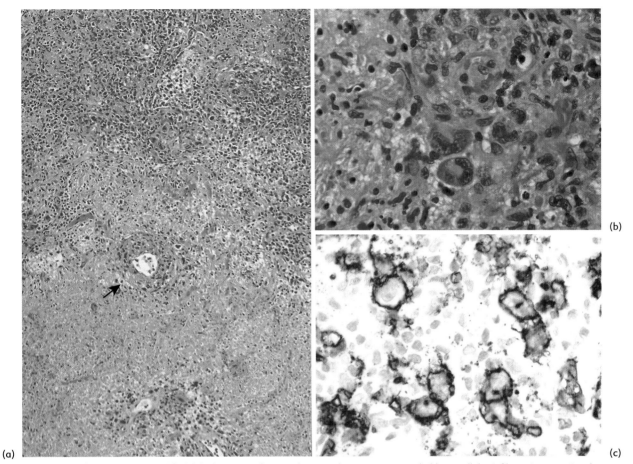

Figure 9–19 Severe atypia in LYG. (a) At low magnification the typical necrosis surrounded by a cellular infiltrate is appreciated. Vascular infiltration is also seen (arrow), and even at low magnification atypical cells can be seen around the blood vessels and near the necrotic zones. **(b)** Higher magnification showing severely atypical cells including multinucleated cells. **(c)** Immunohistochemical stain for CD20 shows positive staining in the large, atypical cells, while the small background lymphoid cells are negative.

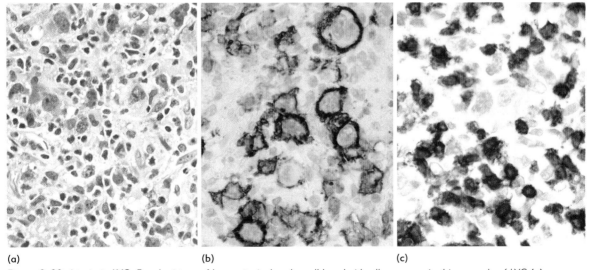

(a) (b) (c)

Figure 9–20 Atypia in LYG. Equal mixture of large atypical and small lymphoid cells are seen in this example of LYG **(a)**. Immunohistochemical staining shows a positive reaction for CD20 in the large lymphoid cells **(b)** and for CD3 in the background small lymphoid cells **(c)**.

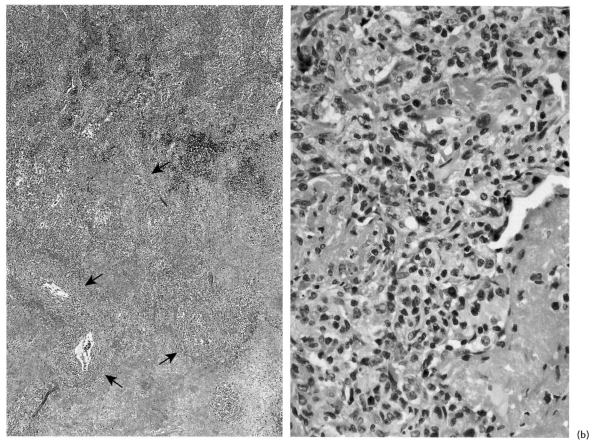

(a)

(b)

Figure 9–21 Variation in cellular infiltrate in LYG. (a) Low magnification showing typical necrosis, vascular infiltration (arrows), and cellular infiltrate. **(b)** Higher magnification of the cellular infiltrate, showing a mixture of mononuclear cells with minimal atypia. Most of the lesion had this appearance (see Fig. 9–22).

least focally in all Grade 2 cases indicates that these also represent lymphomas and should be treated as such with combination chemotherapy. Grade 1 cases are more problematic, but luckily are extremely rare. Although they do not fulfill histologic criteria for malignancy, they can be associated with disseminated disease and rapid progression to overt lymphoma.[61,69,82,89] In our opinion, they also represent a form of lymphoma and should be treated as such. As mentioned earlier, there are reports of response to interferon-α and rituximab in a few patients, but there are no large prospective studies that have compared various treatment options or related them to different grades.[55,68,89]

Differential Diagnosis

Ordinary nodal lymphomas that secondarily involve the lung, especially the large cell variants, are frequently associated with vascular infiltration and necrosis, and they may thus resemble LYG.[58] The diagnosis of LYG should not be made in patients with a history of nodal lymphoma. Other lymphomas, such as anaplastic large cell lymphoma and high-grade B-cell lymphomas in patients with AIDS, can involve the lung primarily.[98,100] They may superficially resemble LYG because of focal necrosis and vascular infiltration, but attention to cytological features of the cells and the lack of a mixed cell infiltrate even focally should suggest the correct diagnosis. The results of immunohistochemical staining, of course, are also important. It should be remembered that necrosis and vascular infiltration are usually prominent in high-grade LYG, and their absence should be a clue that the process represents a lymphoma other than LYG.

Hodgkin's disease also enters the differential diagnosis of LYG. Although pulmonary involvement by Hodgkin's

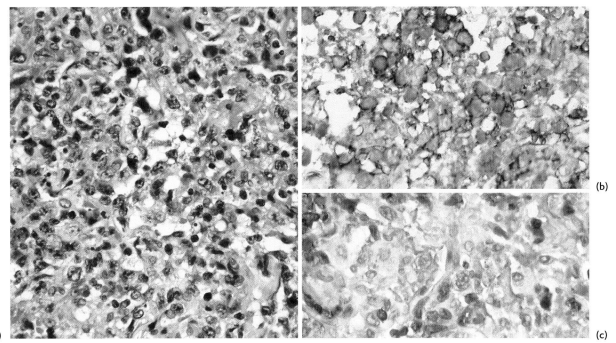

Figure 9–22 Photomicrograph of a small area from the same case shown in Figure 9–21 which contained closely packed atypical cells diagnostic of lymphoma **(a)**. The large cells stain for CD20 **(b)** and are negative for CD3 **(c)**.

disease usually represents contiguous spread from mediastinal disease, rare examples of primary Hodgkin's disease of the lung do occur.[90] A mixed cell infiltrate, necrosis, and vascular infiltration are common in this lesion, but the finding of eosinophils, lacunar cells, and Reed-Sternberg cells should suggest the correct diagnosis. Immunohistochemistry should also help in that Reed-Sternberg cells, in contrast to the large atypical cells of LYG, stain for CD15 and are negative for CD20 and CD3.

The presence of necrosis and vascular invasion in LYG raises the possibility of a primary pulmonary vasculitis, especially *Wegener's granulomatosis*, and the features of those two diseases are contrasted in Table 9–4. Briefly, the purely mononuclear cell infiltrate of LYG without eosinophils, neutrophils, or multinucleated giant cells, the absence of true granulomatous inflammation, the presence of vascular infiltration rather than inflammation, and the absence of a necrotizing vasculitis exclude the diagnosis of Wegener's granulomatosis.

Rarely, cases of *tuberculosis*, especially in the elderly or in immunocompromised persons, can lack well-formed granulomatous inflammation, and they may be characterized by central necrotic zones surrounded by a lymphohistiocytic infiltrate. The organisms can be demonstrated by special stains. This observation emphasizes the importance of examining special stains for organisms in cases lacking definite histologic features of malignancy.

MISCELLANEOUS LYMPHOID LESIONS

Posttransplant Lymphoproliferative Disorder

Lymphoproliferative diseases are uncommon, but serious, complications of organ transplantation, occurring in 1% to 10% of patients.[91,94a,95,97,99,108] Recipients of heart–lung transplants appear to be at highest risk. The lungs, including both native and allograft, are commonly involved and may be the only organ affected. Histologically, posttransplant lymphoproliferative disorder in the lung may be indistinguishable from LYG. Although most are B-cell lymphoproliferative disorders, cases have been reported that contain numerous background small T lymphocytes similar to LYG.[95] There are reports in the older literature of LYG occurring in renal transplant recipients, but these would currently be classified as posttransplant lymphoproliferative disorder.[69,72] In fact, in the study of Myers et al,[79] three patients initially diagnosed as LYG based on histologic findings were subsequently found to have had transplants

Table 9-4　Contrasting Features of Lymphomatoid Granulomatosis and Wegener's Granulomatosis

	LYG	Wegener's Granulomatosis
Radiographic Findings	Multiple nodules	Multiple nodules
Extrapulmonary Involvement		
Upper respiratory tract	No	Common
Glomerulonephritis	No	Common
Other major sites	Skin, nervous system	Skin, nervous system, ears, eyes, joints, etc.
ANCA	No	Usually
Prognosis	Poor	Good
Histologic Findings		
Cellular infiltrate	Mixed mononuclear cells	Acute and chronic inflammation with histiocytes, multinucleated giant cells
Atypical lymphoid cells	Characteristic	No
Necrotizing granulomas	No	Characteristic
Necrotizing vasculitis	No (infiltration of vessel walls but no necrosis)	Characteristic

and were reclassified. Posttransplant lymphoproliferative disorders are associated with EBV infection, and it was the histologic similarity between these lesions and LYG that prompted Katzenstein and Peiper[70] to investigate cases of LYG for EBV infection.

Infectious Mononucleosis and Other Infections

Pulmonary involvement is uncommon in infectious mononucleosis in immunocompetent individuals and is usually of little clinical consequence. An atypical pneumonia with mild respiratory complaints occurs in less than 5% and is usually self-limited. Rarely, rapidly progressive respiratory failure is encountered, and lung biopsy may be needed for diagnosis.[96] A patchy interstitial and perivascular infiltrate of lymphocytes and plasma cells distributed along lymphatic pathways is seen in such cases. An airspace exudate containing similar cells may accompany the interstitial process.

It should be remembered that other infections can also cause prominent lymphoplasmacytic lung infiltrates, especially viral infections. We have seen examples of parainfluenza virus and healing varicella pneumonia with these features. Careful attention to the clinical and radiographic manifestations, as well as the histologic findings, should prevent overdiagnosis of specific lymphoproliferative disorders.

Intravascular Lymphomatosis (Malignant Angioendotheliomatosis)

Intravascular lymphomatosis is a rare form of malignant lymphoma that is characterized by intravascular growth in small vessels. Clinical manifestations are usually related to skin and central nervous system involvement.[92] Although the lung is commonly involved at autopsy, significant respiratory complaints during life are uncommon. Dyspnea, cough, fever, and interstitial infiltrates may occur, and a lung biopsy may be required for diagnosis.[102,107] The main histologic finding is the filling of capillary, small artery, and venule lumens by malignant-appearing lymphoid cells that are usually of B-cell and less frequently of T-cell origin.[93,101,106,107]

Benign Lymphocytic Angiitis and Granulomatosis

Benign lymphocytic angiitis and granulomatosis (BLAG) was first described by Saldana et al[85] in an effort to reclassify the pulmonary angiitis and granulomatosis. They separated this entity from 'malignant angiitis and granulomatosis' (LYG), based mainly on the lack of cytological atypia in the lymphoid cells. There have been few subsequent reports of BLAG, and controversy abounds regarding its existence.[94,103,105] Most cases probably represent Grade 1 LYG, while others comprise a variety of unrelated inflammatory conditions. For these reasons, we prefer not to use this term for diagnosis.

Unclassified Lymphoid Lesions

In a small proportion of biopsy specimens showing lymphoid lesions, the histologic features are not characteristic enough to diagnose a specific disease, and thus we maintain a category for unclassified lymphoid lesions. These lesions can be given various descriptive diagnoses that reflect the composition of the infiltrating cells, such as 'atypical lymphoplasmacytic infiltrate' or 'atypical lymphohistiocytic infiltrate', for example. In such cases, the true nature of the lesion usually declares itself given sufficient time or benefit of additional tissue biopsies.

REFERENCES

Bronchus-Associated Lymphoid Tissue, Follicular Bronchiolitis, and Lymphoid Interstitial Pneumonia

1. Banerjee D, Ahmad D: Malignant lymphoma complicating lymphocytic interstitial pneumonia: A monoclonal B-cell neoplasm arising in a polyclonal lymphoproliferative disorder. Hum Pathol 13:780, 1982.
2. Barberà JA, Hayashi S, Hegele RG, Hogg JC: Detection of Epstein-Barr virus in lymphocytic interstitial pneumonia by in situ hybridization. Am Rev Respir Dis 145:940, 1992.
3. Bonner H Jr, Ennis RS, Geelhoed GW, et al: Lymphoid infiltration and amyloidosis of the lung in Sjögren's syndrome. Arch Pathol 95:42, 1973.
4. Church J, Isaacs H, Saxon A, et al: Lymphoid interstitial pneumonitis and hypogammaglobulinemia in children. Am Rev Respir Dis 124:491, 1981.
5. Grieco M, Chinoy-Acharya P: Lymphocytic interstitial pneumonia associated with the acquired immune deficiency syndrome. Am Rev Respir Dis 131:952, 1985.
6. Herbert A, Walters M, Cawley M, Godfrey R: Lymphocytic interstitial pneumonia identified as lymphoma of mucosa-associated lymphoid tissue. J Pathol 146:129, 1985.
7. Howling SJ, Hansell DM, Wells AU, et al: Follicular bronchiolitis: Thin-section CT and histologic findings. Radiology 212:637, 1999.
8. Julsrud P, Brown L, Li C-Y, et al: Pulmonary processes of mature-appearing lymphocytes: Pseudolymphoma, well-differentiated lymphocytic lymphoma, and lymphocytic interstitial pneumonitis. Radiology 127:289, 1978.
9. Kintzer JS Jr, Rosenow EC III, Kyle RE: Thoracic and pulmonary abnormalities in multiple myeloma. A review of 958 cases. Arch Intern Med 138:777, 1978.
10. Koss M, Hochholzer L, Langloss J, et al: Lymphoid interstitial pneumonia: Clinicopathological and immunopathological findings in 18 cases. Pathology 19:178, 1987.
11. Kradin RL, Mark EJ: Benign lymphoid disorders of the lung, with a theory regarding their development. Hum Pathol 14:857, 1983.
12. Kradin R, Young R, Kradin L, Mark E: Immunoblastic lymphoma arising in chronic lymphoid hyperplasia of the pulmonary interstitium. Cancer 50:1339, 1982.
13. Liebow AA, Carrington CB: Diffuse pulmonary lymphoreticular infiltrations associated with dysproteinemia. Med Clin North Am 57:809, 1973.
14. Malamou-Mitsi V, Tsai MM, Gal AA, Koss MN, O'Leary TJ: Lymphoid interstitial pneumonia not associated with HIV infection: Role of Epstein-Barr virus. Mod Pathol 5:487, 1992.
15. Nicholson AG, Wotherspoon AC, Diss TC, et al: Reactive pulmonary lymphoid disorders. Histopathology 26:405, 1995.
16. Palosaari D, Colby T: Bronchiolocentric chronic lymphocytic leukemia. Cancer 58:1695, 1986.
17. Richmond I, Pritchard GE, Ashcroft T, et al: Bronchus associated lymphoid tissue (BALT) in human lung: Its distribution in smokers and non-smokers. Thorax 48:1130, 1993.
18. Rogers BB, Browning I, Rosenblatt H, et al: A familial lymphoproliferative disorder presenting with primary pulmonary manifestations. Am Rev Respir Dis 145:203, 1992.
19. Rollins S, Colby T: Lung biopsy in chronic lymphocytic leukemia. Arch Pathol Lab Med 112:607, 1988.
20. Schuurman HJ, Gooszen H, Tan I, et al: Low-grade lymphoma of immature T-cell phenotype in a case of lymphocytic interstitial pneumonia and Sjogren's syndrome. Histopathology 11:1193, 1987.
21. Solal-Celigny P, Couderc L, Herman D, et al: Lymphoid interstitial pneumonitis in acquired immunodeficiency syndrome-related complex. Am Rev Respir Dis 131:956, 1985.
22. Strimlan CV, Rosenow EC III, Weiland LH, et al: Lymphocytic interstitial pneumonitis. Review of 13 cases. Ann Intern Med 88:616, 1978.
23. Sue-Chu M, Karjalainen E-M, Altraja A, et al: Lymphoid aggregates in endobronchial biopsies from young elite cross-country skiers. Am J Respir Crit Care Med 158:597, 1998.
24. Swigris JJ, Berry GJ, Raffin TA, et al: Lymphoid interstitial pneumonia: A narrative review. Chest 122:2150, 2002.
25. Teruya-Feldstein J, Kingma, DW, Weiss A, et al: Chemokine gene expression and clonal analysis of B cells in tissues involved by lymphoid interstitial pneumonitis from HIV-infected pediatric patients. Mod Pathol 14:929, 2001.
26. Travis WD, Fox CH, Devaney KO, et al: Lymphoid pneumonitis in 50 adult patients infected with the human immunodeficiency virus: Lymphocytic

interstitial pneumonitis versus nonspecific interstitial pneumonitis. Hum Pathol 23:529, 1992.

27. Yoshizawa Y, Ohdama S, Ikeda A, et al: Lymphoid interstitial pneumonia associated with depressed cellular immunity and polyclonal gammopathy. Am Rev Respir Dis 130:507, 1984.

28. Yousem S, Colby T, Carrington C: Follicular bronchitis/bronchiolitis. Hum Pathol 16:700, 1985.

Nodular Lymphoid Hyperplasia

29. Abbondanza SL, Rush W, Bijwaard KE, et al: Nodular lymphoid hyperplasia of the lung: A clinicopathologic study of 14 cases. Am J Surg Pathol 24:587, 2000.

30. Feoli F, Carbone A, Dina M, et al: Pseudolymphoma of the lung: Lymphoid subsets in the lung mass and in peripheral blood. Cancer 48:2218, 1981.

31. Koss M, Hochholzer L, Nichols P, et al: Primary non-Hodgkin's lymphoma and pseudolymphoma of lung: A study of 161 patients. Hum Pathol 14:1024, 1983.

32. Kradin R, Spirn R, Mark E: Intrapulmonary lymph nodes. Clinical, radiologic and pathologic features. Chest 87:662, 1985.

33. Marchevsky A, Padilla M, Kaneko M, Kleinerman J: Localized lymphoid nodules of lung: A reappraisal of the lymphoma versus pseudolymphoma dilemma. Cancer 51:2070, 1983.

34. Matsubara O, Tan-Liu NS, Kenney RM, Mark EJ: Inflammatory pseudotumors of the lung: Progression from organizing pneumonia to fibrous histiocytoma or to plasma cell granuloma in 32 cases. Hum Pathol 19:807, 1988.

35. Saltzstein SL: Pulmonary malignant lymphomas and pseudolymphomas: Classification, therapy and prognosis. Cancer 16:928, 1963.

Small Lymphocytic Lymphoma

36. Addis BJ, Hyjek E, Isaacson PG: Primary pulmonary lymphoma: A re-appraisal of its histogenesis and its relationship to pseudolymphoma and lymphoid interstitial pneumonia. Histopathology 13:1, 1988.

37. Ahmed S, Kussick SJ, Siddiqui AK, et al: Bronchial-associated lymphoid tissue lymphoma: A clinical study of a rare disease. Eur J Cancer 40:1320, 2000.

38. Bégueret H, Vergier B, Parrens M, et al: Primary lung small B-cell lymphoma versus lymphoid hyperplasia: Evaluation of diagnostic criteria in 26 cases. Am J Surg Pathol 26:76, 2002.

39. Cordier J-F, Chailleux E, Lauque D, et al: Primary pulmonary lymphomas: A clinical study of 70 cases in nonimmunocompromised patients. Chest 103:201, 1993.

40. Evans H: Extranodal small lymphocytic proliferation: A clinicopathologic and immunocytochemical study. Cancer 49:84, 1982.

41. Gephardt G, Tubbs R, Liu A, et al: Pulmonary lymphoid neoplasms. Role of immunohistology in the study of cellular immunotypes and in differential diagnosis. Chest 89:545, 1986.

42. Herbert A, Wright D, Isaacson P, Smith J: Primary malignant lymphoma of the lung: Histopathologic and immunologic evaluation of nine cases. Hum Pathol 15:415, 1984.

43. Kennedy J, Nathwani B, Burke J, et al: Pulmonary lymphomas and other pulmonary lymphoid lesions: A clinicopathologic and immunologic study of 64 patients. Cancer 56:539, 1985.

44. Kurosu K, Yumoto N, Furukawa M, et al: Low-grade pulmonary mucosa-associated lymphoid tissue lymphoma with or without intraclonal variation. Am J Respir Crit Care Med 158:1613, 1998.

45. Kurtin PJ, Myers JL, Adlakha H, et al: Pathologic and clinical features of primary pulmonary extranodal marginal zone B-cell lymphoma of MALT type. Am J Surg Pathol 25:997, 2001.

46. Le Tourneau A, Audouin J, Garbe L, et al: Primary pulmonary malignant lymphoma, clinical and pathological findings, immunocytochemical and ultrastructural studies in 15 cases. Hematol Oncol 1:49, 1983.

47. Li G, Hansmann M-L, Zwingers T, Lennert K: Primary lymphomas of the lung: Morphological, immunohistochemical and clinical features. Histopathology 16:519, 1990.

48. Peterson H, Snider H, Yam L, et al: Primary pulmonary lymphoma: A clinical and immunohistochemical study of six cases. Cancer 56:805, 1985.

49. Shiota T, Chiba W, Ikeda S, Ikei N: Gene analysis of pulmonary pseudolymphoma. Chest 103:335, 1993.

50. Subramanian D, Albrecht S, Gonzalez JM, Cagle PT: Primary pulmonary lymphoma: Diagnosis by immunoglobulin gene rearrangement study using a novel polymerase chain reaction technique. Am Rev Respir Dis 148:222, 1993.

51. Turner R, Colby T, Doggett R: Well-differentiated lymphocytic lymphoma. A study of 47 patients with primary manifestation in the lung. Cancer 54:2088, 1984.

52. Weiss LM, Yousem SA, Warnke RA: Non-Hodgkin's lymphomas of the lung. A study of 19 cases emphasizing the utility of frozen section immunologic studies in differential diagnosis. Am J Surg Pathol 9:480, 1985.

53. Wotherspoon AC, Soosay GN, Diss TC, Isaacson PG: Low-grade primary B-cell lymphoma of the lung: An immunohistochemical, molecular, and cytogenetic study of a single case. Am J Clin Pathol 94:655, 1990.

Lymphomatoid Granulomatosis

54. Anders KH, Latta H, Chang BS, et al: Lymphomatoid granulomatosis and malignant lymphoma of the central nervous system in the acquired immunodeficiency syndrome. Hum Pathol 20:326, 1989.

55. Beaty MW, Toro J, Sorbara L: Cutaneous lymphomatoid granulomatosis: Correlation of clinical and biologic features. Am J Surg Pathol 25:1111, 2001.

56. Bleiweiss IJ, Strauchen JA: Lymphomatoid granulomatosis of the lung: Report of a case and gene rearrangement studies. Hum Pathol 19:1109, 1988.

57. Carlson KC, Gibson LE: Cutaneous signs of lymphomatoid granulomatosis. Arch Dermatol 127:1693, 1991.

58. Colby T, Carrington C: Pulmonary lymphomas simulating lymphomatoid granulomatosis. Am J Surg Pathol 6:19, 1982.

59. Fauci A, Haynes B, Costa J, et al: Lymphomatoid granulomatosis: Prospective clinical and therapeutic experience over 10 years. N Engl J Med 306:68, 1982.

60. Guinee D, Jaffe E, Kingma D, et al: Pulmonary lymphomatoid granulomatosis. Evidence for proliferation of Epstein-Barr virus infected B-lymphocytes with a prominent T-cell component and vasculitis. Am J Surg Pathol 18:753, 1994.

61. Guinee DG, Perkins SL, Travis WD, et al: Proliferation and cellular phenotype in lymphomatoid granulomatosis: Implications of a higher proliferation index in B cells. Am J Surg Pathol 22:1093, 1998.

62. Haque AK, Myers JL, Hudnall SD, et al: Pulmonary lymphomatoid granulomatosis in acquired immunodeficiency syndrome: Lesions with Epstein-Barr virus infection. Mod Pathol 11:347, 1998.

63. Ilowite N, Fligner C, Ochs H, et al: Pulmonary angiitis with atypical lymphoreticular infiltrates in Wiskott-Aldrich syndrome: Possible relationship of lymphomatoid granulomatosis and EBV infection. Clin Immunol Immunopathol 41:479, 1986.

64. Jaffe ES, Lipford EH Jr, Margolick JB, et al: Lymphomatoid granulomatosis and angiocentric lymphoma: A spectrum of post-thymic T-cell proliferations. Semin Respir Med 10:167, 1989.

65. Jaffe ES, Wilson WH: Lymphomatoid granulomatosis: Pathogenesis, pathology and clinical implications. Cancer Surv 30:233, 1997.

66. Jaffe ES, Wilson WH: Lymphomatoid granulomatosis. In: Pathology and Genetics of Tumors of Hematopoetic and Lymphoid Tissues, WHO Classification of Tumors, Lyon, IARC Press, 2001, p. 185.

67. James W, Odom R, Katzenstein A: The cutaneous manifestations of lymphomatoid granulomatosis: Report of forty-four patients and a review of the literature. Arch Dermatol 117:196, 1981.

68. Jordan K, Grothey JK, Grothe A, et al: Successful treatment of mediastinal lymphomatoid granulomatosis with rituximab monotherapy. Eur J Haematol 74:263, 2005.

69. Katzenstein A, Carrington C, Liebow A: Lymphomatoid granulomatosis. A clinicopathologic study of 152 cases. Cancer 43:360, 1979.

70. Katzenstein A-L, Peiper S: Detection of Epstein-Barr virus genomes in lymphomatoid granulomatosis: Analysis of 29 cases using the polymerase chain reaction technique. Mod Pathol 3:435, 1990.

71. Koss M, Hochholzer L, Langloss J, et al: Lymphomatoid granulomatosis: A clinicopathologic study of 42 patients. Pathology 18:283, 1986.

72. Liebow A, Carrington C, Friedman P: Lymphomatoid granulomatosis. Hum Pathol 3:457, 1972.

73. Lipford E Jr, Margolick J, Longo D, et al: Angiocentric immunoproliferative lesions: A clinicopathologic spectrum of post-thymic T-cell proliferations. Blood 72:1674, 1988.

74. McNiff JM, Cooper D, Howe G, et al: Lymphomatoid granulomatosis of the skin and lung: An angiocentric T-cell-rich B-cell lymphoproliferative disorder. Arch Dermatol 132:1464, 1996.

75. Medeiros LJ, Jaffe ES, Chen Y-Y, Weiss LM: Localization of Epstein-Barr viral genomes in angiocentric immunoproliferative lesions. Am J Surg Pathol 16:439, 1992.

76. Medeiros LJ, Peiper SC, Elwood L, et al: Angiocentric immunoproliferative lesions: A molecular analysis of eight cases. Hum Pathol 22:1150, 1991.

77. Mittal K, Neri A, Feiner H, Schinella R, Alfonso F: Lymphomatoid granulomatosis in the acquired immunodeficiency syndrome. Evidence of Epstein-Barr virus infection and B-cell clonal selection without myc rearrangement. Cancer 65:1345, 1990.

78. Morice WG, Kurtin PJ, Myers JL: Expression of cytolytic lymphocyte-associated antigens in pulmonary lymphomatoid granulomatosis. Am J Clin Pathol 118:391, 2002.

79. Myers JL, Kurtin PJ, Katzenstein A-LA, et al: Lymphomatoid granulomatosis: Evidence of immunophenotypic diversity and relationship to Epstein-Barr virus infection. Am J Surg Pathol 19:1300, 1995.

80. Nair BD, Joseph MG, Catton GE, Lach B: Radiation therapy in lymphomatoid granulomatosis. Cancer 64:821, 1989.

81. Nichols P, Koss M, Levine A, et al: Lymphomatoid granulomatosis: A T-cell disorder? Am J Med 72:467, 1982.

82. Nicholson AG, Wotherspoon AC, Diss TC: Lymphomatoid granulomatosis: Evidence that some cases represent Epstein-Barr virus-associated B-cell lymphoma. Histopathology 29:317, 1996.

83. Patton W, Lynch J III: Lymphomatoid granulomatosis. Clinicopathologic study of four cases and literature review. Medicine (Baltimore) 61:1, 1982.

84. Sabourin J-C, Kanavaros P, Briere J, et al: Epstein-Barr virus (EBV) genomes and EBV-encoded latent membrane protein (LMP) in pulmonary lymphomas occurring in nonimunocompromised patients. Am J Surg Pathol 17:995, 1993.

85. Saldana M, Patchefsky A, Israel H, Atkinson G: Pulmonary angiitis and granulomatosis. The relationship between histologic features, organ involvement and response to treatment. Hum Pathol 8:391, 1977.

86. Sordillo P, Epremian B, Koziner B, et al: Lymphomatoid granulomatosis: An analysis of clinical and immunologic characteristics. Cancer 49:2070, 1982.

87. Tanaka Y, Sasaki Y, Kurozumi H, et al: Angiocentric immunoproliferative lesion associated with chronic active Epstein-Barr virus infection in an 11-year-old boy. Am J Surg Pathol 18:623, 1994.

88. Taniere P, Thivolet-Béjui F, Vitrey D, et al: Lymphomatoid granulomatosis – a report on four cases: Evidence for B phenotype of the tumoral cells. Eur Respir J 12:102, 1998.

89. Wilson WH, Kingma DW, Raffild M, et al: Association of lymphomatoid granulomatosis with Epstein-Barr viral infection of B lymphocytes and response to interferon-α2b. Blood 87:4531, 1996.

90. Yousem S, Weiss L, Colby T: Primary pulmonary Hodgkin's disease: A clinicopathologic study of 15 cases. Cancer 57:1217, 1986.

Miscellaneous Lymphoid Lesions

91. Craig FE, Gulley ML, Banks PE: Posttransplantation lymphoproliferative disorders. Am J Clin Pathol 99:265, 1993.

92. Ferreri AJM, Campo E, Seymour JF, et al: Intravascular lymphoma: Clinical presentation, natural history, management and prognostic factors in a series of 38 cases, with special emphasis on the "cutaneous variant". Br J Haematol 127:173, 2004.

93. Ferry JA, Harris NL, Picker LJ, et al: Intravascular lymphomatosis (malignant angioendotheliomatosis): A B-cell neoplasm expressing surface homing receptors. Mod Pathol 1:444, 1988.

94. Gracey D, DeRemee R, Colby T, Unni K, Weiland L: Benign lymphocytic angiitis and granulomatosis: Experience with three cases. Mayo Clin Proc 63:323, 1988.

94a. Halkos ME, Miller JI, Mann KP, et al: Thoracic presentations of post-transplant lymphoproliferative disorders. Chest 126:2013, 2004.

95. Kowal-Vern A, Swinnen L, Pyle J, et al: Characterization of postcardiac transplant lymphomas: Histology, immunophenotyping, immunohistochemistry, and gene rearrangement. Arch Pathol Lab Med. 120:41, 1996.

96. Myers J, Peiper S, Katzenstein A: Pulmonary involvement in infectious mononucleosis: Histopathologic features and detection of Epstein-Barr virus related DNA sequences. Mod Pathol 2:444, 1989.

97. Ramalingam P, Rybicki L, Smith MD, et al: Posttransplant lymphoproliferative disorders in lung transplant patients: The Cleveland Clinic experience. Mod Pathol 15:647, 2002.

98. Ray P, Antoine M, Mary-Krause M, et al: AIDS-related primary pulmonary lymphoma. Am J Respir Crit Care Med 158:1221, 1998.

99. Reams BD, McAdams HP, Howell DN, et al: Posttransplant lymphoproliferative disorder: Incidence, presentation, and response to treatment in lung transplant recipients. Chest 124:1242, 2003.

100. Rush WL, Andriko JW, Taubenberger JK, et al: Primary anaplastic large cell lymphoma of the lung: A clinicopathologic study of five patients. Mod Pathol 13:1285, 2000.

101. Sepp N, Schuler G, Romani N, et al: "Intravascular lymphomatosis" (angioendotheliomatosis): Evidence for a T-cell origin in two cases. Hum Pathol 21:1051, 1990.

102. Snyder LS, Harmon KR, Estensen RD: Intravascular lymphomatosis (malignant angioendotheliomatosis) presenting as pulmonary hypertension. Chest 96:1199, 1989.

103. Tukiainen H, Terho EO, Syrjanen K, Sutinen S: Benign lymphocytic angiitis and granulomatosis. Thorax 43:649, 1988.

104. Vergier B, Capron F, Trojani M, et al. Benign lymphocytic angiitis and granulomatosis: A T-cell lymphoma? Hum Pathol 23:1191, 1992.

105. Weiss M, Rolfes D, Alvira M, Cohen L: Benign lymphocytic angiitis and granulomatosis: A case report with evidence of an autoimmune etiology. Am J Clin Pathol 8:110, 1984.

106. Wick MR, Mills SE, Scheithauer BW, Cooper PH, Davitz MA, Parkinson K: Reassessment of malignant "angioendotheliomatosis": Evidence in favor of its reclassification as "intravascular lymphomatosis". Am J Surg Pathol 10:112, 1986.

107. Yousem SA, Colby TV: Intravascular lymphomatosis presenting in the lung. Cancer 65:349, 1990.

108. Yousem SA, Randhawa P, Locker J, et al: Posttransplant lymphoproliferative disorders in heart-lung transplant recipients: Primary presentation in the allograft. Hum Pathol 20:361, 1989.

10

INFECTION I. UNUSUAL PNEUMONIAS

Most pneumonias are caused by common pyogenic bacteria, respiratory viruses, or mycoplasma and are diagnosed by a combination of clinical and laboratory studies, including sputum cultures and serologic tests. Lung biopsy is usually not needed in these cases. Fulminant, life-threatening pneumonia, especially in immunocompromised patients, however, and pneumonia due to unusual organisms are likely to be biopsied, and selected examples of these infections are discussed in this chapter. Organisms that usually cause granulomatous inflammation are discussed in Chapter 11.

IDENTIFICATION OF ORGANISMS

Cultures

Samples of all lung biopsy specimens should be routinely cultured for organisms. In immunocompromised patients, cultures for all possible organisms need to be obtained, including aerobic and anaerobic bacteria, viruses, fungi, and mycobacteria. In nonimmunocompromised individuals, depending on the clinical situation, cultures can be more selective. Examination of a frozen section can be very helpful in this regard, since certain histologic reactions will indicate or exclude some organisms; that is, if granulomatous inflammation is seen, there is no need for viral or ordinary bacterial cultures. Likewise, if a chronic interstitial pneumonia is found, only viral cultures need to be taken, and one may even argue against the need for this. It should be emphasized, however, *if there is any question about the need for a particular culture, it should be performed.* While histologic techniques, if carefully executed, are an excellent means of demonstrating organisms and more sophisticated methods are available using fixed tissue, cultures remain essential, not only for definitive identification of the organism but also for drug sensitivity testing. For optimal culture results, a representative piece of the involved lung tissue, rather than a cotton swab scraping of the affected area, should be sent to the microbiology laboratory.

Special Stains and Other Techniques for Identifying Organisms in Tissue

Special stains for bacteria, acid-fast bacilli, and fungi should be examined in all cases in which an infectious etiology is suspected either because inflammatory changes are seen histologically or because there is a suggestive history (as in immunocompromised patients).[1,2,6] The Brown–Brenn and Brown–Hopps tissue Gram stains are equally useful for identifying pyogenic bacteria. The authors prefer the Ziehl–Neelsen (AFB) stain for demonstrating acid-fast bacilli, but fluorescent techniques (auramine–rhodamine stain) are equally useful. We consider the Grocott–Gomori methenamine silver (GMS) stain to be most reliable for highlighting fungi and pneumocystis, and modified silver stains that can be performed rapidly are available.[8] The Fontana–Masson stain is useful for identifying melanin-containing fungi, such as cryptococci and dematiaceous organisms, although it is not specific.[4] Other stains such as the PAS–Gridley may also be useful for identifying fungi, but we have found them to produce less consistent results. *The PAS (periodic acid–Schiff) stain without a counterstain should not be used as an initial screening procedure*, however, since it does not adequately differentiate organisms from background necrosis and debris. It can be useful for delineating the internal structural details of some organisms after they have been detected with silver stains. Other techniques utilizing calcofluor white[5] and lectin histochemistry[3] have been described but are not widely used.

Immunohistochemical techniques utilizing specific antibodies can be performed on formalin-fixed tissue and can enhance the pathologist's accuracy in identifying organisms in tissue specimens.[9] The most useful commercially available antibodies include those against cytomegalovirus (CMV), herpes simplex virus, toxoplasma, certain serogroups of *Legionella*, and *Pneumocystis carinii* (see further on). Additional techniques utilizing in situ hybridization and the polymerase chain reaction (PCR) are also available and have been applied to a variety of infections.[7]

PNEUMONIA IN IMMUNO-COMPROMISED PATIENTS

Individuals may be immunocompromised because of a congenital immunologic deficiency or, more commonly,

an acquired defect in the immune system. The presence of an underlying malignancy, another debilitating disease, human immunodeficiency virus (HIV) infection, or the use of steroid or cytotoxic therapy in treating a malignant or autoimmune disease or organ transplantation are the usual causes of acquired immunodeficiency. Immunocompromised patients are susceptible to infection from a wide variety of organisms.[11,13–15] Many infections are due to *opportunistic pathogens* that cause serious disease only in patients with an abnormal immune response and are relatively harmless to immunologically intact individuals. Pyogenic bacteria are the most commonly encountered pathogens and include a variety of Gram-negative and Gram-positive organisms. Pneumonias caused by these bacteria are not likely to require biopsy, however, since the diagnosis can usually be made from smears and cultures of sputum or tracheobronchial secretions. *Malacoplakia* (see Chapter 12) is one exception in which diagnosis is invariably based on tissue examination. It occurs rarely in the lung in immunocompromised patients, and *E. coli*, *Klebsiella*, and *Rhodococcus equi* are the usual causative organisms.[10] Other opportunistic pathogens, such as *P. carinii*, some fungi (especially *Aspergillus*, *Mucor*, and *Candida*), and certain viruses such as herpesvirus and CMV are often diagnosed by lung biopsy, and are discussed in this chapter. In addition to opportunistic pathogens, organisms that are pathogenic in immunologically intact individuals can also infect immunocompromised patients and may require lung biopsy for diagnosis, including mycobacteria and fungi (see Chapter 11). The incidence of these various infectious agents will differ among institutions and depends both on geographic location and on the nature of the patient's underlying immunologic deficiency.[14]

In interpreting lung biopsy specimens from immunocompromised patients, it is important to remember that abnormalities in these patients' immune systems are usually reflected histologically as well as clinically, and, therefore, *inflammatory responses that would be expected in immunologically intact individuals may be altered or absent*.[12] That is, there may be little or no inflammatory reaction to fungi or bacteria which under usual conditions would cause granuloma formation or acute inflammation, for example, and diffuse alveolar damage (DAD) (see Chapter 2) is often the only histologic reaction. It is imperative, therefore, to examine routinely special stains for organisms, including Gram stain, AFB, and GMS, in all immunocompromised patients, regardless of the type or amount of tissue reaction produced.

Identification of the organisms by the pathologist is especially important in this situation, since dissemination may occur rapidly and therapy usually must be instituted before the results of the cultures are known.

VIRAL PNEUMONIAS

Viruses are a common cause of pneumonia in early childhood.[16] They are implicated less frequently in serious lung infections in adults, although they are an important cause of pneumonia in certain groups of immunocompromised individuals. Many viruses can be identified in biopsy material by examining the tissue response and cytopathic changes.[17,19] Immunohistochemistry, in situ hybridization and PCR techniques can be used to identify many viruses and have largely replaced electron microscopy in this function.[9,18,28,82,87] The following sections review selected viral pneumonias that are likely to be encountered on lung biopsy

specimens. The important diagnostic features of these infections are summarized in Table 10–1.

Cytomegalovirus

CMV pneumonia occurs predominantly in immunocompromised patients, among whom recipients of bone marrow transplants, heart–lung, and other solid-organ transplants are especially susceptible.[20,21,24,27,44,46] A high incidence also occurs in HIV-infected individuals, and this situation is discussed further in Chapter 12. Rare cases have been reported in immunocompetent individuals.[26,33,39] Mortality rates are usually high, and rapid diagnosis is necessary so that antiviral therapy can be promptly instituted.

Clinical Features

Patients with CMV pneumonia usually present with fever, dyspnea, nonproductive cough, and diffuse chest infiltrates. Localized infiltrates have been described

Table 10–1 Viral Pneumonias: Diagnostic Light and Electron Microscopic Features

Virus	Inclusions (Nuclear/ Cytoplasmic)	Cellular Alteration	Tissue Reaction	Diagnostic Ultrastructural Features
Cytomegalovirus	Yes/Yes	Cytomegaly	Interstitial pneumonia; DAD	100–200 nm particle with round core, double membrane
Herpes simplex Varicella-zoster	Yes/No	Rare multinucleation	DAD; necrosis	150–200 nm particle with round core, double membrane
Measles	Yes/Yes	Multinucleation	Interstitial pneumonia; DAD	15–20 nm tubular filaments
Adenovirus	Yes/No	Smudge cells	Necrotizing bronchiolitis; DAD	60–90 nm icosahedral particles in crystalline array
Influenza	No/No	None	DAD, necrotizing bronchiolitis, BOOP	–
Respiratory syncytial virus	No/Yes	Occasional multinucleation	Necrotizing bronchiolitis, interstitial pneumonia	–
Parainfluenza virus	No/Yes	Frequent multinucleation	DAD; interstitial pneumonia	–
Hantavirus	No/No	None	Edema, early DAD	–
SARS coronavirus	No/No	None	DAD	60–95 nm spherical particles with spike-like projections

Abbreviations: DAD = diffuse alveolar damage; BOOP = bronchiolitis obliterans–organizing pneumonia; SARS = severe acute respiratory syndrome.

rarely.[33,39] Diagnosis often requires tissue examination, and percutaneous aspirations, transbronchial lung biopsies, and open lung biopsies have all been effective. Examination of bronchoalveolar lavage (BAL) fluids may also establish the diagnosis.[25,30,38,41,49] Although viral cultures are more sensitive for diagnosis than is microscopic examination of tissue, they tend to be relatively slow even with the development of rapid culture techniques.[20,27,28] Additionally, they cannot distinguish between subclinical infection and disease.[49]

Histologic Features

The diagnostic histologic feature of CMV infection is cellular enlargement combined with intranuclear and intracytoplasmic inclusions. The intranuclear inclusions are central, dark purple, Feulgen-positive bodies that are separated from the surrounding chromatin by a clear halo (Fig. 10–1; see also Figs 12–6 and 12–7). The cytoplasmic inclusions that are found in many, but not all, infected cells appear as coarse, basophilic granules. They contain a mucopolysaccharide envelope that stains with PAS and is Feulgen-negative.[21,37] They may also stain positively with GMS and should not be confused with other organisms (Fig. 10–1b).[29] Alveolar macrophages, alveolar lining cells, endothelial cells,

various interstitial cells, and bronchiolar epithelium may all be involved.[24] The number of inclusions seen by light microscopy is thought to roughly correlate with viral titers, but inclusions may be absent from some cases in which viral culture results are positive.[24,36] Ultrastructurally, the intranuclear inclusions are composed of viral particles within a dense reticular matrix (Fig. 10–1b, *inset*). The viral particles measure 100 to 200 nm in diameter and consist of a clear to granular, round core surrounded by a double membrane.[19,34,37]

Most cases of CMV infection show a focal or diffuse interstitial pneumonia in addition to the characteristically altered cells (Fig. 10–2).[20,24,36] DAD with hyaline membranes, a proteinaceous alveolar exudate, and sometimes intraalveolar hemorrhage is a common associated finding. Necrosis is usually not prominent. A necrotizing type of *tracheobronchitis* due to CMV infection has been described in patients with AIDS.[31,51] Sometimes, cytomegaly and inclusions are found without other associated abnormalities, and their significance is uncertain.[20] A variety of other infectious agents, including different types of bacteria, fungi, and even other viruses, may be associated with CMV pneumonia; *P. carinii* (see further on) is especially common.[36,41,44]

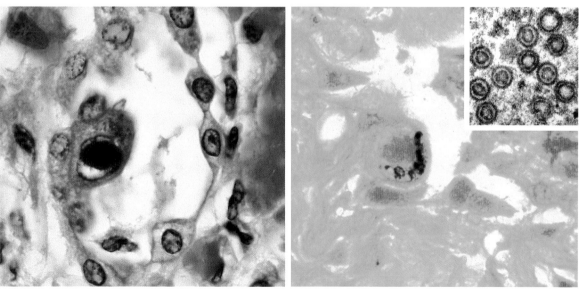

(a)   (b)

Figure 10–1 Cytomegalovirus. (a) High magnification view showing enlarged cell (compare with adjacent normal-sized alveolar pneumocytes) containing intranuclear and intracytoplasmic inclusions. The intranuclear inclusion appears purple and is separated from the nuclear membrane by a clear space. The cytoplasmic inclusions are coarsely granular and basophilic. **(b)** Staining of the cytoplasmic inclusions of a CMV-infected cell with GMS. This staining occurs because the cytoplasmic inclusions have a mucopolysaccharide coat. Inset is an electron micrograph of CMV particles. Note the central core surrounded by a double membrane.

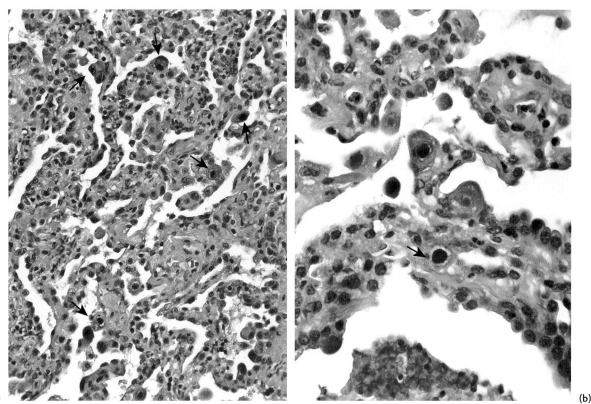

(a)   (b)

Figure 10–2 CMV pneumonia. (a) Low magnification showing nonspecific type of chronic interstitial pneumonia. Enlarged, CMV-infected alveolar pneumocytes can be appreciated even at low magnification (arrows). **(b)** Higher magnification showing typical CMV-infected pneumocytes lining thickened alveolar septa. An infected cell is present in the interstitium as well (arrow).

Monoclonal and polyclonal antibodies to CMV are commercially available, and, therefore, immunofluorescence or immunoperoxidase staining techniques can be used to confirm the diagnosis.[25,41,50] In situ hybridization can also be performed and may be more sensitive.[18,23,30,48] This technique has been used in a few cases to detect CMV infection in asymptomatic patients before cytopathic changes are evident.[47] A combined, two-color staining technique using in situ hybridization followed by immunostaining for CMV antigen has been described.[43,53] The PCR technique has also been utilized.[22,32,35,40,42] It is not at all clear, however, whether any of these techniques offer significantly increased sensitivity over careful examination of hematoxylin and eosin (H and E)-stained sections.[32,45,48,50]

Herpes Simplex Virus

Herpes simplex is an uncommon cause of respiratory tract infection that usually occurs in patients who have an underlying debilitating disease or are immuno-suppressed.[54,56–60] Burn patients are particularly susceptible to this infection.[59] The lungs and/or tracheobronchial tree may be affected by the process.

Herpes pneumonia is a form of necrotizing bronchopneumonia that results from aspiration of the organism into the lungs from the oral cavity or upper airways. Patients with prolonged intubation, for example, may develop herpetic laryngeal ulcers, herpes tracheobronchitis, and eventually bronchopneumonia. Herpes simplex virus is commonly identified in tracheobronchial secretions of patients undergoing mechanical ventilation for the adult respiratory distress syndrome.[62] In immunocompromised individuals, organisms from an oral herpes ulcer may be aspirated into the tracheobronchial tree, with subsequent tracheobronchitis and pneumonia. Mortality rates in patients with herpes pneumonia are high, and most cases are diagnosed at autopsy.

Examples of isolated *herpes tracheobronchitis* without involvement of distal lung parenchyma have been rarely described in patients without a history of prior intubation and with no known underlying disease.[56,61] These individuals may present with wheezing, dyspnea, or fever. *Neonatal pneumonia* due to herpes simplex has also been reported.[55,57] It usually is a component of disseminated herpes viral infection, but rarely it may be seen as an isolated finding.

Histologic Features

Herpes simplex pneumonia is characterized by patchy, nodular, or confluent foci of necrosis that usually are centered around bronchioles (Fig. 10–3).[58,59] Ghosts of alveolar septa are frequently seen in these areas, and an eosinophilic, proteinaceous exudate, containing remnants of karyorrhectic neutrophils and other cellular debris, is present within the necrotic areas. The surrounding alveoli may show DAD with prominent hyaline membranes. Intranuclear inclusions are characteristic and can be found in the alveolar lining cells

or alveolar macrophages at the edge of the necrotic zones, although they may be difficult to identify when necrosis is extensive. The inclusions consist of two morphologic forms (Fig. 10–4). One is characterized by an eosinophilic, ground glass change in the affected nuclei, which are often irregularly shaped and contain a thin, peripheral rim of condensed chromatin. The other is a Cowdry A type inclusion that consists of a round, eosinophilic central body separated from the surrounding nuclear chromatin by a clear halo. Multinucleated giant cells containing characteristic inclusions are occasionally seen but are not common. In contrast to CMV infection, the cells in herpes pneumonia are not enlarged, their nuclear inclusions are red rather than purple or basophilic, and cytoplasmic inclusions are absent. Ultrastructurally, the viral particles are similar to CMV (Fig. 10–4, *right inset*), measuring from 150 to 200 nm and consisting of a

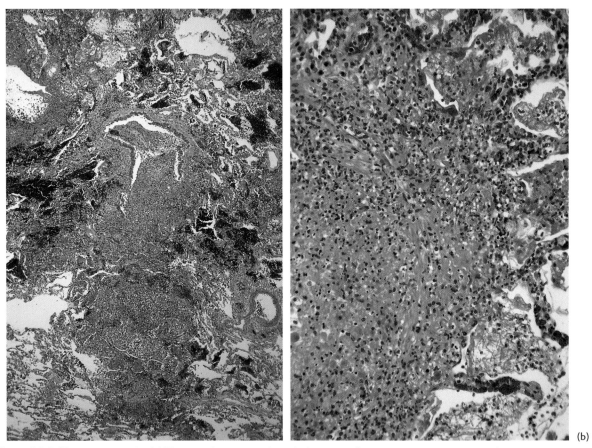

(a)

(b)

Figure 10–3 Herpes pneumonia. (a) The typical necrotizing bronchiolocentric inflammatory reaction is seen in this photomicrograph. Note that the bronchioles in the center are partially destroyed by the inflammatory reaction which extends into adjacent parenchyma. **(b)** Higher magnification showing the prominent karyorrhexis that is typical of this infection.

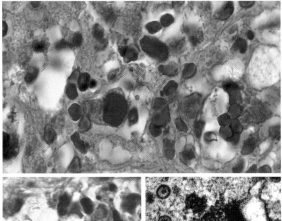
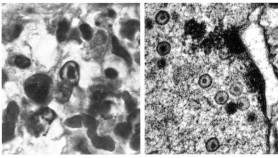

Figure 10–4 **Herpes pneumonia.** Ground glass intranuclear inclusion. Note the peripheral rim of condensed chromatin surrounding the dark purple inclusion. Left inset shows a Cowdry type A intranuclear inclusion characterized by a central eosinophilic inclusion surrounded by a clear zone. The right inset is an electron micrograph showing the typical round particles of herpesvirus.

central core surrounded by a double membrane.[19,57] Immunofluorescent or immunoperoxidase staining using antibodies to herpesvirus may help confirm the diagnosis in difficult cases.[54,57,60] In situ hybridization and the PCR technique are additional methods that can be utilized.[40,48,53]

A necrotizing tracheobronchitis accompanies herpes pneumonia in most cases and rarely occurs as an isolated finding (see previous section).[56,61] This lesion is characterized by ulceration of the airway epithelium and deposition of a fibrinous, purulent exudate over the denuded surface (Fig. 10–5). The characteristic intranuclear inclusions can be identified within viable cells located in adjacent intact mucosa or in underlying mucous glands.

Although most examples of herpes pneumonia show a striking peribronchiolar distribution due to the fact that the infection is spread via the airways, occasional cases lack this distribution.[58] These variants reflect the less common hematogenous spread of infection.

Neonatal pneumonia most commonly occurs by this mechanism.[55,57]

Varicella-Zoster

Varicella virus, the agent of chickenpox, is indistinguishable from the herpes zoster virus that causes herpes zoster, or shingles – hence the name varicella-zoster.[64] Chickenpox predominantly affects young children, whereas herpes zoster occurs only in individuals who have had previous varicella-zoster virus infection (chickenpox).

Clinical Features

Pneumonic infiltrates occur in approximately 15% of patients with chickenpox, most of whom are adults.[71] Children who develop varicella pneumonia usually are immunocompromised or otherwise debilitated, whereas in adults this complication occurs as frequently in immunocompetent as in immunocompromised individuals. In all cases, the generalized skin rash of chickenpox occurs 1 day or more before the onset of pulmonary involvement. Dyspnea, cough, and fever are common presenting complaints, and a diffuse nodular infiltrate is seen on chest roentgenograms. Mortality ranges from 10% to 30%; the higher mortality occurs in immunosuppressed patients and pregnant women.[71]

Disseminated herpes zoster is seen predominantly in immunocompromised patients or in those with underlying malignant disease.[63–65,68,70] Individuals with Hodgkin's disease are particularly predisposed to this condition. It usually is characterized by skin dissemination. Lung involvement is an uncommon complication, and mortality is low.

Histopathologic Features

The histopathologic appearance of varicella-zoster pneumonia is similar to that of herpes simplex pneumonia. Foci of necrosis, often located in peribronchiolar parenchyma, are common, and there is associated DAD with interstitial pneumonia, hyaline membranes, and proteinaceous intraalveolar exudates.[71] Intranuclear inclusions that are indistinguishable from those caused by herpes simplex are found in the alveolar lining cells. Rare cases with giant cell formation have been reported.[69] Healing of the pneumonic process is followed by diffuse pulmonary calcification in some cases.[67] Persistent minute necrotic nodules have also been described following recovery from varicella pneumonia.[66]

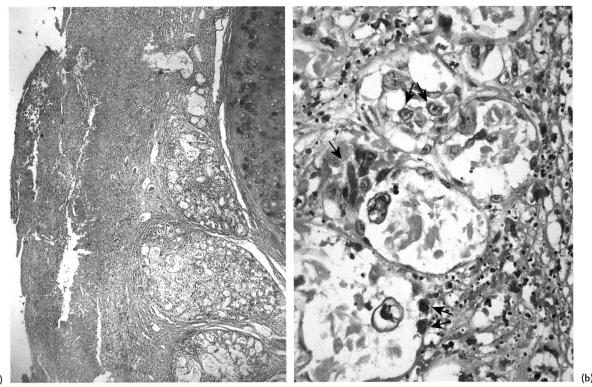

(a)   (b)

Figure 10–5 Herpes tracheobronchitis. (a) Extensive ulceration of tracheal mucosa (left) with thick necrotic exudate covering the surface. **(b)** Higher magnification showing typical inclusions in the tracheal mucous glands (arrows).

Measles Virus

Clinical Features

Clinically apparent pneumonia is an uncommon complication of measles infection, and death in such cases is rare. The disorder usually occurs in immunocompromised children, with a few cases reported in immunocompromised adults.[72,75,76,79] A skin rash is usually present. Occasionally, cases without a rash occur, and are referred to as *giant cell pneumonia*.[77,78]

Histopathologic Features

The most characteristic morphologic feature of measles pneumonia is the presence of large multinucleated giant cells containing eosinophilic, Feulgen-negative intranuclear and intracytoplasmic inclusions (Fig. 10–6).[77–79] These cells, which possess from a few to up to 60 nuclei within abundant pink cytoplasm, are thought to be formed from the fusion of type 2 alveolar lining cells. They are found predominantly in the alveolar spaces and often line the alveolar septa. Ultrastructurally, the viral inclusions are composed of tightly packed tubules measuring from 15 to 20 nm in diameter and having

6-nm cross-striations when viewed longitudinally (see Fig. 10–6b, *inset*).[19,73,75,77] They have been identified within endothelial cells and macrophages in addition to alveolar lining cells. Associated histologic changes include DAD with hyaline membranes and an intra-alveolar proteinaceous exudate.[74,75] Focal necrosis may occur, and squamous metaplasia of bronchial epithelium has also been reported.

Other viruses can occasionally cause pneumonia containing multinucleated giant cells, including varicella-zoster, parainfluenza, and respiratory syncytial virus (RSV).[69,101,106,123,131] Varicella-zoster is distinguished by the lack of intracytoplasmic inclusions, and RSV and parainfluenza by the lack of intranuclear inclusions. Although these pneumonias are sometimes referred to as giant cell pneumonia, this term is generally reserved for cases due to measles.

Adenovirus

Clinical Features

Infection with adenovirus is usually manifested by minor flu-like symptoms and upper respiratory tract

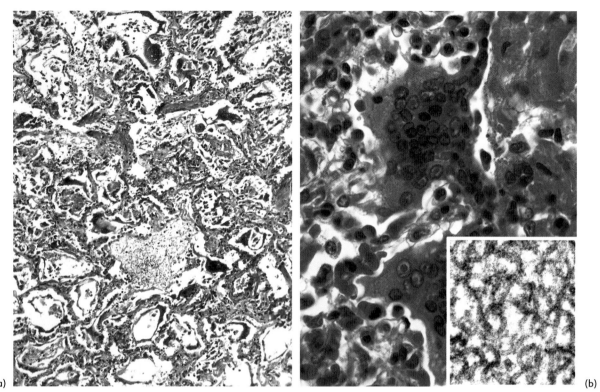

(a)

(b)

Figure 10–6 Measles pneumonia. (a) Low magnification showing DAD with prominent alveolar pneumocyte hyperplasia and remnants of hyaline membranes. A striking additional finding is the presence of numerous large multinucleated giant cells lining alveolar septa. **(b)** Higher magnification of multinucleated cells showing prominent eosinophilic intranuclear inclusions. Inset is an electron micrograph showing the typical tubular structure of the viral particles (×113,000, courtesy of Dr Eduardo Yunis).

involvement suggestive of the 'common cold'. Pneumonia is a rare complication that is fatal in up to 40% of patients. Most fatalities occur in children under 1 year old,[83,93,95,97] but deaths of adults have been reported, including both previously healthy[85,89] and immunocompromised individuals.[88,91,92,99] Neonatal cases have also been reported and are associated with high mortality rates.[81,86,90,94] Some cases of adenovirus, especially in children, may follow a measles infection.[95] Disseminated infection to extrathoracic organs has been described in neonates and immunocompromised patients.[81,88,90]

Histologic Features

The histologic hallmark of adenovirus pneumonia is a combination of bronchiolar necrosis with associated necrotizing bronchopneumonia and characteristic intranuclear inclusions.[83,92,94,95] The bronchiolar epithelium may be sloughed, and the necrosis often extends into the wall and adjacent parenchyma (Fig. 10–7). The bronchiolar lumens may become filled

with granular eosinophilic debris from the necrotic cells, and distal air trapping may occur secondary to bronchiolar occlusion. Necrosis often extends into peribronchiolar alveoli, and DAD with hyaline membranes and intraalveolar proteinaceous exudation is a common accompanying finding (Fig. 10–8).

Two types of intranuclear inclusions occur, and they are found in both bronchiolar epithelium and alveolar lining cells. The most characteristic one is a homogeneous, amphophilic or basophilic, Feulgen-positive mass that almost completely fills the nucleus (see Fig. 10–9). Cells with such inclusions are termed *smudge cells*. They are often enlarged and darkly stained and usually are easily visualized at low magnification. The second type of inclusion is a round, eosinophilic, Feulgen-negative body separated from the surrounding chromatin by a clear halo. It is smaller and less distinctly demarcated than the Cowdry A type inclusion that is characteristic of herpesvirus. Ultrastructurally, the inclusions are composed of hexagonal particles measuring 60 to 90 nm in diameter (Fig. 10–9b).[80,86,91,93,95]

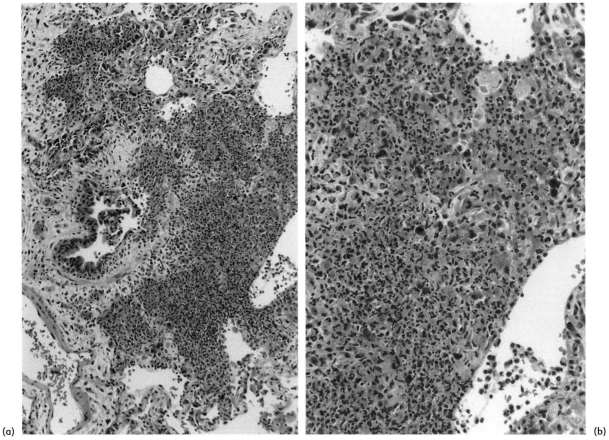

(a) (b)

Figure 10–7 Adenovirus pneumonia. (a) At low magnification the typical bronchiolocentric necrotizing inflammatory process is appreciated. Note the ulceration and partial destruction of the bronchiole in the center. **(b)** Higher magnification showing the acute inflammatory infiltrate with prominent karyorrhexis. Note the prominent 'smudge' cells admixed with the necrotic inflammatory cells.

They have a central dense core and an outer coat, and they are usually arranged in a lattice-like or crystalline pattern. As with other viruses, immunohistochemical techniques using specific antibodies are available, and in situ hybridization or the PCR technique can be used to confirm the diagnosis.[80,82,87,90,92,98]

In some cases, recovery from the acute illness is accompanied by peribronchiolar scarring and the development of constrictive bronchiolitis obliterans (obliterative bronchiolitis, see Chapter 16).[84] Such patients may have prolonged pulmonary impairment, with death occurring many months after the initial illness. There is also some evidence that adenovirus infections may be related to the development of other forms of chronic lung disease, such as bronchiectasis.[82,84,87,96,97]

The tissue reaction to adenovirus is similar to that in herpes pneumonia in that both are bronchiolocentric

necrotizing processes with prominent karyorrhexis. The characteristic smudge cells of adenovirus pneumonia differ from herpes-infected cells in that they are enlarged and the homogenous intranuclear inclusions lack a surrounding rim of condensed chromatin. In difficult cases, immunohistochemical stains or in situ hybridization may be needed to distinguish them. The clinical situation should also help, since herpes pneumonia occurs almost exclusively in immuno-compromised persons while adenovirus pneumonia can affect immunocompetent individuals.

Other Viruses

Influenza

The pathologic features of influenza pneumonia are well described in detailed autopsy studies carried out

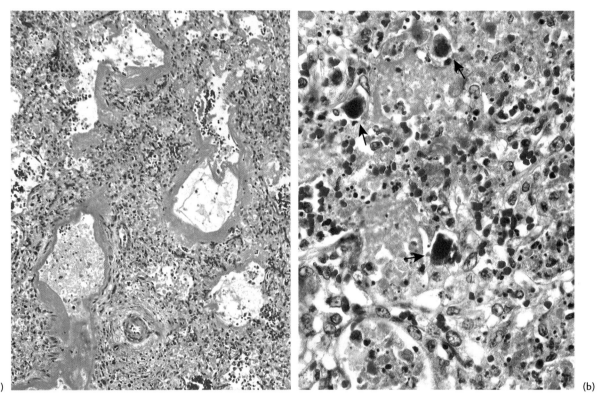

(a)   (b)

Figure 10–8 DAD in adenovirus pneumonia. (a) Prominent hyaline membranes are present along with karyorrhectic debris in the thickened interstitium. **(b)** Higher magnification showing the characteristic infected 'smudge' cells with nuclear inclusions (arrows).

during the 1918, 1957, and 1968 pandemics.[110] Occasionally, lung biopsy is performed for diagnosis, and pathologic findings have been reported in a few cases.[112,116,127,132] In fatal cases, DAD (see Chapter 2) is the usual pathologic finding and is characterized by edema, hemorrhage, and hyaline membranes. Necrotizing bronchitis and bronchiolitis may be prominent features, and secondary bacterial infection frequently occurs. Similar changes are found at lung biopsy, although they tend to be less severe. DAD is the most common finding, while a mild chronic interstitial pneumonia and bronchiolitis obliterans–organizing pneumonia (BOOP) have been noted occasionally.[132] By electron microscopy, filamentous, fibrillar structures have been observed within epithelial and endothelial cell nuclei, and granular inclusions have been described in the cytoplasm of some cells.[116,130] Chronic sequelae, including interstitial fibrosis, bronchiectasis, and bronchiolitis obliterans, have also been reported.[119]

Respiratory Syncytial Virus

RSV is a significant cause of respiratory infections in infants and young children.[100,111,114] Bronchiolitis, which may be severe, is the usual clinical manifestation, and mortality is low. The major histologic changes described at autopsy include necrotizing bronchiolitis and interstitial pneumonia or a combination of both.[100,106,109,117,120] The bronchial epithelium is usually sloughed, and necrotic debris fills the bronchial lumens. Necrosis of the alveolar walls and evidence of DAD may also occur. Histologic changes of giant cell pneumonia have been rarely described.[106] Small, round, eosinophilic intracytoplasmic inclusion bodies surrounded by a clear halo may be seen.[106,120]

Parainfluenza Virus

Parainfluenza virus is structurally similar to RSV and also shares clinical and epidemiologic similarities.[113] Four types have been identified, and type 3 is most often associated with respiratory tract infection.[125] Pulmonary infections occur mainly in infants and children, and tracheobronchitis and bronchiolitis are the usual manifestations. Pneumonia occurs less often and may be severe in immunocompromised individuals, including adults as well as children.[101,123,125,131] Pathologically, DAD and interstitial pneumonia are the most common

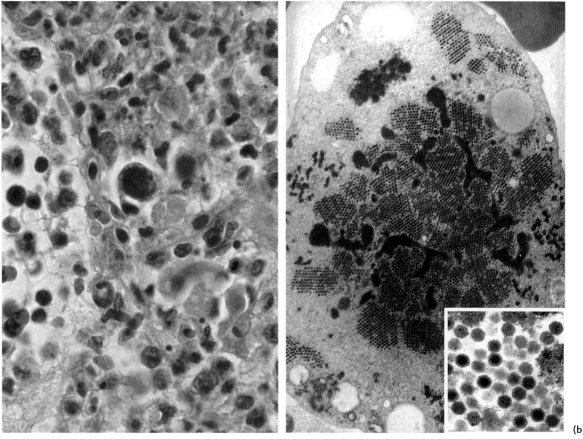

(a)
(b)

Figure 10–9 Adenovirus pneumonia. (a) High magnification of smudge cell. Note the purple inclusion that fills the nucleus. In contrast to the intranuclear inclusion of herpes pneumonia (compare with Fig. 10–4), there is no peripheral rim of condensed chromatin. (b) Electron micrograph showing hexagonal viral particles (inset, ×62,000) arranged in a lattice-like pattern. (Inset courtesy of Dr David Walker.)

findings, and there may be a prominent giant cell reaction. PAS-positive, eosinophilic intracytoplasmic inclusions have been described in most cases. Immunohistochemical staining can be performed with commercially available antibodies.[125]

Hantavirus

A highly publicized outbreak of severe respiratory illness occurred in the southwestern United States in May 1993, and cases have subsequently been reported from elsewhere in the Unites States and South America.[102,108,121,128] Archival studies have documented the existence of isolated cases of this disease as early as 1978.[134] The disease is due to various strains of hantavirus, and the major clinical manifestations are related to pulmonary involvement (hence the name *hantavirus pulmonary syndrome*).

Clinically, patients with hantavirus pulmonary syndrome present with fever, myalgias, and gastrointestinal complaints, followed in a few days by cough and dyspnea.[121] Hematologic abnormalities are often present, including thrombocytopenia, a left shift in the myeloid series, and the presence of large immunoblastic lymphoid cells. Bilateral chest infiltrates and respiratory failure develop rapidly. Mortality rates approach 75% in some series, and death usually occurs within the first 3 days after hospitalization.[108,121]

The main pathologic findings in autopsy cases are pulmonary edema and pleural effusion.[105,108,128] A mild interstitial pneumonia with delicate hyaline membranes has been described and fits with early DAD. Immature lymphoid cells are often seen in small blood vessels. Immunohistochemistry utilizing monoclonal antibodies or immune serum can confirm the diagnosis.[105,133,134]

Severe Acute Respiratory Syndrome (SARS) Coronavirus

An unusual atypical pneumonia was first observed in Guangdong Province in mainland China in November 2002, and within a few months it had spread to Hong Kong, Viet Nam, Singapore, Canada, and more than 30 countries worldwide.[129] The disease was highly infectious, and close contacts, including healthcare workers, were especially susceptible. Worsening respiratory status unresponsive to antibiotics and often culminating in the acute respiratory distress syndrome (ARDS) was the hallmark, and mortality rates approached 10–15%. Within a few months of its emergence, a novel coronavirus was identified as the causative organism and named SARS coronavirus. This virus is endemic in certain wild animals that were considered culinary delicacies in China (raccoon dogs and civets), and it is thought to have been transmitted from the animals to humans.

Clinically, patients generally present with fever, chills, myalgias, and malaise.[118,129] Cough is also common, but usually does not occur until several days after the onset.[124] Watery diarrhea may accompany the other findings, and lymphopenia is common. Ground glass opacities are usually present on chest computed tomography (CT) examinations. The diagnosis can be confirmed by reverse transcriptase polymerase chain reaction (RT-PCR) assays for viral RNA. Seroconversion with rising anti-SARS coronavirus antibodies is found after about 1 week. Although a minority of patients defervesce with resolution of the radiographic changes after a few days, most have persistent fever with increasing shortness of breath and worsening radiographic findings, and about 20–30% develop ARDS. There is some evidence that steroids together with ribavirin, a broad-spectrum antiviral agent, may be beneficial.[115]

Most pathologic studies from patients with SARS have been performed on autopsy specimens, with only a few open lung biopsies examined.[103,107,111,126] DAD is almost uniformly present, and both acute and organizing stages have been described depending on the length of time that elapsed after the onset. Viral inclusions are not observed by light microscopy, but electron microscopy demonstrates viral particles within the cytoplasm of alveolar pneumocytes.[103,107] The viruses are spherical and enveloped with spike-like surface projections, and they range in size from 60 to 95 nm. In situ hybridization techniques have demonstrated viral DNA in alveolar pneumocytes.[104]

FUNGAL PNEUMONIAS

This section reviews important fungal pneumonias that are likely to be encountered on lung biopsy specimens. The differentiating histologic features of the main organisms are summarized in Table 10–2. Although morphologic features can be helpful in distinguishing various fungal hyphae, microbiologic cultures are the most reliable method for definitive identification.[179]

Aspergillosis

Traditionally, aspergillus lung infection is divided into three forms: invasive, saprophytic (mycetomas), and allergic (Table 10–3). Several forms of invasive aspergillosis are recognized and are thought to comprise a spectrum of reactions that depend on a combination of patient immunologic status, underlying lung structure, and nature of exposure.[145,146] The various forms of invasive aspergillosis are discussed in the following

Table 10–2 Fungal Pneumonias: Contrasting Histologic Features

	Aspergillosis	Mucormycosis	Candidiasis	Torulopsis Infection
Organism Morphology				
Hyphae	Thin (3–5 μm), septate	Wide (10–15 μm), nonseptate	–	–
Branching	Dichotomous, 45°	Haphazard, 90°	–	–
Budding yeasts	–	–	+ (3–6 μm)	+ (2–4 μm)
Pseudohyphae	–	–	+	–
Tissue Reaction				
Vascular invasion, infarction	+	+	–	–
Acute inflammation, abscess	–	–	+	+

Table 10–3 Forms of Pulmonary Aspergillosis
Invasive aspergillosis
Aspergillus pneumonia
Necrotizing tracheobronchitis
Necrotizing granulomatous inflammation
Chronic necrotizing aspergillosis
Saprophytic infection
Mycetoma (Aspergilloma)
Allergic reaction
Allergic bronchopulmonary aspergillosis

section, while mycetomas are reviewed later on in this chapter, and allergic reactions are covered in Chapter 6.

Aspergillus Pneumonia

Aspergillus pneumonia is the most common form of invasive aspergillosis, and the two terms are often used synonymously. Aspergillus pneumonia occurs almost exclusively in patients who have an underlying malignancy or other debilitating disease or in patients who are otherwise immunosuppressed.[137,145,146,152,154,155,160,166,171,173,175] Individuals with acute leukemia are particularly susceptible to this infection, especially during periods of granulocytopenia.[160,175] Patients with chronic obstructive pulmonary disease (COPD) and cirrhosis, and individuals receiving prolonged corticosteroid therapy are also at increased risk for invasive aspergillosis.[158] The incidence of aspergillus infections in patients with AIDS appears to be increasing.[162] Rare cases of aspergillus pneumonia have been reported in previously healthy persons,[139,142,144,150,177] however, and saprophytic colonization of infarcted lung parenchyma has also been described.[140] The lung is the primary site of infection in most cases, and inhalation of airborne spores is thought to be the cause. *Aspergillus fumigatus*, *A. niger*, and *A. flavus* are the species most commonly involved. Concurrent infection with other organisms, both bacterial and fungal, is common.[160,163]

Clinical Features: The usual clinical manifestations of aspergillus pneumonia include fever, cough, chest pain, and, occasionally, hemoptysis.[138,160,164,182] Patchy infiltrates that may progress to dense consolidation are seen radiographically. The diagnosis is difficult to establish antemortem, since sputum cultures are usually negative.[137] Even if positive cultures are obtained, their significance may not be appreciated, since aspergillus species are common saprophytes in patients without

invasive disease. Serum enzyme-linked immunosorbent assays (ELISA) for galactomannan antigen, a polysaccharide component of the fungal wall, may be helpful, although a negative test does not exclude the diagnosis and false-positive tests occur.[158,170] PCR testing of BAL fluids for aspergillus DNA can also be performed.[169] It is associated with a high negative predictive value, but a low positive predictive value. A halo sign on chest CT examinations can be helpful but is present in only a minority of cases.[158] Tissue examination is the most reliable method for diagnosis, and the pathologist must be able to recognize the infection, since mortality rates are high and cure is possible only with early institution of antifungal therapy. In some patients following recovery from granulocytopenia, the lung infiltrates may evolve into cavitary lesions resembling fungus balls (see text following).[135,160,165]

Histologic Features: The classic tissue reaction in aspergillus pneumonia is hemorrhagic infarction with a sparse inflammatory cell infiltrate (Fig. 10–10).[145,160,164,182] Fungal hyphae are found invading blood vessel walls and permeating alveolar septa, and arterial lumens can be completely occluded by plugs of fungi. The amount of inflammation depends on the patient's immune status, and, in some cases, necrotizing bronchopneumonia containing a prominent neutrophil infiltrate may be seen.[164] This lesion may have a striking gross appearance characterized by a dark rim surrounding a central yellow–gray region and has been called a 'target lesion'.[164] It is thought to be a precursor of hemorrhagic infarcts, since vascular invasion is often present and progression to classic infarction has occasionally been documented. Invasion by the fungal hyphae through the bronchial walls is thought to be the initial event in aspergillus pneumonia. The organisms then enter the adjacent arteries, causing vascular occlusion and eventual parenchymal infarction.

Aspergillus organisms can be visualized in routine H and E-stained sections, in which they appear as pale blue elements. Also, they are well outlined by GMS and PAS stains. Morphologically, they are long, thin, septate mycelia that average 4 μm in diameter and have dichotomous, 45° branching points (see Table 10–2 and Fig. 10–11). The mycelia are typically arranged in parallel and radiate outward from a central point. Findings have been reported that help distinguish aspergillus species from other pathogenic fungi such as *Fusarium* and related organisms. These include more uniform branching and lack of adventitious sporulation, although the differentiating features may be difficult to

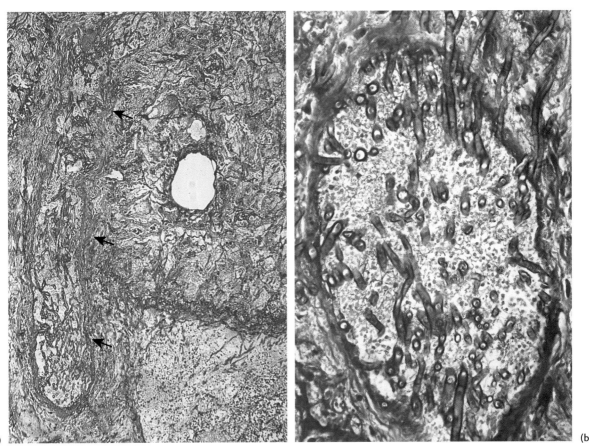

Figure 10–10 Invasive aspergillus pneumonia. (a) Extensive tissue invasion is seen at low magnification, with infarction and minimal inflammation. Note the artery at left (arrows) that is filled with organisms. **(b)** Vascular invasion by the fungal hyphae is seen in this artery at higher magnification.

interpret.[156,179] Immunohistochemistry utilizing monoclonal antibodies may be helpful in identifying them.[168]

Other Forms of Invasive Aspergillosis

Necrotizing tracheobronchitis is a less common form of invasive aspergillosis that, like aspergillus pneumonia, usually occurs in patients with some form of immune compromise.[143,148,153,160,163,167,182] It is characterized by extensive ulceration of the trachea and bronchi and colonization by fungal hyphae, often with superficial invasion of the wall. Sometimes, a pseudomembrane containing numerous organisms is prominent (so-called *pseudomembranous tracheobronchitis*).[148,167] In lung transplant recipients, the changes may be localized to the transplanted side and usually involve the anastomosis line.[153,158] Patients commonly present with fever, dyspnea, wheezing, cough, or hemoptysis, although some are asymptomatic. Chest radiographs may be normal. Respiratory failure and death rapidly ensue in

most cases, although early treatment can be curative. Localized, superficial aspergillus infection of a bronchial stump following lobectomy has also been reported and may represent a related phenomenon.[172]

Rarely, a more limited form of invasive aspergillosis has been described in which *necrotizing granulomas* containing organisms are observed (Fig. 10–12).[161,176,178] This lesion occurs both in immunocompromised and in immunologically intact individuals. The granulomas resemble reactions that commonly occur in tuberculous or fungal infections, and the prognosis is good. A bronchocentric distribution to the granulomas appears to be characteristic, and there may be associated tissue eosinophilia.[157] A similar, often suppurative, granulomatous reaction has also been described in patients with underlying chronic granulomatous disease.[149,152]

Chronic necrotizing aspergillosis (also known as *semi-invasive aspergillosis*) is a chronic, indolent form of invasive aspergillosis that usually occurs in individuals

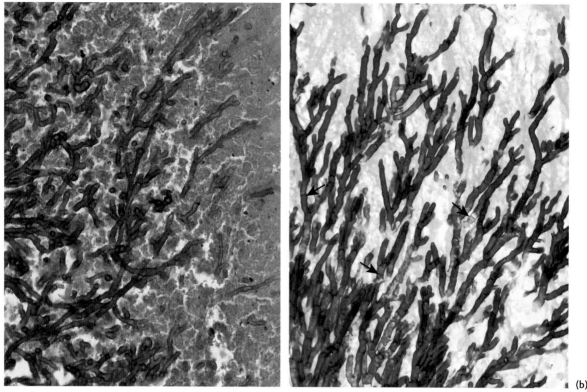

(a) (b)

Figure 10–11 Morphology of aspergillus hyphae. (a) The hyphae are easily seen in H and E-stained sections. Note that they are thin with dichotomous branching and appear relatively uniform. **(b)** The organisms are well outlined with GMS, in which the scattered septations (arrows) are better appreciated.

with underlying chronic lung disease, including COPD, or prior tuberculosis, as well as in persons with mild immune compromise such as diabetes mellitus, alcoholism, or corticosteroid treatment.[136,141,146,147,174,177,180] Patients generally present with fever and cough, and progressive cavitary lung infiltrates are seen radiographically. The course typically spans several months and may mimic tuberculosis clinically. The pathologic features are not well defined but appear to resemble mycetomas with superficial invasion of the wall. Necrotizing granulomatous inflammation is seen in some cases.[183] Vascular invasion and extensive parenchymal necrosis, however, are not features. Some of the cases of *invasive cavitary aspergillosis* in patients with cancer reported by Pai et al[165] and *aspergillosis in AIDS* patients reported by Wright et al[181] may represent variants of this form of aspergillosis.

Mucormycosis (Phycomycosis)

Mucormycosis refers to infection by fungi in the class Zygomycetes (formerly Phycomycetes) and the order Mucorales. The most common agents include the genera *Rhizopus* and *Mucor*. Pulmonary mucormycosis shares many clinical and pathologic features with invasive aspergillus pneumonia. It is found almost exclusively in patients with underlying diseases, especially leukemia, lymphoma, and diabetes mellitus,[185,187–189,191] but has also been reported in previously healthy individuals.[186,190,192] The usual clinical manifestations are fever, chest pain, and patchy pulmonary infiltrates. Massive hemoptysis occurs occasionally, and mortality is high. Sputum cultures are rarely positive, and even direct cultures of lung tissue may be negative.

The characteristic pathologic features are extensive parenchymal and vascular invasion by mycelia, with resultant hemorrhagic infarction and minimal cellular infiltration (see Table 10–2).[188] The organisms can be differentiated from aspergillus because they are wider, averaging 10 to 15 μm in diameter, and are nonseptate (Fig. 10–13). They frequently are fragmented and have irregular branching points, often at 90° angles, which is in contrast to the regular, dichotomous, 45° branching of aspergillus. They also are haphazardly scattered

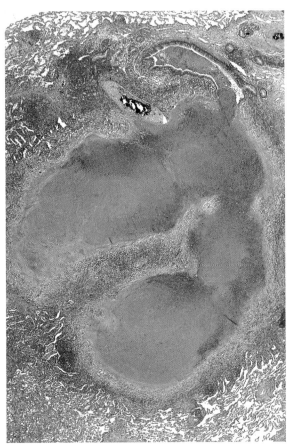

Figure 10–12 Necrotizing granulomatous inflammation in invasive aspergillosis. Note the bronchiolocentric distribution of the process that follows the branching pattern of the parent bronchiole (top).

within the tissues, unlike the more orderly arrangement of aspergillus. Although they stain well with PAS and appear basophilic with H and E stains, they often stain only weakly with silver preparations. Identification can be facilitated by lectin histochemistry or immunofluorescent staining using a specific antibody.[184,185] Occasionally, large, round to oval chlamydoconidia are found in addition to hyphal elements, and they should not be confused with other organisms.[185,186]

Candidiasis

Candida is a common cause of fungal infection in immunocompromised patients, and *C. albicans* or *C. tropicalis* is the usual species that is isolated.[193,194,202,207] The organism may cause either superficial infection of the mucosal surfaces or deep disseminated infection involving multiple organs. Several factors, in addition

to malignancy and cytotoxic chemotherapy with myelosuppression, predispose the patient to the development of deep infections, including indwelling venous catheters, prolonged antibiotic therapy, severe burns, and major abdominal surgery.[194,197,201,204,205] Disseminated candidiasis may also occur in infants.[199,200]

Although the lungs are frequently involved in disseminated candidiasis, clinically significant pulmonary disease is uncommon, and primary candida pneumonia in the absence of disseminated candidiasis is rare.[195,198,202] Dubois et al[195] could attribute antemortem chest infiltrates to candidal infection in only two of 24 patients in whom pulmonary candidiasis was documented at autopsy. Moreover, there are no characteristic clinical features of pulmonary candidiasis. Since candida species frequently are saprophytes in the oral cavity, skin, and respiratory tree, especially in ventilated patients, the only definitive method of diagnosis is to identify the organisms in the tissue.[196]

Histopathologic Features

Two morphologic varieties of pulmonary candidiasis have been described.[195,202,206] One is caused by *hematogenous* spread in cases of disseminated candidiasis and is characterized by small (2 to 4 mm) miliary nodules randomly distributed in the pulmonary parenchyma. The nodules have central necrosis with varying amounts of acute inflammation, depending on whether the patient is granulocytopenic (Fig. 10–14). Clusters of both pseudohyphae and budding yeasts can be found in the center of the nodules (see Table 10–2). The pseudohyphae consist of elongated blastospores that are arranged in chains resembling sausage links, while the yeasts are round, ranging from 3 to 6 μm (Fig. 10–15). The organisms can be seen in H and E-stained slides, but they are better visualized with the GMS or PAS stain. They are also weakly Gram-positive. Immunohistochemical staining utilizing a specific monoclonal antibody may also be used to identify the organism.[203] Although fungal elements are occasionally found within small blood vessels, the extensive vascular invasion and parenchymal infarction characteristic of aspergillus pneumonia and mucormycosis are not seen.

The second form of pulmonary candidiasis is related to *aspiration* and is usually a terminal event of little clinical significance. Such cases are frequently associated with candidiasis involving the oral cavity, esophagus, larynx, or trachea. Distribution of the lesions around bronchioles is considered to be evidence of aspiration, and, frequently, vegetable matter or other gastric contents are also identified. There may

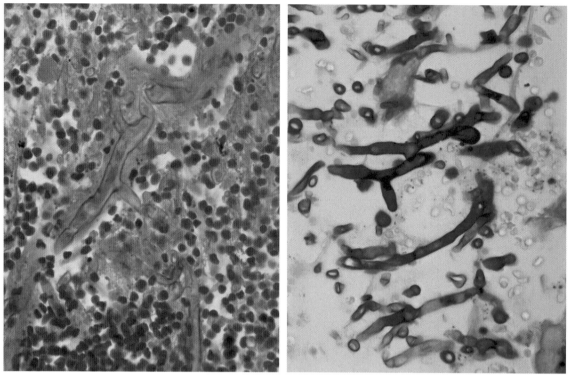

(a)

(b)

Figure 10–13 Mucormycosis. (a) The organisms are easily visible in H and E-stained sections, where they are wide with 90° branching and no septation (compare with aspergillus in Fig. 10–11). **(b)** They are well outlined with GMS, which emphasizes the irregular to 90° branching and the lack of septation.

be an associated acute inflammatory cell infiltrate with bronchopneumonia and abscess formation. In some cases, especially in preterminal aspiration, clusters of organisms are found within the airways with no associated inflammatory reaction.

Other Fungi

Torulopsis glabrata (Candida glabrata)

This organism (not to be confused with *Torula*, which is synonymous with *Cryptococcus neoformans*) is a saprophytic yeast that has been reported to cause fungemia and deep infection in immunocompromised individuals.[208,214] Lung involvement is generally secondary to disseminated disease, although primary pulmonary infection has been described.[208,214] Tissue necrosis with variable amounts of acute or chronic inflammation and, occasionally, microabscess formation are the usual histopathologic findings. The organisms are small, round to oval yeasts measuring 2 to 4 μm in diameter and showing numerous budding forms (see Table 10–2). They appear basophilic with

H and E stain and are well visualized with GMS or PAS stains. They differ from candida species because they are smaller and do not form pseudohyphae. They are also smaller and more uniform in size than *Cryptococcus neoformans*, and they lack its mucinous capsule. Although the organisms are similar in size to *Histoplasma capsulatum*, they show buds more frequently and do not cause the characteristic granulomatous response of this fungus (see Chapter 11).

Pseudallescheria boydii

The usual etiologic agent of *maduromycosis*, this fungus (previously known as *Allescheria boydii*) is a rare cause of pneumonia in immunocompromised or debilitated patients.[209,213,216,217] Parenchymal necrosis and abscess formation are the usual tissue responses. Morphologically, the organisms are septate hyphae that measure 2 to 5 μm in diameter and contain rounded ends. They grow in a disorganized pattern and form dense clusters. It is difficult to differentiate *Pseudallescheria boydii* from certain other fungi, especially aspergillus, on the basis of histologic findings alone, and cultures are necessary for confirmation. Correct identification is important

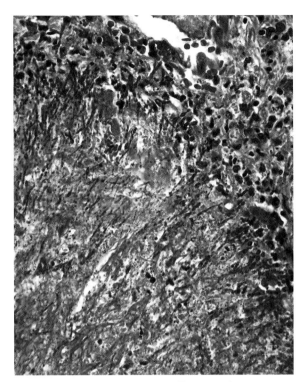

Figure 10–14 Candida pneumonia. This example is characterized by an abscess containing numerous organisms that are visible in the H and E-stained slide. A rim of necrotic inflammatory cells surrounds the central mass of organisms.

since *Pseudallescheria boydii* is often resistant to amphotericin, and treatment with imidazole derivatives may be more effective.[211]

Malassezia furfur

Malassezia furfur is a component of the normal microflora of adult skin, and it also causes the common superficial fungal infection *tinea versicolor*. Its growth requirements are unusual in that it needs an exogenous source of fatty acids. Rare examples of deep infection involving lung and other organs have been described in chronically ill patients.[210,212] All reported individuals had been receiving parenteral alimentation with Intralipid. The organism is a globoid- to elliptical-shaped, 2- to 4-μm yeast with broad-based unipolar buds. Characteristic ultrastructural features include thick multilayered walls with internal corrugations.

Mycetomas

Pulmonary mycetomas, or fungus balls, are generally considered to represent noninvasive or saprophytic growths of mycelia within a preexisting lung cavity.[145,146,182] The cavity may be related to a variety of underlying diseases, including chronic obstructive lung disease, bronchiectasis, healed tuberculosis, sarcoidosis, and infarcts, for example, and patients with ankylosing spondylitis may have an increased incidence of mycetomas.[222] Necrotic carcinomas may also be the site of fungal colonization, although well-developed fungus balls are not always present in such cases.[228,235] Less often, mycetomas develop in patients with previous invasive fungal pneumonia, presumably due to excavation and encapsulation of necrotic zones with residual, persistent, but no longer invasive, organisms.[160,213,233] Many investigators, however, feel that these cases should be considered examples of cavitating pneumonia rather than true mycetomas.[135,145,146,213] Aspergillus is the usual organism identified within mycetomas, although other fungi have also been described, including various phycomycetes,[220,224] *Pseudallescheria boydii*,[213,218,219] *Cladosporium cladosporioides*,[226] *Penicillium decumbens*,[236] and *Coccidioides immitis*.[231,233]

Clinical Features

The most common clinical manifestation of pulmonary mycetoma is hemoptysis, and fatal massive hemoptysis is a well-recognized complication.[182,232,234] Some patients are asymptomatic. Radiographically, the lesions are usually found in the upper lobes. They appear as well-defined cavities containing a central, rounded density, which is separated from the superior border by a crescent-shaped clear space. Most pulmonary mycetomas are encountered by the pathologist at autopsy, although some are resected during life, especially in patients with severe hemoptysis.[222,232]

Pathologic Features

Grossly, the fungus ball consists of a cavity filled with soft, tan-brown, friable material that corresponds to the radiographically apparent central density (Fig. 10–16). Histologically, this material is composed of a tangled mass of mycelia and cellular debris that often exhibits a prominent lamellar arrangement (Fig. 10–17). The wall of the cavity is lined with dense fibrous tissue and chronic inflammation. Granulomatous inflammation is usually not a feature. Invasion of blood vessels and tissue necrosis that are characteristic of invasive fungal infection are not present. The deposition of birefringent calcium oxalate crystals on the edge of the cavity is common in *A. niger* mycetomas (Fig. 10–18).[221,223,225,229,230] Sometimes the oxalate crystals can be identified in sputum cytology preparations and their presence

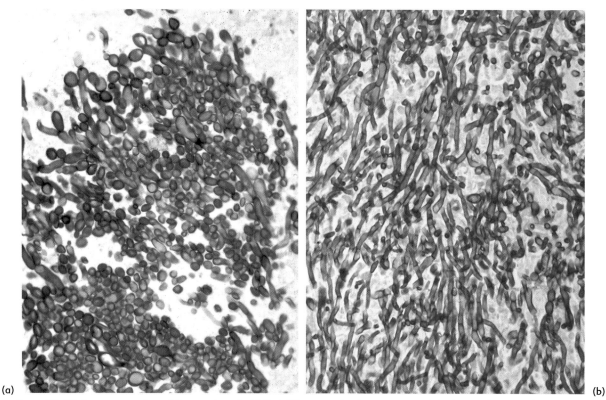

Figure 10–15 Appearance of candida organisms in GMS. (a) Yeasts predominate over pseudohyphae in this example. **(b)** Pseudohyphae predominate in this example. They differ from true hyphae because of rounded ends, giving the appearance of sausage links, in contrast to the perpendicular septations characteristic of aspergillus.

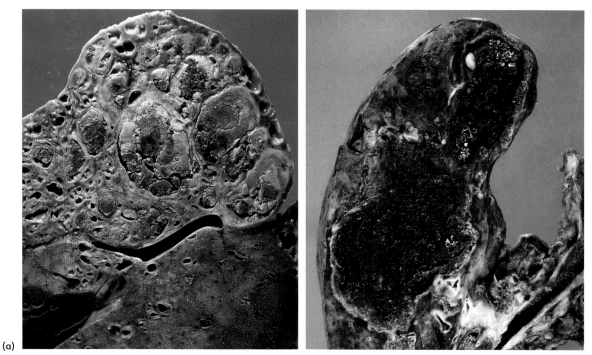

Figure 10–16 Mycetomas. (a) Aspergillus mycetoma arising in honeycomb lung from a patient with end-stage sarcoidosis. **(b)** This mycetoma has a black color due to *Aspergillus niger*.

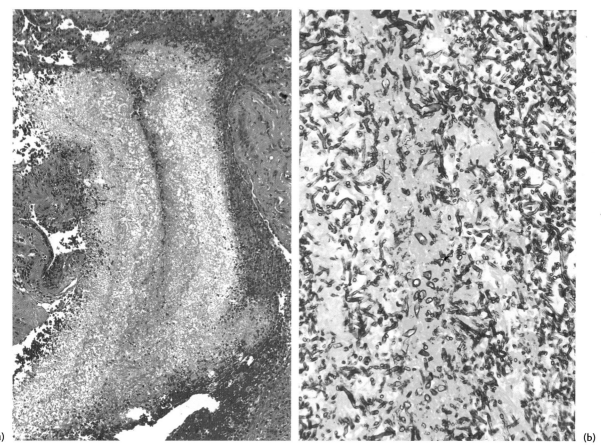

(a)

(b)

Figure 10–17 Aspergillus mycetoma. (a) Low magnification showing the typical lamellated appearance of the mass of organisms comprising the fungus ball. **(b)** GMS stain at higher magnification showing the haphazard arrangement of the organisms within the fungal mass.

should prompt a careful search for the organisms.[227] It is postulated that the oxalic acid produced by the fungus may damage blood vessels and thus contribute to the development of hemoptysis.[223,225] A role has also been proposed for the complexing of iron with the calcium oxalate, leading to subsequent oxidant generation.[221]

NOCARDIOSIS AND ACTINOMYCOSIS

Nocardiosis

Clinical Features

The lung is the most common primary site of infection by *Nocardia*, and *N. asteroides* is the usual species involved.[241,242] Most patients with pulmonary nocardiosis have an underlying disease or other reason for immunocompromise that predisposes them to infection.[248] The clinical symptoms vary from mild chest complaints

to an acute toxic illness. Radiographically, a variety of patterns are seen, ranging from a solitary nodule to extensive, often cavitary, infiltrates.[240] Rarely, endobronchial masses occur, and pleural involvement has been described.[243,253] Hematogenous dissemination, especially to the central nervous system, is common. Response to sulfonamide therapy is usually excellent.

Histologic Features

Lung biopsy is often required for diagnosis of this infection since the organisms frequently cannot be cultured from sputum. The pathologic features are characterized by a necrotizing acute bronchopneumonia with abscess formation (Fig. 10–19).[248] A histiocytic response with poorly formed granulomas may surround the necrotic areas. The organisms cannot be visualized in H and E-stained sections, but they are well outlined with tissue Gram stains (Brown–Hopps or Brown–Brenn), where they appear Gram-positive, and they stain well with

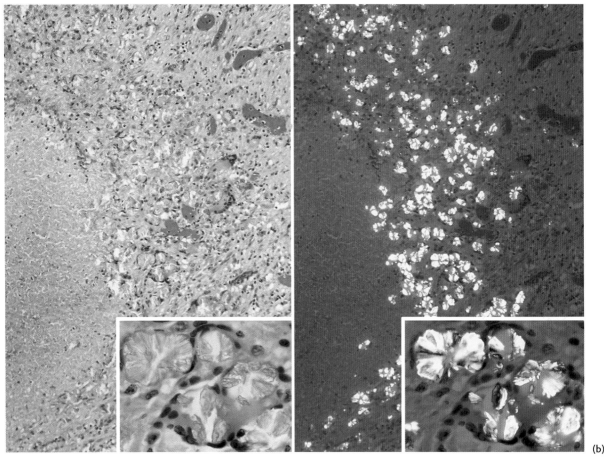

(a)

(b)

Figure 10–18 Calcium oxalate deposition on the periphery of an *Aspergillus niger* mycetoma. **(a)** is an H and E-stained section, and **(b)** is under partially polarized light. The insets are higher magnification views.

GMS (Fig. 10–20). They are also weakly acid-fast, a feature that is best demonstrated in the Fite modification of the Ziehl–Neelsen stain.[250] By these techniques, nocardia appear as long, branching, filamentous rods that measure 0.5 to 1.0 μm in diameter (Fig. 10–21). They usually do not aggregate in granules in lung infections (in contrast to extrapulmonary infections). PCR techniques have been used to identify the organisms in culture-negative cases.[253]

Actinomycosis

Clinical Features

Although most actinomycotic infections involve the soft tissue as chronic suppurative processes with extensive necrosis and fistula formation, the lungs are occasionally involved.[238,248] Pulmonary lesions usually occur in immunologically intact patients, although

emphysema, bronchitis, and bronchiectasis are common associated diseases. The presentation is generally that of an unresolving bronchopneumonia with fever, productive cough, and a chest infiltrate.[244,252] In some cases, a lung mass that mimics carcinoma is seen. Endobronchial lesions have also been reported.[237,239,246] *Actinomyces israelii* is the usual causative agent. It is a fastidious anaerobic organism, and culture results are frequently negative. Infection is thought to result from aspiration of organisms from the oropharynx, and patients with poor dentition are at increased risk.

Histopathologic Features

Histologically, there is extensive tissue destruction by acute inflammation and necrosis. Microabscesses are prominent, and fistula formation is a frequent complication in untreated patients.[238,248] A thick zone of granulation tissue, composed of collagen, fibroblasts,

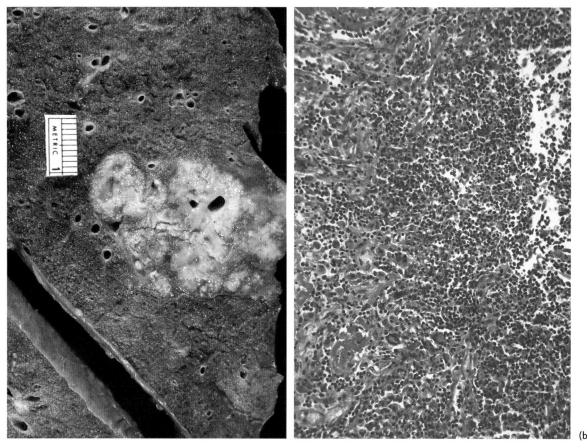

Figure 10–19 Nocardia pneumonia. (a) Gross photograph of abscess due to nocardia. **(b)** Microscopic appearance of abscess cavity (right) with surrounding rim of fibrosis, chronic inflammatory cells, and histiocytes (left). Note the occasional multinucleated giant cells.

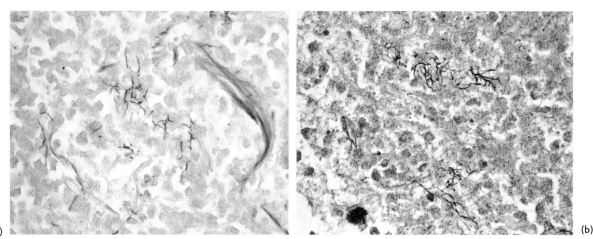

Figure 10–20 Nocardia. (a) High magnification view of Gram stain showing typical long, branching, Gram-positive, filamentous rods. **(b)** GMS stain showing similar morphology.

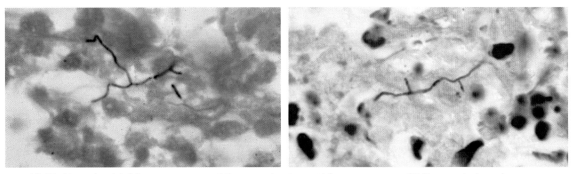

Figure 10–21 Nocardia. (a) Oil immersion view of Fite stain showing acid-fast appearance. **(b)** Gram stain from the same case, showing Gram-positive organism.

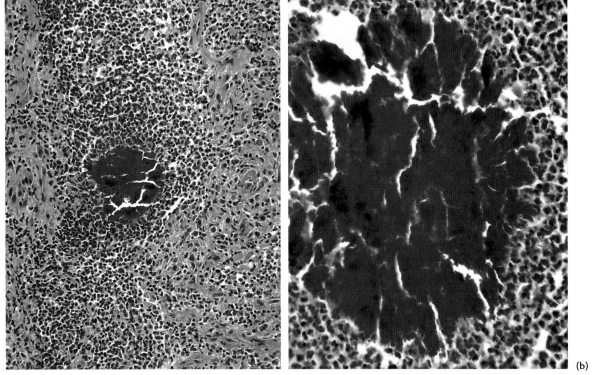

Figure 10–22 Actinomycosis. (a) Low magnification view of a sulfur granule that is present within dense acute inflammation and surrounded by fibrosis. **(b)** Higher magnification view of the sulfur granule showing the club-like projections (Splendore–Hoeppli phenomenon) on the periphery of the granule and the close interaction with the surrounding acute inflammatory cells.

capillaries, and chronic inflammatory cells, surrounds the central, purulent material. Large, foamy macrophages may accumulate around the granulation tissue. Typically, 'sulfur' *granules* or *grains* are found in the abscess cavities (Fig. 10–22).[239] In H and E-stained sections, the granules are large basophilic or amphophilic

structures, averaging 100 to 300 μm in diameter. Prominent eosinophilic, club-like rods radiate from their periphery – a feature known as the *Splendore–Hoeppli phenomenon*.[1,251] It is caused by the accumulation of a proteinaceous exudate on the surface of the organism and is thought to be related to precipitated antigen–

antibody complexes. It is not specific for actinomycosis and is seen surrounding other organisms, including various fungi (classically *Sporothrix*), bacteria, and parasites.[1,247] The granules are generally numerous, although in occasional cases they can be rare and difficult to find. Thin, filamentous, Gram-positive branching rods that are 0.5 μm in diameter can be demonstrated within the granules by means of a Gram stain or a GMS stain (see Fig. 10–23).[239] They are not acid-fast.

Differential Diagnosis

The thin, branching filamentous rods of nocardia and actinomyces are indistinguishable in Gram and silver (GMS) stains, and they cause a similar type of destructive, suppurative inflammatory reaction in tissue. They differ, however, in that nocardia is weakly acid-fast and does not form granules in the lung, while actinomyces is not acid-fast and forms granules (Table 10–4).

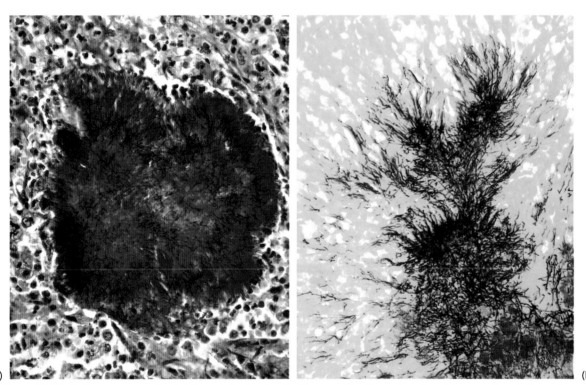

(a)   (b)

Figure 10–23 **Actinomyces granules.** (a) Gram stain showing the Gram-positive filamentous, branching organisms in the center of the granule. (b) Higher magnification of a GMS stain from the same case, showing the typical organisms within a granule.

Table 10–4   Contrasting Features of Actinomycosis, Nocardiosis and Botryomyosis

	Actinomycosis	Nocardiosis	Botryomycosis
Organism morphology	Long, branching filamentous rods Granules present	Long, branching filamentous rods No granules	Cocci or short rods Granules present
Staining properties	Gram-positive Not acid-fast	Gram-positive Weakly acid-fast	Gram-positive or Gram-negative Not acid-fast
Tissue reaction	Suppurative, ± granulomas Fistulas common	Suppurative, ± granulomas	Suppurative

Occasionally, other bacteria, most often staphylococcus or pseudomonas, form clusters resembling the granules of actinomyces, and the resulting pneumonia is referred to as *botryomycosis*.[1,239,245,249] These bacterial clusters are distinguished from true granules by the morphology of the component organisms (cocci or short rods rather than long branching filamentous rods) (see Table 10–4). Gram staining, of course, should help as well.

LEGIONNAIRES' DISEASE AND RELATED PNEUMONIAS

Clinical Features

Although first recognized following a large outbreak among participants in the American Legion convention in Philadelphia in 1976, Legionnaires' disease has subsequently been identified as the cause of several other epidemics both in the United States and abroad.[254,255,263,271,275,288] Sporadic cases also occur.[261,272,274,279] The causative organism, *Legionella pneumophila*, is a small, pleomorphic, Gram-negative bacillus that can be cultured on modified Mueller–Hinton agar. Multiple serogroups have been identified. The usual mode of presentation is an acute pneumonic illness characterized by high fever, chills, cough, and chest pain, associated with malaise and arthralgias. Gastrointestinal symptoms may be prominent, and renal and central nervous system dysfunction are common. The disease occurs in immunocompromised as well as immunologically intact individuals, and renal as well as bone marrow transplant recipients seem to have an increased risk of infection. Radiographs initially show patchy infiltration that often progresses to dense consolidation with multiple-lobe involvement. Pleural effusions are common, but cavitation is unusual. Although mortality as high as 25% has been reported in some series, deaths occur in less than 10% of previously healthy individuals who receive appropriate antibiotic therapy.[261,272] A milder type of illness presenting as a flu-like syndrome without pneumonia has also been reported, and asymptomatic seroconversion may even occur.[272]

Histopathologic Features

The characteristic histopathologic finding is an acute bronchopneumonia similar to other bacterial pneumonias and characterized by a mixture of neutrophils and macrophages within alveolar spaces (see Fig. 10–24).[254,255,266,268,269,279,285,288] Karyorrhexis of the inflammatory cells is usually a striking feature, and this finding, although not specific, should suggest legionella in the etiology. Fibrin, proteinaceous deposits, and erythrocytes are also present within the alveolar spaces. DAD is a common accompanying feature and rarely may be the only finding. Occasionally, coagulative necrosis of the alveolar septa is seen, and abscess formation may occur in a few cases. Although definitive diagnosis requires identification of the organism by culture or other techniques (see further on), the pathologist should suggest the diagnosis in any acute bronchopneumonia encountered on a lung biopsy specimen, since biopsies are unlikely to be performed in other more common bacterial pneumonias.

Extensive intraalveolar fibrosis has been described in a few cases,[254,266] especially at autopsy, and changes of bronchiolitis obliterans–organizing pneumonia (BOOP) have followed episodes of acute pneumonia.[259] Extrathoracic dissemination of the infection can also occur. Hilar and peribronchial lymph nodes are affected most often, although involvement of liver, spleen, kidneys, and bone marrow is observed occasionally.[267,284]

Identification of Organisms in Tissue

Legionella organisms can be demonstrated in tissue by the Dieterle silver impregnation stain, in which they appear as small pleomorphic rods both within cells and free within alveolar spaces.[258,283] This stain, however, can be both difficult to perform and difficult to interpret because of frequent artifactual background staining. Ordinary tissue Gram stains, such as Brown–Brenn or Brown–Hopps, may be positive in some cases, and they are easier to interpret, since they do not stain formalin pigment or other extraneous background material.[273,288] A modified Gimenez stain has been reported to be a reliable method of demonstrating organisms in frozen sections.[264] By electron microscopy, the bacteria can be found within inflammatory cells as well as extracellularly (Fig. 10–25a).[257,268–270,278,282] Although this technique confirms the Gram-negative nature of the bacilli, there are no specific ultrastructural features for definitive identification. Of course, electron microscopy is not a practical screening method for detecting the organisms.

Immunohistochemical techniques using specific antibodies are also available for identifying the organism in tissue (Fig. 10–25b). Either immunofluorescence or immunoperoxidase techniques can be utilized, and an immunoenzyme technique has also

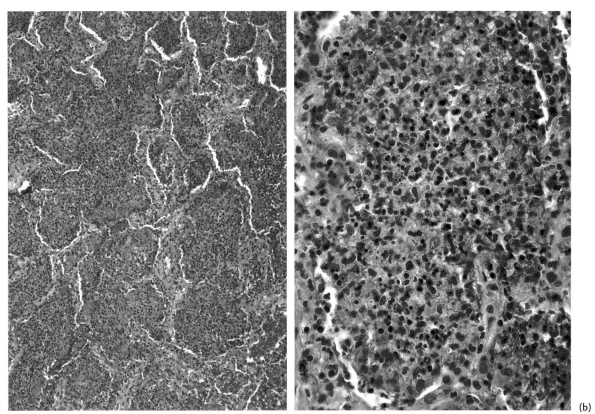

(a)   (b)

Figure 10–24 Legionnaires' disease. (a) Low magnification showing an acute bronchopneumonia characterized by the filling of alveolar spaces by an acute inflammatory cell exudate. (b) Higher magnification showing the prominent karyorrhexis that is characteristic of this infection.

been described.[256,267,280,281,282,284,287] These methods can be applied to formalin-fixed, paraffin-embedded tissue as well as to frozen sections, and they have also been used in evaluating smears from sputum, tracheal aspirates, or BAL fluids. The main drawback of these immunohistologic methods is that antibodies are not commercially available for all legionella serogroups, and therefore some infections may be missed.[281] Also, there is a significant false-negative rate even when antibodies to the correct serogroup are used. In situ hybridization using RNA probes is another technique that can be employed to identify the organisms.[260]

Related Bacteria of the Legionellaceae Family

A number of other organisms have been identified that require similar growth media and share certain metabolic and biochemical features with *L. pneumophila*.[262] They also produce a clinically and pathologically similar acute pneumonia and are grouped with *L. pneumophila*

in the family Legionellaceae. The most common ones include the Legionella-like organisms (*L. bozemanii*, *L. dumoffii*, *L. longbeachae*), *L. feeleii*, the causative agent of Pontiac fever;[277] and the Pittsburgh pneumonia agent *L. micdadei* (also termed *L. pittsburgensis*).[276,288] Some of these organisms are weakly acid-fast.[288] Ultrastructurally, a distinct electron-dense band has been demonstrated within the periplastic space of the Pittsburgh pneumonia agent, which is thought to be related to the variable acid-fast-staining properties of this organism.[265]

ANTHRAX

Anthrax is an often fatal bacterial infection caused by *Bacillus anthracis*, a Gram-positive aerobic rod that is present in the soil.[291,293] Most cases occur in animals, usually cattle, sheep, horses, or goats. Human infection is rare, most cases being related to agricultural (hence the name *wool-sorters' disease*[289,294]) or industrial (as

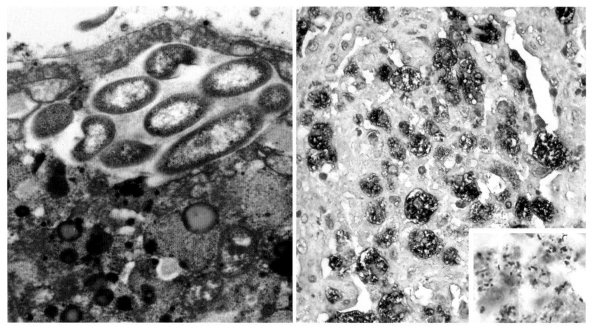

(a)   (b)

Figure 10-25 Legionnaires' disease. (a) Electron micrograph showing bacilli within a phagocytic vacuole in the cytoplasm of an alveolar macrophage (×18,500, courtesy of Dr Michael T Mazur). **(b)** Immunohistochemical stain using a commercial antibody to *Legionella pneumophila*, showing the characteristic granular staining in macrophage cytoplasm. Inset is a Dieterle stain showing typical small pleomorphic rods.

in Sverdlovsk, Russia in 1979[292]) exposures, and, more recently, bioterrorism.[290] The most common form of anthrax involves the skin (*cutaneous anthrax*) and is usually curable. Systemic disease, however, is usually fatal and occurs following ingestion (*gastrointestinal anthrax*) or inhalation (*inhalational anthrax*) of the organism, and it occasionally complicates cutaneous disease. Virulence is thought to be due both to the presence of a protective capsule on the organism and the production of toxins.

Most pathologic descriptions of inhalational anthrax have been from autopsy studies.[289,292,294] The usual thoracic finding is a necrotizing, hemorrhagic media-stinitis in which organisms are generally numerous. Lung findings are characterized mainly by pulmonary edema. Although acute bronchopneumonia is seen in about half of patients, it is overshadowed by the mediastinal hemorrhage and pulmonary edema. Hemorrhagic meningitis and intestinal hemorrhage are common accompanying features. These findings reflect the pathogenesis of the disease, in which inhaled spores are phagocytosed by alveolar macrophages and transported to regional lymph nodes where they germinate. Release of organisms and toxins causes local tissue destruction, and entrance into the bloodstream

results in massive septicemia and toxemia with secondary involvement of multiple organs.

PNEUMOCYSTIS PNEUMONIA

Pneumocystis pneumonia is an important pulmonary infection in immunocompromised individuals. It was first recognized as a cause of serious lung disease in institutionalized, malnourished infants in Europe during World War II.[302,313] This form of the disease was known as *interstitial plasma cell pneumonia* because of a prominent plasma cell infiltrate in alveolar septa. Although this neonatal illness is now rare in Europe, it is still seen in some underdeveloped parts of the world. In more recent years, pneumocystis pneumonia has emerged as an important infection in individuals receiving immunosuppressive therapy for malignant or autoimmune disease or following organ transplanta-tion. It also is a significant infection in patients with AIDS (see Chapter 12). Although rare cases have been reported in persons without known immunologic defects, adequate documentation appears lacking in these cases.[305,324,346]

Although originally considered a protozoa, current evidence based on the sequencing analysis of ribosomal

RNA and other techniques favors fungus.[314,317] It is now known that the organism is genetically diverse and host-species-specific. The type causing disease in humans has been renamed *P. girovecii*, while *P. carinii* is used for the organism in rats.[336] The acronym PCP, previously referring to '*Pneumocystis carinii* pneumonia', now refers to 'pneumocystis pneumonia'. Propagation of the organism has been achieved in tissue culture, but cultivation on cell-free media has not been successful.[351]

Clinical Features

Clinically, the onset of pneumocystis pneumonia is usually either acute or subacute.[313,340] Fever, dyspnea, and dry cough develop and may progress to respiratory failure if left untreated. Bilateral alveolar and interstitial infiltrates radiating out from the hila are the most common radiographic manifestations, although atypical localized infiltrates or nodules, as well as upper lobe infiltrates suggestive of tuberculosis, have also been reported.[297,308,337,345] Patients with AIDS tend to have a less acute form of illness, and examples with a prolonged, but stable, clinical course have been reported in this patient population.[330,352] Mortality rates are significantly higher for non-HIV-infected patients than for patients with AIDS.[334] Atypical radiographic manifestations are more frequent in AIDS patients and include pleural effusions and pneumothorax in addition to unusual parenchymal infiltrates.[298,322] Extrapulmonary dissemination to multiple organs is occasionally seen and is also more common in patients with AIDS.[306,309,320,335,342,348] Rarely, in HIV-infected patients receiving inhaled pentamidine prophylaxis, extrapulmonary disease has occurred in the absence of clinically apparent lung involvement.[311,343]

The most direct means of diagnosis is a lung biopsy, and percutaneous needle and transbronchial lung biopsy techniques are successful, in addition to open lung biopsy.[302,323,340] In AIDS patients, however, organisms are often so numerous that they can be visualized in sputum or BAL specimens, and lung biopsy may not be necessary (see Chapter 12).

Histologic Features

A variety of histologic findings can be observed in pneumocystis pneumonia (Table 10–5).[333,350] The classically described manifestation is a frothy, foamy, or honeycomb exudate within the alveolar spaces, associated with an interstitial pneumonia.[1,302,341] This exudate, which can be seen in the H and E-stained

Table 10–5   Histologic Manifestations of Pneumocystis Pneumonia
* Intraalveolar froth and interstitial pneumonia (classic)
* Diffuse alveolar damage
Granulomatous inflammation
Fibrosis
Intraalveolar macrophage accumulation
Interstitial pneumonia
Calcification
Necrosis
Vasculitis
Pulmonary alveolar proteinosis-like areas
No histologic reaction

* Most common findings accounting for the majority of cases.

sections, is diagnostic of pneumocystis infection, even without special stains (Fig. 10–26; see also Fig. 12–3). It is the most common tissue manifestation of pneumocystis infection in AIDS patients and reflects the presence of large numbers of cysts. It is found less often in non-AIDS patients.[296,308,350,354]

DAD (see Chapter 2) with prominent hyaline membrane formation is the next most common histologic manifestation of pneumocystis pneumonia, and it is most often seen in non-AIDS patients (Fig. 10–27).[296,308,354] Typically, the organisms are found within the hyaline membranes. Less often, the organisms are associated with the organizing stage of DAD (Fig. 10–28). Other less frequent manifestations include granulomatous inflammation, giant cells, interstitial pneumonia, fibrosis, vasculitis, necrosis, calcification, foci of pulmonary alveolar proteinosis, and increased numbers of intraalveolar macrophages.[307,327,328,332,333,339,349,350,354] The granulomatous inflammation may consist of necrotizing or non-necrotizing granulomas, but more often there is a poorly formed granulomatous response with loose aggregates of histiocytes and lymphocytes (Fig. 10–29).[307,325,328,350,354] Fibrosis may affect the interstitium or airspaces and represents a form of organizing pneumonia in many cases. Vasculitis is rare and may be associated with parenchymal necrosis.[332] Tissue invasion by the organisms has been documented in cases with necrosis and may be etiologic in the development of vasculitis as well.[339] Lung cysts may evolve from necrotic zones and rupture can lead to pneumothorax.[298] Rare cases of pneumocystis infection unassociated with any histologic response have also been reported, and their significance is uncertain.[308]

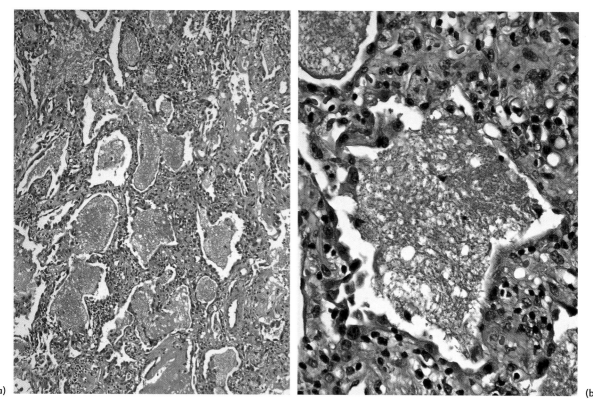

Figure 10–26 Pneumocystis pneumonia. (a) Low magnification showing the filling of alveolar spaces by an eosinophilic frothy-appearing exudate. The alveolar septa show nonspecific thickening by mild chronic inflammation and fibrosis. **(b)** Higher magnification view showing the characteristic frothy or honeycomb appearance to the intraalveolar exudate. Note the minute dot-like structures within the spaces in the exudate.

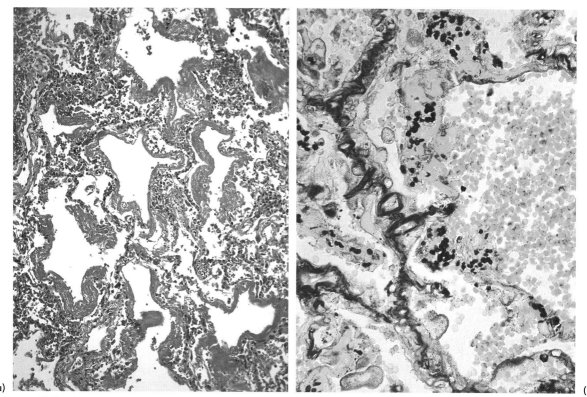

Figure 10–27 Acute DAD in pneumocystis pneumonia. (a) Prominent hyaline membranes line alveolar septa in this example. **(b)** GMS staining showing the organisms within the hyaline membranes.

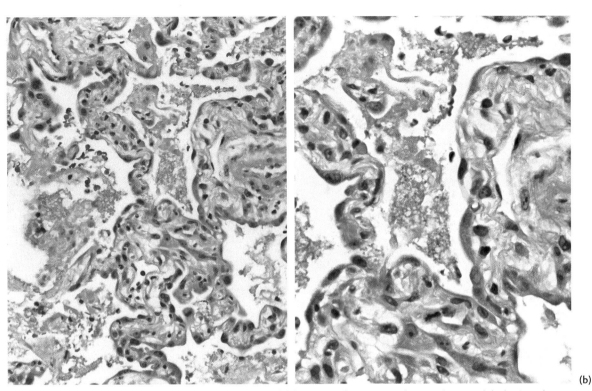

(a)   (b)

Figure 10–28 Organizing DAD in pneumocystis pneumonia. **(a)** Low magnification view showing the typical thickening of alveolar septa by fibroblasts and alveolar pneumocyte hyperplasia that is characteristic of the organizing stage of DAD. Additionally, the frothy exudates of pneumocystis are seen in alveolar spaces. **(b)** Higher magnification view of the intraalveolar frothy exudate. This appearance is pathognomonic of pneumocystis, even without special stains.

It should be remembered that pneumocystis pneumonia is accompanied by other infections, most commonly CMV, in about 10% of cases.[350] Therefore, especially when atypical histologic features are encountered, the possibility of an accompanying infection should be considered and excluded by carefully examining special stains and searching for viral inclusions.

Identification of Organisms

The variation in histologic pattern produced by pneumocystis infection underscores the importance of using special stains to identify this organism, especially in the absence of alveolar froth. The organisms consist of a mixture of *cysts* containing intracystic bodies (*sporozoites*), and free *trophozoites*, and stains are available that outline either the cysts or the sporozoites and trophozoites.[300] The GMS stain is the most useful means of identifying organisms, provided that a control slide, containing pneumocystis rather than other fungal organisms, is prepared in order to avoid false-negatives.[310] This stain colors the cysts, which are round, often indented, or helmet-shaped and measure 4 to 6 μm in diameter (Fig. 10–30; see also Fig. 12–2). One or two dot-like foci of enhanced staining are often seen within the cysts and can be useful in their identification.[353] Pneumocystis organisms are distinguished from fungal yeasts by their lack of budding forms and location within the alveolar spaces. Rare examples of pneumocystis pneumonia have been reported in which the organisms failed to stain with GMS despite a positive control slide.[315] This lack of staining was attributed to the presence of numerous trophozoites rather than cysts.

Cresylecht violet and toluidine blue O are other stains that outline the cysts, and they can be prepared quickly on frozen sections or smears.[301,303,351] A rapid-acting GMS stain has also been described. PAS alone does not adequately differentiate the cysts from the background exudate, but the organisms can be demonstrated with the PAS–Gridley technique.[331] Calcofluor white is another rapid stain, but it requires fluorescence

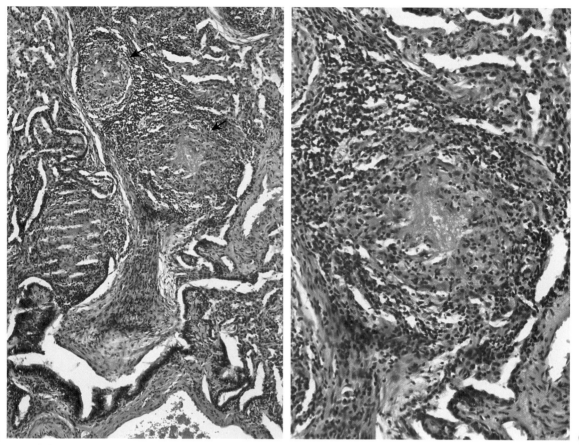

(a)   (b)

Figure 10–29 Granulomatous inflammation in pneumocystis pneumonia. (a) Low magnification view showing granulomas (arrows) within airspaces where they are associated with airspace organization (bronchiolitis obliterans). **(b)** Higher magnification view showing the epithelioid histiocytes surrounding the typical frothy exudate of pneumocystis.

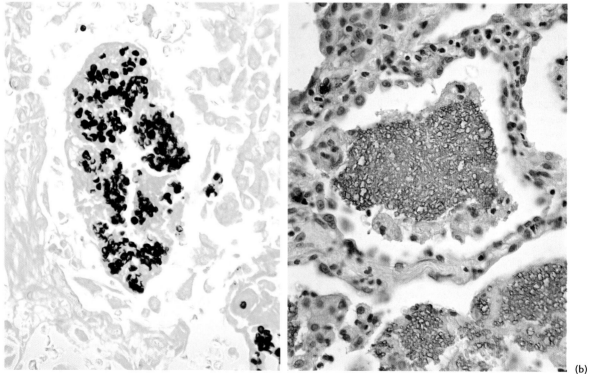

(a)   (b)

Figure 10–30 Staining of pneumocystis. (a) GMS stain showing the round and sometimes indented or helmet-shaped organisms within the intraalveolar exudate. **(b)** Immunohistochemical stain using a commercial antibody to the organism.

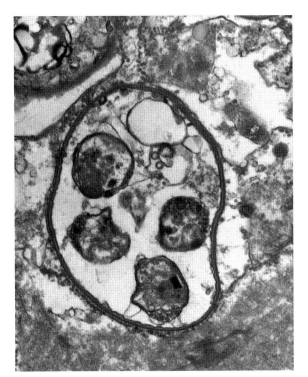

Figure 10–31 Electron micrograph of pneumocystis, showing a cyst containing multiple sporozoites. Note the membranotubular material on the surface at the top.

microscopy.[316] The organisms can also be seen under polarized light in hematoxylin-stained sections following pepsin pretreatment.[295] Other staining methods such as Giemsa, polychrome methylene blue (Wright's), or Wright–Giemsa (Diff-Quik) outline the small, 1- to 2-μm intracystic forms (sporozoites) or trophozoites but not the cysts (see Fig. 12–2).[312,341] These stains are more difficult to interpret than the techniques that outline the larger cyst walls, and we do not recommend them for use in tissue sections. A method has also been described for simultaneous demonstration of cyst wall and sporozoites using plastic-embedded specimens.[344]

Monoclonal antibodies to pneumocystis are commercially available and readily applicable to tissue sections, using immunoperoxidase or immunofluorescence techniques (Fig. 10–30b).[306,329,342,350] There is little evidence, however, that they offer significant diagnostic advantage over the GMS stain in tissue, although they appear to add increased sensitivity in smears and fluids.[321,326] In situ hybridization utilizing probes to ribosomal RNA and PCR using DNA primers are additional techniques that have been described to identify the organism.[299,319,338]

Ultrastructure

By electron microscopy, a mixture of cysts and trophozoites is seen within the alveolar spaces.[302,304,317,318,323,347] The cysts are thick walled, measure from 4 to 6 μm in diameter, and contain up to eight sporozoites that measure 1 to 1.5 μm in diameter (Fig. 10–31). Some of the cysts appear to be empty and partially collapsed. Abundant membranotubular material typically is present on their surface. The trophozoites are thin walled, smaller, and more variable in size, ranging from 1 to 5 μm.

REFERENCES

General

1. Binford C, Connor D, eds: *Pathology of Tropical and Extraordinary Diseases*, Washington, DC, Armed Forces Institute of Pathology, 1976.
2. Chandler F, Watts J: *Pathologic Diagnosis of Fungal Infections*, Chicago, ASCP Press, 1987.
3. Karayannopoulou G, Weiss J, Danjanov I: Detection of fungi in tissue sections by lectin histochemistry. Arch Pathol Lab Med 112:746, 1988.
4. Kimura M, McGinnis MR: Fontana-Masson-stained tissue from culture-proven mycoses. Arch Pathol Lab Med 122:1107, 1998.
5. Monheit JE, Cowan DF, Moore DG: Rapid detection of fungi in tissues using calcofluor white and fluorescence microscopy. Arch Pathol Lab Med 108:616, 1984.
6. Renshaw AA: The relative sensitivity of special stains and culture in open lung biopsies. Am J Clin Pathol 102:736, 1994.
7. Schluger NW, Rom WN: The polymerase chain reaction in the diagnosis and evaluation of pulmonary infections. Am J Respir Crit Care Med 152:11, 1995.
8. Shimono L, Hartman B: A simple and reliable rapid methenamine silver stain for *Pneumocystis carinii* and fungi. Arch Pathol Lab Med 110:855, 1986.
9. Taylor CR, Cote RJ: *Immunomicroscopy: A Diagnostic Tool for the Surgical Pathologist*, Vol. 19, *Major Problems in Pathology*, 3rd ed, Philadelphia, WB Saunders, 2005.

Infections in Immunocompromised Patients

10. de Peralta-Venturina MN, Clubb FJ, Kielhofner MA: Pulmonary malacoplakia associated with *Rhodococcus equi* infection in a patient with acquired immunodeficiency syndrome. Am J Clin Pathol 102:459, 1994.
11. Lurie H, Duma R: Opportunistic infections of the lung. Hum Pathol 1:233, 1970.
12. Myerowitz RL: *The Pathology of Opportunistic Infections with Pathogenetic, Diagnostic, and Clinical Correlations*, New York, Raven Press, 1983.
13. Rosenow EC III, Wilson WR, Cockerill FR III: Pulmonary disease in the immunocompromised host. I. Mayo Clin Proc 60:473, 1985.

14. Shelhamer JH, Toews GB, Masur H, et al: Respiratory disease in the immunosuppressed patient. Ann Intern Med 117:415, 1993.

15. Wilson WR, Cockerill FR III, Rosenow EC III: Pulmonary disease in the immunocompromised host. II. Mayo Clin Proc 60:610, 1985.

Viral Infections

General

16. Reichman R, Dolin R: Viral pneumonias. Med Clin North Am 64:491, 1980.

17. Strano A: Light microscopy of selected viral diseases (morphology of viral inclusion bodies). Pathol Annu 11:53, 1976.

18. Weiss LM, Movahed LA, Berry GJ, Billingham ME: In situ hybridization studies for viral nucleic acids in heart and lung allograft biopsies. Am J Clin Pathol 93:675, 1990.

19. Yunis E, Hashida Y, Haas J: The role of electron microscopy in the identification of viruses in human disease. Pathol Annu 12:311, 1977.

Cytomegalovirus

20. Beschorner W, Hutchins G, Burns W, et al: Cytomegalovirus pneumonia in bone marrow transplant recipients: Miliary and diffuse patterns. Am Rev Respir Dis 122:107, 1980.

21. Browning J, More I, Boyd A: Adult pulmonary cytomegalic inclusion disease: Report of a case. J Clin Pathol 33:11, 1980.

22. Burgart LJ, Heller MJ, Reznicek MJ, Greiner TC, Teneyck CJ, Robinson RA: Cytomegalovirus detection in bone marrow transplant patients with idiopathic pneumonitis: A clinicopathologic study of the clinical utility of the polymerase chain reaction on open lung biopsy specimen tissue. Am J Clin Pathol 96:572, 1991.

23. Cao M, Beckstead JH: Localization of cytomegalovirus DNA in plastic-embedded sections by in situ hybridization. A methodologic study. Am J Pathol 134:457, 1989.

24. Craighead L: Pulmonary cytomegalovirus infection in the adult. Am J Pathol 63:487, 1971.

25. Crawford S, Bowden R, Hackman R, et al: Rapid detection of cytomegalovirus pulmonary infection by bronchoalveolar lavage and centrifugation culture. Ann Intern Med 108:180, 1988.

26. Eddleston M, Peacock S, Juniper M, et al. Severe cytomegalovirus infection in immunocompetent patients. Clin Infect Dis 24:52, 1997.

27. Fend F, Prior C, Margreiter R, Mikuz G: Cytomegalovirus pneumonitis in heart-lung transplant recipients: Histopathology and clinicopathologic considerations. Hum Pathol 21:918, 1990.

28. Gleaves CA, Smith TF, Wold AD, Wilson WR: Detection of viral and chlamydial antigens in open-lung biopsy specimens. Am J Clin Pathol 83:371, 1985.

29. Gorelkin L, Chandler FW, Ewing EP: Staining qualities of cytomegalovirus inclusions in the lungs of patients with the acquired immunodeficiency syndrome: A potential source of diagnostic misinterpretation. Hum Pathol 17:926, 1986.

30. Hilborne LH, Nieberg RK, Cheng L, Lewin KJ: Direct in situ hybridization for rapid detection of cytomegalovirus in bronchoalveolar lavage. Am J Clin Pathol 87:766, 1987.

31. Imoto EM, Stein RM, Shellito JE, Curtis JL: Central airway obstruction due to cytomegalovirus-induced necrotizing tracheitis in a patient with AIDS. Am Rev Respir Dis 142:884, 1990.

32. Jiwa M, Steenberger RDM, Zwaan FE, Kluin PM, Raap AK, Van der Ploeg M: Three sensitive methods for the detection of cytomegalovirus in lung tissue of patients with interstitial pneumonitis. Am J Clin Pathol 93:491, 1990.

33. Karakelides H, Aubry M-C, Ryu JH: Cytomegalovirus pneumonia mimicking lung cancer in an immunocompetent host. Mayo Clin Proc 78:488, 2003.

34. Kasnic G Jr, Sayeed A, Azar HA: Nuclear and cytoplasmic inclusions in disseminated human cytomegalovirus infection. Ultrastruct Pathol 3:229, 1982.

35. Kotsimbos AT, Sinickas V, Glare EM, et al; Quantitative detection of human cytomegalovirus DNA in lung transplant recipients. Am J Respir Crit Care Med 156:1241, 1997.

36. Macasaet F, Holley K, Smith T, Keys T: Cytomegalovirus studies of autopsy tissue. II. Incidence of inclusion bodies and related pathologic data. Am J Clin Pathol 63:859, 1975.

37. Martin A Jr, Kurtz S: Cytomegalic inclusion disease. An electron microscopic histochemical study of the virus at necropsy. Arch Pathol 82:27, 1966.

38. Masih AS, Woods GL, Thiele GM, et al: Detection of cytomegalovirus in bronchoalveolar lavage: A comparison of techniques. Mod Pathol 1:108, 1991.

39. Mera JR, Whimbey E, Elting L, et al: Cytomegalovirus pneumonia in adult non-transplantation patients with cancer: Review of 20 cases occurring from 1964 through 1990. Clin Infect Dis 22:1046, 1996.

40. Oda Y, Katsuda S, Yasunori O, et al: Detection of human cytomegalovirus, Epstein-Barr virus, and herpes simplex virus in diffuse interstitial pneumonia by polymerase chain reaction and immunohistochemistry. Am J Clin Pathol 102:495, 1994.

41. Paradis IL, Grgurich WF, Dummer JS, et al: Rapid detection of cytomegalovirus pneumonia from lung lavage cells. Am Rev Respir Dis 138:697, 1988.

42. Persons DL, Moore JA, Fishback JL: Comparison of polymerase chain reaction, DNA hybridization, and histology with viral cultures to detect cytomegalovirus in immunosuppressed patients. Mod Pathol 4:149, 1991.

43. Rimsza LM, Vela EE, Frutiger YM, et al. Rapid automated combined in situ hybridization and immunohistochemistry for sensitive detection of cytomegalovirus in paraffin-embedded tissue biopsies. Am J Clin Pathol 141:102, 1996.

44. Rosen P, Hajdu S: Cytomegalovirus inclusion disease at

autopsy of patients with cancer. Am J Clin Pathol 55:749, 1971.

45. Shibata M, Terashima M, Kimura H, et al: Quantitation of cytomegalovirus DNA in lung tissue of bone marrow transplant recipients. Hum Pathol 23:911, 1992.

46. Sissons JGT, Borysiewicz LK: Human cytomegalovirus infection. Thorax 44:241, 1989.

47. Solans EP, Garrity ER Jr, McCabe M, et al. Early diagnosis of cytomegalovirus pneumonitis in lung transplant patients. Arch Pathol Lab Med 119:33, 1995.

48. Strickler JG, Manivel JD, Copenhaver CM, Kubic VL: Comparison of in situ hybridization and immunohistochemistry for detection of cytomegalovirus and herpes simplex virus. Hum Pathol 21:443, 1990.

49. Tamm M, Traenkle P, Grilli B, et al: Pulmonary cytomegalovirus infection in immunocompromised patients. Chest 119:838, 2001.

50. Theise ND, Haber MM, Grimes MM: Detection of cytomegalovirus in lung allografts: Comparison of histologic and immunohistochemical findings. Am J Clin Pathol 96:762, 1991.

51. Vasudevan VP, Mascarenhas DAN, Klapper P, Lomvardias S: Cytomegalovirus necrotizing bronchiolitis with HIV infection. Chest 97:483, 1990.

52. Wolber RA, Lloyd RV: Cytomegalovirus detection by nonisotopic in situ DNA hybridization and viral antigen immunostaining using a two-color technique. Hum Pathol 19:736, 1988.

Herpes Simplex Virus

53. Geradts J, Warnock M, Yen TSB: Use of the polymerase chain reaction in the diagnosis of unsuspected herpes simplex viral pneumonia: Report of a case. Hum Pathol 21:118, 1990.

54. Graham BS, Snell JD Jr: Herpes simplex virus infection of the adult lower respiratory tract. Medicine (Baltimore) 62:384, 1983.

55. Greene GR, King D, Romansky SG, Marble RD: Primary herpes simplex pneumonia in a neonate. Am J Dis Child 137:464, 1983.

56. Legge RH, Thompson AB, Linder J, et al: Acyclovir-responsive herpetic tracheobronchitis. Am J Med 85:561, 1988.

57. Nakamura Y, Yamamoto S, Tanaka S, et al: Herpes simplex viral infection in human neonates: An immunohistochemical and electron microscopic study. Hum Pathol 16:1091, 1985.

58. Nash G: Necrotizing tracheobronchitis and bronchopneumonia consistent with herpetic infection. Hum Pathol 3:283, 1972.

59. Nash G, Foley F: Herpetic infection of the middle and lower respiratory tract. Am J Clin Pathol 54:857, 1970.

60. Ramsey PG, Fife KH, Hackman RC, et al: Herpes simplex virus pneumonia. Ann Intern Med 97:813, 1982.

61. Sherry MK, Klainer AS, Wolff M, Gerhard H: Herpetic tracheobronchitis. Ann Intern Med 109:229, 1988.

62. Tuxen D, Cade J, McDonald M, et al: Herpes simplex virus from the lower respiratory tract in adult respiratory distress syndrome. Am Rev Respir Dis 126:416, 1982.

Varicella-Zoster Virus

63. Charles RE, Katz RL, Ordonez NG, Mackay, B: Varicella-zoster infection with pleural involvement. A cytological and ultrastructural study of a case. Am J Clin Pathol 85:522, 1986.

64. Dolin R, Reichman R, Mazur M, Whitley R: Herpes zoster-varicella infections in immunosuppressed patients. Ann Intern Med 89:375, 1978.

65. Feldman S, Hughes W, Kim H: Herpes zoster in children with cancer. Am J Dis Child 126:178, 1973.

66. Meyer B, Stalder H, Wegmann W: Persistent pulmonary granulomas after recovery from varicella pneumonia. Chest 89:457, 1986.

67. Raider L: Calcification in chickenpox pneumonia. Chest 60:504, 1971.

68. Reboul F, Donaldson S, Kaplan H: Herpes zoster and varicella infections in children with Hodgkin's disease. An analysis of contributing factors. Cancer 41:95, 1978.

69. Saito F, Yutani C, Imakita M, et al: Giant cell pneumonia caused by varicella zoster virus in a neonate. Arch Pathol Lab Med 113:201, 1989.

70. Schimpff S, Serpick A, Stoler B, et al: Varicella-zoster infections in patients with cancer. Ann Intern Med 76:241, 1972.

71. Triebwasser J, Harris R, Bryant R, Rhoades E: Varicella pneumonia in adults. Report of seven cases and a review of literature. Medicine (Baltimore) 46:409, 1967.

Measles Virus

72. Akhtar M, Young I: Measles giant cell pneumonia in an adult following long-term chemotherapy. Arch Pathol 96:145, 1973.

73. Archibald R, Weller R, Meadow S: Measles pneumonia and the nature of the inclusion bearing giant cells: A light and electron microscope study. J Pathol 103:27, 1971.

74. Becroft D, Osborne D: The lungs in fatal measles infection in childhood: Pathological, radiological and immunological correlations. Histopathology 4:401, 1980.

75. Breitfeld V, Hashida Y, Sherman F, et al: Fatal measles infection in children with leukemia. Lab Invest 28:279, 1973.

76. Gremillion DH, Crawford GE: Measles pneumonia in young adults. An analysis of 106 cases. Am J Med 71:539, 1981.

77. Joliat G, Abetel G, Schindler A, Kapanci Y: Measles giant cell pneumonia without rash in a case of lymphocytic lymphosarcoma. An electron microscopic study. Virchows Arch A Pathol Pathol Anat 358:215, 1973.

78. Lewis M, Cameron A, Shah K: Giant-cell pneumonia caused by measles and methotrexate in childhood leukemia in remission. Br Med J 1:330, 1978.

Adenovirus

79. Sobonya R, Hiller C, Pingleton W, Watanabe I: Fatal measles (Rubeola) pneumonia in adults. Arch Pathol Lab Med 102:366, 1978.

80. Abbondanzo SL, English CK, Kagan E, et al: Fatal adenovirus pneumonia in a newborn identified by electron microscopy and in situ hybridization. Arch Pathol Lab Med 113:1349, 1989.

81. Abzug MJ, Levin MJ: Neonatal adenovirus infection: Four patients and review of the literature. Pediatrics 87:890, 1991.

82. Bateman ED, Hagashi S, Kuwano K, et al: Latent adenoviral infection in follicular bronchiectasis. Am J Respir Crit Care Med 115:170, 1995.

83. Becroft D: Histopathology of fatal adenovirus infection of the respiratory tract in young children. J Clin Pathol 20:561, 1967.

84. Becroft D: Bronchiolitis obliterans, bronchiectasis, and other sequelae of adenovirus type 21 infection in young children. J Clin Pathol 24:72, 1971.

85. Dudding B, Wagner S, Zeller J, et al: Fatal pneumonia associated with adenovirus Type 7 in three military trainees. N Engl J Med 286:1289, 1972.

86. Green WR, Williams AW: Neonatal adenovirus pneumonia. Arch Pathol Lab Med 113:190, 1989.

87. Hogg JC, Irving WL, Porter H, et al: In situ hybridization studies of adenoviral infections of the lung and their relationship to follicular bronchiectasis. Am Rev Respir Dis 139:1531, 1989.

88. Landry M, Fong C, Neddermann K, et al: Disseminated adenovirus infection in an immunocompromised host. Pitfalls in diagnosis. Am J Med 83:555, 1987.

89. Loker E Jr, Hodges G, Kelley D: Fatal adenovirus pneumonia in a young adult associated with ADV-7 vaccine administered 15 days earlier. Chest 66:197, 1974.

90. Matsuoka T, Naito T, Kubota Y, et al: Disseminated adenovirus (type 19) infection in a neonate: Rapid detection of the infection by immunofluorescence. Acta Paediatr Scand 79:568, 1990.

91. Myerowitz R, Stalder H, Oxman M, et al: Fatal disseminated adenovirus infection in a renal transplant recipient. Am J Med 59:591, 1975.

92. Ohori NP, Michaels MG, Jaffe R, et al: Adenovirus pneumonia in lung transplant recipients. Hum Pathol 26:1073, 1995.

93. Pinkerton H, Carroll S: Fatal adenovirus pneumonia in infants. Am J Pathol 65:543, 1971.

94. Pinto A, Beck R, Jadavji T: Fatal neonatal pneumonia caused by adenovirus type 35: Report of one case and review of the literature. Arch Pathol Lab Med 116:95, 1992.

95. Schonland M, Strong M, Wesley A: Fatal adenovirus pneumonia. Clinical and pathological features. S Afr Med J 50:1748, 1976.

96. Simila S, Linna O, Lanning P, et al: Chronic lung damage caused by adenovirus type 7: A ten-year follow-up study. Chest 80:127, 1981.

97. Wenman WM, Pagtakhan RD, Reed MH, et al: Adenovirus bronchiolitis in Manitoba. Epidemiologic, clinical, and radiologic features. Chest 81:605, 1982.

98. Wu T-C, Kanayama MD, Hruban RH, Au W-C, Askin FB, Hutchins GM: Virus-associated RNAs (VA-I and VA-II): An efficient target for the detection of adenovirus infections by in situ hybridization. Am J Pathol 140:991, 1992.

99. Zahradnik J, Spencer M, Porter D: Adenovirus infection in the immunocompromised patient. Am J Med 68:725, 1980.

Other Viruses

100. Aherne W, Bird T, Court S, et al: Pathological changes in virus infections of the lower respiratory tract in children. J Clin Pathol 23:7, 1970.

101. Akizuki S, Nasu N, Setoguchi M, et al: Parainfluenza virus in an adult. Arch Pathol Lab Med 115:824, 1991.

102. Castillo C, Naranjo J, Sepulveda A, et al. Hantavirus pulmonary syndrome due to Andes virus in Temuco, Chile. Clinical experience with 16 adults. Chest 120:548, 2001.

103. Cheung OY, Chan JWM, Ng CK, Koo CK: The spectrum of pathological changes in severe acute respiratory syndrome (SARS). Histopathology 45:119, 2004.

104. Chow K-C, Hsiao C-H, Lin T-Y, et al: Detection of severe acute respiratory syndrome-associated coronavirus in pneumocytes. Am J Clin Pathol 121:574, 2004.

105. Colby TV, Zaki SR, Feddersen RM, et al. Hantavirus pulmonary syndrome is distinguishable from acute interstitial pneumonia. Arch Pathol Lab Med 124:1463, 2000.

106. Delage G, Brochu P, Robillard L, et al: Giant cell pneumonia due to respiratory syncytial virus. Arch Pathol Lab Med 108:623, 1984.

107. Ding Y, Wang H, Shen H, et al: The clinical pathology of severe acute respiratory syndrome (SARS): A report from China. J Pathol 200:282, 2003.

108. Duchin J, Koster FT, Peters CJ, et al: Hantavirus pulmonary syndrome: A clinical description of 17 patients with a newly recognized disease. N Engl J Med 330:949, 1994.

109. Englund JA, Sullivan CJ, Jordan C, et al: Respiratory syncytial virus infection in immunocompromised adults. Ann Intern Med 109:203, 1988.

110. Feldman P, Cohan M, Hierholzer W: Fatal Hong Kong influenza: A clinical, microbiological and pathological analysis of nine cases. Yale J Biol Med 45:49, 1972.

111. Franks TJ, Chong PY, Chui P, et al. Lung pathology of severe acute respiratory syndrome (SARS): A study of 8 autopsy cases from Singapore. Hum Pathol 34:743, 2003.

112. Garantziotis S, Howell DN, McAdams HP, et al. Influenza pneumonia in lung transplant recipients: Clinical features and association with bronchiolitis obliterans syndrome. Chest 119:1277, 2001.

113. Hall CB. Respiratory syncytial virus and parainfluenza virus. N Engl J Med 344:1917, 2001.

114. Hall C, Kopelman A, Douglas R Jr, et al: Neonatal respiratory syncytial virus infection. N Engl J Med 300:393, 1979.

115. Ho JC, Ooi GC, Mok TY, et al. High-dose pulse versus nonpulse corticosteroid regimens in severe acute respiratory syndrome. Am J Respir Crit Care Med 168:1449, 2003.

116. Klimek J, Lindenberg L, Cole S, et al: Fatal case of influenza pneumonia with superinfection by multiple bacteria and herpes simplex virus. Am Rev Respir Dis 113:683, 1976.

117. Kurlandsky LE, French G, Webb PM, et al: Fatal respiratory syncytial virus pneumonia in a previously healthy child. Am Rev Respir Dis 138:468, 1988.

118. Lam M-F, Ooi GC, Lam B, et al. An indolent case of severe acute respiratory syndrome. Am J Respir Crit Care Med 169:125, 2004.

119. Laraya-Cuasay L, DeForest A, Huff D, et al: Chronic pulmonary complications of early influenza virus infection in children. Am Rev Respir Dis 116:617, 1977.

120. Levenson RM, Kantor OS: Fatal pneumonia in an adult due to respiratory syncytial virus. Arch Intern Med 147:791, 1987.

121. Levy H, Simpson SQ: Hantavirus pulmonary syndrome. Am J Respir Crit Care Med 149:1710, 1994.

122. Lewis VA, Champlin R, Enflund J, et al: Respiratory disease due to parainfluenza virus in adult bone marrow transplant recipients. Clin Infect Dis 23:1033, 1996.

123. Little BW, Tihen WS, Dickerman JD, Craighead JE: Giant cell pneumonia associated with parainfluenza virus type 3 infection. Hum Pathol 12:478, 1981.

124. Liu C-L, Lu Y-T, Peng M-J, et al: Clinical and laboratory features of severe acute respiratory syndrome vis-à-vis onset of fever. Chest 126:509, 2004.

125. Madden JF, Burchette JL, Hale LP: Pathology of parainfluenza virus infection in patients with congenital immunodeficiency syndromes. Hum Pathol 35:594, 2004.

126. Nicholls JM, Poon LL, Lee KC, et al. Lung pathology of fatal severe acute respiratory syndrome. Lancet 361:1773, 2003.

127. Noble R, Lillington G, Kempson R: Fatal diffuse influenzal pneumonia: Premortem diagnosis by lung biopsy. Chest 63:644, 1973.

128. Nolte KB, Feddersen RM, Foucar K, et al: Hantavirus pulmonary syndrome in the United States. A pathological description of a disease caused by a new agent. Hum Pathol 26:110, 1995.

129. Peiris JSM, Yuen KY, Osterhaus ADME, Stohr K: The severe acute respiratory syndrome. N Engl J Med 349:2431, 2003.

130. Tamura H, Aronson B: Intranuclear fibrillary inclusions in influenza pneumonia. Arch Pathol Lab Med 102:252, 1978.

131. Weintrub PS, Sullender WM, Lombard C, et al: Giant cell pneumonia caused by parainfluenza type 3 in a patient with acute myelomonocytic leukemia. Arch Pathol Lab Med 111:569, 1987.

132. Yeldandi AV, Colby TV: Pathologic features of lung biopsy specimens from influenza pneumonia cases. Hum Pathol 25:47, 1994.

133. Zaki SR, Greer PW, Coffield LM, et al. Hantavirus pulmonary syndrome: Pathogenesis of an emerging infectious disease. Am J Pathol 146:552, 1995.

134. Zaki SR, Khan AS, Goodman RA, et al: Retrospective diagnosis of hantavirus pulmonary syndrome, 1978–1993. Implications for emerging infectious diseases. Arch Pathol Lab Med 120:134, 1996.

Fungal Pneumonias

Aspergillosis

135. Albelda SM, Talbot GH, Gerson SL, et al: Pulmonary cavitation and massive hemoptysis in invasive pulmonary aspergillosis. Influence of bone marrow recovery in patients with acute leukemia. Am Rev Respir Dis 131:115, 1985.

136. Binder RE, Faling J, Pugatch RD, et al: Chronic necrotizing pulmonary aspergillosis: A discrete clinical entity. Medicine (Baltimore) 61:109, 1982.

137. Boon AP, O'Brien D, Adams DH: 10 year review of invasive aspergillosis detected at necropsy. J Clin Pathol 44:452, 1991.

138. Borkin M, Arena F, Brown A, Armstrong D: Invasive aspergillosis with massive fatal hemoptysis in patients with neoplastic disease. Chest 78:835, 1980.

139. Brown E, Freedman S, Arbeit R, Come S: Invasive pulmonary aspergillosis in an apparently nonimmunocompromised host. Am J Med 69:624, 1980.

140. Buchanan DR, Lamb D: Saprophytic invasion of infarcted pulmonary tissue by *Aspergillus* species. Thorax 37:693, 1982.

141. Caras WE, Pluss JL: Chronic necrotizing pulmonary aspergillosis: Pathologic outcome after itraconazole therapy. Mayo Clin Proc 71:25, 1996.

142. Clancy CJ, Nguyen MH: Acute community-acquired pneumonia due to aspergillus in presumably immunocompetent hosts: Clues for recognition of a rare but fatal disease. Chest 114:629, 1998.

143. Clarke A, Skelton J, Fraser RS: Fungal tracheobronchitis. Report of 9 cases and review of the literature. Medicine (Baltimore) 70:1, 1991.

144. Emmons R, Able E, Tenenberg D, Schachter J: Fatal pulmonary psittacosis and aspergillosis. Case report of dual infection. Arch Intern Med 140:697, 1980.

145. Fraser R: Pulmonary aspergillosis: Pathologic and pathogenetic features. Pathol Ann 28(Pt 1):231, 1993.

146. Gefter WB: The spectrum of pulmonary aspergillosis. J Thorac Imaging 7:56, 1992.

147. Gefter WB, Weingrad TR, Epstein DM, et al: "Semi-invasive" pulmonary aspergillosis. Radiology 140:313, 1981.

148. Hines DW, Haber MH, Yaremko L, Britton C, McLawhon RW, Harris AA: Pseudomembranous tracheobronchitis caused by *Aspergillus*. Am Rev Respir Dis 143:1408, 1991.

149. Hotchi M, Fujiwara M, Hata S, Nasu T: Chronic granulomatous disease associated with peculiar *Aspergillus* lesions. Patho-anatomical report based on two autopsy cases and a brief review of all autopsy cases reported in Japan. Virchows Arch A Pathol Anat Histol 387:1, 1980.

150. Karam G, Griffin F Jr: Invasive pulmonary aspergillosis in nonimmunocompromised, non-neutropenic hosts. Rev Infect Dis 8:357, 1986.

151. Kato T, Usami I, Morita H, et al: Chronic necrotizing pulmonary aspergillosis in pneumoconiosis: Clinical and radiologic findings in 10 patients (clinical investigations). Chest 121:118, 2004.

152. Kelly JK, Pinto A, Whitelaw WA, et al: Fatal aspergillus pneumonia in chronic granulomatous disease. Am J Clin Pathol 86:235, 1986.

153. Kramer MR, Denning DW, Marshall SE, et al: Ulcerative tracheobronchitis after lung transplantation: A new form of invasive aspergillosis. Am Rev Respir Dis 144:552, 1991.

154. Lake KB, Browne PM, Van Dyke JJ, Ayers L: Fatal disseminated aspergillosis in an asthmatic patient treated with corticosteroids. Chest 83:136, 1983.

155. Lewis M, Kallenbach J, Ruff P, et al: Invasive pulmonary aspergillosis complicating influenza A pneumonia in a previously healthy patient. Chest 87:691, 1985.

156. Liu K, Howell DN, Perfect JR, Schell WA: Morphologic criteria for the preliminary identification of *Fusarium, Paecilomyces*, and *Acremonium* species by histopathology. Am J Clin Pathol 109:45, 1998.

157. Meeker DP, Gephardt GN, Cordasco EM Jr, Wiedemann HP: Hypersensitivity pneumonitis versus invasive pulmonary aspergillosis: Two cases with unusual pathologic findings and review of the literature. Am Rev Respir Dis 143:431, 1991.

158. Meersseman W, Vandecasteele SJ, Wilmer A, et al: Invasive aspergillosis in critically ill patients without malignancy. Am J Respir Crit Care Med 170:621, 2004.

159. Mehrad B, Paciocco G, Martinez FJ, et al: Spectrum of aspergillus infection in lung transplant recipients: Case series and review of the literature. Chest 119:169, 2001.

160. Meyer R, Young L, Armstrong D, Yu B: Aspergillosis complicating neoplastic disease. Am J Med 54:6, 1973.

161. Nagata N, Sueishi K, Tanaka K, Iwata Y: Pulmonary aspergillosis with bronchocentric granulomas. Am J Surg Pathol 14:485, 1990.

162. Nash G, Irvine R, Kerschmann RL, et al: Pulmonary aspergillosis in acquired immune deficiency syndrome: Autopsy study of an emerging pulmonary complication of human immunodeficiency virus infection. Hum Pathol 28:1268, 1997.

163. Niimi T, Kajita M, Saito H: Necrotizing bronchial aspergillosis in a patient receiving neoadjuvant chemotherapy for non-small cell lung carcinoma. Chest 100:277, 1991.

164. Orr D, Myerowitz R, Dubois P: Pathoradiologic correlation of invasive pulmonary aspergillosis in the compromised host. Cancer 41:2028, 1978.

165. Pai U, Blinkhorn RJ Jr, Tomashefski JF Jr: Invasive cavitary pulmonary aspergillosis in patients with cancer: A clinicopathologic study. Hum Pathol 25:293, 1994.

166. Patterson TF, Kirkpatrick WR, White M, et al: Invasive aspergillosis: Disease spectrum, treatment practices, and outcomes. Medicine (Baltimore) 79:250, 2000.

167. Pervez NK, Kleinerman J, Kattan M, et al: Pseudomembranous necrotizing bronchial aspergillosis. A variant of invasive aspergillosis in a patient with hemophilia and acquired immune deficiency syndrome. Am Rev Respir Dis 131:961, 1985.

168. Phillips P, Weiner MH: Invasive aspergillosis diagnosed by immunohistochemistry with monoclonal and polyclonal reagents. Hum Pathol 18:1015, 1987.

169. Raad I, Hanna H, Huaringa A, et al: Diagnosis of invasive pulmonary aspergillosis using polymerase chain reaction-based detection of aspergillus in BAL. Chest 121:1171, 2002.

170. Reichenberger F, Habicht JM, Gratwohl A, Tamm M: Diagnosis and treatment of invasive pulmonary aspergillosis in neutropenic patients. Eur Respir J 19:743, 2002.

171. Robertson M, Larson R: Recurrent fungal pneumonias in patients with acute nonlymphocytic leukemia undergoing multiple courses of intensive chemotherapy. Am J Med 84:233, 1988.

172. Roig J, Ruiz J, Puig X, et al: Bronchial stump aspergillosis four years after lobectomy. Chest 104:295, 1993.

173. Rose H, Varkey B: Deep mycotic infection in the hospitalized adult. A study of 123 patients. Medicine (Baltimore) 54:499, 1975.

174. Saraceno JL, Phelps DT, Ferro TJ, et al. Chronic necrotizing pulmonary aspergillosis: Approach to management. Chest 112:541, 1997.

175. Spearing RL, Pamphilon DH, Prentice AG: Pulmonary aspergillosis in immunosuppressed patients with haematological malignancies. Q J Med 59:611, 1986.

176. Tazelaar HD, Baird AM, Mill M, Grimes MM, Schulman LL, Smith CR: Bronchocentric mycosis occurring in transplant recipients. Chest 96:92, 1989.

177. Thommi G, Bell G, Liu J, Nugent K: Spectrum of invasive pulmonary aspergillosis in immunocompetent patients with chronic obstructive pulmonary disease. South Med J 84:828, 1991.

178. Tron V, Churg A: Chronic necrotizing pulmonary aspergillosis mimicking bronchocentric granulomatosis. Pathol Res Pract 181:621, 1986.

179. Watts JC, Chandler FW: Morphologic identification of mycelial pathogens in tissue sections: A caveat. Am J Clin Pathol 109:1, 1998.

180. Wiggins J, Clark TJH, Corrin B: Chronic necrotising pneumonia caused by *Aspergillus niger*. Thorax 44:440, 1989.

181. Wright JL, Lawson L, Chan N, Filipenko D: An unusual form of pulmonary aspergillosis in two patients with the acquired immunodeficiency syndrome. Am J Clin Pathol 100:57, 1993.

182. Young R, Bennett J, Vogel C, et al: Aspergillosis. The spectrum of the disease in 98 patients. Medicine (Baltimore) 49:147, 1970.

183. Yousem SA: The histological spectrum of chronic necrotizing forms of pulmonary aspergillosis. Hum Pathol 28:650, 1997.

Mucormycosis

184. Benbow EW, Delamore IW, Stoddart RW, Reid H: Disseminated zygomycosis associated with erythroleukaemia: Confirmation by lectin stains. J Clin Pathol 38:1039, 1985.

185. Chandler FW, Watts JC, Kaplan W, et al: Zygomycosis. Report of four cases with formation of chlamydoconidia in tissue. Am J Clin Pathol 84:99, 1985.

186. Espinoza C, Halkias D: Pulmonary mucormycosis as a complication of chronic salicylate poisoning. Am J Clin Pathol 80:508, 1983.

187. Lehrer R, Howard D, Sypherd P, et al: Mucormycosis. Ann Intern Med 93(Pt I):93, 1980.

188. Meyer R, Rosen P, Armstrong D: Phycomycosis complicating leukemia and lymphoma. Ann Intern Med 77:871, 1972.

189. Murray, H: Pulmonary mucormycosis with massive fatal hemoptysis. Chest 68:65, 1975.

190. Record N Jr, Ginder D: Pulmonary phycomycosis without obvious predisposing factors. JAMA 235:1256, 1976.

191. Ventura GJ, Kantarjian HM, Anaissie E, et al: Pneumonia with *Cunninghamella* species in patients with hematologic malignancies. A case report and review of the literature. Cancer 58:1534, 1986.

192. Zeilender S, Drenning D, Glauser FL, Bechard D: Fatal *Cunninghamella bertholletiae* infection in an immunocompetent patient. Chest 97:1482, 1990.

Candidiasis

193. Buff SJ, McLelland R, Gallis HA, et al: *Candida albicans* pneumonia: Radiographic appearance. AJR Am J Roentgenol 138:645, 1982.

194. Cho S, Choi H: Opportunistic fungal infection among cancer patients. An autopsy study. Am J Clin Pathol 72:617, 1979.

195. Dubois P, Myerowitz R, Allen C: Pathoradiologic correlation of pulmonary candidiasis in immunosuppressed patients. Cancer 40:1026, 1977.

196. El-Ebiary M, Torres A, Fàbregas N, et al. Significance of the isolation of *Candida* species from respiratory samples in critically ill, non-neutropenic patients: an immediate portmortem histologic study. Am J Respir Crit Care Med 156:583, 1997.

197. Gaines J, Remington J: Disseminated candidiasis in the surgical patient. Surgery 72:730, 1972.

198. Haron E, Vartivarian S, Anaissie E, et al: Primary *Candida* pneumonia: Experience at a large cancer center and a review of the literature. Medicine (Baltimore) 72:137, 1993.

199. Kassner EG, Kauffman SL, Yoon JJ, et al: Pulmonary candidiasis in infants: Clinical, radiologic, and pathologic features. AJR Am J Roentgenol 137:707, 1981.

200. Knox WF, Hooton VN, Barson AJ: Pulmonary vascular candidiasis and use of central venous catheters in neonates. J Clin Pathol 40:559, 1987.

201. Law E, Kim O, Stieritz D, McMillan B: Experience with systemic candidiasis in the burned patient. J Trauma 12:543, 1972.

202. Masur H, Rosen P, Armstrong D. Pulmonary disease caused by *Candida* species. Am J Med 63:914, 1977.

203. Montcagudo C, Marcilla A, Mormenco S, Llombart-Bosch A, Sentandreu R: Specific immunohistochemical identification of *Candida albicans* in paraffin-embedded tissue with a new monoclonal antibody (1B12). Am J Clin Pathol 103:130, 1995.

204. Myerowitz R, Pazin G, Allen C: Disseminated candidiasis. Changes in incidence, underlying diseases and pathology. Am J Clin Pathol 68:29, 1977.

205. Parker J Jr, McCloskey J, Knauer K: Pathobiologic features of human candidiasis. A common deep mycosis of the brain, heart and kidney in the altered host. Am J Clin Pathol 65:991, 1976.

206. Rose H, Sheth N: Pulmonary candidiasis. A clinical and pathological correlation. Arch Intern Med 138:964, 1978.

207. Wingard J, Merz W, Saral R: *Candida tropicalis*: A major pathogen in immunocompromised patients. Ann Intern Med 91:539, 1979.

Other Fungi

208. Aisner J, Schimpff S, Sutherland J, et al: *Torulopsis glabrata* infections in patients with cancer. Increasing incidence and relationship to colonization. Am J Med 61:23, 1976.

209. Alture-Werber E, Edberg S, Singer J: Pulmonary infection with *Allescheria boydii*. Am J Clin Pathol 66:1019, 1976.

210. Dankner WM, Spector SA, Fierer J, Davis CE: Malassezia fungemia in neonates and adults: Complication of hyperalimentation. Rev Infect Dis 9:743, 1987.

211. Nonaka D, Yfantis H, Southall P, Sun C-C: Pseudallescheriasis as an aggressive opportunistic infection in a bone marrow transplant recipient. Arch Pathol Lab Med 126:207, 2002.

212. Redline RW, Redline SS, Boxerbaum B, Dahms BB: Systemic *Malassezia furfur* infections in patients receiving Intralipid therapy. Hum Pathol 16:815, 1985.

213. Schwartz DA: Organ-specific variation in the morphology of the fungomas (fungus balls) of *Pseudallescheria boydii*: Development within necrotic host tissue. Arch Pathol Lab Med 113:476, 1989.

214. Srivastava S, Kleinman G, Manthous CA: Torulopsis pneumonia: A case report and review of the literature. Chest 110:858, 1996.

215. Valdivieso M, Luna M, Bodey G, et al: Fungemia due to *Torulopsis glabrata* in the compromised host. Cancer 38:1750, 1976.

216. Walker D, Adamec T, Krigman M: Disseminated petriellidosis (allescheriosis). Arch Pathol Lab Med 102:158, 1978.

217. Winston D, Jordan M, Rhodes J: *Allescheria boydii* infections in the immunosuppressed host. Am J Med 63:830, 1977.

Mycetomas
218. Arnett J, Hatch H Jr: Pulmonary allescheriasis. Report of a case and review of the literature. Arch Intern Med 135:1250, 1975.
219. Bakerspigel A, Wood T, Burke S: Pulmonary allescheriasis. Report of a case from Ontario, Canada. Am J Pathol 68:299, 1977.
220. Cohen M, Brook C, Naylor B, et al: Pulmonary phycomycetoma in a patient with diabetes mellitus. Am Rev Respir Dis 116:519, 1977.
221. Ghio AJ, Peterseim DS, Roggli VL, Piantadosi CA: Pulmonary oxalate deposition associated with *Aspergillus niger* infection. An oxidant hypothesis of toxicity. Am Rev Respir Dis 145:1499, 1992.
222. Jewkes J, Kay PH, Paneth M, Citron KM: Pulmonary aspergilloma: Analysis of prognosis in relation to haemoptysis and survey of treatment. Thorax 38:572, 1983.
223. Kimmerling EA, Fedrick JA, Tenholder MF: Invasive *Aspergillus niger* with fatal pulmonary oxalosis in chronic obstructive pulmonary disease. Chest 101:870, 1992.
224. Kirkpatrick M, Pollock H, Wimberley N: An intracavitary fungus ball composed of Syncephalastrum. Am Rev Respir Dis 120:943, 1979.
225. Kurrein F, Green G, Rowles S: Localized deposition of calcium oxalate around a pulmonary *Aspergillus niger* fungus ball. Am J Clin Pathol 64:556, 1975.
226. Kwon-Chung K, Schwartz I, Rybak B: A pulmonary fungus ball produced by *Cladosporium cladosporioides*. Am J Clin Pathol 64:564, 1975.
227. Lee SH, Barnes WG, Schaetzel WP: Pulmonary aspergillosis and the importance of oxalate crystal recognition in cytology specimens. Arch Pathol Lab Med 110:1176, 1986.
228. McGregor DH, Papasian CJ, Pierce PD: Aspergilloma within cavitating pulmonary adenocarcinoma. Am J Clin Pathol 91:100, 1989.
229. Metzger J, Garagusi V, Kerwin D: Pulmonary oxalosis caused by *Aspergillus niger*. Am Rev Respir Dis 129:501, 1984.
230. Nime F, Hutchins G: Oxalosis caused by *Aspergillus* infection. Johns Hopkins Med J 133:183, 1973.
231. Putnam J, Harper W, Greene J Jr, et al: *Coccidioides immitis*. A rare cause of pulmonary mycetoma. Am Rev Respir Dis 112:733 1975.
232. Rafferty P, Biggs B-A, Crompton GK, Grant IWB: What happens to patients with pulmonary aspergilloma? Analysis of 23 cases. Thorax 38:579, 1983.
233. Rohatgi PK, Schmitt RG: Pulmonary coccidioidal mycetoma. Am J Med Sci 287:27, 1984.
234. Shapiro MJ, Albeda SM, Mayock RL, McLean GK: Severe hemoptysis associated with pulmonary aspergilloma. Percutaneous intracavitary treatment. Chest 94:1225, 1988.

235. Smith FB, Beneck D: Localized aspergillus infestation in primary lung carcinoma. Clinical and pathological contrasts with post-tuberculous intracavitary aspergilloma. Chest 100:554, 1991.
236. Yoshida K, Hiraoka T, Ando M, et al: *Penicillium decumbens*. A new cause of fungus ball. Chest 101:1152, 1992.

Nocardia and Actinomycosis
237. Ariel I, Breuer R, Kamal NS, Ben-Dov I, Mogle P, Rosenmann E: Endobronchial actinomycosis simulating bronchogenic carcinoma: Diagnosis by bronchial biopsy. Chest 99:493, 1991.
238. Brown J: Human actinomycosis. A study of 181 subjects. Hum Pathol 4:319, 1973.
239. de Montpreville VT, Nashashibi N, Dulmet EM: Actinomycosis and other bronchopulmonary infections with bacterial granules. Ann Diagn Pathol 3:67, 1999.
240. Feigen DS: Nocardiosis of the lung: Chest radiographic findings in 21 cases. Radiology 159:9, 1986.
241. Frazier A, Rosenow E III, Roberts G: Nocardiosis. A review of 25 cases occurring during 24 months. Mayo Clin Proc 50:657, 1975.
242. Gorevic P, Katler E, Agus B: Pulmonary nocardiosis. Occurrence in men with systemic lupus erythematosus. Arch Intern Med 140:361, 1980.
243. Henkle JQ, Nair SV: Endobronchial pulmonary nocardiosis. JAMA 256:1331, 1986.
244. Hsieh M-J, Liu H-P, Chang J-P, Chang C-H: Thoracic actinomycosis. Chest 104:366, 1993.
245. Katapadi K, Pujol F, Vuletin JC, et al: Pulmonary botryomycosis in a patient with AIDS. Chest 109:276, 1996.
246. Lau K-Y: Endobronchial actinomycosis mimicking pulmonary neoplasm. Thorax 47:664, 1992.
247. Mamlok V, Cowan WT Jr, Schnadig V: Unusual histopathology of mucormycosis in acute myelogenous leukemia. Am J Clin Pathol 88:117, 1987.
248. Oddo D, Gonzalez S: Actinomycosis and nocardiosis. A morphologic study of 17 cases. Pathol Res Pract 181:320, 1986.
249. Paz HL, Little BJ, Ball WC Jr, et al: Primary pulmonary botryomycosis: A manifestation of chronic granulomatous disease. Chest 101:1160, 1992.
250. Robboy S, Vickery A: Tinctorial and morphologic properties distinguishing actinomycosis and nocardiosis. N Engl J Med 282:593, 1970.
251. Rodig SJ, Dorfman DM: Splendore-Hoeppli phenomenon. Arch Pathol Lab Med 125:1515, 2001.
252. Sarodia BD, Farver C, Erzurum S, Maurer JR: A young man with two large lung masses. Chest 116:814, 1999.
253. Wada R, Itabashi C, Nakayama Y, et al: Chronic granulomatous pleuritis caused by nocardia: PCR based diagnosis by nocardial 16S rDNA in pathological specimens. J Clin Pathol 56:966, 2003.

Legionnaires' Disease and Related Pneumonias
254. Blackmon J, Chandler F, Cherry W, et al: Legionellosis. Am J Pathol 103:429, 1981.

255. Boyd J, Buchanan W, MacLeod T, et al: Pathology of five Scottish deaths from pneumonic illnesses acquired in Spain due to Legionnaire's disease agent. J Clin Pathol 31:809, 1978.

256. Broome C, Cherry W, Winn W, McPherson B: Rapid diagnosis of Legionnaire's disease by direct immunofluorescent staining. Ann Intern Med 90:1, 1979.

257. Chandler F, Blackmon J, Hicklin M, et al. Ultrastructure of the agent of Legionnaire's disease in the human lung. Am J Clin Pathol 71:43, 1979.

258. Chandler F, Hicklin M, Blackmon J: Demonstration of the agent of Legionnaire's disease in tissue. N Engl J Med 297:1218, 1977.

259. Chastre J, Raghu G, Soler P, et al: Pulmonary fibrosis following pneumonia due to acute Legionnaire's disease. Clinical, ultrastructural, and immunofluorescent study. Chest 91:57, 1987.

260. Fain JS, Bryan RN, Cheng L, Lewin KJ, Porter DD, Grody WW: Rapid diagnosis of Legionella infection by a nonisotopic in situ hybridization method. Am J Clin Pathol 95:719, 1991.

261. Falco V, de Sevilla TF, Alegre J, Ferrer A, Vazquez JMM: Legionella pneumonia: A cause of severe community-acquired pneumonia. Chest 100:1007, 1991.

262. Fang G-D, Yu VL, Vickers RM: Disease due to the Legionellaceae (other than Legionella pneumophila): Historical, microbiological, clinical, and epidemiological review. Medicine (Baltimore) 68:116, 1989.

263. Fraser D, Tsai T, Orenstein W, et al: Legionnaire's disease. Description of an epidemic pneumonia. N Engl J Med 297:1189, 1977.

264. Greer P, Chandler F, Hicklin M: Rapid demonstration of Legionella pneumophila in unembedded tissue. An adaptation of the Gimenez stain. Am J Clin Pathol 73:788, 1980.

265. Gress F, Myerowitz R, Pasculle A, et al: The ultrastructural morphologic features of Pittsburgh pneumonia agent. Am J Pathol 101:63, 1980.

266. Hernandez F, Kirby B, Stanley T, Edelstein P: Legionnaire's disease. Postmortem pathologic findings of twenty cases. Am J Clin Pathol 73:488, 1980.

267. Hicklin M, Thomason B, Chandler F, Blackmon J: Pathogenesis of acute Legionnaire's disease pneumonia. Immunofluorescent microscopic study. Am J Clin Pathol 73:480, 1980.

268. Kariman K, Shelburne J, Gough W, et al: Pathologic findings and long-term sequelae in Legionnaire's disease. Chest 75:736, 1979.

269. Katz S, Brodsky I, Kahn B: Legionnaire's disease. Ultrastructural appearance of the agent in a lung biopsy specimen. Arch Pathol Lab Med 103:261, 1979.

270. Katz S, Nash P: The morphology of the Legionnaire's disease organism. Am J Pathol 90:701, 1978.

271. Keys T: Legionnaire's disease. A review of the epidemiology and clinical manifestations of a newly recognized infection. Mayo Clin Proc 55:129, 1980.

272. Kirby B, Snyder K, Meyer R, Finegold S: Legionnaire's disease: Report of sixty-five nosocomially acquired cases and review of the literature. Medicine (Baltimore) 59:188, 1980.

273. Liu F, Wright DN: Gram stain in Legionnaires' disease. Am J Med 77:549, 1984.

274. Marshall W, Foster R Jr, Winn W: Legionnaire's disease in renal transplant patients. Am J Surg 141:423, 1981.

275. McDade J, Shepard C, Fraser D, et al: Legionnaire's disease. Isolation of a bacterium and demonstration of its role in other respiratory disease. N Engl J Med 297:1197, 1977.

276. Muder RR, Yu VL, Zuravleff JJ: Pneumonia due to the Pittsburgh pneumonia agent: New clinical perspective with a review of the literature. Medicine (Baltimore) 62:120, 1983.

277. Palutke WA, Crane LR, Wentworth BB, et al: Legionella feeleii-associated pneumonia in humans. Am J Clin Pathol 86:348, 1986.

278. Rodgers F: Ultrastructure of Legionella pneumophila. J Clin Pathol 32:1195, 1979.

279. Schurmann D, Ruf B, Fehrenbach FJ, Jautzke G, Pohle HD: Fatal Legionnaires' pneumonia: Frequency of legionellosis in autopsied patients with pneumonia from 1969 to 1985. J Pathol 155:35, 1988.

280. Suffin S, Kaufmann A, Whitaker B, et al: Legionella pneumophila. Identification in tissue sections by a new immunoenzymatic procedure. Arch Pathol Lab Med 104:283, 1980.

281. Theaker JM, Tobin O'HJ, Jones SEC, et al: Immuno-histological detection of Legionella pneumophila in lung sections. J Clin Pathol 40:143, 1987.

282. van den Bergen H, Meenhorst P, Ruiter D, et al: Legionnaire's disease: Case report with special emphasis on electron microscopy and potential risk of infection at autopsy. Histopathology 3:523, 1979.

283. Van Orden A, Greer P: Modification of the Dieterle spirochete stain. J. Histotechnol. 1:51, 1977.

284. Watts J, Hicklin M, Thomason B, et al: Fatal pneumonia caused by Legionella pneumophila, serogroup 3: Demonstration of the bacilli in extrathoracic organs. Ann Intern Med 92:186, 1980.

285. Weisenburger D, Helms C, Renner E: Sporadic Legionnaire's disease. A pathologic study of 23 fatal cases. Arch Pathol Lab Med 105:130, 1981.

286. Weisenberger D, Rappaport H, Ahluwalia M, et al: Legionnaire's disease. Am J Med 69:476, 1980.

287. White H, Felton W, Sun C: Extrapulmonary histopathologic manifestations of Legionnaire's disease. Arch Pathol Lab Med 104:287, 1980.

288. Winn W Jr, Myerowitz R: The pathology of the Legionella pneumonias: A review of 74 cases and the literature. Hum Pathol 12:401, 1981.

Anthrax

289. Albrink WS, Brooks SM, Biron RE, Kopel M: Human inhalation anthrax: A report of three fatal cases. Am J Pathol 36:457, 1960.

290. Bush LM, Abrams BH, Beall A, Johnson CC: Index case of fatal inhalational anthrax due to bioterrorism in the United States. N Engl J Med 345:1607, 2001.

291. Dixon TC, Meselson M, Guillemin J, Hanna PC: Anthrax. N Engl J Med 341:815, 1999.

292. Grinberg LM, Abramova FA, Yampolskaya OV, et al: Quantitative pathology of inhalational anthrax I: Quantitative microscopic findings. Mod Pathol 14:482, 2001.

293. Shafazand S, Doyle R, Ruoss S, et al: Inhalational anthrax: Epidemiology, diagnosis, and management. Chest 116:1369, 1999.

294. Suffin SC, Carnes WH, Kaufmann AF: Inhalation anthrax in a home craftsman. Hum Pathol 9:594, 1978.

Pneumocystis Pneumonia

295. An T, Tabaczka P: The use of polarization microscopy in the diagnosis of pneumocystis pneumonia. Arch Pathol Lab Med 128:363, 2004.

296. Askin F, Katzenstein A: Pneumocystis infection masquerading as diffuse alveolar damage: A potential source of diagnostic error. Chest 79:420, 1981.

297. Barrio JL, Suarez M, Rodriguez JL, et al: *Pneumocystis carinii* pneumonia presenting as cavitating and noncavitating solitary pulmonary nodules in patients with the acquired immunodeficiency syndrome. Am Rev Respir Dis 134:1094, 1986.

298. Beers MP, Sohn M, Swartz M: Recurrent pneumothorax in AIDS patients with pneumocystis pneumonia: A clinicopathologic report of three cases and review of the literature. Chest 98:266, 1990.

299. Blumenfeld W, McCook O, Holodniy M, Katzenstein DA: Correlation of morphologic diagnosis of *Pneumocystis carinii* with the presence of pneumocystis DNA amplified by the polymerase chain reaction. Mod Pathol 5:103, 1992.

300. Blumenfeld W, Miller CN, Chew KL, Mayall BH, Griffiss JM: Correlation of *Pneumocystis carinii* cyst density with mortality in patients with acquired immunodeficiency syndrome and pneumocystis pneumonia. Hum Pathol 23:612, 1992.

301. Bowling M, Smith M, Wescott S: A rapid staining procedure for *Pneumocystis carinii*. Am J Med Technol 39:267, 1973.

302. Burke B, Good R: *Pneumocystis carinii* infection. Medicine (Baltimore) 52:23, 1973.

303. Cameron R, Watts J, Kasten B: *Pneumocystis carinii* pneumonia. An approach to rapid laboratory diagnosis. Am J Clin Pathol 72:90, 1979.

304. Campbell W Jr: Ultrastructure of pneumocystis in human lung. Life cycle in human pneumocystosis. Arch Pathol 93:312, 1972.

305. Cano S, Capote F, Pereira A, Calderon E, Castillo J: *Pneumocystis carinii* pneumonia in patients without predisposing illnesses: Acute episode and follow-up of five cases. Chest 104:376, 1993.

306. Cote RJ, Rosenblum M, Telzak EE, May M, Unger PD, Cartun RW: Disseminated *Pneumocystis carinii* infection causing extrapulmonary organ failure: Clinical, pathologic, and immunohistochemical analysis. Mod Pathol 3:25, 1990.

307. Cruickshank B: Pulmonary granulomatous pneumocystosis following renal transplantation. Report of a case. Am J Clin Pathol 63:384, 1975.

308. Dee P, Winn W, McKee K: *Pneumocystis carinii* infection of the lung: Radiologic and pathologic correlation. AJR Am J Roentgenol 132:741, 1979.

309. Dembinski AS, Smith DM, Goldsmith JC, Woods GL: Widespread dissemination of *Pneumocystis carinii* infection in a patient with acquired immune deficiency syndrome receiving long-term treatment with aerosolized pentamidine. Am J Clin Pathol 95:96, 1991.

310. Demicco W, Stein A, Urbanetti J, Fanburg B: False negative biopsy of *Pneumocystis carinii* pneumonia. Chest 75:389, 1979.

311. DeRoux SJ, Adsay NV, Ioachim HL: Disseminated pneumocystosis without pulmonary involvement during prophylactic aerosolized pentamidine therapy in a patient with the acquired immunodeficiency syndrome. Arch Pathol Lab Med 115:1137, 1991.

312. Domingo J, Waksal HW: Wright's stain in rapid diagnosis of *Pneumocystis carinii*. Am J Clin Pathol 81:511, 1984.

313. Dutz W: *Pneumocystis carinii* pneumonia. Pathol Annu 5:309, 1970.

314. Edman JC, Kovacs JA, Masur H, et al: Ribosomal RNA sequence shows *Pneumocystis carinii* to be a member of the fungi. Nature 334:519, 1988.

315. El-Sadr W, Sidhu G: Persistence of trophozoites after successful treatment of *Pneumocystis carinii* pneumonia. Ann Intern Med 105:889, 1986.

316. Fraire AE, Kemp B, Greenberg D, et al: Calcofluor white stain for the detection of *Pneumocystis carinii* in transbronchial lung biopsy specimens: A study of 68 cases. Mod Pathol 9:861, 1996.

317. Haque AU, Plattner SB, Cook RT, Hart MH: *Pneumocystis carinii*. Taxonomy as viewed by electron microscopy. Am J Clin Pathol 87:504, 1987.

318. Hasleton PS, Curry A, Rankin EM: *Pneumocystis carinii* pneumonia: A light microscopical and ultrastructural study. J Clin Pathol 34:1138, 1981.

319. Hayashi Y, Watanabe J-I, Nakata K, Fukayama M, Ikeda H: A novel diagnostic method of *Pneumocystis carinii*: In situ hybridization of ribosomal ribonucleic acid with biotinylated oligonucleotide probes. Lab Invest 63:576, 1990.

320. Hennessey NP, Parro EL, Cockerell CJ: Cutaneous *Pneumocystis carinii* infection in patients with acquired immunodeficiency syndrome. Arch Dermatol 127:1699, 1991.

321. Homer KS, Wiley EL, Smith AL, et al: Monoclonal antibody to *Pneumocystis carinii*. Comparison with silver stain in bronchial lavage specimens. Am J Clin Pathol 97:619, 1992.

322. Horowitz ML, Schiff M, Samuels J, Russo R, Schnader J: *Pneumocystis carinii* pleural effusion: Pathogenesis and pleural fluid analysis. Am Rev Respir Dis 148:232, 1993.

323. Huang S, Marshall K: *Pneumocystis carinii* infection. A cytologic, histologic, and electron microscopic study of the organism. Am Rev Respir Dis 102:623, 1970.

324. Jacobs JL, Libby DM, Winters RA, et al: A cluster of *Pneumocystis carinii* pneumonia in adults without predisposing illnesses. N Engl J Med 324:246, 1991.

325. Klein JS, Warnock M, Webb WR, Gamsu G: Cavitating and noncavitating granulomas in AIDS patients with *Pneumocystis* pneumonitis. AJR Am J Roentgenol 152:753, 1989.

326. Kovacs JA, Ng VL, Masur H, et al: Diagnosis of *Pneumocystis carinii* pneumonia: Improved detection in sputum with use of monoclonal antibodies. N Engl J Med 318:589, 1988.

327. Lee MM, Schinella RA: Pulmonary calcification caused by *Pneumocystis carinii* pneumonia. A clinicopathological study of 13 cases in acquired immune deficiency syndrome patients. Am J Surg Pathol 15:376, 1991.

328. LeGolvan D, Heidelberger, K: Disseminated granulomatous *Pneumocystis carinii* pneumonia. Arch Pathol 95:344, 1973.

329. Levin M, McLeod R, Young Q, et al: Pneumocystis pneumonia: Importance of gallium scan for early diagnosis and description of a new immunoperoxidase technique to demonstrate *Pneumocystis carinii*. Am Rev Respir Dis 128:182, 1983.

330. Limper AH, Offord KP, Smith TF, Martin WJ II: *Pneumocystis carinii* pneumonia: Differences in lung parasite number and inflammation in patients with and without AIDS. Am Rev Respir Dis 140:1204, 1989.

331. Lindley RP, Mooney P: A rapid stain for Pneumocystis. J Clin Pathol 40:811, 1987.

332. Liu YC, Tomashefski JF, Tomford FW, Green H: Necrotizing *Pneumocystis carinii* vasculitis associated with lung necrosis and cavitation in a patient with acquired immunodeficiency syndrome. Arch Pathol Lab Med 113:494, 1989.

333. Luna MA, Cleary KR: Spectrum of pathologic manifestations of *Pneumocystis carinii* pneumonia in patients with neoplastic diseases. Semin Diagn Pathol 6:262, 1989.

334. Mansharamani NG, Garland R, Delaney D, Kaziel H: Management and outcome patterns for adult *Pneumocystis carinii* pneumonia, 1985 to 1995: Comparison of HIV-associated cases to other immunocompromised states. Chest 118:704, 2000.

335. Matsuda S, Urata Y, Shiota T, et al: Disseminated infection of *Pneumocystis carinii* in a patient with the acquired immunodeficiency syndrome. Virchows Arch A Cell Pathol 414:523, 1989.

336. Miller R, Huang L: *Pneumocystis jirovecii* infection. Thorax 59:731, 2004.

337. Milligan S, Stulbarg M, Gamsu G, Golden J: *Pneumocystis carinii* pneumonia radiographically simulating tuberculosis. Am Rev Respir Dis 132:1124, 1985.

338. Morris A, Sciurba FC, Lebedeva IP, et al: Association of chronic obstructive pulmonary disease severity and *Pneumocystis* colonization. Am J Respir Crit Care Med 170:408, 2004.

339. Murry CE, Schmidt RA: Tissue invasion by *Pneumocystis carinii*: A possible cause of cavitary pneumonia and pneumothorax. Hum Pathol 23:1380, 1992.

340. Peters SG, Prakash UBS: *Pneumocystis carinii* pneumonia. Review of 53 cases. Am J Med 82:73, 1987.

341. Price R, Hughes W: Histopathology of *Pneumocystis carinii* infestation and infection in malignant disease in childhood. Hum Pathol 5:737, 1974.

342. Radio SJ, Hansen S, Goldsmith J, Linder J: Immunohistochemistry of *Pneumocystis carinii* infection. Mod Pathol 3:462, 1990.

343. Ragni MV, Dekker A, DeRubertis FR, et al: *Pneumocystis carinii* infection presenting as necrotizing thyroiditis and hypothyroidism. Am J Clin Pathol 95:489, 1991.

344. Schwartz DA, Munger RG, Katz SM: Plastic embedding evaluation of *Pneumocystis carinii* pneumonia in AIDS. Am J Surg Pathol 11:304, 1987.

345. Sterling RP, Bradley BB, Khalil KG, et al: Comparison of biopsy-proven *Pneumocystis carinii* pneumonia in acquired immune deficiency syndrome patients and renal allograft recipients. Ann Thorac Surg 38:494, 1984.

346. Stiller RA, Paradis IL, Dauber JH: Subclinical pneumonitis due to *Pneumocystis carinii* in a young adult with elevated antibody titers to Epstein-Barr virus. J Infect Dis 166:926, 1992.

347. Sueishi K, Hisano S, Sumiyoshi A, Tanaka K: Scanning and transmission electron microscopic study of pulmonary *Pneumocystosis*. Chest 72:213, 1977.

348. Telzak EE, Cote RJ, Gold JWM, Campbell SW, Armstrong D: Extrapulmonary *Pneumocystis carinii* infections. Rev Infect Dis 12:380, 1990.

349. Tran Van Nhieu J, Vojtek A-M, Bernaudin J-F, Escudier E, Fleury-Feith J: Pulmonary alveolar proteinosis associated with *Pneumocystis carinii*: Ultrastructural identification in bronchoalveolar lavage in AIDS and immunocompromised non-AIDS patients. Chest 98:801, 1990.

350. Travis WD, Pittaluga S, Lipschik GY, et al: Atypical pathologic manifestations of *Pneumocystis carinii* pneumonia in the acquired immune deficiency syndrome. Review of 123 lung biopsies from 76 patients with emphasis on cysts, vascular invasion, vasculitis, and granulomas. Am J Surg Pathol 14:615, 1990.

351. Walzer PD: Diagnosis of *Pneumocystis carinii* pneumonia. J Infect Dis 157:629, 1988.

352. Wassermann K, Pothoff G, Kirn E, Fätkenheuer G, Krueger GRF: Chronic *Pneumocystis carinii* pneumonia in AIDS. Chest 104:667, 1993.

353. Watts JC, Chandler FW: *Pneumocystis carinii* pneumonitis. The nature and diagnostic significance of

the methenamine silver-positive "intracystic bodies". Am J Surg Pathol 9:744, 1985.

354. Weber W, Askin F, Dehner L: Lung biopsy in *Pneumocystis carinii* pneumonia. Am J Clin Pathol 67:11, 1977.

355. Yale SH, Limper AH: *Pneumocystis carinii* pneumonia in patients without acquired immunodeficiency syndrome: Associated illnesses and prior corticosteroid therapy. Mayo Clin Proc 71:5, 1996.

INFECTION II. GRANULOMATOUS INFECTIONS

The evaluation of granulomatous lung inflammation is a common task for the surgical pathologist. Most necrotizing granulomas are caused by infection, usually fungal or mycobacterial, and the responsible organism is usually demonstrable in the tissue. A number of important noninfectious lesions, however, especially various pulmonary vasculitides and sarcoidosis, can also cause pulmonary granulomas. Although ideally all specimens should be cultured, in practice this procedure is not always possible, since the tissue may be immersed in formalin before being received by the pathology laboratory. Furthermore, in acutely ill patients, a diagnosis may be needed before the results of cultures are available. The pathologist, therefore, rather than the microbiologist, must assume primary responsibility for identifying infectious organisms in lung granulomas.[6]

Helpful guidelines for evaluating necrotizing granulomas are summarized in Table 11–1. Not only can the pathologist be expected to document the presence or absence of organisms in granulomas, but also he or she

Table 11–1   Guidelines for Identifying Organisms in Necrotizing Granulomas

- Use the H and E in addition to special stains to identify fungi (both the tissue reaction and organism morphology are important).

- Begin the search for organisms in the center of necrotic zones rather than in the surrounding viable inflammatory areas.

- Perform special stains (AFB, GMS) on at least two blocks that contain active, necrotic granulomatous areas.

- Remember that organisms may not be identifiable in up to one-third of solitary necrotizing granulomas. Absence of organisms does not by itself imply a noninfectious condition.

Table 11–2 Contrasting Morphologic Features of Common Fungi Causing Granulomatous Inflammation in the Lung

	Histoplasma	Coccidioides	Cryptococcus	Blastomyces
Average size	3 μm (range, 1 to 5 μm)	30 to 60 μm (spherules); 2 to 5 μm (endospores)	4 to 7 μm (range, 2 to 15 μm)	8 to 15 μm (range, 2 to 30 μm)
Morphology	Oval, budding yeast; uniform in size, buds uncommon	Spherules, endospores; no budding forms	Round, budding yeast; variation in size, fragmentation common	Round, budding yeast; uniform in size
Distinguishing structural features (H and E)	Single nucleus, perinuclear clear zone (intracellular organisms only)*	Thick wall, central basophilic endospores (spherule only)	Pale, thin cell wall; extracellular clear zone (halo)	Thick cell wall, basophilic protoplasm, multiple nuclei
Mucicarmine staining	Negative	Negative	Usually positive	Negative
Type of granulomas	Necrotizing	Necrotizing; early lesions suppurative; eosinophils common	Necrotizing, non-necrotizing	Necrotizing with suppuration

*Intracellular organisms are seen only in disseminated histoplasmosis. Histoplasma cannot be visualized within caseous necrosis in lung granulomas without special stains.

can, with good accuracy, specifically identify many fungi (Table 11–2).

IDENTIFICATION OF ORGANISMS

Special stains for acid-fast bacilli and fungi should be examined in all cases.[2,3,5,6] We prefer the Ziehl–Neelsen (AFB) stain for mycobacteria and Grocott–Gomori methenamine silver (GMS) stain for fungi, although the auramine–rhodamine and PAS–Gridley stains are also satisfactory. Use of the periodic acid–Schiff (PAS) stain without a counterstain is not recommended when searching for fungi in necrotizing granulomas, because it fails to adequately differentiate the organisms from the background necrosis and debris. However, it can be helpful in delineating the internal structural detail of a fungus that already has been located by other staining methods. Other stains that are useful include the Fontana–Masson (FM) stain and the combined FM–alcian blue, FM–mucicarmine, and alcian blue–PAS stains, especially for identifying cryptococci.[35,36,40] Rarely, ordinary bacteria have been reported to cause necrotizing, usually suppurative, granulomatous reactions.[1,4] Examples include *Burkholderia pseudomallei* (melioidosis), *Brucella suis* (tularemia), and other rare organisms (*Burkholderia cepacia*, *Pseudomonas andersonii*).

Gram stains or silver impregnation techniques (Warthin Starry stain) can sometimes outline the organisms, but more often the diagnosis depends on cultures.

The importance of an ordinary hematoxylin and eosin (H and E) stain cannot be overemphasized in evaluating necrotizing granulomas. Several fungi, including blastomyces, cryptococcus, and coccidioides, for example, are easily visualized with H and E and show distinct morphologic features in this stain. The combination of the H and E appearance and the special stain findings can greatly facilitate identification. The appearance of the tissue reaction can provide additional clues to the organism. For example, suppurative granulomas are characteristic of blastomycosis and coccidioidomycosis, non-necrotizing granulomas are common in cryptococcosis, and eosinophilia may be prominent in coccidioidomycosis. In some cases, immunofluorescence or immunoperoxidase techniques using specific antibodies can help in identifying the organism. More sophisticated methods utilizing the polymerase chain reaction (PCR) have been utilized in tuberculosis cases.[73,81,83,87,89]

It should be remembered that organisms are almost always located in the central necrotic zones of caseating granulomas rather than in surrounding viable tissue or non-necrotizing granulomas.[6,92] In the study by Ulbright and Katzenstein,[6] acid-fast bacilli and histoplasma were found almost exclusively within such an area. Although cryptococcus and coccidioides occasionally were found in surrounding viable histiocytes, they were mainly present in necrotic zones. To conserve time and energy, therefore, the pathologist should begin his or her search for organisms in the central, most necrotic portion of the granuloma.

In most cases, the examination of sections from two tissue blocks is sufficient to identify an infectious agent, provided that the blocks include areas containing the most active and preferably most necrotic granulomatous inflammation. With this technique, an infectious agent will be identifiable in most necrotizing granulomas. It should be remembered, however, that a small but significant proportion of otherwise typical necrotizing granulomas (one-third in Ulbright and Katzenstein's study[6] of radiographically solitary lesions) will be negative for organisms by special stains and sometimes cultures. These cases likely represent infectious granulomas in which organisms have been removed by the inflammatory process, and the diagnosis

of other diseases, especially pulmonary vasculitides, should not be considered unless specific diagnostic features are present (see Chapter 8).

GENERAL FEATURES OF INFECTIOUS GRANULOMAS

Infectious granulomas share some features with the pulmonary vasculitides (see Chapter 8), which may make diagnosis difficult.[5,6] Irregular, 'geographic'-shaped necrosis, a characteristic finding in Wegener's granulomatosis, occasionally occurs in infections (Fig. 11–1a). Remnants of inflamed blood vessels and ghosts of alveolar septa are sometimes seen in the necrotic zones (so-called infarct-like necrosis, Fig. 11–1b). Vasculitis, which is a hallmark of Wegener's granulomatosis and other vasculitides, is common in both fungal and mycobacterial infections (Fig. 11–2). The vasculitis of infection is not necrotizing, however, and is generally characterized by a mural infiltrate of lymphocytes and

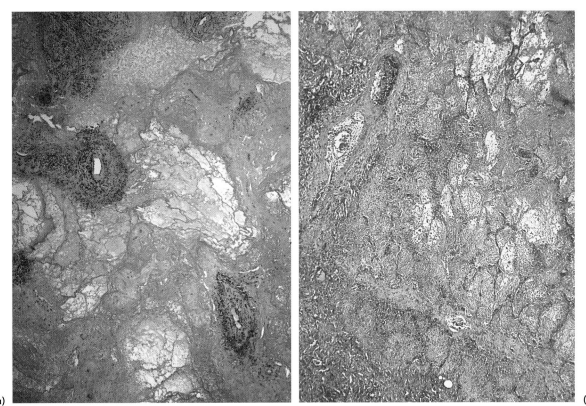

(a)   (b)

Figure 11–1 Infectious granulomas. (a) Irregular, geographic-shaped necrosis is seen in this example of tuberculosis. Inflammation in blood vessels is also prominent. **(b)** Infarct-like necrosis is prominent in this example of histoplasmosis. Note the remnants of alveolar septa in the necrotic zone. An adjacent artery is also inflamed (left).

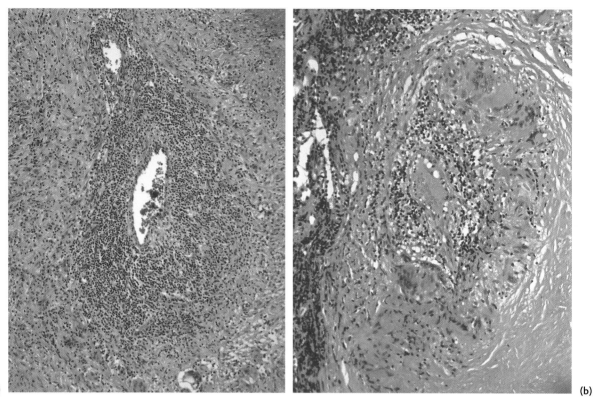

(a)   (b)

Figure 11–2 Vasculitis in infectious granulomas. (a) A dense chronic inflammatory cell infiltrate is present in the wall of this artery and narrows the lumen. The artery is located on the edge of a necrotizing granuloma (right), in which histoplasma were identified. **(b)** This artery from a case of tuberculosis shows granulomatous inflammation in its wall. The necrotic center of the granuloma is on the right.

plasma cells. The intima may be expanded by the cellular infiltrate, and, sometimes, epithelioid histiocytes, and even non-necrotizing granulomas, accompany the other chronic inflammatory cells. A transmural neutrophil infiltrate with necrosis that is characteristic of Wegener's granulomatosis, however, is not a feature of infection-related vasculitis. Bronchocentric granulomas, the characteristic finding in bronchocentric granulomatosis (see Chapter 6), are common in infections. In these lesions, bronchiolar mucosa is partially or completely replaced by palisading epithelioid histiocytes (Fig. 11–3). The former instance is easy to recognize because the necrotizing granuloma is partly surrounded by bronchiolar epithelium. When there is no residual epithelium, the bronchocentric location of the granulomatous inflammation is inferred by the presence of a nearby pulmonary artery (see Fig. 6–20). These observations underscore the need to carefully exclude an infectious etiology by means of special stains and cultures before considering a diagnosis of noninfectious granulomatous diseases. The differential diagnosis

of granulomatous infections and the noninfectious pulmonary vasculitides is discussed in more detail in Chapter 8.

The following sections concentrate mainly on fungal organisms that are common in the United States. Histologic features that aid in their recognition and differentiation are summarized in Table 11–2. Dirofilarial infections are also discussed, since they are an important cause of solitary lung nodules in certain areas of the United States, and aspects of tuberculosis and nontuberculous mycobacteria that are relevant to the surgical pathologist are briefly reviewed.

HISTOPLASMOSIS

Histoplasma capsulatum is a widespread fungus whose natural habitat is the soil. It exists in the mycelial form in nature but assumes the yeast phase at body temperature. The organism is endemic primarily in the central United States, but cases of histoplasmosis may occur well outside of this area.

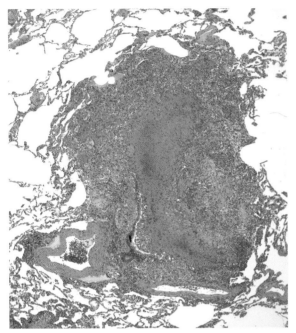

Figure 11–3 Bronchocentric granuloma in tuberculosis. A necrotizing granuloma partially replaces the bronchiole in the center.

Clinical Features

The vast majority of histoplasma infections in humans do not produce symptoms. Their existence is documented by the subsequent development of skin or serologic reactivity to histoplasma-related antigens or by the presence of characteristic radiographic calcifications. Several clinical syndromes occur, however, including *acute pulmonary histoplasmosis, disseminated histoplasmosis*, and *chronic histoplasmosis*.[7,8] *Histoplasmoma* is an important complication of acute pulmonary histoplasmosis which may be encountered by the surgical pathologist.

Acute Pulmonary Histoplasmosis

Acute pulmonary histoplasmosis encompasses the forms of the disease previously termed *primary histoplasmosis* and *acute histoplasmosis*.[7,8] Primary histoplasmosis is considered a misnomer since, unlike primary tuberculosis, which is followed by life-long tuberculin hypersensitivity, histoplasmosis is not necessarily associated with lasting histoplasmin sensitivity, and, therefore, infection and reinfection are common in endemic areas. Clinically, most patients are asymptomatic. The uncommon symptomatic form of the disease occurs predominantly in infants or children, and fever and cough are the usual clinical manifestations. Hilar and mediastinal lymph node enlargement and a patchy parenchymal infiltrate are seen radiographically. The course is usually self-limited, although sometimes dissemination occurs (see text following). Occasionally, inhalation of a large number of spores causes symptomatic disease, a form of infection previously termed *acute histoplasmosis*. These patients present with influenza-like symptoms accompanied by patchy, soft infiltrates or nodules that can be seen on chest radiographs. This form of the disease can represent a type of primary infection, or it can occur in previously infected individuals (reinfection type). It is usually self-limited, and the diagnosis is based on clinical, laboratory, and radiographic findings. Occasionally, in acutely ill patients in whom the diagnosis is unsuspected clinically, a lung biopsy will be performed.

Disseminated Histoplasmosis

This entity usually occurs in patients with abnormal immune systems, although otherwise apparently healthy individuals can be affected as well.[7,10,12] Approximately a third of the cases involve infants younger than 1 year old. This form of the disease is characterized by widespread parasitization of macrophages by the organisms, and multiple organs, especially reticuloendothelial, are affected. Interstitial lung infiltrates are often seen radiographically. The diagnosis is usually established from urine or blood cultures or by liver or bone marrow biopsy. Bronchoalveolar lavage specimens and lung biopsy specimens may be used in some cases.

Chronic Histoplasmosis

This type of histoplasmosis usually occurs in patients with emphysema or other chronic lung disease.[9] White males are affected more frequently than women or blacks, and the symptoms resemble those of tuberculosis. Pneumonic infiltrates and cavitary lesions are seen radiographically. The diagnosis is usually based on recovery of the organisms from sputum cultures, although lung biopsy occasionally may be necessary. Elevated complement-fixation titers can also help to establish the diagnosis in some cases. Skin tests are not useful, because false-negative results can occur, and positive results are found in the majority of healthy persons in endemic areas.[7]

Histoplasmomas

Histoplasmomas are thought to develop around a healing or healed focus of acute pulmonary histoplasmosis.[7] They appear radiographically as well-circumscribed masses, and they may slowly enlarge. Patients are usually asymptomatic, the lesions being found on a routine chest radiograph. This is the form of histoplasmosis most frequently encountered by the surgical pathologist, since the nodules are often excised.

Pathologic Features

The gross appearance of most forms of pulmonary histoplasmosis resembles that of any other necrotizing granulomatous process. Pulmonary histoplasmomas tend to be distinct, however, because their caseous central portion is often composed of multiple concentric lamellae, resembling the growth rings of a tree (Fig. 11–4). Although this lamellated appearance is characteristic of a histoplasmoma, it is not pathognomonic and may also be produced by other organisms. Disseminated histoplasmosis differs grossly in that necrotizing granulomas are usually not seen.

Microscopically, histoplasmomas and other forms of histoplasmosis (except disseminated histoplasmosis, see text following) are indistinguishable from necrotizing granulomas caused by other fungi and mycobacteria.[6]

Usually, the granulomas are well circumscribed and often contain a layer of laminated acellular collagen that is external to a rim of active granulomatous inflammation (Fig. 11–4b). Central calcification is common. In occasional cases, the granulomas are poorly circumscribed, and the inflammatory process may invade and destroy the pulmonary parenchyma in an irregular pattern. The frequent occurrence of infarct-like necrosis and vasculitis (see Fig. 11–1b) in such cases initially may suggest Wegener's granulomatosis. The correct diagnosis is established, however, when organisms are demonstrated in special stains or cultures. GMS is the most useful stain for identifying histoplasma in lung granulomas. Numerous organisms can usually be found within the central necrotic zones, although they may be sparse in the poorly circumscribed lesions (Fig. 11–5).[6] They appear as small, uniform, oval-shaped yeasts ranging in size from 1 to 5 μm (average, 3 μm). Budding forms can be found but usually are not numerous. The organisms cannot be seen in routine H and E stains unless they are present within histiocytes, a finding usually observed only in disseminated histoplasmosis (see text following). Rarely, hyphae have been described

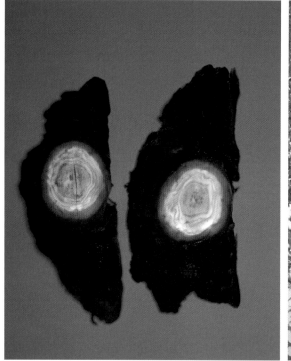
(a)

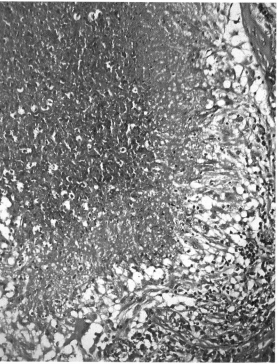
(b)

Figure 11–4 Histoplasmoma. (a) Gross appearance of a necrotizing granuloma due to histoplasma. Note the lamellated, tree-ring appearance of the necrotic zone. This appearance, although characteristic of histoplasmoma, is not specific and can be seen in other fungal as well as mycobacterial granulomas. **(b)** Microscopic appearance of necrotizing granuloma, showing the characteristic epithelioid histiocytes surrounding central necrosis.

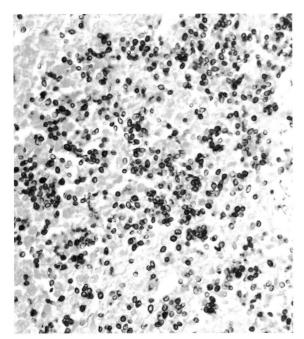

Figure 11–5 **GMS stain of histoplasma from the center of a necrotizing granuloma.** Note the small, uniform, oval-shaped yeasts. Buds are not numerous.

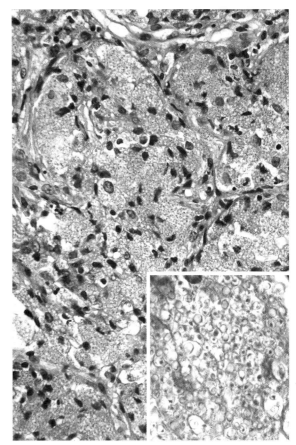

Figure 11–6 **Disseminated histoplasmosis.** Alveolar spaces in this example are packed with histiocytes containing abundant finely vacuolated cytoplasm. The inset is a higher magnification view showing the typical oval-shaped intracellular organisms with a single nucleus. Histoplasma can be visualized in H and E-stained sections only when they are present within cell cytoplasm.

in tissue, most commonly in cases of endocarditis with intravascular growth.[11]

In one case of acute histoplasmosis biopsied early in its course, granulomas were said to be absent, and the main finding was an intraalveolar mononuclear inflammatory cell exudate, containing organisms.[14] That patient, however, was an intravenous drug user and may have had underlying immune compromise (AIDS) that altered the inflammatory response. In our experience, active granulomatous inflammation is seen even in early acute histoplasmosis, although the granulomas may have purulent centers.

Disseminated histoplasmosis differs microscopically from other forms of histoplasmosis in that well-formed, necrotizing granulomas are usually absent, and the organisms are present extensively within histiocytes.[10,13] In the lung, the interstitium is the main site of involvement, although histiocytes accumulate within alveolar spaces as well (Fig. 11–6). At low magnification, the alveolar septa and peribronchiolar tissue appear expanded by sheets of plump histiocytes with granular cytoplasm, and organism-filled macrophages may pack alveolar spaces. The typical morphology of the intracellular organisms is readily appreciated when the slides are examined under higher magnification. In contrast to the granulomatous forms of the disease, in which the organism usually cannot be visualized in H and E stains, the intracellular yeasts in disseminated histoplasmosis are readily visible in routine H and E stains. They appear as small, ovoid bodies with a single, often eccentric nucleus and a characteristic perinuclear clear zone resulting from shrinkage of protoplasm from the cell walls (Fig. 11–6, *inset*).

Staining Techniques

Sometimes, histoplasma stains only faintly with GMS, even when a control slide using another fungus (usually candida or aspergillus) stains strongly.[6] For this reason, a control slide containing histoplasma should be prepared when histoplasmosis is suspected in a biopsy specimen. The PAS stain outlines the organisms well when they are located intracellularly, but it is not useful in evaluating necrotizing granulomas, since the stain does not adequately differentiate the red-staining organisms from the pink–red background necrosis. An immunoperoxidase technique using a rabbit antibody to histoplasma has been described.[13]

COCCIDIOIDOMYCOSIS

Coccidioides immitis is another saprophytic fungus that occurs naturally in the soil. It is restricted to the western hemisphere and is highly endemic in the southwestern United States. The fungus is dimorphic and grows in nature and on most artificial media as a mold; in vivo, it forms a spherule and reproduces by endosporulation.[18,24] Occasionally, mycelia are also found in tissue specimens.[22,25]

Clinical Features

Pulmonary involvement by coccidioides takes several forms, including primary pulmonary coccidioidomycosis, persistent primary coccidioidomycosis, and disseminated coccidioidomycosis.[15,18,24] *Primary pulmonary coccidioidomycosis* is generally asymptomatic or mildly symptomatic and causes patchy, soft, or hazy chest infiltrates. Occasionally, the major manifestations include erythema nodosum, erythema multiforme, and arthralgias. This symptom complex is known as *valley fever*, which is a reference to the San Joaquin Valley, where the infection is highly endemic. Peripheral eosinophilia is common in this syndrome.[19,23] Primary pulmonary coccidioidomycosis is usually self-limited and clears within 2 or 3 weeks. Rarely, respiratory failure may occur.[20]

In *persistent primary coccidioidomycosis*, the disease persists for more than 6 to 8 weeks and has several different manifestations, including persistent coccidioidal pneumonia, chronic progressive pneumonia, miliary infiltrates, and nodules (coccidioidoma). Patients with *persistent coccidioidal pneumonia* are usually quite ill, with fever, chest pain, cough, and large pulmonary infiltrates that may take many months to clear. *Chronic progressive pneumonia* is an uncommon variant of coccidioidomycosis that is characterized by biapical fibronodular lesions resembling tuberculosis. *Miliary pulmonary lesions* occur in a small percentage of patients, and the clinical manifestations are varied.[15] Mild chest symptoms are most common, but, in

immunocompromised individuals, the disease may be fulminant with respiratory failure. Occasionally, an area of pneumonia evolves into a well-circumscribed spherical density (*coccidioidoma* or *coccidioidal nodule*) or cavity. These lesions may be noted on a routine chest radiograph long after the antecedent pneumonic infiltrate has cleared, and there may be few associated symptoms.

Disseminated coccidioidomycosis occurs infrequently, and immunocompromised patients, pregnant women, blacks, Mexicans, and Filipinos appear predisposed to this complication.[18,26] Any organ can be involved, but skin, bone and joints, meninges, and the genitourinary system are the sites most often associated with clinically significant disease. The clinical course varies from chronic or relapsing to fulminant. Although the lung is the source of initial infection, a history of prior symptomatic pulmonary infection is not always present, since dissemination can follow an asymptomatic primary infection.

Most cases of coccidioidomycosis are diagnosed by means of positive cultures; skin tests are also useful for diagnosis, and serologic tests aid in both diagnosis and assessment of prognosis.[16,18] The solitary coccidioidal nodule, because it may masquerade clinically as a neoplasm, is commonly excised for diagnosis.

Histopathologic Features

Necrotizing granulomatous inflammation is the characteristic tissue reaction in coccidioidomycosis.[6,17] The granulomas often contain purulent central zones, and larger suppurative areas are common, especially early in the course of the pneumonic form and in extrapulmonary lesions.[18] This mixed granulomatous and suppurative reaction is thought to be related to the presence of both spherules (that elicit a granulomatous reaction) and endospores (that cause an acute inflammatory reaction). Eosinophils are often prominent in the inflammatory reactions, and areas resembling eosinophilic pneumonia have been described in the surrounding parenchyma (Fig. 11–7).[19,21] Organisms are generally present in moderate to large numbers, and they are found in both necrotic and viable zones and occasionally within histiocytes. Both spherules and endospores are typically present. The spherules are easily visible in H and E-stained sections and form the basis for identifying the fungus in tissue sections (Fig. 11–8). They are large round structures ranging from 30 to 60 μm and are rimmed by a thick, brown, somewhat refractile cell wall. The cell wall surrounds

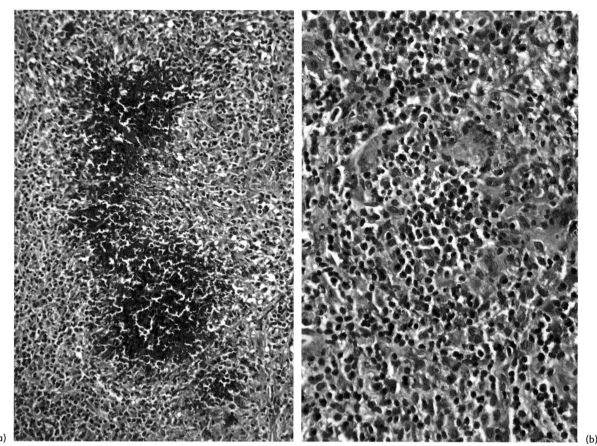

(a)   (b)

Figure 11–7 Coccidioidomycosis. (a) Necrotizing granuloma containing necrotic eosinophils in its center. **(b)** Higher magnification view showing the prominent eosinophil infiltrate among the epithelioid histiocytes.

a central zone that either appears empty or contains small basophilic endospores ranging in size from 2 to 5 μm. The endospores are released when the spherules rupture, and therefore they may also be present within necrotic zones. Free endospores stain poorly with H and E, but they are well visualized in the GMS stain (Fig. 11–8c). Mycelial forms are occasionally found, in addition to the more characteristic elements.[2,17,18,22,25]

The characteristic spherules distinguish coccidioides from other commonly encountered fungal organisms. However, when there are numerous endospores and only a few spherules, coccidioides may superficially resemble fungi such as histoplasma and cryptococci. A search for budding forms should clarify the issue, since coccidioides, in contrast to the yeasts, does not form buds. Also, a careful search should uncover at least a few characteristic spherules. Sometimes, small coccidioides spherules may be difficult to distinguish from large blastomyces yeasts (see further on).[59] The

presence (or absence) of budding forms will also be important in this differential diagnosis.

CRYPTOCOCCOSIS

Cryptococcus neoformans is a ubiquitous yeast whose natural habitat is the soil, especially that containing pigeon droppings. Most organisms are surrounded by a thick mucinous capsule, a feature that helps to distinguish cryptococcus from other fungal yeasts.

Clinical and Radiographic Features

Pulmonary cryptococcosis manifests a variety of clinical and radiographic features.[29,34,41] The disease occurs in both immunocompromised and immunocompetent individuals, most often between the ages of 30 and 50 years, although it has been reported in persons of all ages. White males are affected more frequently than

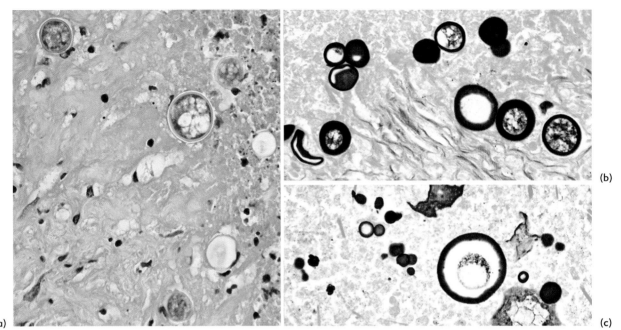

(a)

(b)

(c)

Figure 11–8 Morphologic features of coccidioidomyces. (a) H and E appearance of organisms within a necrotic granuloma. Note the large round spherules with refractile walls surrounding basophilic endospores. Some spherules appear empty. **(b)** GMS stain showing varying sized spherules, some containing endospores, some empty. **(c)** GMS stain showing numerous small, round endospores as well as an empty spherule. Note the absence of buds.

blacks or women. Approximately a third of patients are asymptomatic; the others present with a spectrum of symptoms ranging from a mild cough and low-grade fever to a severe, life-threatening illness. The chest radiographic findings are variable and include single or multiple well-demarcated masses, areas of segmental consolidation, and poorly defined nodular densities.[29,34,37] Cavitation occurs in 10–15% of cases, and hilar lymph node enlargement is common. Miliary infiltrates are seen occasionally, and pleural effusion occurs rarely.[42] A primary complex characterized by involvement of the tracheobronchial lymph nodes, as well as the lung, has been described in a few cases.[27,41] The diagnosis of cryptococcosis is established either by culture or by microscopic examination of the tissue; other laboratory procedures such as skin tests and serologic studies are generally not helpful. Lung resection may be curative in solitary granulomas as long as there is not meningeal involvement. Amphotericin or other antifungal therapy is indicated when the lung lesions progress and cannot be resected, when patients are immunosuppressed, and when there is proven dissemination.[33] Observation alone may be sufficient in non-immunocompromised patients without extrapulmonary involvement or significant symptoms.[39]

Histologic Features

A wide spectrum of histologic features occurs in cryptococcosis, varying from no reaction to necrotizing granulomatous inflammation. In immunologically intact individuals, a granulomatous reaction is usually found.[27,28,32] The process may resemble an ordinary well-circumscribed necrotizing granuloma (Fig. 11–9). Non-necrotizing granulomas are usually prominent accompanying features, and the granulomatous reaction often is completely non-necrotizing (Fig. 11–10). In the latter situation, large numbers of multinucleated histiocytes are characteristic, and they are loosely aggregated in a background of chronic inflammation and fibrosis. Rarely, bronchiolitis obliterans–organizing pneumonia (BOOP) is the main histologic finding (see Chapter 2). Usually, loose aggregates of epithelioid histiocytes or multinucleated histiocytes can be found at least focally in these cases, and their presence in this situation should alert the pathologist to carefully search for organisms.

Cryptococci appear as pale blue or gray round yeasts in H and E-stained slides (Fig. 11–11). They vary considerably in size, with an average diameter of 4 to 7 μm and a range from 2 to 15 μm. Fragmentation is

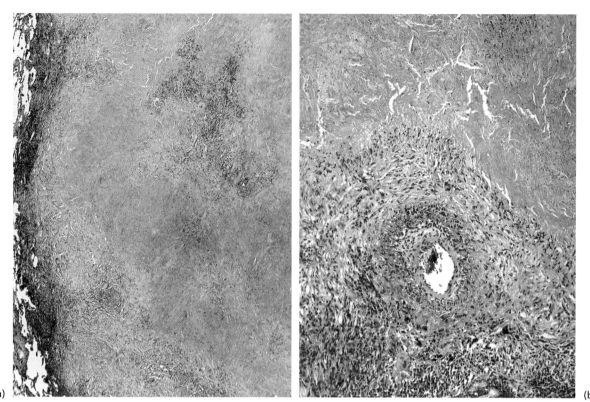

(a) (b)

Figure 11–9 Necrotizing granuloma due to cryptococcus. (a) Low magnification showing irregular-shaped necrosis bounded by epithelioid histiocytes and chronic inflammation. (b) Vascular inflammation was prominent adjacent to the necrotic zone in this example.

a prominent feature. The yeasts are usually separated from surrounding necrotic debris by an unstained clear space, an artifact that is caused by retraction of their thick mucinous capsule (see Fig. 11–12, inset). A similar clear zone can usually also be appreciated when the yeasts are present within cells and it imparts a characteristic bubbly appearance to the cell cytoplasm at low magnification (see Fig. 11–10b). The organism's capsule stains bright red with mucicarmine, and this staining characteristic is considered to be diagnostic of cryptococcus (see Figs 11–11b, inset, and 11–12a). Although blastomyces (see further on) may sometimes stain weakly with mucicarmine, it differs from cryptococcus because it is larger and more uniform, and contains a characteristic thick wall surrounding multiple basophilic nuclei. Combined FM–alcian blue or FM–mucicarmine stains can also help identify cryptococcus. With those stains the cell wall appears black and is surrounded by a blue or red capsule.[35,36] Occasionally, examples of cryptococcal forms that lack the mucinous capsule have been reported.[28,30,31]

Because of their small size and failure to stain with mucicarmine, these forms may be confused morphologically with histoplasma. The shape of the organisms (round for cryptococcus and oval for histoplasma) and the presence of fragmented forms (not a feature of histoplasma) should help in diagnosis. An FM stain may also help in such cases, although sometimes a culture of the organism may be necessary for definite diagnosis.[40]

Immunocompromised patients with pulmonary cryptococcosis frequently do not manifest a granulomatous reaction to the organisms.[38] In such cases, sheets of organisms fill the alveolar spaces, and there is little, if any, cellular reaction (see Fig. 11–12). Interstitial and intracapillary location of the organisms has also been described in examples of disseminated disease.[38] The gross appearance is often mucoid, owing to the presence of confluent masses of the encapsulated yeasts. Although the absent cellular reaction in these cases has been attributed by some to the presence of a mucinous capsule on the organism, it seems more likely that severe immune compromise is responsible.

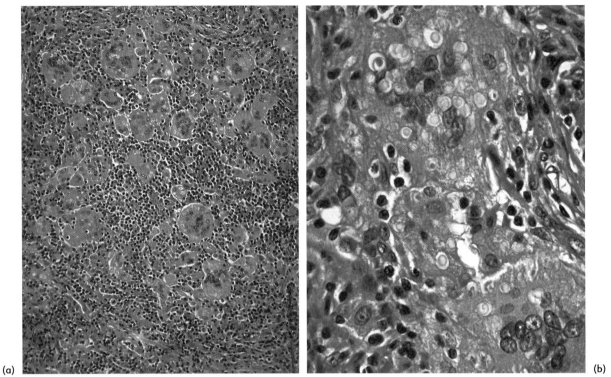

(a) (b)

Figure 11–10 Non-necrotizing granulomatous inflammation due to cryptococcus. (a) Low magnification showing loosely formed non-necrotizing granulomas containing numerous multinucleated giant cells, many of which have bubbly cytoplasm. **(b)** Higher magnification of the giant cells, showing the typical round, lightly staining intracellular organisms separated by a clear zone from the cell cytoplasm.

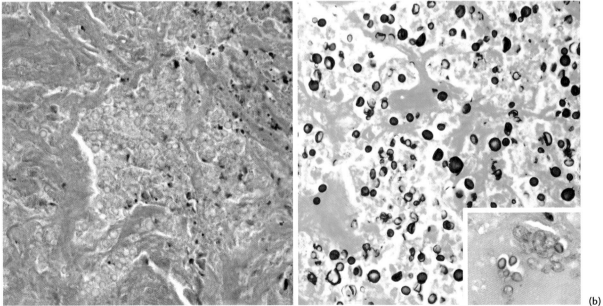

(a) (b)

Figure 11–11 Morphologic features of cryptococcus. (a) H and E appearance showing lightly colored, gray, round organisms within necrotic granuloma. A clear halo (see Fig.11–10b) is not present around the organisms in this example. **(b)** GMS stain showing round yeasts with variation in size and numerous fragmented forms. Inset is a mucicarmine stain showing weakly positive staining of the organisms.

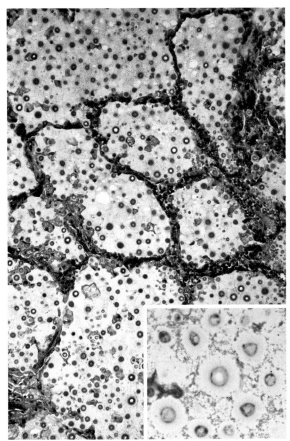

Figure 11–12 Cryptococcal pneumonia in an immunocompromised patient. At low magnification the alveolar spaces are filled with numerous organisms that stain red in this mucicarmine stain. There is no associated inflammatory reaction. Inset is an H and E stain at higher magnification, showing sheets of organisms surrounded by a prominent clear halo.

NORTH AMERICAN BLASTOMYCOSIS

Blastomyces dermatitidis is a dimorphic fungus that grows as a mycelium in the laboratory at room temperature and as a yeast at 37°C. The yeast phase is the usual form found in infected tissue, although hyphae have been reported rarely.[43,48]

The endemic area for North American blastomycosis includes the South, South Central, and Great Lakes areas of the United States, as well as parts of Canada; cases in Africa and South America have also been reported.[53] The natural habitat of the fungus is not definitely known, since the organism has only rarely been isolated from soil or other possible environmental sources. Skin tests and serologic studies do not reliably indicate infection, and, therefore, epidemiologic study of this disease has been difficult and often incomplete.[53,54]

Clinical Features

Pulmonary blastomycosis generally affects young to middle-aged adults, and men are affected more often than women.[53,54,57] The disease frequently is acquired by individuals who engage in outdoor activities, such as hunting, and thus the apparent male predominance may be related more to different avocational preferences than to real differences in susceptibility.

Like several other fungi, blastomyces causes a variety of clinical syndromes.[45,47,53,54] *Acute pneumonia* may occur and is characterized by the abrupt onset of high fever, chills, and cough associated with patchy chest infiltrates. This form of the disease is generally self-limited, and most patients recover without therapy. An *asymptomatic acute pneumonia* that is analogous to asymptomatic primary histoplasmosis or coccidioidomycosis has been documented in a few cases in local epidemics.[44,53] Although most investigators believe that asymptomatic infection is common, it is difficult to document because of the lack of reliable skin and serologic tests.[45,53] In a few patients, *progressive pulmonary blastomycosis* may follow the acute pneumonic form. It is characterized by a rapid spread throughout both lungs. The clinical course in some patients resembles that of the acute respiratory distress syndrome (ARDS).[46,51,55] Distant organ involvement may occur, and mortality is high despite treatment. *Chronic blastomycosis (recurrent* or *reactivation)* may develop in the lung or extrapulmonary sites, especially the skin, months or years following recovery from acute pneumonia. This form of the disease has also been noted rarely in previously healthy patients with no history of antecedent acute pneumonia, and such patients are presumed to have had a clinically unrecognized asymptomatic acute pneumonia.[50]

The chest radiographic findings in blastomycosis are varied.[43,47,52,56] Most commonly, mass-like nodular densities or areas of consolidation are found. Occasionally there may be interstitial opacities or even a miliary pattern. A few lesions undergo cavitation. Evidence of pleural involvement is common and pleural effusions may occur.[49]

Histologic Features

The initial tissue reaction in the lung to blastomyces is an acute inflammatory cell infiltrate followed by a

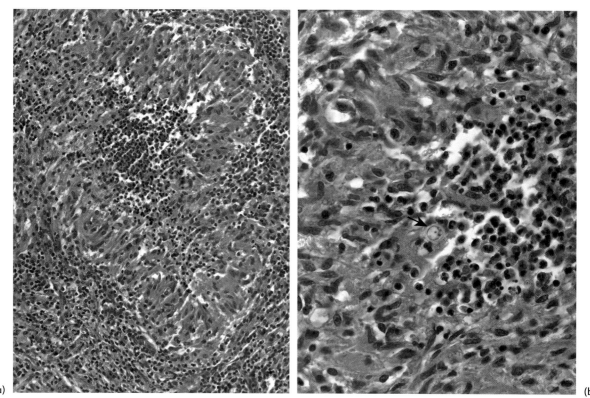

(a)　　　　　　　　　　　　　　　　　　　　　　　　　　　　　　(b)

Figure 11–13 Blastomycosis. (a) Necrotizing granuloma with suppurative center. **(b)** Higher magnification showing blastomyces organism within a histiocyte (arrow) at the edge of the suppurative necrosis. Note the refractile wall surrounding the central basophilic nuclei.

histiocytic response and granuloma formation.[53,57] In biopsy material, necrotizing granulomatous inflammation is usually found. The granulomas are typically suppurative with central necrotic neutrophils surrounded by epithelioid histiocytes (Fig. 11–13). Non-necrotizing granulomas are often found in the surrounding parenchyma as well. The yeasts are present within the purulent centers of the granulomas and within the histiocytes, and are readily visible in routine H and E-stained sections (Figs 11–13b and 11–14). They are round and relatively uniform in size, averaging from 8 to 15 μm in diameter, and possess single broad-based buds. Rarely, large forms ranging up to 40 μm have been reported.[59] A thick, refractile, light brown cell wall surrounds the central protoplasm, which contains multiple nuclei. Similar morphologic features are appreciated in the PAS stain, except that the cell wall appears red. The GMS stain colors blastomyces solid black, and although it facilitates locating the fungi, it tends to obscure the characteristic internal morphologic findings (Fig. 11–14b). Rarely, mycelial forms are also present in tissue.[43,48]

Differential Diagnosis

Blastomyces is larger than cryptococcus, and it does not show the variability in size or the numerous fragmented forms common to the latter organism. Also, cryptococcus lacks the multiple nuclei and central basophilic cytoplasm of blastomyces that are seen in H and E, and it usually contains a mucinous capsule that stains with mucicarmine. In H and E- and PAS-stained sections, blastomyces can sometimes be confused with small spherules of coccidioides.[59] The presence of budding forms and the lack of free endospores in cases of blastomycosis will distinguish between the two organisms. Blastomyces differs from *Paracoccidioides brasiliensis*, the agent of South American blastomycosis, because the latter yeast forms multiple, narrow-necked buds, in contrast to the single, wide-necked bud of blastomyces. The use of the Ziehl–Neelsen acid-fast stain has been advocated to distinguish some forms of blastomyces from certain other fungal organisms, and combined FM stains may help in some cases.[36,58]

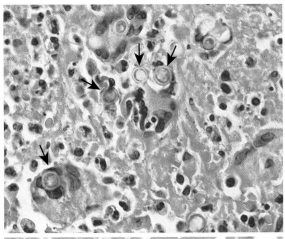

(a)

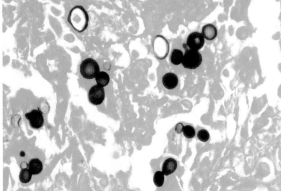

(b)

Figure 11–14 Morphologic features of blastomyces. (a) H and E appearance showing uniform-sized yeasts with thick refractile walls surrounding basophilic nuclei (arrows). Compare with coccidioides at the same magnification (Fig. 11–8a). **(b)** GMS stain showing relatively uniform round yeasts. Compare with cryptococcus (Fig. 11–11b). Note that the internal structure is obscured by this stain.

MISCELLANEOUS FUNGAL INFECTIONS

Sporothrix schenckii, the fungus that produces cutaneous *sporotrichosis*, is a rare cause of granulomatous lung inflammation.[61,63,64,67,70,71] Necrotizing granulomas, often containing central suppuration, have been reported in such cases.[61,67,71] The organisms can be visualized with GMS, PAS, and other routine fungal stains. They appear either as round yeast forms 2 to 3 μm in diameter or as elongated, 1–2 μm by 4–5 μm, 'cigar'-shaped forms. Rarely, so-called asteroid bodies are found. They are star-shaped eosinophilic structures that are produced by the accumulation of spicules

of proteinaceous material around the yeast forms (so-called *Splendore–Hoeppli phenomenon*).[2]

Adiaspiromycosis is another rare fungal infection in the lung.[65,66,69] It is caused by inhalation of spores of the saprophytic soil fungus *Chrysosporium parvum* var. *crescens* (previously known as *Emmonsia crescens*). The disease is usually self-limited, although fatal cases have been reported. Reticulonodular infiltrates are the most common radiographic manifestations, with localized infiltrates occurring occasionally. The organisms are large spherules (mean diameter, >200 μm; range, 50–500 μm) that have trilaminar walls surrounding empty centers. They differ from coccidioides by their large size and lack of endospores. They should not be confused with parasites and miscellaneous structures such as vegetable matter or corpora amylacea.

Alternaria is another fungus that has been reported rarely to cause necrotizing lung granulomas.[68] *Paracoccidioides brasiliensis*, the agent of South American blastomycosis, may also cause lung granulomas in North America.[60,62]

TUBERCULOSIS

The number of tuberculosis cases had steadily declined in the United States since the 1950s, except for a transient increase in annual cases between 1985 and 1992 largely due to increased incidence among HIV-infected individuals, immigration of individuals from countries with a high incidence of tuberculosis, and the development of multidrug-resistant stains. The diagnosis in most cases is established by skin testing and microbiologic cultures. Pathologic examination of tissue remains an important means of diagnosis, however, especially in clinically unsuspected cases, and in sputum-negative or acutely ill patients.[76,77,88,93] Surgically resected portions of lung from patients not responsive to medical therapy are also occasionally encountered by the pathologist.

Clinical Features

The various forms of tuberculosis are well known.[79,86,91] *Primary tuberculosis* occurs following first exposure to the organism. It is usually self-limited and characterized by an area of necrotizing granulomatous inflammation in the lung and in draining lymph nodes (so-called *Ghon focus*). Patients are generally asymptomatic, and the diagnosis is based on positive skin tests. Although the lesions of primary tuberculosis eventually heal, they can contain viable organisms for years. *Progressive primary tuberculosis* occurs in less than 10% of patients, most of whom have some type of underlying immune compromise. Enlarging infiltrates are seen radiographically, and pulmonary and systemic symptoms are common. *Postprimary (chronic, secondary) tuberculosis* is usually due to reactivation of a dormant focus of primary infection, although reinfection may occur in areas where the incidence of tuberculosis is high.[74,85,94] Symptoms such as cough, fever, weight loss, and malaise are common, and apical infiltrates are usually evident radiographically. *Miliary tuberculosis* reflects hematogenous spread of organisms and is usually a manifestation of postprimary infection. A spectrum of clinical findings occurs, ranging from few symptoms to an acute, fulminant febrile illness. Because this form of the disease can mimic other types of interstitial lung disease and because sputum samples are often negative for organisms, diagnosis frequently requires lung biopsy.[88] *Tuberculomas* or solitary granulomas are probably the most common form of tuberculosis encountered by the surgical pathologist. These patients are generally asymptomatic and the lesions excised because of the radiographic suspicion of malignancy.

Pathologic Features

Necrotizing granulomatous inflammation with varying numbers of accompanying non-necrotizing granulomas is the usual histologic reaction in tuberculosis (see Figs 11–1a and 11–3). The appearance is no different from that caused by various fungal or other mycobacterial infections.[86,91,92] In immunocompromised patients, the inflammatory reaction may not be as well developed, and poorly organized histiocytic infiltrates, acute inflammation, or bland necrosis are sometimes seen.[75,82] A spindle cell histiocytic proliferation similar to that described in lymph nodes from immunocompromised persons with nontuberculous mycobacterial infections has been rarely reported.[90]

The organisms are well demonstrated in the Ziehl–Neelsen stain, where they appear as thin, red bacilli with a beaded configuration, although there is some evidence that formalin fixation and xylene use may decrease the sensitivity of this stain.[78] In a minority of cases they remain viable even after formalin fixation.[80] The organisms are usually found within the central, most necrotic zone of the granulomas. The auramine–rhodamine fluorescent stain is also satisfactory for outlining the organisms, and immunohistochemical

methods using antibodies to various constituent proteins of *Mycobacterium tuberculosis* have been described.[72,84] The PCR technique can be used to identify the organisms in paraffin-embedded tissues and can reliably distinguish *M. tuberculosis* from other acid-fast bacilli.[73,81,83,87,89]

NONTUBERCULOUS MYCOBACTERIAL INFECTIONS

Nontuberculous (atypical) mycobacteria are an increasingly important cause of pulmonary, as well as extrapulmonary, infection, a trend that is related in part to a high incidence in patients with AIDS and in part due to increasing recognition of their role in certain chronic lung diseases.[111,112,136] Most non-AIDS patients with pulmonary involvement have evidence of underlying chronic lung disease, malignancy, or immunosuppression, although individuals with no known immunologic defects can also be affected.[100,101,105,127] Patients with cystic fibrosis or abnormal α-1 antitrypsin gene seem to be predisposed.[111,134] The most common atypical mycobacterial agent of human infection is *M. avium-intracellulare complex (MAC)*, and it is the most difficult to treat.[102,103,106,109,110,117,136] *M. kansasii* is another important cause of nontuberculous mycobacteriosis,[103,114] whereas pulmonary infection by other bacilli such as *M. abscessus*,[114] *M. chelonei*,[137] *M. fortuitum*,[114,122,125,137] *M. xenopi*,[105–107,130] *M. malmoense*,[96] *M. bovis*,[123,133,139] *M. terrae*,[121] *M. asiaticum*,[98] *M. simiae*,[97,105,129,135,140] *M. gordoneae*,[104] and *M. haemophilum*[138] has rarely been reported.

Clinically and radiographically, nontuberculous mycobacterial infections often mimic tuberculosis.[100,102,103,107,113,138,139] Bronchiectasis is common, especially in women.[111,113] A unique syndrome due to MAC that resembles the middle lobe syndrome has been reported in elderly women (*Lady Windermere syndrome*).[127]

The spectrum of pathologic changes characteristic of nontuberculous mycobacterial infection is similar to that seen in ordinary tuberculosis.[100,106,109,110,113,120,122,129,131,138] Necrotizing granulomatous inflammation is the most common reaction, and non-necrotizing granulomas are usually present as well. Less commonly, nonspecific inflammatory reactions may be seen, especially in immunocompromised patients, and they include poorly organized histiocytic infiltrates, acute and chronic inflammation, fibrosis, and organizing pneumonia (see Fig. 12–4).[101,110,122,138] Eosinophilic pneumonia has been reported in one patient who subsequently died of *M. simiae* infection.[140] In patients with AIDS, an inflammatory reaction may be completely absent.[136]

The staining characteristics of nontuberculous mycobacteria are similar to those of *M. tuberculosis*.[120] Although certain nontuberculous mycobacteria, especially *M. kansasii*, have been reported to be longer than *M. tuberculosis* and to have a characteristic curved or S shape,[131,132] cultures are necessary for reliable, specific identification. The PCR technique can also be utilized to distinguish these organisms.[81]

Hot Tub Lung

Several reports have linked MAC lung infection with hot tub exposure.[99,108,118,119,128] The organism grows well in water, especially hot water, and infection is thought to occur through aerosol exposure. Patients present with dyspnea, cough, low-grade fever, and, often, hypoxia. Diffuse interstitial infiltrates, sometimes with a miliary nodular pattern, are seen radiographically. Treatment of reported cases is varied and has included

antimicrobials, steroids, a combination of antimicrobials and steroids, or no therapy, and all patients have recovered. Hot tub use can continue provided that the water is appropriately disinfected. Controversy exists whether hot tub lung represents an infection or a hypersensitivity reaction.

The pathologic findings in hot tub lung are sufficiently distinct that the diagnosis can be suggested from the histologic changes in most cases. Typically, a combination of well-formed non-necrotizing granulomas and organizing pneumonia is present, and the changes affect mainly peribronchiolar parenchyma (Fig. 11–15). The granulomas occur both within the interstitium and within airspaces, and they are distinct, well-circumscribed aggregates of epithelioid histiocytes. Necrotizing granulomas are uncommon but are occasionally present. Bronchiolitis obliterans frequently accompanies the organizing pneumonia, and non-specific chronic inflammation may be prominent. Special stains for organisms are negative in most cases.

The differential diagnosis includes both hypersensitivity pneumonia and sarcoidosis. The changes

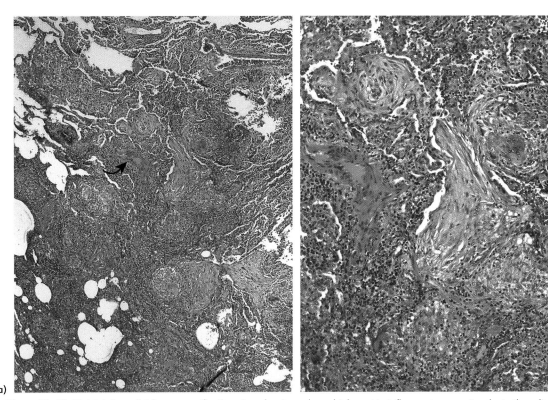

(a)   (b)

Figure 11–15 Hot tub lung. (a) Low magnification view showing a bronchiolocentric inflammatory reaction (note the adjacent pulmonary artery, arrow) characterized by a mixture of non-necrotizing granulomas and intraluminal organization (bronchiolitis obliterans–organizing pneumonia). **(b)** A higher magnification highlights the bronchiolitis obliterans and adjacent non-necrotizing granulomas.

differ from hypersensitivity pneumonia in that the granulomas are well-formed, tight aggregates of epithelioid histiocytes rather than loose aggregates as in hypersensitivity pneumonia. Also, an accompanying cellular chronic interstitial pneumonia that is characteristic of hypersensitivity pneumonia is not present away from the granulomas. The findings differ from sarcoidosis because granulomas are found in airspaces in addition to the interstitium. Also, organizing pneumonia that is common in hot tub lung is not a feature of sarcoidosis.

M. bovis Infection

Pulmonary granulomas have been reported in patients receiving Bacillus Calmette-Guérin (BCG) immuno-

therapy for cancer,[115,116,126] and disseminated infection has occurred rarely following BCG vaccination in immunodeficient individuals.[95] BCG consists of an attenuated strain of *M. bovis*, and the organism has been cultured from lung granulomas in one case.[123] Radiographically, these patients present with solitary nodules or diffuse reticulonodular infiltrates. Both necrotizing and non-necrotizing granulomas have been found histologically, although special stains for acid-fast bacilli are only rarely positive.[124]

DIROFILARIASIS

Canine heartworm disease, caused by *Dirofilaria immitis*, is highly endemic to the southeastern seaboard and

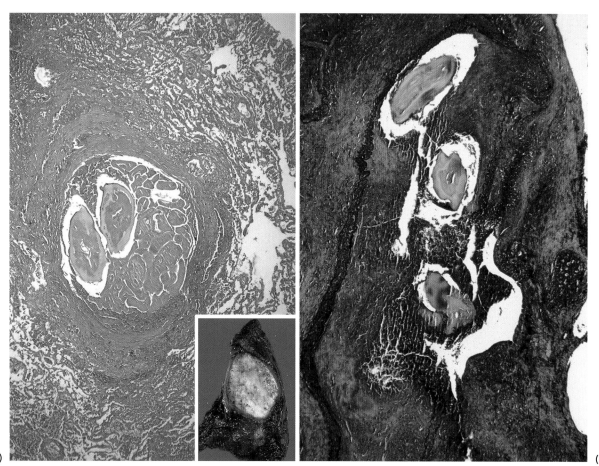

(a) (b)

Figure 11–16 Dirofilarial nodule. (a) At low magnification two organisms are seen within the remnants of an artery in the necrotic center of a nodule. Note the large size of the organisms. Inset shows the gross appearance of the dirofilarial nodule with central necrosis that is surrounded by a thin rim of viable tissue. (b) Elastic tissue stain outlines the elastic tissue in the wall of an artery that contains three dirofiliarial organisms in its lumen.

Gulf Coast states; cases have also been reported from northern and inland United States and from Brazil.[142,145,147,151,153-155] Dogs, as well as cats, foxes, and other mammals, are natural hosts, and mosquitoes are vector-intermediate hosts. In the dog, mature adult worms reside in the right ventricle and shed microfilaria into the bloodstream. The microfilaria are taken up by a mosquito and enter the skin of a second host by a mosquito bite. At that time, they migrate into the subcutaneous tissues, and, after several months, they enter the venous circulation and move to the right ventricle. Humans are dead-end hosts, and those forms that do reach the right ventricle die. Pulmonary lesions are caused by the embolization of dead organisms to the lungs.

Clinical Features

Most patients with pulmonary nodules caused by *D. immitis* are asymptomatic. Cough or chest pain may occasionally occur, and hemoptysis and fever are less common manifestations.[142,145,153-155] Peripheral blood eosinophilia is present in approximately 15% of patients.[155] The radiographic findings are usually characterized by a solitary, well-circumscribed nodule, or 'coin' lesion. The nodule measures less than 2 cm at its greatest dimension, and calcification rarely occurs.[145] Occasionally, multiple nodules are present.[143,145,147,149,150] Although serologic methods are available that may aid in the diagnosis in some cases,[144,148] surgery is generally performed to rule out a malignancy.

Pathologic Features

Grossly, the dirofilarial nodule is a well-demarcated, gray–yellow, necrotic lesion (Fig. 11–16a, inset). It is usually spherical and often surrounded by a thin fibrous capsule. Sometimes the worm can be appreciated grossly.[144,149]

Histologically, the dirofilarial nodule resembles an infarct with surrounding granulomatous inflammation.[143,144,146,149,152,154] There is extensive central necrosis enclosed by a rim composed of variable numbers of epithelioid histiocytes. Dense fibrosis, containing chronic inflammatory cells, is prominent in some cases, and eosinophils may be numerous. The organisms are found within the central necrotic tissue, where they are usually located within the lumen of a necrotic artery (see Fig. 11–16). They are easily recognized without special stains and are large, round to oval

structures, averaging 200 μm (range, 100 to 350 μm) in cross-sectional diameter (Fig. 11–17). They have a characteristically thick (5 to 25 μm), multilayered cuticle that contains transverse striations. A complex internal structure that includes prominent somatic muscle bands can sometimes be seen. In old lesions, the organisms may calcify. Although the internal morphologic features in such cases will be obscured, the cuticle often remains identifiable, and the organisms can be recognized by their large size and typical intravascular location. Because of the vascular involvement, arteries adjacent to the necrotic nodule are often inflamed, and eosinophils may be prominent in the cellular infiltrate. These latter findings may initially suggest a pulmonary vasculitis, but the lack of a necrotizing vasculitis and careful search for organisms should clarify the situation.

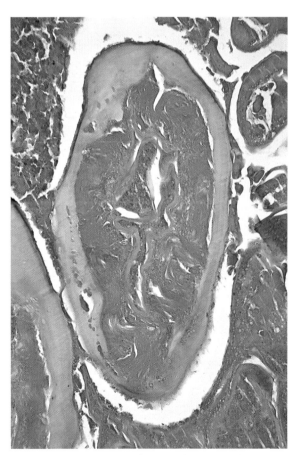

Figure 11–17 Morphologic features of dirofilaria. A characteristic thick cuticle surrounds the complex internal structure.

REFERENCES

General

1. Belchis DA, Simpson E, Colby T: Histopathologic features of *Burkholderia cepacia* pneumonia in patients without cystic fibrosis. Mod Pathol 13:369, 2000.
2. Binford C, Connor D, eds: *Pathology of Tropical and Extraordinary Diseases*, Washington, DC, Armed Forces Institute of Pathology, 1976.
3. Chandler F, Watts J: *Pathologic Diagnosis of Fungal Infections*, Chicago, ASCP Press, 1987.
4. Han XY, Pham AS, Nguyen KU, et al: Pulmonary granuloma caused by *Pseudomonas andersonii sp nov*. Am J Clin Pathol 116:347, 2001.
5. Katzenstein A: The histologic spectrum and differential diagnosis of necrotizing granulomatous inflammation in the lung. In: Fenoglio C, Wolff M, eds: *Progress in Surgical Pathology*, Vol. II, 1980, pp. 41–70.
6. Ulbright T, Katzenstein A: Solitary necrotizing granulomas of the lung. Differentiating features and etiology. Am J Surg Pathol 4:13, 1980.

Histoplasmosis

7. Goodwin R Jr, Des Prez R: Histoplasmosis. Am Rev Respir Dis 117:929, 1978.
8. Goodwin R, Lloyd J, Des Prez R: Histoplasmosis in normal hosts. Medicine (Baltimore) 60:231, 1981.
9. Goodwin R Jr, Owens F, Snell J, et al: Chronic pulmonary histoplasmosis. Medicine (Baltimore) 55:413, 1976.
10. Goodwin R, Shapiro J, Thurman G, et al: Disseminated histoplasmosis: Clinical and pathologic correlations. Medicine (Baltimore) 59:1, 1980.
11. Hutton JP, Durham JB, Miller DP, Everett ED: Hyphal forms of *Histoplasma capsulatum*. A common manifestation of intravascular infections. Arch Pathol Lab Med 109:330, 1985.
12. Kauffman C, Israel K, Smith J, et al: Histoplasmosis in immunosuppressed patients. Am J Med 64:923, 1978.
13. Klatt EC, Cosgrove M, Meyer PR: Rapid diagnosis of disseminated histoplasmosis in tissues. Arch Pathol Lab Med 110:1173, 1986.
14. Reynolds RJ III, Penn RL, Grafton WD, George RB: Tissue morphology of *Histoplasma capsulatum* in acute histoplasmosis. Am Rev Respir Dis 130:317, 1984.

Coccidioidomycosis

15. Arsura EL, Kilgore WB: Miliary coccidioidomycosis in the immunocompetent. Chest 117:404, 2000.
16. Bayer A, Yoshikawa T, Guze I: Chronic progressive coccidioidal pneumonitis. Report of six cases with clinical, roentgenographic, serologic and therapeutic features. Arch Intern Med 139:536, 1979.
17. Deppisch L, Donowho E: Pulmonary coccidioidomycosis. Am J Clin Pathol 58:489, 1972.
18. Drutz D, Cantanzaro A: Coccidioidomycosis. Am Rev Respir Dis 117:559,727, 1978.
19. Echols RM, Palmer DL, Long GW: Tissue eosinophilia in human coccidioidomycosis. Rev Infect Dis 4:656, 1982.
20. Larsen RA, Jacobson JA, Morris AH, et al: Acute respiratory failure caused by primary pulmonary coccidioidomycosis. Two case reports and a review of the literature. Am Rev Respir Dis 131:797, 1985.
21. Lombard CM, Tazelaar HD, Krasne DL: Pulmonary eosinophilia in coccidioidal infections. Chest 91:734, 1987.
22. Putnam J, Harper W, Greene J Jr, et al: *Coccidioides immitis*. A rare cause of pulmonary mycetoma. Am Rev Respir Dis 112:733, 1975.
23. Schermoly MJ, Hinthorn DR: Eosinophilia in coccidioidomycosis. Arch Intern Med 148:895, 1988.
24. Stevens DA: Coccidioidomycosis. N Engl J Med 332:1077, 1996.
25. Thadepalli H, Salem F, Mandal A, et al: Pulmonary mycetoma due to *Coccidioides immitis*. Chest 71:429, 1977.
26. Wack EE, Ampel NM, Galgiani JN, Bronnimann DA: Coccidioidomycosis during pregnancy. An analysis of 10 cases among 47,120 pregnancies. Chest 94:376, 1988.

Cryptococcosis

27. Baker R: The primary pulmonary lymph node complex of *Cryptococcus*. Am J Clin Pathol 65:83, 1976.
28. Farmer S, Komorowski R: Histologic response to capsule-deficient *Cryptococcus neoformans*. Arch Pathol 96:383, 1973.
29. Feigin DS: Pulmonary cryptococcosis: Radiologic-pathologic correlates of its three forms. AJR Am J Roentgenol 141:1263, 1983.
30. Gutierrez F, Fu Y, Lurie H: *Cryptococcosis* histologically resembling *Histoplasmosis*. A light and electron microscopic study. Arch Pathol 99:347, 1975.
31. Harding S, Scheld W, Feldman P, Sande M: Pulmonary infection with capsule-deficient *Cryptococcus neoformans*. Virchows Arch [Pathol Anat] 382:113, 1979.
32. Kahn FW, England DM, Jones JM: Solitary pulmonary nodule due to *Cryptococcus neoformans* and *Mycobacterium tuberculosis*. Am J Med 78:677, 1985.
33. Kerkering T, Duma R, Shadomy S: The evolution of pulmonary cryptococcosis. Clinical implications from a study of 41 patients with and without compromising host factors. Ann Intern Med 94:611, 1981.
34. Khoury MB, Godwin JD, Ravin CE, et al: Thoracic cryptococcosis: Immunologic competence and radiologic appearance. AJR Am J Roentgenol141:893, 1984.
35. Lazcano O, Speights VO Jr, Bilbao J, et al: Combined Fontana-Masson-mucin staining of *Cryptococcus neoformans*. Arch Pathol Lab Med 115:1145, 1991.
36. Lazcano O, Speights VO Jr, Strickler J, et al: Combined histochemical stains in the differential diagnosis of *Cryptococcus neoformans*. Mod Pathol 6:80, 1993.
37. Lee L-N, Yang P-C, Kuo S-H, et al: Diagnosis of pulmonary cryptococcosis by ultrasound guided percutaneous aspiration. Thorax 48:75, 1993.
38. McDonnell JM, Hutchins GM: Pulmonary cryptococcosis. Hum Pathol 16:121, 1985.

39. Nadrous HF, Antonios VS, Terrell CL, Ryu JH: Pulmonary cryptococcosis in nonimmunocompromised patients. Chest 124:2143, 2003.

40. Ro JY, Lee SS, Ayala AG: Advantage of Fontana-Masson stain in capsule-deficient cryptococcal infection. Arch Pathol Lab Med 111:53, 1987.

41. Salyer W, Salyer D, Baker R: Primary complex of *Cryptococcus* and pulmonary lymph nodes. J Infect Dis 130:74, 1974.

42. Young E, Hirsch D, Fainstein V, Williams T: Pleural effusions due to *Cryptococcus neoformans*: A review of the literature and report of two cases with cryptococcal antigen determinations. Am Rev Respir Dis 121:743, 1980.

North American Blastomycosis

43. Atkinson JB, McCurley TL: Pulmonary blastomycosis: Filamentous forms in an immunocompromised patient with fulminating respiratory failure. Hum Pathol 14:186, 1983.

44. Brown LR, Swensen SJ, Van Scoy RE, Prakash UBS, Coles DT, Colby TV: Roentgenologic features of pulmonary blastomycosis. Mayo Clin Proc 66:29, 1991.

45. Cush R, Light R, George R: Clinical and roentgenographic manifestations of acute and chronic blastomycosis. Chest 69:345, 1976.

46. Evans ME, Haynes JB, Atkinson JB, et al: *Blastomyces dermatitidis* and the adult respiratory distress syndrome. Case reports and review of the literature. Am Rev Respir Dis 126:1099, 1982.

47. Halvorsen RA, Duncan JD, Merten DF, et al: Pulmonary blastomycosis: Radiologic manifestations. Radiology 150:1, 1984.

48. Hardin H, Scott D: Blastomycosis: Occurrence of filamentous forms in vivo. Am J Clin Pathol 60:104, 1974.

49. Kinasewitz GT, Penn RL, George RB: The spectrum and significance of pleural disease in blastomycosis. Chest 86:580, 1984.

50. Laskey W, Sarosi G: Endogenous activation in blastomycosis. Ann Intern Med 88:50, 1978.

51. Lemos LB, Baliga M, Guo M: Acute respiratory distress syndrome and blastomycosis: Presentation of nine cases and review of the literature. Ann Diagn Pathol 5:1, 2001.

52. Rabinowitz J, Busch J, Buttram W: Pulmonary manifestations of blastomycosis. Radiological support of a new concept. Radiology 120:25, 1976.

53. Sarosi G, Davies S: Blastomycosis. Am Rev Respir Dis 120:901, 1979.

54. Schwarz J, Salfelder K: Blastomycosis. A review of 152 cases. Curr Top Pathol 65:165, 1977.

55. Skillrud DM, Douglas WW: Survival in adult respiratory distress syndrome caused by blastomycosis infection. Mayo Clin Proc 60:266, 1985.

56. Stelling CB, Woodring JH, Rehm SR, et al: Miliary pulmonary blastomycosis. Radiology 150:7, 1984.

57. Vanek J, Schwarz J, Hakim S: North American blastomycosis. A study of ten cases. Am J Clin Pathol 54:384, 1970.

58. Wages DS, Wear DJ: Acid-fastness of fungi in blastomycosis and histoplasmosis. Arch Pathol Lab Med 106:440, 1982.

59. Watts JC, Chandler FW, Mihalov ML, Kammeyer PL, Armin A-R: Giant forms of *Blastomyces dermatitidis* in the pulmonary lesions of blastomycosis: Potential confusion with *Coccidioides immitis*. Am J Clin Pathol 93:575, 1990.

Miscellaneous Fungal Infections

60. Agia G, Hurst D, Rogers W: Paracoccidioidomycosis presenting as a cavitating pulmonary mass. Chest 78: 650, 1980.

61. Berson S, Brandt F: Primary pulmonary sporotrichosis with unusual fungal morphology. Thorax 32:505, 1977.

62. Bowler S, Woodcock A, Da Costa P, Turner-Warwick M: Chronic pulmonary paracoccidioidomycosis masquerading as lymphangitis carcinomatosa. Thorax 41:72, 1986.

63. England DM, Hochholzer L: Primary pulmonary sporotrichosis. Report of eight cases with clinicopathologic review. Am J Surg Pathol 9:193, 1985.

64. England DM, Hochholzer L: Sporothrix infection of the lung without cutaneous disease. Primary pulmonary sporotrichosis. Arch Pathol Lab Med 111:298, 1987.

65. England DM, Hochholzer L: Adiaspiromycosis: An unusual fungal infection of the lung. Report of 11 cases. Am J Surg Pathol 17:876, 1993.

66. Filho JVB, Amato MBP, Deheinzelin D, Saldiva RHN, de Carvalho CRR: Respiratory failure caused by adiaspiromycosis. Chest 97:1171, 1990.

67. Jay S, Platt M, Reynolds R: Primary pulmonary sporotrichosis. Am Rev Respir Dis 115:1051, 1977.

68. Lobritz R, Roberts T, Marraro R, et al: Granulomatous pulmonary disease secondary to *Alternaria*. JAMA 241:596, 1979.

69. Peres LC, Figueiredo F, Peinado M, Soares FA: Fulminant disseminated pulmonary adiaspiromycosis in humans. Am J Trop Med Hyg 46:146, 1992.

70. Pluss JL, Opal SM: Pulmonary sporotrichosis: Review of treatment and outcome. Medicine (Baltimore) 65:143, 1986.

71. Smith A, Morgan W, Hornick R, Funk A: Chronic pulmonary sporotrichosis: Report of a case, including morphologic and mycologic studies. Am J Clin Pathol 54:401, 1970.

Tuberculosis

72. Barbolini G, Bisetti A, Colizzi V, et al: Immunohistologic analysis of mycobacterial antigens by monoclonal antibodies in tuberculosis and mycobacteriosis. Hum Pathol 20:1078, 1989.

73. Bocart D, Lecossier D, Lassence AD, et al: A search for mycobacterial DNA in granulomatous tissues from

patients with sarcoidosis using the polymerase chain reaction. Am Rev Respir Dis 145:1142, 1992.

74. Caminero JA, Pena MJ, Campos-Herrero MI, et al: Exogenous reinfection with tuberculosis on a European island with a moderate incidence of disease. Am J Respir Crit Care Med 163:717, 2001.

75. Chaisson RE, Schecter GF, Theuer CP, et al: Tuberculosis in patients with the acquired immunodeficiency syndrome. Clinical features, response to therapy, and survival. Am Rev Respir Dis 136:570, 1987.

76. Chan CHS, Chan RCY, Arnold M, et al: Bronchoscopy and tuberculostearic acid assay in the diagnosis of sputum smear-negative pulmonary tuberculosis: A prospective study with the addition of transbronchial biopsy. Q J Med 82:15, 1992.

77. Epstein DM, Kline LR, Albelda SM, Miller WT: Tuberculous pleural effusions. Chest 91:106, 1987.

78. Fukunaga H, Murakami T, Gondo T, et al: Sensitivity of acid-fast staining for *Mycobacterium tuberculosis* in formalin-fixed tissue. Am J Respir Crit Care Med 166:994, 2002.

79. Geppert E, Leff A: The pathogenesis of pulmonary and miliary tuberculosis. Arch Intern Med 139:1381, 1979.

80. Gerston KF, Blumberg L, Tshabalala VA, Murray J: Viability of mycobacteria in formalin-fixed lungs. Hum Pathol 35:571, 2004.

81. Ghossein RA, Ross DG, Salomon RN, Rabson AR: Rapid detection and species identification of mycobacteria in paraffin-embedded tissues by polymerase chain reaction. Diagn Mol Pathol 1:185, 1992.

82. Handwerger S, Mildvan D, Senie R, McKinley FW: Tuberculosis and the acquired immunodeficiency syndrome at a New York City Hospital: 1978–1985. Chest 91:176, 1987.

83. Hardman WJ, Benian GM, Howard T, et al: Rapid detection of mycobacteria in inflammatory necrotizing granulomas from formalin-fixed, paraffin-embedded tissue by PCR in clinically high-risk patients with acid-fast stain and culture-negative tissue biopsies. Am J Clin Pathol 106:384, 1996.

84. Humphrey DM, Weiner MH: Mycobacterial antigen detection by immunohistochemistry in pulmonary tuberculosis. Hum Pathol 18:701, 1987.

85. Jasmer RM, Bozeman L, Schwartzman K, et al: Recurrent tuberculosis in the United States and Canada. Relapse or reinfection? Am J Respir Crit Care Med 170:1360, 2004.

86. Nayak N, Sabharwal B, Bhathena D: The pulmonary tuberculous lesion in North India. I. Incidence, nature and evolution. Am Rev Respir Dis 101:1, 1970.

87. Rish JA, Eisenach KD, Cave MD, et al: Polymerase chain reaction detection of *Mycobacterium tuberculosis* in formalin-fixed tissue. Am J Respir Crit Care Med 153:1419, 1996.

88. Sahn S, Levin D: Diagnosis of miliary tuberculosis by transbronchial lung biopsy. Br Med J 2:667, 1975.

89. Salian NV, Rish JA, Eisenach KD, et al: Polymerase chain reaction to detect *Mycobacterium tuberculosis* in histologic specimens. Am J Respir Crit Care Med 158:1150, 1998.

90. Sekosan M, Cleto M, Senseng C, Farolan M, Sekosan J: Spindle cell pseudotumors in the lungs due to *Mycobacterium tuberculosis* in a transplant patient. Am J Surg Pathol 18:1065, 1994.

91. Slavin R, Walsh T, Pollack A: Late generalized tuberculosis: A clinical pathologic analysis and comparison of 100 cases in the preantibiotic and antibiotic eras. Medicine (Baltimore) 59:352, 1980.

92. Tang Y-W, Procop GW, Zheng X, et al: Histologic parameters predictive of mycobacterial infection. Am J Clin Pathol 109:331, 1998.

93. Van den Brande PM, Van de Mierop F, Verbeken EK, Demedts M: Clinical spectrum of endobronchial tuberculosis in elderly patients. Arch Intern Med 150:2105, 1990.

94. Van Rie A, Warren R, Richardson M, et al: Exogenous reinfection as a cause of recurrent tuberculosis after curative treatment. N Engl J Med 341:1174, 1999.

Nontuberculous Mycobacterial Infection

95. Abramowsky C, Gonzalez B, Sorensen RU: Disseminated bacillus Calmette-Guerin infections in patients with primary immunodeficiencies. Am J Clin Pathol 100:52, 1993.

96. Alberts WM, Chandler KW, Solomon DA, Goldman AL: Pulmonary disease caused by *Mycobacterium malmoense*. Am Rev Respir Dis 135:1375, 1987.

97. Bell RC, Higuchi JH, Donovan WN, et al: *Mycobacterium simiae*. Clinical features and follow-up of twenty-four patients. Am Rev Respir Dis 127:35, 1983.

98. Blacklock ZM, Dawson DJ, Kane DW, McEvoy D: *Mycobacterium asiaticum* as a potential pulmonary pathogen for humans. A clinical and bacteriologic review of five cases. Am Rev Respir Dis 127:241, 1983.

99. Cappelluti E, Fraire AE, Schaefer OP: A case of "hot tub lung" due to *Mycobacterium avium* complex in an immunocompetent host. Arch Intern Med 163:845, 2003.

100. Chapman JS: The atypical mycobacteria. Am Rev Respir Dis 125:119, 1982.

101. Chester AC, Winn WC Jr: Unusual and newly recognized patterns of nontuberculous mycobacterial infection with emphasis on the immunocompromised host. Pathol Ann 21(Pt 1):251, 1986.

102. Christensen E, Dietz G, Ahn C, et al: Pulmonary manifestations of *Mycobacterium intracellularis*. AJR Am J Roentgenol 133:59, 1979.

103. Christensen EE, Dietz GW, Ahn CH, et al: Initial roentgenographic manifestations of pulmonary *Mycobacterium tuberculosis*, *M. kansasii*, and *M. intracellularis* infections. Chest 80:132, 1981.

104. Collop NA: A solitary pulmonary nodule due to *Mycobacterium gordonae*. Respiration 57:351, 1990.

105. Contreras MA, Cheung OT, Sanders DE, Goldstein RS: Pulmonary infection with nontuberculous mycobacteria. Am Rev Respir Dis 137:149, 1988.

106. Costrini AM, Mahler DA, Gross WM, et al: Clinical and roentgenographic features of nosocomial pulmonary disease due to *Mycobacterium xenopi*. Am Rev Respir Dis 123:104, 1981.

107. Dornetzhuber V, Martis R, Burjanova B, et al: Pulmonary mycobacteriosis caused by *Mycobacterium xenopi*. Eur J Respir Dis 63:293, 1982.

108. Embil J, Warren P, Yakrus M, et al: Pulmonary illness associated with exposure to *Mycobacterium-avium* complex in hot tub water. Hypersensitivity pneumonia or infection? Chest 111:813, 1997.

109. Engbaek HC, Vergmann B, Bentzon MW: Lung disease caused by *Mycobacterium avium/Mycobacterium intracellulare*. An analysis of Danish patients during the period 1962–1976. Eur J Respir Dis 62:72, 1981.

110. Farhi DC, Mason UG III, Horsburgh CR Jr: Pathologic findings in disseminated *Mycobacterium avium-intracellulare* infection. Am J Clin Pathol 85:67, 1986.

111. Field SK, Fisher D, Cowie RL: *Mycobacterium avium* complex pulmonary disease in patients without HIV infection. Chest 126:566, 2004.

112. Fournier AM, Dickinson GM, Erdfrocht IR, et al: Tuberculosis and nontuberculous mycobacteriosis in patients with AIDS. Chest 93:772, 1988.

113. Fujita J, Ohtsuki Y, Suemitsu I, et al: Pathological and radiological changes in resected lung specimens in *Mycobacterium avium intracellulare* complex disease. Eur Respir J 13:535, 1999.

114. Griffith DE, Girard WM, Wallace RJ Jr: Clinical features of pulmonary disease caused by rapidly growing mycobacteria: An analysis of 154 patients. Am Rev Respir Dis 147:1271, 1993.

115. Gupta RC, Lavengood R Jr, Smith JP: Miliary tuberculosis due to intravesical bacillus Calmette-Guerin therapy. Chest 94:1296, 1988.

116. Hatzitheofilou C, Obenchain DF, Porter DD, Morton DL: Granulomas in melanoma patients treated with BCG immunotherapy. Cancer 49:55, 1982.

117. Horsburgh CR Jr, Mason UG III, Farhi DC, Iseman MD: Disseminated infection with *Mycobacterium avium-intracellulare*. A report of 13 cases and a review of the literature. Medicine (Baltimore) 64:36, 1985.

118. Kehana LM, Kay JM, Yakrus MA, Waserman S: *Mycobacterium avium* complex infection in an immunocompetent young adult related to hot tub exposure. Chest 111:242, 1997.

119. Khour A, Leslie KO, Tazelaar HD, et al: Diffuse pulmonary disease caused by nontuberculous mycobacteria in immunocompetent people (hot tub lung). Am J Clin Pathol 115:755, 2001.

120. Kommareddi S, Abramowsky CR, Swinehart GL, Hrabak L: Nontuberculous mycobacterial infections: Comparison of the fluorescent auramine-O and Ziehl-Neelsen techniques in tissue diagnosis. Hum Pathol 15:1085, 1984.

121. Kuze F, Mitsuoka A, Chiba W, et al: Chronic pulmonary infection caused by *Mycobacterium terrae* complex: A resected case. Am Rev Respir Dis 128:561, 1983.

122. Marchevsky A, Damsker B, Gribetz A, et al: The spectrum of pathology of nontuberculous mycobacterial infections in open-lung biopsy specimens. Am J Clin Pathol 78:695, 1982.

123. McParland C, Cotton DJ, Gowda KS, et al: Miliary *Mycobacterium bovis* induced by intravesical bacille Calmette-Guérin immunotherapy. Am Rev Respir Dis 146:1330, 1992.

124. Palayew M, Briedis D, Libman M, Michel RP, Levy RD: Disseminated infection after intravesical BCG immunotherapy: Detection of organisms in pulmonary tissue. Chest 104:307, 1993.

125. Pesce RR, Fejka S, Colodny SM: *Mycobacterium fortuitum* presenting as an asymptomatic enlarging pulmonary nodule. Am J Med 91:310, 1991.

126. Quesada J, Libshitz H, Hersh E, Gutterman J: Pulmonary abnormalities in patients intravenously receiving the methanol extraction residue (MER) of bacillus Calmette-Guérin. Cancer 45:1340, 1980.

127. Reich JM, Johnson RE: *Mycobacterium avium* complex pulmonary disease presenting as an isolated lingular or middle lobe pattern. The Lady Windermere syndrome. Chest 101:1605, 1992.

128. Rickman OB, Ryu JH, Fidler ME, Kalra S: Hypersensitivity pneumonitis associated with *Mycobacterium avium* complex and hot tub use. Mayo Clin Proc 77:1233, 2002.

129. Rose HD, Dorff GJ, Lauwasser M, Sheth NK: Pulmonary and disseminated *Mycobacterium simiae* infection in humans. Am Rev Respir Dis 126:1110, 1982.

130. Simor AE, Salit IE, Vellend H: The role of *Mycobacterium xenopi* in human disease. Am Rev Respir Dis 129:435, 1984.

131. Smith MB, Molina CP, Schnadig VJ, et al: Pathologic features of *Mycrobacterium kansasii* infection in patients with acquired immunodeficiency syndrome. Arch Pathol Lab Med 127:554, 2003.

132. Snijder J: Histopathology of pulmonary lesions caused by atypical mycobacteria. J Pathol Bacteriol 90:65, 1965.

133. Thompson PJ, Cousins DV, Gow BL, et al: Seals, seal trainers, and mycobacterial infection. Am Rev Respir Dis 147:164, 1993.

134. Tomashefski JF, Stern RC, Demko CA, Doershuk CF: Nontuberculous mycobacteria in cystic fibrosis: An autopsy study. Am J Respir Crit Care Med 154:523, 1996.

135. Valero G, Peters J, Jorgensen JH, Graybill JR: Clinical isolates of *Mycobacterium simiae* in San Antonio, Texas. An 11-year review. Am J Respir Crit Care Med 152:1555, 1995.

136. Wallace JM, Hannah JB: *Mycobacterium avium* complex infection in patients with the acquired immunodeficiency syndrome. A clinicopathologic study. Chest 93:926, 1988.

137. Wallace RJ, Swenson JM, Silcox VA, et al: Spectrum of disease due to rapidly growing mycobacteria. Rev Infect Dis 5:657, 1983.

138. White DA, Kiehn TE, Bondoc AY, Massarella SA: Pulmonary nodule due to M*ycobacterium haemophilum* in an immunocompetent host. Am J Respir Crit Care Med 160:1366, 1999.
139. Wilkins EGL, Griffiths RJ, Roberts C: Pulmonary tuberculosis due to *Mycobacterium bovis*. Thorax 41:685, 1986.
140. Wright JL, Pare PD, Hammond M, Donevan RE: Eosinophilic pneumonia and atypical mycobacterial infection. Am Rev Respir Dis 127:497, 1983.
141. Zvetina JR, Demos TC, Maliwan N, et al: Pulmonary cavitations in *Mycobacterium kansasii*: Distinctions from *M. tuberculosis*. AJR Am J Roentgenol 143:127, 1984.

Dirofilariasis

142. Asimacopoulos PJ, Katras A, Christie B: Pulmonary dirofilariasis: The largest single-hospital experience. Chest 102:851, 1992.
143. Awe R, Mattox K, Alvarez A, et al: Solitary and bilateral pulmonary nodules due to *Dirofilaria immitis*. Am Rev Respir Dis 112:445, 1975.
144. Chesney TM, Martinez LC, Painter MW: Human pulmonary dirofilarial granuloma. Ann Thorac Surg 36:214, 1983.
145. Ciferri F: Human pulmonary dirofilariasis in the United States: A critical review. Am J Trop Med Hyg 31:302, 1982.
146. Dayal Y, Neafie R: Human pulmonary dirofilariasis. A case report and review of the literature. Am Rev Respir Dis 112:437, 1975.
147. de Campos JRM, Barbas CSV, Filomeno LTB, et al: Human pulmonary dirofilariasis: Analysis of 24 cases from São Paulo, Brazil. Chest 112:729, 1997.
148. Glickman LT, Grieve RB, Schantz PM: Serologic diagnosis of zoonotic pulmonary dirofilariasis. Am J Med 80:161, 1986.
149. Kochar AS: Human pulmonary dirofilariasis. Report of three cases and brief review of the literature. Am J Clin Pathol 84:19, 1985.
150. Levinson E, Ziter F Jr, Westcott J: Pulmonary lesions due to *Dirofilaria immitis* (dog heartworm). Radiology 131:305, 1979.
151. Merrill J, Otis J, Logan W Jr, Davis M: The dog heartworm (*Dirofilaria immitis*) in man. An epidemic pending or in progress? JAMA 243:1066, 1980.
152. Nicholson CP, Allen MS, Trastek VF, Tazelaar HD, Pairolero PC: *Dirofilaria immitis*: A rare, increasing cause of pulmonary nodules. Mayo Clin Proc 67:646, 1992.
153. Risher WH, Crocker EF Jr, Beckman EN, et al: Pulmonary dirofilariasis. The largest single-institution experience. J Thorac Cardiovasc Surg 97:303, 1989.
154. Ro JY, Tsakalakis PJ, White VA, et al: Pulmonary dirofilariasis: The great imitator of primary or metastatic lung tumor. A clinicopathologic analysis of seven cases and a review of the literature. Hum Pathol 20:69, 1989.
155. Robinson N, Chavez C, Conn J: Pulmonary dirofilariasis in man. J Thorac Cardiovasc Surg 74:403, 1977.

12

LUNG INVOLVEMENT IN ACQUIRED IMMUNODEFICIENCY SYNDROME (AIDS)

The first cases of acquired immunodeficiency syndrome (AIDS) were recognized in 1981, when outbreaks of pneumocystis pneumonia occurred in seemingly healthy men with no known immunologic deficits. Since that time, AIDS has been proven to be caused by a retrovirus, human immunodeficiency virus-1 (HIV-1), that infects mainly T lymphocytes and macrophages expressing CD24 receptor molecules with resultant severe deficits of both cell-mediated and humoral immunity.[1] The virus is transmitted primarily by sexual contact or by blood products in a manner much like the transmission of the hepatitis B virus. Homosexuals, intravenous drug abusers, hemophiliacs, female sex partners of men in the latter groups, and residents of certain underdeveloped countries, especially Haiti, comprise the majority of patients with AIDS. A small proportion of cases occur in children, most of whom acquire the disease transplacentally or by blood transfusion.[15,21,26,37] Pulmonary involvement is a major source of morbidity and mortality.[2,7,8,11,13,14,16,17,20,21,23,24,26–30,32,34,35,38,39] Infections are the most important cause of lung infiltrates and may be ascribed to a wide variety of opportunistic and pathogenic organisms. Less often, noninfectious lesions are encountered, such as various interstitial pneumonias, lymphoid infiltrates, or malignancies, for example. The major pulmonary manifestations of AIDS are summarized in Table 12–1. The following sections discuss each lesion, although the pathologic features are described in detail only when they have not been covered in other chapters.

HANDLING OF SPECIMENS

The most common techniques for diagnosing pulmonary infiltrates in AIDS patients include bronchoalveolar lavage (BAL) and transbronchial lung biopsy

Table 12–1　Pulmonary Involvement in AIDS

I. **Infections**
Pneumocystis pneumonia
Bacterial
(M. avium complex, M. tuberculosis, pyogenic
bacteria, nocardia, malacoplakia, etc.)
Fungal
(Candida, aspergillus, and other opportunistic fungi;
cryptococcus, histoplasma, coccidioides,
blastomyces and other pathogenic fungi)
Viral
(Cytomegalovirus, herpesvirus)
Parasitic
(Toxoplasma, strongyloides, cryptosporidia,
microsporidia)

II. **Noninfectious Lesions**
Interstitial pneumonias
(Lymphoid interstitial pneumonia, nonspecific chronic
interstitial pneumonia, diffuse alveolar damage)
Pulmonary alveolar proteinosis
Pulmonary hypertension
Bronchiolitis obliterans–organizing pneumonia

III. **Malignancies**
Kaposi's sarcoma
Lymphoma
Carcinoma

(TBB).[3,5,10,12,18,25,33] The sensitivity of BAL specimens rivals and, according to some reports, may be superior to TBB in diagnosing infections.[12,42] Induced sputum specimens and nonbronchoscopic tracheal aspirates may also be useful,[4,19,22,31,36] whereas open lung biopsies and percutaneous fine needle aspirations are usually not advocated.[9,40,41] The guidelines issued by the Centers for Disease Control (CDC) for prevention of HIV transmission in healthcare settings are widely appreciated and should be carefully followed when handling specimens.[6] They include use of gloves, protective eyewear, and gowns when handling fluids and tissues, and the cleaning of all exposed surfaces with an appropriate disinfectant. Because of the danger of accidental cuts, the use of frozen sections in evaluating open lung biopsies or TBB specimens should be discouraged.

BAL Fluids and Smears

Cytocentrifuge slides prepared from aliquots of BAL fluids should be routinely stained with Papanicolaou, Diff-Quik, Gomori's methenamine silver (GMS), and

Ziehl–Neelsen (AFB) stains. Periodic acid–Schiff (PAS) or hematoxylin and eosin (H and E) stains can be additionally examined. A similar battery of stains is performed on all smears, such as sputum or bronchial washings and brushings. For the GMS control, a separate cytocentrifuge preparation or a smear containing pneumocystis is preferable to a tissue section containing pneumocystis, since smear preparations often need to be overstained compared with tissue sections in order to demonstrate the organisms adequately.

TBB Specimens

For TBBs, three H and E-stained step sections should be examined initially, and additional slides routinely stained with GMS and AFB. A control slide containing pneumocystis (rather than other fungi) should always be used with the GMS stain, since this organism may be more difficult to stain than other fungi.

INFECTIONS

Pneumocystis Pneumonia

The incidence of pneumocystis pneumonia in AIDS patients has decreased in recent years due to the use of antimicrobial prophylaxis and antiretroviral therapy, but this infection remains an important cause of morbidity and mortality in these patients.[7,8,16,23,27,38] The clinical and pathologic features of pneumocystis pneumonia have been reviewed in detail in Chapter 10. The following sections will highlight the features characteristic of the disease in AIDS patients.

Clinical and Radiographic Features

As in non-AIDS patients, fever, cough, and shortness of breath are common symptoms. Individuals with AIDS, however, are more often asymptomatic, and tend to have a less acute onset and more chronic course.[75,76] Atypical radiographic features are seen more frequently, including solitary or multiple nodules (which may cavitate), upper lobe infiltrates resembling tuberculosis, honeycomb change, thin-walled cysts (interstitial emphysema or pneumatoceles), and pneumothorax.[43–45,54,65,71,72,80,88] Pleural effusion and hilar lymphadenopathy occur rarely.[43,70] Occasionally, chest radiographs are normal.[54,80]

Cases of disseminated pneumocystis infection occur with increased frequency in AIDS patients.[43,51,53,56,63,66, 68,78,84,85,90,93,96] A wide variety of organs may be involved, including lymph nodes, liver, middle ear, gastrointestinal tract, thyroid, skin, brain, and bone marrow, for example. Rarely, extrapulmonary dissemination occurs in the absence of lung involvement and can be explained by prior prophylactic treatment with inhaled pentamidine.[57,86] Prolonged persistence of organisms following treatment has been observed in some cases, and recurrences are common.[55] Acute respiratory failure has been reported following highly active antiretroviral therapy (HAART) in patients initially responding to antimicrobial and steroid therapy.[98] This reaction is thought to be a heightened inflammatory response rather than recurrent or resistant infection.

Microscopic Features

Cytologic Preparations: In BAL, bronchial washings or brushings, and sputum specimens, pneumocystis organisms are generally easily recognized in routine Papanicolaou stains.[46,49,59,60,64,67,82,83,87,99] At low magnification, characteristic, large, round to oval, light blue to pink clumps are seen that are of similar size and shape to alveolar ducts and spaces (Fig. 12–1).[59,60,64,67,83,87] These clumps are distinguished from proteinaceous exudates or cellular debris at higher magnification by identifying the typical granular, frothy, or honeycomb appearance characteristic of pneumocystis (see Chapter 10).[59,87] Distinct cyst walls can be appreciated, and they surround multiple basophilic dot-like structures that correspond to the nuclei of sporozoites (Fig. 12–2).

The GMS stain and its rapid variants[76,89] are all effective in confirming the presence of pneumocystis, as are a number of other stains reviewed in Chapter 10. GMS outlines the cyst walls, and in lightly colored preparations, single small, round areas of enhanced staining can often be identified within the cysts or along their walls. Diff-Quik, a modified Wright's stain, is another stain that is easily and rapidly performed and can be applied to cytologic preparations.[49,82,94] It is more difficult to interpret than the GMS stain, however, because it outlines the multiple intracystic sporozoites or free trophozoites but not the larger cyst walls (see Fig. 12–2). Fluorescence of cyst walls in Papanicolaou preparations has been reported but is not a reliable feature.[62,92] Immunoperoxidase or immunofluorescent staining using a specific antibody to pneumocystis is a useful adjunct for diagnosis.[50,53,58,69,73,79,85,91]

Histologic Sections: The histologic appearance of pneumocystis pneumonia in biopsy specimens is variable, as noted in Chapter 10.[61,95] The most common finding in AIDS patients is an intraalveolar frothy or

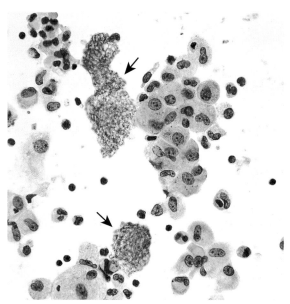

Figure 12–1 Pneumocystis in BAL fluid. Papanicolaou stain showing round- to oval-shaped clusters of organisms (arrows) dispersed among alveolar macrophages. Note the granular, frothy appearance even at low magnification.

foamy exudate, often associated with an interstitial pneumonia. This frothy material is readily visible in H and E-stained slides and is characterized by a distinct honeycomb pattern (due to cyst walls) within which basophilic dot-like structures (sporozoite nuclei) are visible (Fig. 12–3). Its presence is pathognomonic of pneumocystis infection even in those rare cases where the GMS stain is negative. The frothy exudate reflects the presence of large numbers of organisms and is more frequently observed in AIDS than in non-AIDS patients.[75]

Less often, other histologic features are present and are similar to those encountered in non-AIDS patients.[95] Diffuse alveolar damage (DAD) with prominent hyaline membranes is common. A nonspecific type of interstitial pneumonia, granulomatous inflammation, or calcification occurs occasionally.[47,48,74] Parenchymal necrosis with cavitation has been reported in several cases and was associated with necrotizing vasculitis in one.[44,52,77,81]

It should be remembered that various other organisms, especially cytomegalovirus and nontuberculous mycobacteria, are commonly found along with pneumocystis.[20,38] Therefore, the pathologist must carefully examine all pieces of tissue and all special stains, and he or she should not be content to stop looking for organisms after one agent has been identified.

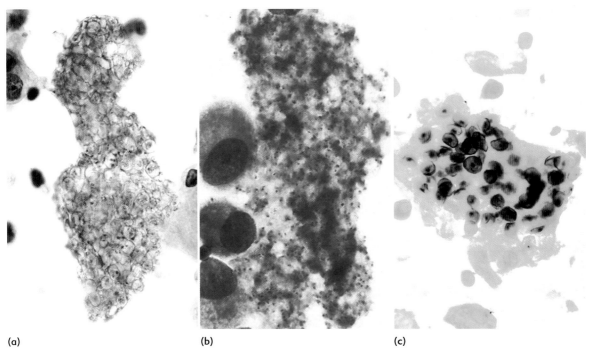

(a)   (b)   (c)

Figure 12–2 Pneumocystis in BAL fluid. (a) High magnification of a Papanicolaou stain showing closely packed cysts containing multiple dot-like structures (sporozoites). **(b)** Diff-Quik stain highlights the sporozoites and free trophozoites (darkly staining dot-like structures) rather than the cysts. **(c)** GMS stain outlines the cyst walls not the sporozoites. A dot-like area of enhanced staining is often present and corresponds to focal thickening along the cyst wall.

Bacterial Infections

Mycobacterium avium Complex (MAC) and Other Nontuberculous Mycobacterial Infections

Mycobacterium avium complex (MAC) is commonly isolated from patients with AIDS.[8,14,100,101,105,110–113] Typically, this infection occurs late in the course of HIV infection, at the time of severe immunosuppression, and it is widely disseminated. Gastrointestinal symptoms usually overshadow respiratory complaints, and generalized lymphadenopathy, hepatosplenomegaly, and anemia are frequently present. Chest radiographs are usually normal, although endobronchial masses have been reported rarely.[107,108] The most characteristic histologic finding is the presence of foamy histiocytes whose cytoplasm is packed with sheets of acid-fast bacilli.[103,105,112] Poorly formed granulomatous inflammation with a mixture of epithelioid histiocytes and acute and chronic inflammation is also common (Fig. 12–4). In a few cases, little or no cellular reaction occurs. The organisms are usually numerous in acid-fast stains. They may appear as negatively stained intracytoplasmic rod-shaped spaces in Diff-Quik-stained cytologic preparations.[102,106]

Nontuberculous mycobacteria other than MAC, including *M. kansasii, M. gordonae,* and *M. scrofulaceum,* have also been reported to cause disease in the AIDS population.[104,109–111] *M. kansasii* is the second most common mycobacterium after MAC in AIDS patients, and it causes clinical and radiographic features similar to tuberculosis.[104,109] It occurs late in the course of HIV infection and responds well to antituberculous therapy. Pathologically, a poorly formed, often suppurative, granulomatous reaction with numerous acid-fast bacilli is characteristic. Other less common reactions include areas of eosinophilic necrosis, abscesses, and a spindle cell infiltrate. Presumptive diagnosis of *M. kansasii* can be made based on morphology, since this organism is said to be longer than MAC, with more prominent beading and a tendency to have folded or bent ends.[109]

Tuberculosis

Tuberculosis remains an important infection in patients with AIDS, especially among intravenous drug users and Haitians, and in patients in nonindustrialized

Since many of the characteristic histologic features of tuberculous infection represent an immunologically mediated response, it is not surprising that the tissue reaction in AIDS patients is often atypical. Granuloma formation may be absent in some cases, whereas only non-necrotizing or poorly formed granulomas may be seen in others.

Miscellaneous Bacterial Pneumonia

Ordinary pathogenic bacteria remain an important cause of pneumonia in AIDS patients.[29,126–129] Gram-negative organisms, including pseudomonas, *E. coli,* klebsiella, enterobacter, and hemophilus species, are encountered most often, but staphylococcus and streptococcus are also common. The diagnosis is usually established by culture of sputum or BAL fluid without the need for biopsy.

Legionnaire's disease and *nocardial pneumonia* are examples of uncommon lung infections in AIDS patients that, as in non-AIDS patients, may require a lung biopsy for diagnosis.[123–125,129] The pathologic findings are similar to those described in patients without AIDS (see Chapter 10). A case of *bacillary angiomatosis* presenting as intrabronchial polyps has been reported.[122]

Rhodococcus equi Pneumonia and Malacoplakia

Rhodococcus equi is a Gram-positive, weakly acid-fast coccobacillus that can be a pathogen in immunocompromised individuals, especially those with HIV infection.[138] Clinically, an indolent, necrotizing pneumonia that progresses over weeks to months is characteristic. The most common radiographic findings include one or more cavitating mass-like nodular densities or areas of lobar consolidation.[135,136]

The pathologic features of *Rhodococcus equi* pneumonia are variable.[134,137,138] Centrally the lesion often resembles an acute, necrotizing bronchopneumonia with neutrophil infiltration and abscess formation, while at the periphery there is a striking histiocyte infiltrate (Fig. 12–5). The histiocytes form dense sheets, and they possess eosinophilic to foamy cytoplasm that contains strongly PAS-positive, granular inclusions similar to those seen in Whipple's disease. The histiocyte infiltrate may be the predominant finding in some cases, and the histiocytes often contain laminated intracytoplasmic inclusions typical of *Michaelis–Gutmann bodies* (Fig. 12–5, inset).[139] In such cases, the diagnosis of *malacoplakia* can be made. Numerous intracellular organisms can be visualized with tissue Gram stains or with the GMS stain. Although the organism is weakly acid-fast in

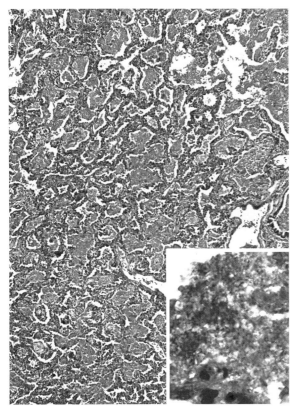

Figure 12–3 Pneumocystis pneumonia. Low magnification view showing the filling of airspaces with a granular eosinophilic exudate accompanied by mild alveolar septal thickening. Inset is a high magnification showing the characteristic frothy appearance of the airspace exudate. (See also Fig. 10–26.)

countries.[8,14,16,17,29,114,115,118–120] The occurrence of multiple drug-resistant strains of *M. tuberculosis* is an accompanying problem in certain urban areas.[116,117] It appears in general that tuberculin-positive persons with AIDS have a high risk for developing active tuberculosis. Unlike nontuberculous mycobacterial infections, tuberculosis can occur early or late in the course of the disease.

As with other infectious diseases in patients with AIDS, the clinical, radiographic, and even pathologic features of tuberculosis are often atypical.[29,114] Infiltrates may be found in any lobe, and mediastinal and/or hilar lymphadenopathy are common, whereas upper lobe cavitary disease is infrequent. There is an increased incidence of extrapulmonary infection, involving especially the peripheral lymph nodes, central nervous system, and bone marrow.[114,120] Endobronchial disease has also been reported.[121]

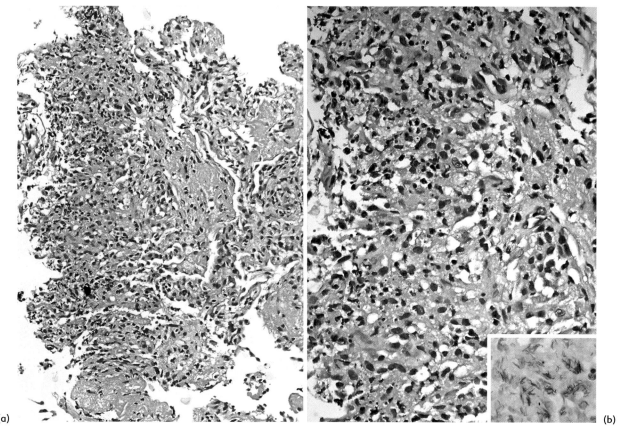

(a)

(b)

Figure 12–4 MAC infection on a transbronchial biopsy (TBB) specimen. (a) An ill-defined granulomatous reaction is seen in this example. (b) Higher magnification shows loosely aggregated epithelioid histiocytes along with acute and chronic inflammation. Sheets of acid-fast bacilli are seen with the Ziehl–Neelsen stain (inset).

culture, acid-fast stains are usually negative in tissue sections. Sometimes the histiocytes become spindle shaped, and the lesion resembles the so-called pseudo-tumor that has been described occasionally in mycobacterial infections (see Chapter 11).

Pulmonary malacoplakia is extremely rare and usually occurs in immunocompromised patients.[130–133,137] Although HIV infection is the most common cause of the immunosuppression, cases have also been described in transplant recipients and in patients with underlying malignancies. Organisms other than rhodococcus have been implicated occasionally, especially *E. coli*.

Fungal Infections

Fungal pneumonias constitute important infectious complications in AIDS patients.[2,13,20,31,32,35] They tend to occur late in the course of disease, frequently disseminate to extrapulmonary sites, and are associated

with high mortality.[16,29,149,162] Tissue reactions, as in all immunocompromised persons, are generally less developed than those expected in individuals with normal immune systems. Coinfection with other organisms, including mycobacteria, pyogenic bacteria, pneumocystis, and cytomegalovirus, is common.[141,147,148]

Cryptococcal pneumonia, either alone or as part of disseminated infection, is an important invasive fungal infection in AIDS.[140–142,145,146,152,154,161] Fever, cough, and dyspnea are its most typical clinical manifestations. Radiographic findings vary from localized densities to nodular interstitial opacities. Hilar lymph node enlargement is common. The same spectrum of tissue reactions to cryptococcus occurs in patients with AIDS as in other individuals (see Chapter 11).[141,146] Necrotizing or non-necrotizing granulomas may be seen, but a granulomatous reaction is often poorly developed or absent. In the latter cases, sheets of yeasts may be found free in alveolar spaces and in alveolar macrophages.

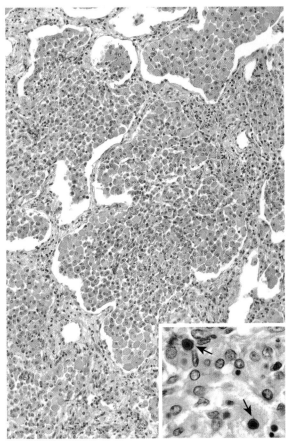

Figure 12–5 Malacoplakia. At low magnification, sheets of histiocytes are seen filling alveolar spaces. Inset is a higher magnification view of the histiocytes, some of which contain intracytoplasmic laminated inclusions typical of Michaelis–Gutmann bodies (arrows).

Organisms may also be found in the interstitium, where they fill alveolar septa, capillaries, and even lymphatic spaces. Several stains, including mucicarmine, alcian blue, and colloidal iron, are helpful in demonstrating the characteristic capsule. Unencapsulated or poorly encapsulated forms also occur, and in that situation the Fontana–Masson stain may be useful.[153] However, as emphasized in Chapter 11, the characteristic features of cryptococcus can usually be appreciated in routine H and E-stained sections and the diagnosis readily confirmed by the GMS stain.

Disseminated *histoplasmosis* (see Chapter 11) is another common fungal infection in AIDS patients, and lung involvement occurs in most cases.[143,148,150,159,160,164] The chest radiograph usually shows nodular interstitial infiltrates, but it may be normal. In microscopic sections, sheets of histiocytes filled with the typical

small, oval-shaped yeasts are seen in alveolar spaces and in the interstitium. Well-formed granulomas are usually not present. Histiocytes containing intracytoplasmic organisms are usually also numerous in BAL fluids or even sputum, and their recognition in these specimens will obviate the need for more invasive diagnostic procedures.

In the southwestern United States, *coccidioidomycosis* (Chapter 11) is an important complication in AIDS patients, either as a primary pulmonary infection or as disseminated disease.[147] Histologically, large numbers of spherules are usually present within necrotic debris, and there may be little associated inflammatory reaction.

Blastomycosis is the least common invasive fungal infection in AIDS patients.[157] It may occur in isolated pulmonary or disseminated forms. As with the other invasive fungal infections, mortality rates are high. Recognition of the organism in cytologic preparations or biopsy specimens is important, since culture may require several weeks (see Chapter 11).

Although mucocutaneous candidiasis is a frequent complication in AIDS patients, invasive infections due to opportunistic fungi are not common. There is some evidence, however, that their incidence may be increasing.[16,29,144] Aspergillus infections, in particular, have become more frequent since the 1990s, possibly since patients with AIDS are living longer with low CD4 counts and may develop chronic lung disease that predisposes them to this infection.[144,149,151,155,156,161] Additional predisposing factors include steroid therapy, prolonged antibiotic therapy, neutropenia, and other infections.[155] The pathologic manifestations are similar to those in non-AIDS patients (see Chapter 10). Invasive aspergillosis with tissue necrosis and vascular invasion is the most common finding. Changes resembling chronic necrotizing aspergillosis have been described as well, as have mycetomas. An ulcerative tracheobronchitis can also occur and is characterized by extensive ulceration of the tracheobronchial tree. There may be a pseudomembrane covering the ulcerated area that contains numerous organisms.[158] Patients with this form of the disease may present with bronchial obstruction and expectorate bronchial casts containing organisms (so-called obstructing bronchial aspergillosis).[144] Involvement of the small bronchi and bronchioles associated with cavitary disease has also been described.[165]

Invasive *candida pneumonia* is diagnosed only rarely during life, but is found more often at autopsy, usually as part of disseminated candidiasis, and it is frequently associated with other infections.[29,30,32,39]

Viral Infections

Cytomegalovirus

Cytomegalovirus (CMV) infections were among the earliest recognized complications of AIDS, and they remain a significant cause of morbidity.[8,169,171,172,176] Intravenous drug users appear to be at highest risk.[166] There is a controversy, however, regarding the true pathogenicity of this organism, since CMV infection is usually accompanied by other diseases, including both pneumonias (especially due to pneumocystis, cryptococcus, MAC, and pyogenic bacteria) and neoplasms (especially Kaposi's sarcoma).[29,173] Also, in some patients, infection, as evidenced by cytopathic effects, occurs in the absence of other pathologic changes. Although the presence of CMV infection in lung should be documented pathologically, only those cases with definite tissue reactions (see text following)

and no other organisms should be considered examples of *CMV pneumonia*.

The diagnostic histologic feature of CMV infection is the presence of enlarged cells (cytomegaly) that contain both nuclear and cytoplasmic inclusions (Figs 12–6 and 12–7; see also Chapter 10). Alveolar macrophages, type 2 pneumocytes, bronchial and bronchiolar epithelium, and capillary endothelial cells may be affected. The cytoplasmic inclusions stain positively with GMS (Fig. 12–7, *inset*) and should not be misinterpreted as fungi.[167] The associated tissue reaction in the lung varies from a mild interstitial pneumonia to extensive areas of DAD.[166,176] Airway involvement characterized by *necrotizing tracheitis* or *bronchiolitis* has been described rarely.[168,175,176] As mentioned, CMV infection can also occur in the absence of a tissue reaction. The significance of those cases is uncertain, but they should not be considered examples of CMV pneumonia.

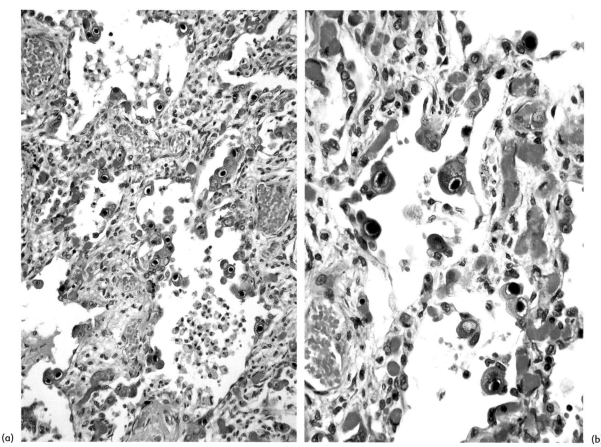

(a) (b)

Figure 12–6 CMV pneumonia. (a) At low magnification, large numbers of CMV-infected cells are seen lining alveolar septa. There is an associated chronic interstitial pneumonia characterized by chronic inflammation and fibrosis in alveolar septa. **(b)** The typical intranuclear and intracytoplasmic inclusions are better appreciated at higher magnification. Compare the size of the infected cells with that of adjacent noninfected alveolar pneumocytes.

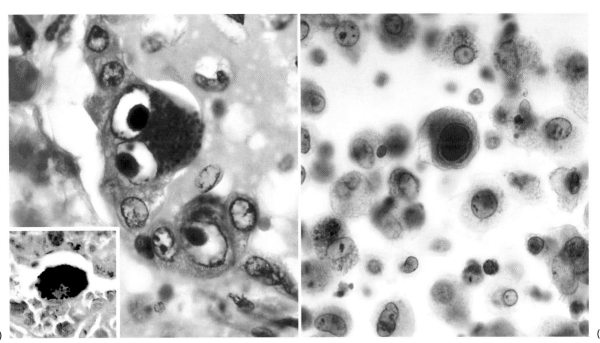

(a)　　　　　　　　　　　　　　　　　　　　　　　　　　　　　　　　　　(b)

Figure 12–7 CMV-infected cells. (a) High magnification showing the prominent darkly staining intranuclear inclusions separated by a clear zone from the nuclear membrane. Numerous coarsely granular intracytoplasmic inclusions are also present. Inset shows positive staining of the intracytoplasmic inclusions in a GMS stain. **(b)** Papanicolaou stain of CMV-infected cell in BAL fluid.

Both BAL and TBB specimens are effective diagnostic modalities for CMV pneumonia (Fig. 12–7).[2,5,10,18,33] The application of immunohistochemical stains using monoclonal antibodies and of in situ hybridization or PCR techniques using CMV-specific DNA probes may help to confirm the diagnosis in difficult cases (see Chapter 10).[170]

Herpes Simplex Virus

Herpes simplex lung infections are considerably less common than CMV infection in AIDS.[20,32] This virus produces a spectrum of histologic reactions ranging from patchy necrosis and DAD to ulcerative tracheo-bronchitis (see Chapter 10). Characteristic intranuclear inclusions can be found in epithelial cells in both lung tissue and BAL specimens. Antibodies to the organism are available for immunohistochemical staining, and in situ hybridization and PCR techniques can also be used.

Epstein-Barr Virus

Not surprisingly, Epstein-Barr virus (EBV) infections can occur in HIV-infected individuals. In one case of fatal disseminated infection, DAD was the main pulmonary finding.[174]

Parasitic Infections

Toxoplasmosis

Toxoplasmosis usually causes encephalitis in patients with AIDS, but disseminated disease with lung involvement also occurs.[179,190,194] Occasionally, pneumonia is the presenting feature of disseminated toxoplasmosis, and it may be the cause of death.[186] As with CMV pneumonia, toxoplasmosis appears to be more common in intravenous drug users.[166]

Histologically, there are varying combinations of an interstitial pneumonia, DAD, and necrotizing pneumonia (Fig. 12–8). The latter is characterized by patchy foci of parenchymal necrosis with prominent karyorrhexis and an associated proteinaceous exudate with minimal inflammation. In active infections, rapidly multiplying tachyzoites are numerous and are found in and around the necrotic zones (Fig. 12–8, inset).[177] They may lie free within airspace exudates, or they may form groups within cytoplasmic vacuoles in alveolar macrophages or interstitial cells. Although tachyzoites appear crescentic in fresh preparations, in fixed tissue specimens they are round to oval and average 2 to 4 µm in greatest dimension. When numerous, they can be visualized in H and E-stained sections, although they may be difficult

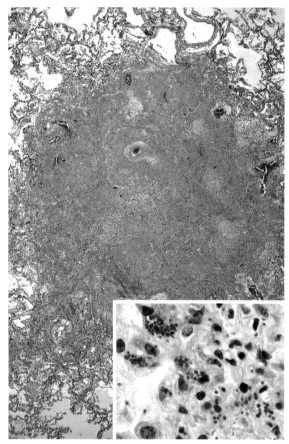

Figure 12–8 Toxoplasmosis characterized by a paucicellular, bronchiolocentric necrotizing pneumonia. Inset is a high magnification showing numerous, uniform-appearing basophilic tachyzoites that are present within cells and lying free.

inclusions. The tachyzoites are similar in size and shape to histoplasma. They can be distinguished from this organism by means of the GMS stain, which outlines histoplasma but fails to stain toxoplasma.

Strongyloidiasis

Strongyloides stercoralis is an intestinal nematode that is widely distributed throughout the world. Infections may last for years, and most patients are asymptomatic or have only minimal symptoms. In immunocompromised patients, however, large numbers of organisms may proliferate and spread via lymphohematogenous routes to extraintestinal organs, especially the lungs.[178,181,182,184,191] In addition to patients with AIDS, this *hyperinfection syndrome* has been reported in persons with underlying malignancy, in organ transplant recipients, and in individuals receiving chronic corticosteroid therapy. The clinical presentation typically is characterized by cough, dyspnea, wheezing, and hemoptysis, and interstitial lung infiltrates are usually seen radiographically. Pathologically, there are areas of acute bronchopneumonia, and scattered, poorly formed granulomas are found within the interstitium in most cases. DAD is a common accompanying feature, and patchy interstitial fibrosis, especially within interlobular septa, has been described. Filariform larvae can be found within the granulomas or surrounded by neutrophils in the areas of bronchopneumonia. They may also occur within the airspaces without an associated inflammatory response (Fig. 12–9). The diagnosis can sometimes be made by identifying the

to distinguish from necrotic debris. They do not stain with GMS or PAS. In chronic infections, cysts containing slowly multiplying bradyzoites are formed. The cysts can be seen in H and E-stained preparations, where they have a granular basophilic appearance due to the presence of the tightly clustered bradyzoites. The internal structure can be highlighted by the PAS stain since the bradyzoites store PAS-positive material. Immunohistochemistry using specific antibodies is the most reliable technique to outline the organisms,[186] and electron microscopy can also help to confirm the diagnosis.[189]

The intracytoplasmic clusters of toxoplasma should not be confused with the intracytoplasmic inclusions of CMV (see Fig. 12–7). The latter are smaller and have less well-defined borders, and they are usually, of course, also accompanied by other features of CMV infection, including cytomegaly and intranuclear

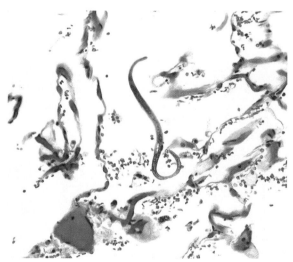

Figure 12–9 Strongyloides larva within an alveolar space with no associated inflammatory reaction.

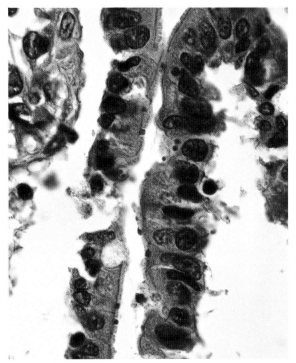

Figure 12–10 Cryptosporidiosis on a TBB specimen. Uniform round basophilic organisms are present along the luminal surface of the bronchial epithelium.

organisms in sputum or BAL specimens.[181,193] Other opportunistic infections commonly accompany the strongyloides infection.[178,181]

Miscellaneous Parasitic Diseases

Lung involvement by *cryptosporidiosis* is a rare complication in AIDS patients.[180,183,185] The organisms are found lining the luminal surface of tracheobronchial epithelial cells, similar to the growth pattern characteristic of the more common gastrointestinal form of the disease (Fig. 12–10). They appear basophilic and are typically round and uniform in size and shape, averaging 2 to 4 μm in diameter. *Isospora* have also been rarely reported in lungs in AIDS patients.[187] *Microsporidiosis* also occurs in this population. Most infections involve the gastrointestinal tract or biliary tree, while keratoconjunctivitis has also been described. Rare examples of disseminated disease involving the lung have been reported.[188,192] Characteristic spores are oval shaped, averaging 2 μm in greatest dimension, and they are Gram-positive. They are found within bronchial epithelial cells and free within airspace exudates. An associated bronchiolitis has been noted in biopsy specimens.

NONINFECTIOUS CAUSES OF LUNG DISEASE

Interstitial Pneumonias

Although the majority of pulmonary infiltrates in AIDS patients are due to infection, interstitial pneumonias are occasionally encountered in which extensive search for organisms is negative.[223] Those lesions are similar clinically and pathologically to their counterparts in patients without evidence of AIDS.

Lymphoid Interstitial Pneumonia and Related Conditions

Lymphoid interstitial pneumonia (LIP) is a rare form of chronic interstitial pneumonia that was originally described before the AIDS epidemic (see Chapter 9). An association with Sjögren's disease and dysproteinemias has been noted. Pathologically it is characterized by diffuse interstitial infiltration by a dense lympho-plasmacytic infiltrate causing widening and distortion of alveolar septa. Germinal centers are often prominent, and poorly formed granulomas may be present. LIP is currently more commonly encountered in AIDS than in non-AIDS patients, and children and Haitians appear to be at greatest risk.[15,21,26,37,196,203,205,207,210,214,220,222,223] In HIV-positive children, in fact, the finding of LIP is considered diagnostic of AIDS. There is also some evidence that the HIV virus may be involved in the pathogenesis of this lesion.[222]

Follicular bronchiolitis, a more limited form of lymphoid infiltration, has also been reported in AIDS patients. It is characterized by a dense lymphoid infiltrate with prominent germinal centers that is confined to the peribronchiolar interstitium (see Chapter 9) rather than being diffuse as in LIP.[199,218] Like LIP, this lesion is not specific for AIDS and has been reported with other types of immunodeficiency, as well as with rheumatoid arthritis and various hypersensitivity reactions.[224] It also occurs more frequently in children with AIDS than in adults with AIDS. Follicular bronchiolitis and LIP may represent two ends of a spectrum of lymphoid infiltration rather than representing separate disease entities.

Many reported cases of LIP have been diagnosed on TBB specimens.[214,222] The diagnosis of LIP on this type of biopsy has to be questioned, however, both because nonspecific chronic inflammation is frequently present in the peribronchial interstitium and also because the distribution of the changes (and thus the distinction from follicular bronchiolitis) cannot be adequately assessed. Accurate diagnosis of LIP, as well as follicular bronchiolitis, therefore, requires surgical lung biopsy.

Other Interstitial Pneumonias

Perhaps the most common interstitial pneumonia encountered in AIDS patients in the absence of infection is a nonspecific type of *chronic interstitial pneumonia*.[213,221–223] This lesion is characterized by a peribronchial or peribronchiolar interstitial chronic inflammatory cell infiltrate, often containing lymphoid follicles. Most reported cases have been diagnosed on TBB specimens, and, therefore, whether the changes represent focal, nonspecific chronic inflammation related to the airways or whether they are part of a diffuse interstitial pneumonia is not clear. Many patients, however, are asymptomatic with normal chest radiographs and, at least in these individuals, the finding is likely a localized reaction.[213,222] In a few cases, the process may represent an early manifestation of LIP.[222] Although the terminology is similar, this lesion should not be confused with the diffuse form of idiopathic chronic interstitial pneumonia that occurs in immunocompetent persons (*nonspecific interstitial pneumonia*, see Chapter 3).

DAD, unassociated with identifiable infection, not surprisingly, also occurs in AIDS patients and is identical to cases in patients without AIDS (see Chapter 2).[26,216,222] Both the acute stage with prominent hyaline membranes and the organizing stage with interstitial fibroblast proliferation have been described.

Desquamative interstitial pneumonia (DIP) has been reported rarely in children with AIDS, although subsequent autopsy studies failed to support the diagnosis in some cases.[15,223]

Miscellaneous Noninfectious Lung Diseases

Pulmonary Alveolar Proteinosis

Rare examples of a pulmonary alveolar proteinosis (PAP)-like lesion (*secondary PAP*) have been reported in AIDS patients.[211,219] All have had associated infections, most commonly pneumocystis pneumonia, and occasionally tuberculosis or CMV pneumonia. Importantly, PAP has not been described in AIDS patients in the absence of infection. The pathogenesis of PAP-like changes in AIDS may be related to impaired clearance mechanisms due to severe immunocompromise. Lung lavage has not been advocated in treating AIDS patients, although the presence of PAP may worsen respiratory distress in patients with pulmonary infections.

Bronchiolitis obliterans–organizing pneumonia (BOOP) has been reported in HIV-positive persons with AIDS.[195,204] BOOP is a common lesion in both immunocompetent and immunocompromised individuals (see Chapter 2), and its occurrence in an HIV-positive individual is likely coincidental. Caution should be exercised in diagnosing this lesion in AIDS patients, however, especially on TBB specimens, since it is frequently a nonspecific reactive finding on the periphery of another lesion (especially infection).

Pulmonary hypertension has been reported in a number of patients with HIV infection.[197,198,200,202,208,209,212,215] Pathologically, changes are similar to those in primary pulmonary hypertension, including the presence of plexiform lesions (see Chapter 13). The pulmonary hypertension has been attributed to HIV, although direct evidence of HIV involvement has not been demonstrated.[197,202,209] An association with membranoproliferative glomerulonephritis was noted in two cases.[198]

There is some evidence that the incidence of *bronchiectasis* may be increased in AIDS patients.[206]

MALIGNANCIES

The association of immune deficiency states with the development of neoplasia in a variety of sites is well documented, and AIDS patients provide no exception.[241] Kaposi's sarcoma, malignant lymphoma, and squamous cell carcinoma comprise the majority of reported lesions, but other neoplasms have been seen as well. Kaposi's sarcoma, however, is the only malignancy to involve the respiratory tract with any frequency in patients with AIDS, although the incidence has decreased considerably due to the advent of HAART.[225]

Kaposi's Sarcoma

Kaposi's sarcoma occurs most often in homosexual or bisexual men with AIDS.[223] Approximately 20% to 30% of AIDS patients with extrapulmonary Kaposi's sarcoma develop respiratory tract involvement during life, although the incidence of pulmonary involvement is higher at autopsy.[233,244] Pulmonary Kaposi's sarcoma can also occur in the absence of extrapulmonary mucocutaneous lesions.[237] Pathologically, three distinct forms involve the lung: (1) nodular submucosal lesions in the tracheobronchial tree, (2) nodular interstitial disease, and (3) diffuse interstitial growth along lymphatic routes.[229,233,244,252,255] The diagnosis often requires open lung biopsy, but it can be made by TBB.[235,236]

The radiographic picture varies with the histopathologic pattern.[229,233,237,244,252,255] Nodular interstitial lesions are usually randomly distributed and appear as poorly outlined densities. Diffuse interstitial infiltrates often start in the hilar area and spread peripherally. Hilar lymphadenopathy and pleural effusion are frequently also present. Tracheobronchial lesions typically occur as multiple nodules, and they are usually accompanied by other forms of lung involvement. Their bronchoscopic appearance is distinct and is characterized by the presence of raised, erythematous, mucosa-covered lesions.[255]

Histologically, the bronchial submucosal as well as interstitial nodular lesions usually resemble classic Kaposi's sarcoma, with interlacing bundles of plump spindle cells, extravasated erythrocytes, and hemosiderin deposits (Fig. 12–11).[229,235,244,247,250,252] Intracytoplasmic

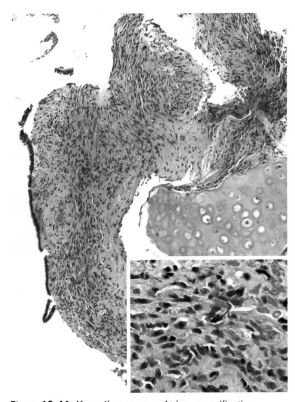

Figure 12–11 Kaposi's sarcoma. At low magnification, marked widening of the bronchial submucosal space by a cellular infiltrate is seen in this TBB. At higher magnification (inset), the infiltrating cells are fairly uniform, spindle shaped, and there are thin-walled vascular spaces and extravasated erythrocytes.

hyaline globules are often seen as well. In the diffuse interstitial pattern, the lesions tend to be more polymorphous, with plasma cells and lymphocytes admixed among the spindle cells. Bland-appearing, slit-like vascular spaces are often interspersed among the other elements, and there may be abundant stromal collagen. The infiltrate follows a distinct lymphangitic distribution with growth around bronchovascular bundles, along interlobular septa, and within the pleura as well as along alveolar septa. Distinct thickening of vascular adventitia and bronchiole walls is produced by the infiltrate. Evidence of intraalveolar hemorrhage with erythrocytes and hemosiderin in airspaces often accompanies the infiltrate. Typically in this form of the disease, cytologic atypia may be difficult to find, and the lymphangitic growth pattern is often more of a clue to the diagnosis than are the high magnification microscopic features.[250] Immunohistochemical staining for endothelial markers, including CD31, CD34 and factor VIII, may facilitate diagnosis.

Kaposi's sarcoma is often associated with various pulmonary infections, especially pneumocystis and CMV pneumonia. An elevated serum lactate dehydrogenase (LDH) level and a chest radiograph with granular opacities or cystic spaces are suggestive of concomitant infection.[237]Although a role had been suggested for CMV in the pathogenesis of this vascular neoplasm, this relationship has not been supported.[234] Rather, there is now good evidence for human herpesvirus 8 (HHV8) infection in the pathogenesis of this neoplasm.[246] Identification of HHV8 by immunohistochemistry or PCR techniques may facilitate diagnosis in difficult cases.[251,253]

Malignant Lymphoma

Lymphoma is the second most common HIV-related neoplasm after Kaposi's sarcoma.[223,249] Most cases are diffuse, high-grade variants of B-cell origin.[230,239–243,248,249] Occasional cases of low-grade B-cell lymphoma of mucosa-associated lymphoid tissue (MALT) have been described.[207,254] Disseminated disease, often with extranodal involvement, is usually present, although pulmonary involvement is uncommon, occurring in only 10% or less of patients.[231,249] Primary pulmonary lymphoma is rare.[217] Most reported cases were high-grade B-cell neoplasms associated with EBV infection. Lymphomatoid granulomatosis has also rarely been reported in patients with AIDS, and, as in non-AIDS patients, an association with EBV has been demonstrated (see Chapter 9).[201,226,245]

Lung Carcinoma

Lung carcinoma occurs occasionally in HIV-infected individuals. It is not clear whether these patients have an increased incidence of lung carcinoma, although the neoplasm appears to occur at a younger age and to be associated with a more fulminant course in HIV-infected persons.[227,228,232,238] Adenocarcinoma is the subtype most often reported.

REFERENCES

General

1. Agostini C, Trentin L, Zambello R, Semenzato G: HIV-1 and the lung: Infectivity, pathogenic mechanisms, and cellular immune responses taking place in the lower respiratory tract. Am Rev Respir Dis 147:1038, 1993.
2. Amberson JB, DiCarlo EF, Metroka CE, et al: Diagnostic pathology in the acquired immunodeficiency syndrome: Surgical pathology and cytology experience with 67 patients. Arch Pathol Lab Med 109:345, 1985.
3. Barrio J, Harcup C, Baier H, Pitchenik A: Value of repeat fiberoptic bronchoscopies and significance of nondiagnostic bronchoscopic results in patients with the acquired immunodeficiency syndrome. Am Rev Respir Dis 135:422, 1987.
4. Bigby T, Margolskee D, Curtis J, et al: The usefulness of induced sputum in the diagnosis of *Pneumocystis carinii* pneumonia in patients with the acquired immunodeficiency syndrome. Am Rev Respir Dis 133: 515, 1986.
5. Broad C, Dake M, Stulbarg M, et al: Bronchoalveolar lavage and transbronchial biopsy for the diagnosis of pulmonary infections in the acquired immunodeficiency syndrome. Ann Intern Med 102:747, 1985.
6. Centers for Disease Control, U.S. Department of Health and Human Services: Guidelines for prevention of transmission of human immunodeficiency virus and hepatitis B virus to health-care and public-safety workers. MMWR Morb Mortal Wkly Rep 38 (Nos. 5 and 6), 1989.
7. Concepcion L, Markowitz GS, Borczuk AC, et al: Comparison of changing autopsy trends in the Bronx population with acquired immunodeficiency syndrome. Mod Pathol 9:1001, 1996.
8. Cury PM, Pulido CF, Furtado VMG, et al: Autopsy findings in AIDS patients from a reference hospital in Brazil: Analysis of 92 cases. Pathol Res Pract 199:811, 2003.
9. Fitzgerald W, Bevelaqua FA, Garay SM, Oranda CP: The role of open lung biopsy in patients with the acquired immunodeficiency syndrome. Chest 91:659, 1987.
10. Francis ND, Golden RD, Forster SM, et al: Diagnosis of lung disease in acquired immune deficiency syndrome: Biopsy or cytology and implications for management. J Clin Pathol 40:1269, 1987.
11. Gal AA, Koss MN, Hartman B, Strigle S: A review of pulmonary pathology in the acquired immune deficiency syndrome. Surg Pathol 1:325, 1988.
12. Griffiths MH, Kocjan G, Miller RF, Godfrey-Faussett P: Diagnosis of pulmonary disease in human immunodeficiency virus infection: Role of transbronchial biopsy and bronchoalveolar lavage. Thorax 44:554, 1989.
13. Guarda LA, Luna MA, Smith JL, et al: Acquired immune deficiency syndrome: Postmortem findings. Am J Clin Pathol 81:549, 1984.
14. Hofman P, Saint-Paul MC, Battaglione V, et al: Autopsy findings in the acquired immunodeficiency syndrome (AIDS). A report of 395 cases from the south of France. Pathol Res Pract 195:209, 1999.
15. Joshi VV, Oleske JM, Minnefor AB, et al: Pathologic pulmonary findings in children with the acquired immunodeficiency syndrome: A study of ten cases. Hum Pathol 16:241, 1985.
16. Klatt EC, Nichols L, Noguchi TT: Evolving trends revealed by autopsies of patients with the acquired immunodeficiency syndrome: 565 autopsies in adults with the acquired immunodeficiency syndrome, Los Angeles, Calif, 1992–1993. Arch Pathol Lab Med 118:884, 1994.
17. Lanjewar DN, Duggal R: Pulmonary pathology in patients with AIDS: An autopsy study from Mumbai. HIV Med 2:266, 2001.
18. Linder J, Vaughn WP, Armitage JO, et al: Cytopathology of opportunistic infection in bronchoalveolar lavage. Am J Clin Pathol 88:421, 1987.
19. Mann J, Altus C, Webber C, et al: Nonbronchoscopic lung lavage for diagnosis of opportunistic infection in AIDS. Chest 91:319, 1987.
20. Marchevsky A, Rosen MJ, Crystal G, Kleinerman J: Pulmonary complications of the acquired immunodeficiency syndrome: A clinicopathologic study of 70 cases. Hum Pathol 16:659, 1985.
21. Marolda J, Pace B, Bonforte RJ, et al: Pulmonary manifestations of HIV infection in children. Pediatr Pulmonol 10:231, 1991.
22. Martin WR, Albertson TE, Siegel B: Tracheal catheters in patients with acquired immunodeficiency syndrome for the diagnosis of *Pneumocystis carinii* pneumonia. Chest 98:29, 1990.
23. Masliah E, DeTeresa RM, Mallory ME, Hanson LA: Changes in pathological findings at autopsy in AIDS cases for the last 15 years. AIDS 14:69, 2000.
24. Miller-Catchpole R, Variakojis D, Anastasi J, et al: The Chicago AIDS autopsy study: Opportunistic infection, neoplasms, and findings from selected organ systems with a comparison to national data. Mod Pathol 2:277, 1989.
25. Milligan SA, Luce JM, Golden J, et al: Transbronchial biopsy without fluoroscopy in patients with diffuse roentgenographic infiltrates and the acquired immunodeficiency syndrome. Am Rev Respir Dis 137:486, 1988.
26. Moran CA, Suster S, Pavlova Z, Mullick FG, Koss MN: The spectrum of pathological changes in the lung in

children with the acquired immunodeficiency syndrome. Hum Pathol 25:877, 1994.

27. Morgello S, Mahboob F, Yakoushina T, et al: Autopsy findings in a human immunodeficiency virus-infected population over 2 decades. Arch Pathol Lab Med 126:182, 2002.

28. Moskovitz L, Hensley GT, Chan JC, Adams K: Immediate causes of death in acquired immunodeficiency syndrome. Arch Pathol Lab Med 109:735, 1985.

29. Murray JF, Mills J: Pulmonary infectious complications of human immunodeficiency virus infection. Am Rev Respir Dis 141:1356, 1582, 1990.

30. Nash G, Fligiel S: Pathologic features of the lung in the acquired immunodeficiency syndrome: An autopsy study of seventeen homosexual males. Am J Clin Pathol 81:6, 1984.

31. Ng VL, Gartner I, Weymouth LA, et al: The use of mucolysed sputum for the identification of pulmonary pathogens associated with human immunodeficiency virus infection. Arch Pathol Lab Med 113:488, 1989.

32. Niedt GW, Schinella RA: Acquired immunodeficiency syndrome. Clinicopathologic study of 56 autopsies. Arch Pathol Lab Med 109:727, 1985.

33. Orenstein M, Webber CA, Cash M, et al: Value of bronchoalveolar lavage in the diagnosis of pulmonary infection in acquired immune deficiency syndrome. Thorax 41:345, 1986.

34. Pass HI, Potter DA, Machec AM, et al: Thoracic manifestations of the acquired immune deficiency syndrome. J Thorac Cardiovasc Surg 88:654, 1984.

35. Reichert CM, O'Leary TJ, Levens DL, et al: Autopsy pathology in the acquired immune deficiency syndrome. Am J Pathol 112:357, 1983.

36. Rolston KVI, Rodriguez S, McRory L, et al: Diagnostic value of induced sputum in patients with the acquired immunodeficiency syndrome. Am J Med 85:269, 1988.

37. Rubinstein A, Morecki R, Silverman B, et al: Pulmonary disease in children with acquired immune deficiency syndrome and AIDS-related complex. J Pediatr 108:498, 1986.

38. Sehonanda A, Choi YJ, Blum S: Changing patterns of autopsy findings among persons with acquired immunodeficiency syndrome in an inner-city population: A 12-year retrospective study. Arch Pathol Lab Med 120:459, 1996.

39. Stover DE, White DA, Romano PA, et al: Spectrum of pulmonary disorders associated with the acquired immune deficiency syndrome. Am J Med 78:429, 1985.

40. Stulbarg MS, Golden JA: Open lung biopsy in the acquired immunodeficiency syndrome (AIDS). Chest 91:639, 1987.

41. Wallace JM, Batra P, Gong H Jr, Ovenfors C-O: Percutaneous needle lung aspiration for diagnosing pneumonitis in the patient with acquired immunodeficiency syndrome (AIDS). Am Rev Respir Dis 131:389, 1985.

42. Weldon-Linne CM, Rhone DP, Bourassa R: Bronchoscopy specimens in adults with AIDS: Comparative yields of cytology, histology and culture for diagnosis of infectious agents. Chest 98:24, 1990.

Pneumocystis Pneumonia

43. Afessa B, Green WR, Williams WA, et al: *Pneumocystis carinii* pneumonia complicated by lymphadenopathy and pneumothorax. Arch Intern Med 148:2651, 1988.

44. Barrio JL, Suarez M, Rodriquez JL, et al: *Pneumocystis carinii* pneumonia presenting as cavitating and noncavitating solitary pulmonary nodules in patients with the acquired immunodeficiency syndrome. Am Rev Respir Dis 134:1094, 1986.

45. Beers MF, Sohn M, Swartz M: Recurrent pneumothorax in AIDS patients with pneumocystis pneumonia: A clinicopathologic report of three cases and review of the literature. Chest 98:266, 1990.

46. Bigby TD, Margolskee D, Curtis JL, et al: The usefulness of induced sputum within diagnosis of *Pneumocystis carinii* pneumonia in patients with the acquired immunodeficiency syndrome. Am Rev Respir Dis 133:515, 1986.

47. Bleiweiss IJ, Jagirdar JS, Klein MJ, et al: Granulomatous *Pneumocystis carinii* pneumonia in three patients with the acquired immune deficiency syndrome. Chest 94:580, 1988.

48. Blumenfeld W, Basgoz N, Owen WF Jr, Schmidt DM: Granulomatous pulmonary lesions in patients with the acquired immunodeficiency syndrome (AIDS) and *Pneumocystis carinii* infection. Ann Intern Med 109:505, 1988.

49. Blumenfeld W, Griffiss JM: *Pneumocystis carinii* in sputum: Comparable efficacy of screening stains and determination of cyst density. Arch Pathol Lab Med 112:816, 1988.

50. Blumenfeld W, Kovacs JA: Use of a monoclonal antibody to detect *Pneumocystis carinii* in induced sputum and bronchoalveolar lavage fluid by immunoperoxidase staining. Arch Pathol Lab Med 112:1233, 1988.

51. Carter TR, Cooper PH, Petri WA Jr, et al: *Pneumocystis carinii* infection of the small intestine in a patient with acquired immune deficiency syndrome. Am J Clin Pathol 89:679, 1988.

52. Chechani V, Zanan MK, Finch PJP: Chronic cavitary *Pneumocystis carinii* pneumonia in a patient with AIDS. Chest 95:1347, 1989.

53. Cote RJ, Rosenblum M, Telzak EE, May M, Unger PD, Cartun RW: Disseminated *Pneumocystis carinii* infection causing extrapulmonary organ failure: Clinical, pathologic, and immunohistochemical analysis. Mod Pathol 3:25, 1990.

54. DeLorenzo LJ, Huang CT, Maguire GP, Stone DJ: Roentgenographic patterns of *Pneumocystis carinii* pneumonia in 104 patients with AIDS. Chest 91:323, 1987.

55. DeLorenzo LJ, Maguire GP, Wormser GP, et al: Persistence of *Pneumocystis carinii* pneumonia in the acquired immunodeficiency syndrome. Evaluation of therapy by follow-up transbronchial lung biopsy. Chest 88:79, 1988.

56. Dembinski AS, Smith DM, Goldsmith JC, Woods GL: Widespread dissemination of *Pneumocystis carinii* infection in a patient with acquired immune deficiency syndrome receiving long-term treatment with aerosolized pentamidine. Am J Clin Pathol 95:96, 1991.

57. Devoux SJ, Volkan Adsay N, Ioachim HL: Disseminated pneumocystosis without pulmonary involvement during prophylactic aerosolized pentamidine therapy in a patient with the acquired immunodeficiency syndrome. Arch Pathol Lab Med 115:1137, 1991.

58. Elvin KM, Bjorkman E, Heurlin N, Hjerpe A: *Pneumocystis carinii* pneumonia: Detection of parasites in sputum and bronchoalveolar lavage fluid by monoclonal antibodies. Br Med J 297:381, 1988.

59. Flint A, Beckwith AL, Naylor B: *Pneumocystis carinii* pneumonia. Cytologic manifestations and rapid diagnosis in routinely prepared Papanicolaou-stained preparations. Am J Med 81:1009, 1986.

60. Gal AA, Klatt EC, Koss MN, et al: The effectiveness of bronchoscopy in the diagnosis of *Pneumocystis carinii* and cytomegalovirus pulmonary infections in acquired immunodeficiency syndrome. Arch Pathol Lab Med 111:238, 1987.

61. Gal AA, Koss MN, Strigle S, Augritt P: *Pneumocystis carinii* infection in the acquired immune deficiency syndrome. Semin Diagn Pathol 6:787, 1989.

62. Ghali VS, Garcia RL, Skolom J: Fluorescence of *Pneumocystis carinii* in Papanicolaou smears. Hum Pathol 15:907, 1984.

63. Gherman CR, Ward RR, Bassis ML: *Pneumocystis carinii* otitis media and mastoiditis as the initial manifestation of the acquired immunodeficiency syndrome. Am J Med 85:250, 1988.

64. Golden JA, Hollander H, Stulbarg MS, et al: Bronchoalveolar lavage as the exclusive diagnostic modality for *Pneumocystis carinii* pneumonia. A prospective study among patients with acquired immunodeficiency syndrome. Chest 90:18, 1986.

65. Goodman PC, Daley C, Minagi H: Spontaneous pneumothorax in AIDS patients with *Pneumocystis carinii* pneumonia. AJR Am J Roentgenol 147:29, 1986.

66. Grimes MM, La Pook JD, Bar MH, et al: Disseminated *Pneumocystis carinii* infection in a patient with acquired immunodeficiency syndrome. Hum Pathol 18:307, 1987.

67. Hartman B, Koss M, Hui A, et al: *Pneumocystis carinii* pneumonia in the acquired immunodeficiency syndrome (AIDS). Diagnosis with bronchial brushings, biopsy, and bronchoalveolar lavage. Chest 87:603, 1985.

68. Hennessey NP, Parro EL, Cockerell CJ: Cutaneous *Pneumocystis carinii* infection in patients with acquired immunodeficiency syndrome. Arch Dermatol 127:1699, 1991.

69. Homer KS, Wiley EL, Smith AL, et al: Monoclonal antibody to *Pneumocystis carinii*. Comparison with silver stain in bronchial lavage specimens. Am J Clin Pathol 97:619, 1992.

70. Horowitz ML, Schiff M, Samuels J, Russo R, Schnader J: *Pneumocystis carinii* pleural effusion: Pathogenesis and pleural fluid analysis. 148:232, 1993.

71. Joe L, Gordan F, Parker RH: Spontaneous pneumothorax with *Pneumocystis carinii* infection. Occurrence in patients with acquired immunodeficiency syndrome. Arch Intern Med 146:1816, 1986.

72. Klein JS, Warnock M, Webb WR, Gamsu G: Cavitating and noncavitating granulomas in AIDS patients with Pneumocystis pneumonitis. AJR Am J Roentgenol 152:753, 1985.

73. Kovacs JA, Ng VL, Nasur H, et al: Diagnosis of *Pneumocystis carinii* pneumonia: Improved detection in sputum with use of monoclonal antibodies. N Engl J Med 318:589, 1988.

74. Lee MM, Schinella RA: Pulmonary calcification caused by *Pneumocystis carinii* pneumonia. A clinicopathological study of 13 cases in acquired immune deficiency syndrome patients. Am J Surg Pathol 15:376, 1991.

75. Limper AH, Offord KP, Smith TF, Martin WJ II: *Pneumocystis carinii* pneumonia: Differences in lung parasite number and inflammation in patients with and without AIDS. Am Rev Respir Dis 140:1204, 1989.

76. Lindley RP, Mooney P: A rapid stain for pneumocystis. J Clin Pathol 40:811, 1987.

77. Liu YC, Tomashefski JF Jr, Tomford JW, Green H: Necrotizing *Pneumocystis carinii* vasculitis associated with lung necrosis and cavitation in a patient with acquired immunodeficiency syndrome. Arch Pathol Lab Med 113:494, 1989.

78. Matsuda S, Urata Y, Shiota T, et al: Disseminated infection of *Pneumocystis carinii* in a patient with the acquired immunodeficiency syndrome. Virchows Arch A Cell Pathol 414:523, 1989.

79. Millard PR, Heryet AR: Observations favoring *Pneumocystis carinii* pneumonia as a primary infection: A monoclonal antibody study on paraffin sections. J Pathol 154:365, 1988.

80. Mones JM, Saldana MJ, Oldham SA: Diagnosis of *Pneumocystis carinii* pneumonia. Roentgenographic-pathologic correlates based on fiberoptic bronchoscopy specimens from patients with the acquired immunodeficiency syndrome. Chest 89:522, 1986.

81. Murry CE, Schmidt RA: Tissue invasion by *Pneumocystis carinii*: A possible cause of cavitary pneumonia and pneumothorax. Hum Pathol 23:1380, 1992.

82. O'Brien RF, Quinn JL, Miyahara BT, et al: Diagnosis of *Pneumocystis carinii* pneumonia by induced sputum in a city with moderate incidence of AIDS. Chest 95:136, 1989.

83. Pitchenik AE, Ganjei P, Torres A, et al: Sputum examination for the diagnosis of *Pneumocystis carinii* pneumonia in the acquired immunodeficiency syndrome. Am Rev Respir Dis 133:226, 1986.

84. Poblite RB, Rodriguez K, Foust RT, et al: *Pneumocystis carinii* hepatitis in the acquired immunodeficiency syndrome (AIDS). Ann Intern Med 110:737, 1989.

85. Radso SJ, Hansen S, Goldsmith J, Linder J: Immunohistochemistry of *Pneumocystis carinii* infection. Mod Pathol 3:462, 1990.

86. Ragni MV, Dekker A, DeRubertis FR, et al: *Pneumocystis carinii* infection presenting as necrotizing thyroiditis and hypothyroidism. Am J Clin Pathol 95:489, 1991.

87. Rorat E, Garcia RL, Skolom J: Diagnosis of *Pneumocystis carinii* pneumonia by cytologic examination of bronchial washings. JAMA 254:1950, 1985.

88. Sherman M, Levin D, Breidbart D: *Pneumocystis carinii* pneumonia with spontaneous pneumothorax. A report of three cases. Chest 90:609, 1986.

89. Shimono LH, Hartman B: A simple and reliable rapid methenamine silver stain for *Pneumocystis carinii* and fungi. Arch Pathol Med 110:855, 1986.

90. Smith MA, Hirschfield LS, Zahtz G, Siegal FP: *Pneumocystis carinii* otitis media. Am J Med 85:745, 1988.

91. Stager CE, Fraire AE, Kim H-S, et al. Modification of the fungi-fluor and the genetic systems fluorescent antibody methods for detection of *Pneumocystis carinii* in bronchoalveolar lavage specimens. Arch Pathol Lab Med 119:142, 1995.

92. Sun T, Chess O: Fluorescence not specific for *Pneumocystis carinii*. Acta Cytol 30:549, 1986.

93. Telzak EE, Cote RJ, Gold JWM, Campbell SW, Armstrong D: Extrapulmonary *Pneumocystis carinii* infections. Rev Infec Dis 12:380, 1990.

94. Tollerud DJ, Wesseler TA, Kim CK, Baughman RP: Use of a rapid differential stain for identifying *Pneumocystis carinii* in bronchoalveolar lavage fluid. Diagnostic efficacy in patients with AIDS. Chest 95:494, 1989.

95. Travis WD, Pittaluga S, Lipschik GY, et al: Atypical pathologic manifestations of *Pneumocystis carinii* pneumonia in the acquired immune deficiency syndrome. Review of 123 lung biopsies from 76 patients with emphasis on cysts, vascular invasion, vasculitis, and granulomas. Am J Surg Pathol 14:615, 1990.

96. Unger PD, Rosenblum M, Krown SE: Disseminated *Pneumocystis carinii* infection in a patient with acquired immunodeficiency syndrome. Hum Pathol 19:113, 1988.

97. Wasserman K, Pothoff G, Kirn E, Fatkenheuer G, Krueger GRF: Chronic *Pneumocystis carinii* pneumonia in AIDS. Chest 104:667, 1993.

98. Wislez M, Bergot E, Antoine M, et al: Acute respiratory failure following HAART introduction in patients treated for *Pneumocystis carinii* pneumonia. Am J Respir Crit Care Med 164:847, 2001.

99. Zaman MK, Wooten OJ, Suprahmanya B, et al: Rapid noninvasive diagnosis of *Pneumocystis carinii* from induced liquefied sputum. Ann Intern Med 109:7, 1988.

Mycobacterium avium Complex and Other Nontuberculous Mycobacterial Infections

100. Chaisson RE, Hopewell PC: Mycobacteria and AIDS mortality. Am Rev Respir Dis 139:1, 1989.

101. Horsburgh CR Jr, Selik RM: The epidemiology of disseminated nontuberculous mycobacterial infection in the acquired immunodeficiency syndrome (AIDS). Am Rev Respir Dis 139:4, 1989.

102. Jannotta FS, Sidawy MK: The recognition of mycobacterial infections by intraoperative cytology in patients with acquired immunodeficiency syndrome. Arch Pathol Lab Med 113:1120, 1989.

103. Klatt EC, Jensen DF, Meyer PR: Pathology of *Mycobacterium avium-intracellulare* in the acquired immunodeficiency syndrome. Hum Pathol 18:709, 1987.

104. Levine B, Chaisson RE: *Mycobacterium kansasii*: A cause of treatable pulmonary disease associated with advanced human immunodeficiency virus (HIV) infection. Ann Intern Med 114:861, 1991.

105. Marinelli DL, Albelda SM, Williams TM, et al: Nontuberculous mycobacterial infection in AIDS: Clinical, pathologic, and radiographic features. Radiology 160:77, 1986.

106. Maygarden SJ, Flanders EL: Mycobacteria can be seen as "negative images" in cytology smears from patients with acquired immunodeficiency syndrome. Mod Pathol 2:239, 1989.

107. Mehle ME, Adamo JP, Mehta AC, et al: Endobronchial *Mycobacterium avium-intracellulare* infection in a patient with AIDS. Chest 96:119, 1989.

108. Packer SJ, Cesario T, Williams JH Jr: *Mycobacterium avium* complex infection presenting as endobronchial lesions in immunosuppressed patients. Ann Intern Med 109:389, 1988.

109. Smith MB, Molina CP, Schnadig VJ, et al: Pathologic features of *Mycobacterium kansasii* infection in patients with acquired immunodeficiency syndrome. Arch Pathol Lab Med 127:554, 2003.

110. Snider DE Jr, Hopewell PC, Mills J, Reichman LB: Mycobacterioses and the acquired immunodeficiency syndrome. Am Rev Respir Dis 136:492, 1987.

111. Tenholder MF, Moser RJ III, Tellis CJ: Mycobacteria other than tuberculosis. Pulmonary involvement in patients with acquired immunodeficiency syndrome. Arch Intern Med 148:953, 1988.

112. Wallace JM, Hannah JB: *Mycobacterium avium* complex infection in patients with the acquired immunodeficiency syndrome. A clinicopathologic study. Chest 93:926, 1988.

113. Young LS: *Mycobacterium avium* complex infection. J Infect Dis 157:863, 1988.

Tuberculosis

114. Chaisson RE, Schecter GF, Theuer CP, et al: Tuberculosis in patients with the acquired immunodeficiency syndrome. Clinical features, response to therapy and survival. Am Rev Respir Dis 136:570, 1987.

115. Chaisson RE, Slutkin G: Tuberculosis and human immunodeficiency virus infection. J Infect Dis 159:96, 1989.

116. Fischl MA, Uttamchandani RB, Daikos GL, et al: An outbreak of tuberculosis caused by multiple-drug-

resistant tubercle bacilli among patients with HIV infection. Ann Intern Med 117:177, 1992.

117. FitzGerald JM, Grzybowski S, Allen EA: The impact of human immunodeficiency virus infection on tuberculosis and its control. Chest 100:191, 1991.

118. Handwerger S, Mildvan D, Senie R, McKinley FW: Tuberculosis and the acquired immunodeficiency syndrome at a New York City hospital: 1978–1985. Chest 91:176, 1987.

119. Pitchenik AE, Burr J, Suarez M, et al: Human T-cell lymphotropic virus-III (HTLV-III) seropositivity and related disease among 71 consecutive patients in whom tuberculosis was diagnosed. A prospective study. Am Rev Respir Dis 135:875, 1987.

120. Sunderam G, McDonald RJ, Maniatis T, et al: Tuberculosis as a manifestation of the acquired immunodeficiency syndrome (AIDS). JAMA 256:362, 1986.

121. Wasser LS, Shaw GW, Talavera W: Endobronchial tuberculosis in the acquired immunodeficiency syndrome. Chest 94:1240, 1988.

Pyogenic Bacterial Infections

122. Foltzer MA, Guiney WB Jr, Wager GC, Alpern HD: Bronchopulmonary bacillary angiomatosis. Chest 104:973, 1993.

123. Javaly K, Horowitz HW, Wormser GP: Nocardiosis in patients with human immunodeficiency virus infection: Report of 2 cases and review of the literature. Medicine (Baltimore) 71:128, 1992.

124. Kim J, Minamoto GY, Grieco MH: Nocardial infection as a complication of AIDS: Report of six cases and review. Rev Infect Dis 13:624, 1991.

125. Kramer MR, Uttamchandani RB: The radiographic appearance of pulmonary nocardiosis associated with AIDS. Chest 98:382, 1990.

126. Nichols L, Balogh K, Silverman M: Bacterial infections in the acquired immunodeficiency syndrome. Am J Clin Pathol 92:787, 1989.

127. Polsky B, Gold JWM, Whimbey E, et al: Bacterial pneumonia in patients with acquired immunodeficiency syndrome. Ann Intern Med 104:38, 1986.

128. Schlamm HT, Yancovitz SR: *Haemophilus influenzae* pneumonia in young adults with AIDS, ARC, or risk of AIDS. Am J Med 86:11, 1989.

129. Witt DJ, Craven DE, McCabe WR: Bacterial infections in adult patients with the acquired immune deficiency syndrome (AIDS) and AIDS-related complex. Am J Med 82:900, 1987.

Malacoplakia

130. Byard RW, Bourne AJ, Thorner PS: Malacoplakia of the lung – a review. Surg Pathol 4:301, 1991.

131. Colby TV, Hunt S, Pelzmann K, Carrington CB: Malakoplakia of the lung: A report of two cases. Respiration 39:295, 1980.

132. Crouch E, Wright J, White V, Churg A: Malakoplakia mimicking carcinoma metastatic to lung. Am J Surg Pathol 8:151, 1984.

133. de Peralta-Venturina MN, Clubb FJ, Kielhofner MA: Pulmonary malacoplakia associated with *Rhodoccus equi* infection in a patient with acquired immunodeficiency syndrome. Am J Clin Pathol 102:459, 1994.

134. Kwon KY, Colby TV: *Rhodococcus equi* pneumonia and pulmonary malakoplakia in acquired immunodeficiency syndrome. Pathologic features. Arch Pathol Lab Med 118:744, 1994.

135. MacGregor JH, Samuelson WM, Sane DC, et al: Opportunistic lung infection caused by *Rhodococcus (Corynbacterium) equi*. Radiology 160:83, 1986.

136. Samies JH, Hathaway BN, Echols RM, et al: Lung abscess due to *Corynebacterium equi*. Report of the first case in a patient with acquired immune deficiency syndrome. Am J Med 80:685, 1986.

137. Schwartz DA, Ogden PO, Blumberg HM, Honig E: Pulmonary malakoplakia in a patient with the acquired immunodeficiency syndrome: Differential diagnostic considerations. Arch Pathol Lab Med 114:1267, 1990.

138. Scott MA, Graham BS, Verrall R, et al: *Rhodococcus equi* – an increasingly recognized opportunistic pathogen: Report of 12 cases and review of 65 cases in the literature. Am J Clin Pathol 103:649, 1995.

139. Yuoh G, Hove MGM, Wen J, Haque AK: Pulmonary malakoplakia in acquired immunodeficiency syndrome. An ultrastructural study of morphogenesis of Michaelis-Gutmann bodies. Mod Pathol 9:976, 1996.

Fungal Infections

140. Cameron ML, Bartlett JA, Gallis HA, Waskin HA: Manifestations of pulmonary cryptococcosis in patients with acquired immunodeficiency syndrome. Rev Infect Dis 13:64, 1991.

141. Chechani V, Kamholz SL: Pulmonary manifestations of disseminated cryptococcosis in patients with AIDS. Chest 98:1060, 1990.

142. Chuck SL, Sande MA: Infections with *Cryptococcus neoformans* in the acquired immunodeficiency syndrome. N Engl J Med 321:794, 1989.

143. Conces DJ Jr, Stockberger SM, Tarver RD, Wheat LJ: Disseminated histoplasmosis in AIDS: Findings on chest radiographs. AJR Am J Roentgenol 160:15, 1993.

144. Denning DW, Follansbee SE, Scolaro M, et al.: Pulmonary aspergillosis in the acquired immunodeficiency syndrome. N Engl J Med 324:654, 1991.

145. Eng RH, Bishburg E, Smith SM, et al.: Cryptococcal infections in patients with acquired immune deficiency syndrome. Am J Med 81:19, 1986.

146. Gal AA, Kiss MM, Hawkins J, et al: The pathology of pulmonary cryptococcal infections in the acquired immunodeficiency syndrome. Arch Pathol Lab Med 110:502, 1986.

147. Graham AR, Sobonya RE, Bronnimann DA, Galgiani JN: Quantitative pathology of coccidioidomycosis in acquired immunodeficiency syndrome. Hum Pathol 19:800, 1988.

148. Graybill JR: Histoplasmosis and AIDS. J Infect Dis 158:623, 1988.

149. Holmberg K, Meyer RD: Fungal infections in patients with AIDS and AID-related complex. Scand J Infect Dis 18:179, 1986.

150. Johnson PC, Khardori N, Najjar AF, et al: Progressive disseminated histoplasmosis in patients with acquired immunodeficiency syndrome. Am J Med 85:152, 1988.

151. Klapholz A, Salomon N, Perlman DC, Talavera W: Aspergillosis in the acquired immunodeficiency syndrome. Chest 100:1614, 1991.

152. Kovacs JA, Kovacs AA, Polis M, et al: Cryptococcosis in the acquired immunodeficiency syndrome. Ann Intern Med 103:533, 1985.

153. Kwon-Chung KJ, Hill WB, Bennett JE: New, special stain for histopathological diagnosis of cryptococcosis. J Clin Microbiol 13:383, 1981.

154. Miller WT Jr, Edelman JM, Miller WT: Cryptococcal pulmonary infection in patients with AIDS: Radiographic appearance. Radiology 175:725, 1990.

155. Mylonakis E, Barlam TF, Flanigan T, Rich JD: Pulmonary aspergillosis and invasive disease in AIDS. Review of 342 cases. Chest 114:251, 1998.

156. Nash G, Irvine R, Kerschmann RL, Herndier B: Pulmonary aspergillosis in acquired immune deficiency syndrome: Autopsy study of an emerging pulmonary complication of human immunodeficiency virus infection. Hum Pathol 28:1268, 1997.

157. Pappas PG, Pottage JC, Powderly WG, et al: Blastomycosis in patients with the acquired immunodeficiency syndrome. Ann Intern Med 116:847, 1992.

158. Pervez NK, Kleinerman J, Kattan M, et al: Pseudomembranous necrotizing bronchial aspergillosis. Am Rev Respir Dis 131:961, 1985.

159. Salzman SH, Smith RL, Aranda CP: Histoplasmosis in patients at risk for the acquired immunodeficiency syndrome in a nonendemic setting. Chest 93:916, 1988.

160. Sarosi GA, Johnson PC: Disseminated histoplasmosis in patients infected with human immunodeficiency virus. Clin Infect Dis 14(Suppl 1):S60, 1992.

161. Shibuya K, Coulson WF, Wollman JS, et al: Histopathology of cryptococcosis and other fungal infections in patients with acquired immunodeficiency syndrome. Int J Infect Dis 5:78, 2001.

162. Stansell JD: Pulmonary fungal infections in HIV-infected persons. Semin Respir Infect 8:116, 1993.

163. Tomita T, Chiga M: Disseminated histoplasmosis in acquired immunodeficiency syndrome. Light and electron microscopic observations. Hum Pathol 19:438, 1988.

164. Wheat LJ, Connolly-Stringfield PA, Baker RL, et al: Disseminated histoplasmosis in the acquired immune deficiency syndrome: Clinical findings, diagnosis and treatment, and review of the literature. Medicine (Baltimore) 69:361, 1990.

165. Wright JL, Lawson L, Chan N, Filipenko D: An unusual form of pulmonary aspergillosis in two patients with the acquired immunodeficiency syndrome. Am J Clin Pathol 100:57, 1993.

Viral Infections

166. Ambros RA, Lee E-Y, Sharer LR, et al: The acquired immunodeficiency syndrome in intravenous drug abusers and patients with a sexual risk: Clinical and postmortem comparisons. Hum Pathol 18:1109, 1987.

167. Gorelkin L, Chandler FW, Ewing EP: Staining qualities of cytomegalovirus inclusions in the lungs of patients with the acquired immunodeficiency syndrome: A potential diagnostic misinterpretation. Hum Pathol 17:926, 1986.

168. Imoto EM, Stein RM, Shellito JE, Curtis JL: Central airway obstruction due to cytomegalovirus-induced necrotizing tracheitis in a patient with AIDS. Am Rev Respir Dis 142:884, 1990.

169. Jacobson MA, Mills J: Serious cytomegalovirus disease in the acquired immunodeficiency syndrome (AIDS). Ann Intern Med 108:585, 1988.

170. Keh WC, Gerber MA: In situ hybridization for cytomegalovirus DNA in AIDS patients. Am J Pathol 131:490, 1988.

171. Klatt EC, Shibata D: Cytomegalovirus infection in the acquired immunodeficiency syndrome: Clinical and autopsy findings. Arch Pathol Lab Med 112:540, 1988.

172. McGuinness G, Scholes JV, Garay SM, et al: Cytomegalovirus pneumonitis: Spectrum of parenchymal CT findings with pathologic correlation in 21 AIDS patients. Radiology 192:451, 1994.

173. Millar AB, Patou G, Millar RF, et al: Cytomegalovirus in the lungs of patients with AIDS: Respiratory pathogen or passenger? Am Rev Respir Dis 141:1474, 1990.

174. Stopyra GA, Multhaupt HAB, Alexa L, et al: Epstein-Barr virus-associated adult respiratory distress syndrome in a patient with AIDS: A case report and review. Mod Pathol 12:984, 1999.

175. Vasudevan VP, Mascarenhas DAN, Klapper P, Lombardias S: Cytomegalovirus necrotizing bronchiolitis with HIV infection. Chest 97:483, 1990.

176. Wallace JM, Hannah J: Cytomegalovirus pneumonitis in patients with AIDS. Findings in an autopsy series. Chest 92:198, 1987.

Parasitic Infections

177. Binford C, Connor D, eds: *Pathology of Tropical and Extraordinary Diseases*, Washington, DC, Armed Forces Institute of Pathology, 1976, pp 284–300.

178. Byard RW, Bourne AJ, Matthews N, et al: Pulmonary strongyloidiasis in a child diagnosed on open lung biopsy. Surg Pathol 5:55, 1993.

179. Catteral JR, Hofflin JM, Remington JS: Pulmonary toxoplasmosis. Am Rev Respir Dis 133:704, 1986.

180. Forgacs P, Tarshis A, Ma P, et al: Intestinal and bronchial cryptosporidiosis in an immunodeficient homosexual man. Ann Intern Med 99:793, 1983.

181. Haque AK, Schnadig V, Rubin SA, Smith JM: Pathogenesis of human strongyloidiasis: Autopsy and quantitative parasitological analysis. Mod Pathol 7:276, 1994.

182. Lin AL, Kessimian N, Benditt JO: Restrictive pulmonary disease due to interlobular septal fibrosis associated with disseminated infection by *Strongyloides stercoralis*. Am J Respir Crit Care Med 151:205, 1995.

183. Ma P, Villanueva TG, Kaufman D, Gillooley JF: Respiratory cryptosporidiosis in the acquired immune deficiency syndrome. JAMA 252:1298, 1984.

184. Maayan S, Wormser GP, Widerhorn J, et al: *Strongyloides stercoralis* hyperinfection in a patient with the acquired immune deficiency syndrome. Am J Med 83:945, 1987.

185. Moore JA, Frenkel JK: Respiratory and enteric cryptosporidiosis in humans. Arch Pathol Lab Med 115:1160, 1991.

186. Nash G, Kerschmann RL, Herndier B, Dubey JP: The pathological manifestations of pulmonary toxoplasmosis in the acquired immunodeficiency syndrome. Hum Pathol 25:652, 1994.

187. Restrepo G, Macher AM, Radany EH: Disseminated extraintestinal isosporiasis in a patient with acquired immune deficiency syndrome. Am J Clin Pathol 87:536, 1987.

188. Schwartz DA, Visvesvara GS, Leitch GJ, et al: Pathology of symptomatic microsporidial (*Encephalitozoon hellem*) bronchiolitis in the acquired immunodeficiency syndrome: A new respiratory pathogen diagnosed from lung biopsy, bronchoalveolar lavage, sputum, and tissue culture. Hum Pathol 24:937, 1993.

189. Tang T, Harb J, Dunne WM Jr, et al: Cerebral toxoplasmosis in an immunocompromised host. A precise and rapid diagnosis by electron microscopy. Am J Clin Pathol 85:104, 1986.

190. Tschirhart D, Klatt EC: Disseminated toxoplasmosis in the acquired immunodeficiency syndrome. Arch Pathol Lab Med 112:1237, 1988.

191. Vieyra-Herrera G, Becerril-Carmona G, Padua-Gabriel A, et al: *Strongyloides stercoralis* hyperinfection in a patient with the acquired immune deficiency syndrome. Acta Cytol 2:277, 1988.

192. Weber R, Kuster H, Keller R, et al: Pulmonary and intestinal microsporidiosis in a patient with the acquired immunodeficiency syndrome. Am Rev Respir Dis 146:1603, 1992.

193. Williams J, Dralle W, Verghese A: Diagnosis of pulmonary strongyloidiasis by bronchoalveolar lavage. Chest 94:643, 1988.

194. Yermakov V, Rashid RK, Vuletin JC, et al: Disseminated toxoplasmosis. Case report and review of the literature. Arch Pathol Lab Med 106:524, 1982.

Noninfectious Causes of Lung Disease

195. Allen JN, Wewers MD: HIV-associated bronchiolitis obliterans organizing pneumonia. Chest 96:197, 1989.

196. Colclough AB: Interstitial pneumonia in human immunodeficiency virus infection: A report of a fatal case in childhood. Histopathology 12:211, 1988.

197. Coplan NL, Shimony RY, Ioachim HL, et al: Primary pulmonary hypertension associated with human immunodeficiency viral infection. Am J Med 89:96, 1990.

198. de Chadarevian J-P, Lischner HW, Karmazin N, et al: Pulmonary hypertension and HIV infection: New observations and review of the syndrome. Mod Pathol 7:685, 1994.

199. Ettensohn DB, Mayer KH, Kessimian N, Smith PS: Lymphocytic bronchiolitis associated with HIV infection. Chest 93:201, 1988.

200. Goldsmith GH Jr, Baily RG, Brettler DB, et al: Primary pulmonary hypertension in patients with classic hemophilia. Ann Intern Med 108:797, 1988.

201. Haque AK, Myers JL, Hudnall SD, et al: Pulmonary lymphomatoid granulomatosis in acquired immunodeficiency syndrome: Lesions with Epstein-Barr virus infection. Mod Pathol 11:347, 1998.

202. Jacques C, Richmond G, Tierney L, et al: Primary pulmonary hypertension and human immunodeficiency virus infection in a non-hemophiliac man. Hum Pathol 23:191, 1992.

203. Joshi VV, Kauffman S, Oleske JM, et al: Polyclonal polymorphic B-cell lymphoproliferative disorder with prominent pulmonary involvement in children with acquired immune deficiency syndrome. Cancer 59:1455, 1987.

204. Khater FJ, Moorman JP, Myers JW, et al: Bronchiolitis obliterans organizing pneumonia as a manifestation of AIDS: Case report and literature review. J Infect 49:159, 2004.

205. Kornstein MJ, Pietra GG, Hoxie JA, Conley ME: The pathology and treatment of interstitial pneumonitis in two infants with AIDS. Am Rev Respir Dis 133:1196, 1986.

206. McGuinness G, Naidich DP, Garay S, et al: AIDS associated bronchiectasis: CT features. J Comput Assist Tomogr 17:260, 1993.

207. McGuinness G, Scholes JV, Jagirdar JS, et al: Unusual lymphoproliferative disorders in nine adults with HIV or AIDS: CT and pathologic findings. Radiology 190:59, 1995.

208. Mehta NJ, Khan IA, Mehta RN, Sepkowitz DA: HIV-related pulmonary hypertension: Analytic review of 131 cases. Chest 118:1133, 2000.

209. Mette SA, Palevsky HI, Pietra GG, et al: Primary pulmonary hypertension in association with human immunodeficiency virus infection. Am Rev Respir Dis 145:1196, 1992.

210. Morris JC, Rosen MJ, Marchevsky A, Teirstein AS: Lymphocytic interstitial pneumonia in patients at risk for the acquired immune deficiency syndrome. Chest 91:63, 1987.

211. Nhieu JTV, Vojtek A-M, Bernaudin J-F, et al: Pulmonary alveolar proteinosis associated with *Pneumocystis carinii*: Ultrastructural identification in bronchiolar lavage in AIDS and immunocompromised non-AIDS patients. Chest 98:801, 1990.

212. Nunes H, Humbert M, Sitbon O, et al: Prognostic factors for survival in human immunodeficiency virus-

associated pulmonary arterial hypertension. Am J Respir Crit Care Med 167:1433, 2003.

213. Ognibene FP, Masur H, Rogers P, et al: Nonspecific interstitial pneumonitis without evidence of *Pneumocystis carinii* in asymptomatic patients infected with human immunodeficiency virus (HIV). Ann Intern Med 109:874, 1988.

214. Oldham SAA, Castillo M, Jacobson FJ, et al: HIV-associated lymphocytic interstitial pneumonia: Radiologic manifestations and pathologic correlation. Radiology 170:83, 1989.

215. Polos PG, Wolfe D, Harley RA, et al: Pulmonary hypertension and human immunodeficiency virus infection: Two reports and a review of the literature. Chest 101:474, 1992.

216. Ramaswamy G, Jagadha V, Tchertkoff V: Diffuse alveolar damage and interstitial fibrosis in acquired immunodeficiency syndrome patients without concurrent pulmonary infection. Arch Pathol Lab Med 109:408, 1985.

217. Ray P, Antoine M, Mary-Krause M, et al: AIDS-related primary pulmonary lymphoma. Am J Respir Crit Care Med 158:1221, 1998.

218. Rogers J, Langston C, Guerra IC: Pulmonary follicular lymphoid hyperplasia in a child with HTLV-III-related immunodeficiency. Pediatr Pulmonol 2:175, 1986.

219. Ruben FL, Talamo TS: Secondary pulmonary alveolar proteinosis occurring in two patients with acquired immune deficiency syndrome. Am J Med 80:1187, 1986.

220. Solal-Celigny P, Couderc LJ, Herman D, et al: Lymphoid interstitial pneumonitis in acquired immunodeficiency syndrome (AIDS) related complex. Am Rev Respir Dis 131:956, 1985.

221. Suffredini AF, Ognibene FP, Lack EE, et al: Nonspecific interstitial pneumonitis: A common cause of pulmonary disease in the acquired immunodeficiency syndrome. Ann Intern Med 107:7, 1987.

222. Travis WD, Fox CH, Devaney KO, et al: Lymphoid pneumonitis in 50 adult patients infected with the human immunodeficiency virus: Lymphocytic interstitial pneumonitis versus nonspecific interstitial pneumonitis. Hum Pathol 23:529, 1992.

223. White DA, Matthay RA: Noninfectious pulmonary complications of infection with the human immunodeficiency virus. Am Rev Respir Dis 140:1763, 1989.

224. Yousem SA, Colby TV, Carrington CB: Follicular bronchitis/bronchiolitis. Hum Pathol 16:700, 1985.

Kaposi's Sarcoma and Other Malignancies

225. Aboulafia DM: The epidemiologic, pathologic, and clinical features of AIDS-associated pulmonary Kaposi's sarcoma. Chest 117:1128, 2000.

226. Anders KH, Latta H, Chang BS, et al: Lymphomatoid granulomatosis and malignant lymphoma of the central nervous system in the acquired immunodeficiency syndrome. Hum Pathol 20:236, 1989.

227. Braun MA, Killam DA, Remick SC, Ruckdeschel JC: Lung cancer in patients seropositive for human immunodeficiency virus. Radiology 175:341, 1990.

228. Chan TK, Aranda CP, Rom WN: Bronchogenic carcinoma in young patients at risk for acquired immunodeficiency syndrome. Chest 103:862, 1993.

229. Davis SD, Henschke CI, Chamides BK, Westcott JL: Intrathoracic Kaposi sarcoma in AIDS patients: Radiographic-pathologic correlation. Radiology 163:495, 1987.

230. Di Carlo EF, Amberson JB, Metroka CE, et al: Malignant lymphomas and the acquired immunodeficiency syndrome. Evaluation of 30 cases using a working formulation. Arch Pathol Lab Med 110:1012, 1986.

231. Eisner MD, Kaplan LD, Herndier B, Stulbarg MS: The pulmonary manifestations of AIDS-related non-Hodgkin's lymphoma. Chest 110:729, 1996.

232. Fraire AE, Awe RJ: Lung cancer in association with human immunodeficiency virus infection. Cancer 70:432, 1992.

233. Garay SM, Belenko M, Fazzini E, Schinella R: Pulmonary manifestations of Kaposi's sarcoma. Chest 91:39, 1987.

234. Grody WW, Lewin KJ, Naeim F: Detection of cytomegalovirus DNA in classic and epidemic Kaposi's sarcoma by in situ hybridization. Hum Pathol 19:524, 1988.

235. Hamm PG, Judson MA, Aranda CP: Diagnosis of pulmonary Kaposi's sarcoma with fiberoptic bronchoscopy and endobronchial biopsy. A report of five cases. Cancer 59:807, 1987.

236. Hanson PJV, Harcourt-Webster JN, Gazzard BG, Collins JV: Fiberoptic bronchoscopy in diagnosis of bronchopulmonary Kaposi's sarcoma. Thorax 42:269, 1987.

237. Huang L, Schnapp LM, Gruden JF, et al: Presentation of AIDS-related pulmonary Kaposi's sarcoma diagnosed by bronchoscopy. Am J Respir Crit Care Med 153:1385, 1996.

238. Karp J, Profeta G, Marantz PR, Karpel JP: Lung cancer in patients with immunodeficiency syndrome. Chest 103:410, 1993.

239. Khojasteh A, Reynolds RD, Khojasteh CA: Malignant lymphoreticular lesions in patients with immune disorders resembling acquired immunodeficiency syndrome (AIDS): review of 80 cases. South Med J 79:1070, 1986.

240. Knowles DM, Chamulak, GA, Subar M, et al: Lymphoid neoplasia associated with the acquired immunodeficiency syndrome (AIDS). The New York University Medical Center experience with 105 patients (1981–1986). Ann Intern Med 108:744, 1988.

241. Levine AM, Gill P-S, Muggia F: Malignancies in the acquired immunodeficiency syndrome. Curr Probl Cancer 11:209, 1987.

242. Loureiro C, Gill PS, Meyer PR, et al: Autopsy findings in AIDS-related lymphoma. Cancer 62:735, 1988.

243. Lowenthal DA, Straus DJ, Campbell SW, et al: AIDS-related lymphoid neoplasia. The Memorial Hospital experience. Cancer 61:2325, 1988.

244. Meduri GU, Stover DE, Lee M, et al: Pulmonary Kaposi's sarcoma in the acquired immune deficiency syndrome. Clinical, radiographic, and pathologic manifestations. Am J Med 81:11, 1986.

245. Mittal K, Neri A, Feiner H, et al: Lymphomatoid granulomatosis in the acquired immunodeficiency syndrome. Cancer 65:1345, 1990.

246. Moore PS, Chang Y: Detection of herpesvirus-like DNA sequences in Kaposi's sarcoma in patients with and without HIV infection. N Engl J Med 332:1181, 1995.

247. Nash G, Fligiel B: Kaposi's sarcoma presenting as pulmonary disease in the acquired immune deficiency syndrome. Diagnosis by lung biopsy. Hum Pathol 15:999, 1984.

248. Poelzleitner D, Huebsch P, Mayerhoffer S, et al: Primary pulmonary lymphoma in a patient with the acquired immune deficiency syndrome. Thorax 44:438, 1989.

249. Polish LB, Cohn DL, Ryder JW, et al: Pulmonary non-Hodgkin's lymphoma in AIDS. Chest 96:1321, 1989.

250. Purdy LJ, Colby TV, Yousem SA, Battifora H: Pulmonary Kaposi's sarcoma: Premortem histologic diagnosis. Am J Surg Pathol 10:301, 1986.

251. Si MW, Jagirdar J, Zhang Y-J, et al: Detection of KSHV in transbronchial biopsies in patients with Kaposi sarcoma. Appl Immunohistochem Mol Morphol 13:61, 2005.

252. Sivit CJ, Schwartz AM, Rockoff SD: Kaposi's sarcoma of the lung in AIDS: Radiologic-pathologic analysis. AJR Am J Roentgenol 148:25, 1987.

253. Tamm, M, Reichenberger F, McGandy CE, et al: Diagnosis of pulmonary Kaposi's sarcoma by detection of human herpes virus 8 in bronchoalveolar lavage. Am J Respir Crit Care Med. 157:458, 1998.

254. Teruya-Feldstein J, Temeck BK, Sloas MM, et al: Pulmonary malignant lymphoma of mucosa-associated lymphoid tissue (MALT) arising in a pediatric HIV-positive patient. Am J Surg Pathol 19:357, 1995.

255. Zibrak JD, Silvestri RC, Costello P, et al: Bronchoscopic and radiologic features of Kaposi's sarcoma involving the respiratory system. Chest 90:476, 1986.

13

PULMONARY HYPERTENSION AND OTHER VASCULAR DISORDERS

This chapter concentrates on the general morphologic features of pulmonary hypertension and includes discussions of important specific subtypes. Other vascular lesions that may be encountered by the surgical pathologist, including emboli, infarcts, arteriovenous fistulas, and aneurysms, are also briefly covered. A knowledge of the normal morphologic features of the pulmonary vasculature is essential in order to understand and recognize the pathologic alterations of blood vessels, and these will be reviewed first.

THE PULMONARY VASCULATURE

The pulmonary vasculature consists of a mixture of pulmonary and systemic (bronchial) vessels. An understanding of the normal structure and location of these vessels is crucial to the recognition and diagnosis of the diseases that arise from them. In evaluating the pulmonary vasculature, an elastic tissue stain is extremely helpful, since it both outlines normal structural characteristics and helps in determining if an abnormality exists.

Table 13–1 summarizes the important morphologic features of the vessels comprising the pulmonary vasculature. *Pulmonary arteries* are classified according to their size and structure, and they include *elastic arteries*, *muscular arteries*, and *arterioles*. *Elastic arteries* constitute the main pulmonary arteries and their intrapulmonary branches. Their external diameter measures greater than 1.0 mm. They are located adjacent to bronchi, and their walls are composed of multiple, generally parallel, elastic laminae. Smaller arteries with an external diameter of between 0.1 and 1.0 mm are termed *muscular arteries*. They are located adjacent to bronchioles and are characterized by media composed of circularly oriented smooth muscle fibers located between internal and external elastic membranes. The mean thickness of the media in these vessels normally

Table 13–1   Morphologic Features of the Pulmonary Vasculature

	Location	Diameter (mm)	Structural Features
Pulmonary Arterial System			
Elastic arteries	Adjacent to bronchi	>1.0	Media containing multiple parallel elastic laminae
Muscular arteries	Adjacent to bronchioles and alveolar ducts	0.1–1.0	Media lined by internal and external elastic laminae
Arterioles	Alveolar septa	<0.1	Endothelial cells apposed to single elastic lamina; no smooth muscle
Capillaries	Alveolar septa	0.008	Endothelial cells covering basement membrane
Pulmonary Venous System			
Veins	Interlobular septa	>0.1	Media lined by single distinct inner elastic lamina, irregular peripheral fibers
Venules	Alveolar septa	<0.1	Endothelial cells apposed to single elastic lamina
Bronchial Vasculature			
Bronchial arteries	Bronchial wall	Variable, smaller than pulmonary arteries	Thick media lined by prominent elastic lamina; thin or indistinct external elastic lamina
Bronchial veins	Bronchial wall	Variable	Thin media lined by single internal elastic lamina, contain valves

averages 5–10% of their external diameter (see later on) and may range up to 20%. They are generally the same size or slightly smaller than the adjacent airway. Arterial vessels that are less than 0.1 mm in external diameter occur within alveolar septa and are termed *arterioles*. By light microscopy, these vessels consist of a layer of endothelial cells directly apposed to a single elastic lamina. Electron microscopy, however, reveals an 'intermediate' cell, presumably a myofibroblast, that lies between the endothelium and the elastic lamina.

Although this classification of pulmonary arteries is practical, it is somewhat oversimplified. The data suggest, for example, that there are long segments of transition from elastic to muscular arteries.[16,60] Furthermore, there is a portion between the muscular artery and the arteriole in which the disappearing muscle has a spiral arrangement, so that, on cross-section, only one segment of the arterial circumference will show a muscular media.[19,20] For practical purposes, however, terminology of individual vessels is less important than understanding normal morphology and recognizing abnormalities. In examining lung biopsy specimens, the muscular arteries and arterioles are the main vessels to be evaluated. For muscular arteries,

their size relative to the adjacent airway should be assessed, and the relative thickness of the intima and media should be evaluated by using an elastic tissue stain.[8,11] Muscularization of arterioles (see further on) is another change to recognize, since it is an important morphologic feature of pulmonary hypertension.

Pulmonary capillaries are found in the alveolar septa and measure approximately 0.008 mm in external diameter. These vessels consist of a layer of endothelium covering a basement membrane.

Pulmonary veins measure greater than 0.1 mm in diameter and are found in the interlobular septa. The venous wall is thinner than that of an artery of the same size and has a distinct inner elastic lamina with a peripheral layer of irregularly distributed elastic fibers. The presence of a single elastic lamina distinguishes veins from arteries, which contain two (internal and external) elastic layers. Large veins near the hilum may have cardiac muscle in their walls. *Pulmonary venules* measure less than 0.1 mm and are histologically indistinguishable from arterioles. They can be clearly identified only by tracing the small vessel to its connecting vein.

The *bronchial arteries* are systemic vessels with a muscular media and a distinct, often thickened, internal elastic lamina.[6] The external elastic lamina is generally thin and indistinct. Bronchial arteries are usually located in the wall of the bronchi that they supply and are smaller than nearby pulmonary arteries. Their media is also thicker than that of pulmonary arteries and may contain an internal longitudinally oriented muscle layer in addition to a circular smooth muscle layer. The lumens often appear narrowed by the prominent medial muscular layers. Numerous anastomosing branches form a plexus of small vessels that extends from the peribronchial connective tissue to the mucosa. Bronchial vessels follow the airways distally as far as terminal bronchioles. Anastomoses between the bronchial and pulmonary microvasculature are common. Bronchial arteries may become markedly hypertrophied in inflammatory bronchial diseases such as bronchiectasis. *Bronchial veins* form networks around the bronchial wall and in the submucosa. Bronchial veins have the same general structure as *pulmonary veins* although they possess thinner walls and contain valves.

Pulmonary lymphatics are found in the interlobular septa accompanying veins, in the bronchovascular bundles, and in the subpleural connective tissue. They do not contain an elastic lamina. Pulmonary lymphatics have valves, whereas the pulmonary veins do not. Larger lymphatics may contain irregular masses of smooth muscle in their walls.

PULMONARY HYPERTENSION

General

Pulmonary hypertension is defined clinically as a mean pulmonary artery pressure greater than 25 mmHg at rest or greater than 30 mmHg during exercise.[40,47,52] It is traditionally divided into *primary* and *secondary* categories, depending upon whether or not a cause can be identified. The more recent World Health Organization (WHO) classification, however, divides pulmonary hypertension into five groups based on mechanisms rather than associated conditions (Table 13–2).[2,7] The rationale for this classification relates to the fact that the histopathologic findings depend more on the mechanism of the hypertension than on whether the hypertension is primary or secondary. In fact, the findings in many different forms of secondary hypertension are identical to those in primary hypertension.

The secondary forms of pulmonary hypertension are most often encountered by the pathologist since they are common incidental findings in specimens examined

Table 13–2 Modified WHO Classification of Pulmonary Hypertension*

I. Pulmonary Arterial Hypertension
  Idiopathic (Primary) – Sporadic/familial
  Associated with specific conditions/agents
    (congenital left-to-right shunts, collagen vascular disease, portal hypertension, HIV infection, drugs and toxins, etc.)
  Persistent pulmonary hypertension of newborn

II. Pulmonary Venous Hypertension
  Due to obstruction of intrapulmonary veins
    (pulmonary venoocclusive disease, capillary hemangiomatosis)
  Due to cardiac abnormality (left-sided atrial or ventricular heart disease or left-sided valvular disease)
  Due to extrinsic compression of central pulmonary veins (fibrosing mediastinitis, tumors)

III. Pulmonary Hypertension Associated with Lung Disease and/or Hypoxemia
  (COPD, interstitial lung disease, sleep apnea, alveolar hypoventilation, high altitude, developmental abnormalities)

IV. Pulmonary Hypertension Due to Chronic Thrombotic and/or Embolic Disease
  Chronic thromboembolic occlusion of proximal pulmonary artery
  Obstruction of distal pulmonary arteries (thrombi, thromboemboli, tumor, foreign material, parasites)

V. Miscellaneous (sarcoidosis, lymphangiomyomatosis, eosinophilic granuloma)

*This classification is a modification of the WHO classification as presented in references 2 and 7.

because of other diseases such as interstitial lung disease, emphysema, or cancer, for example. Sometimes, also, lung biopsy is utilized to assess the feasibility of corrective surgery in patients with congenital heart disease and secondary pulmonary hypertension (see text following). Less commonly, clinically unsuspected cases of pulmonary hypertension will be first recognized by the pathologist. Although lung biopsy is sometimes used to evaluate cases of clinically diagnosed idiopathic pulmonary hypertension, it is usually not recommended, since related morbidity and mortality are considerable, treatment may not be affected, and the biopsy may make subsequent transplantation difficult.[2,40,45] The following sections will concentrate on the general morphologic features of pulmonary hypertension with brief discussions of specific forms of the disease as they pertain to the surgical pathologist.

Histologic Features

The main pathologic findings in pulmonary hypertension occur in muscular pulmonary arteries and arterioles. Elastic tissue stains are especially helpful in evaluating pulmonary hypertension because they can identify the type of blood vessel involved, and they can distinguish medial and intimal abnormalities.[18] Changes also occur in the larger elastic pulmonary arteries, but these vessels are less likely to be encountered by the surgical pathologist. They generally show atherosclerosis rather than medial or intimal hypertrophy.[17] If there has been hypertension since early childhood, the walls also may be thickened and show an 'aortic' configuration of the elastic lamina. This appearance is characterized by closely apposed, parallel elastic fibrils instead of the more widely separated elastic tissue that is seen in the normal pulmonary trunk of older children and adults.

Muscular hypertrophy in the media of small pulmonary arteries is a constant finding in pulmonary hypertension, and, if present by itself, usually correlates with mild to moderate degrees of hypertension (Fig. 13–1). This abnormality should be initially suspected when the lumen appears narrowed and surrounded by an unusually thick media, and it can be confirmed by measuring the medial thickness and the external vessel diameter.[8,11] Multiplying the medial thickness by two and dividing the product by the external diameter of the vessel yields the medial thickness to diameter percentage. Normally this figure should be less than 10–20%.[20] Practically speaking, a rough estimate can be made of the ratio of medial thickness to artery radius without requiring quantitative measurements. A helpful feature that is sometimes present and should suggest pulmonary hypertension is the appearance of increased numbers of medial smooth muscle fibers in artery walls, characterized by closely spaced nuclei arranged in parallel.

Muscularization of arterioles is another feature present early in pulmonary hypertension. It is characterized by extension of smooth muscle into arterioles, so that these vessels develop a distinct muscular media (Fig. 13–2).[10,20] Muscularized arterioles can be identified histologically by finding small muscular arteries within alveolar septa. Normally, muscular arteries in adults are present adjacent to bronchioles and alveolar ducts but not in the more peripheral alveolated parenchyma.

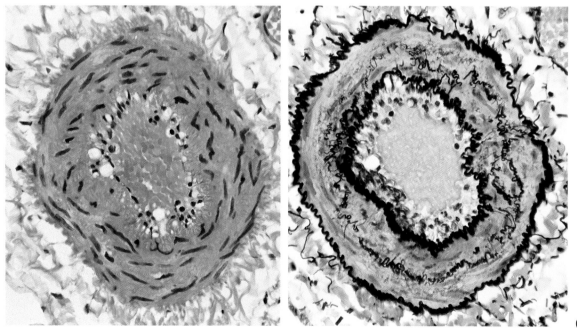

(a)

(b)

Figure 13–1 Medial hypertrophy in mild pulmonary hypertension. (a) The medial thickness is about 50% of the total artery diameter. Note the increased numbers of elongated smooth muscle cells that are present within the media. **(b)** Elastic tissue stain of the same artery, clearly outlining the internal and external elastic lamina.

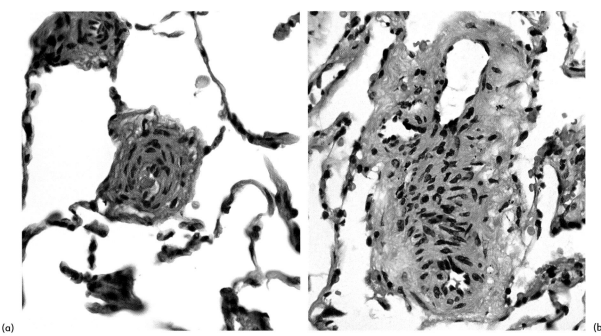

(a)   (b)

Figure 13–2 Muscularization of arterioles. (a) This arteriole situated in an alveolar septum has acquired a smooth muscle coat, and the lumen is narrowed by the hyperplastic small muscle. **(b)** Another arteriole showing the prominent smooth muscle hyperplasia and luminal narrowing.

Elastic tissue stains confirm that the vessels are arterioles, because they contain a single elastic layer.

Changes in the intima often accompany the medial hypertrophy. Early on, there is cellular proliferation in the intima of small muscular arteries that is best appreciated in elastic tissue stains (Fig. 13–3). Although the proliferating cells were originally thought to be endothelial, ultrastructural examination suggests that some are either smooth muscle cells or a specialized cell related to the myofibroblast and referred to by Heath and associates as a 'vasoformative reserve cell'.[13] There is some evidence that the development of proliferative intimal lesions may depend to some degree on thickness of the internal elastic lamina.[1]

In severe pulmonary hypertension, intimal fibrosis becomes prominent and may completely occlude the lumens of small arteries (Fig. 13–4). A distinctive *concentric laminar fibrosis* may be seen that is characterized by marked thickening of the intima by collagen and variable numbers of spindle-shaped cells arranged concentrically around the lumen (Fig. 13–5). Elastin deposition with reduplication of the internal elastic lamina may accompany these changes – hence the synonymous term *fibroelastosis*. Concentric laminar fibrosis should not be confused with the patchy, irregularly distributed intimal fibrosis that occurs as a

normal anatomic feature of small pulmonary arteries in older individuals.[26] The latter lesion appears smooth or homogeneous instead of laminar, and, of course, these patients lack other morphologic stigmata of pulmonary hypertension.

Plexiform lesions occur in many forms of severe pulmonary hypertension.[5,14,27] Although most investigators feel that plexiform lesions represent a late stage in pulmonary hypertension, some have proposed that they precede the formation of occlusive concentric intimal lesions.[4] Plexiform lesions are found in small muscular arteries, usually just distal to their origin from a larger vessel in which there is medial hypertrophy and often fibrous intimal thickening or occlusion (Fig. 13–6).[5] The plexiform lesion consists of an aneurysmal expansion in the vessel wall that, in early-occurring lesions, contains a distinctive proliferation of tiny, thick-walled vascular channels lined by cells resembling endothelium (Fig. 13–7). Small fibrin thrombi and foci of necrosis may be seen in the vascular channels and in the wall of the parent vessel. In older lesions, collagen appears between the vascular channels, and the resulting structure may be difficult to distinguish from a recanalized thromboembolus. Staining for nitric oxide synthetase (NOS) isomers has been demonstrated in plexiform lesions.[3] Nitric oxide has a role in both vasodilation and angiogenesis.

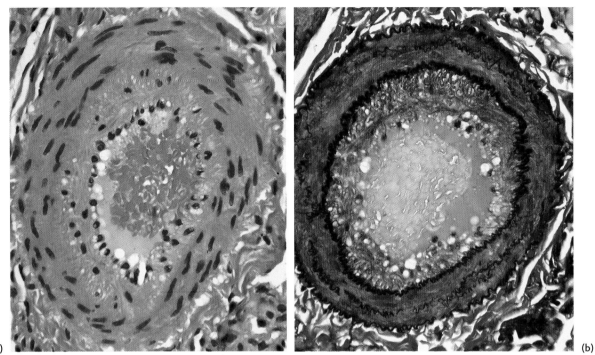

(a)   (b)

Figure 13–3 Intimal proliferation in pulmonary hypertension. (a) Medial hypertrophy is apparent in this artery in the routine H and E stain, but the intimal thickening is more difficult to appreciate. **(b)** An elastic tissue stain of the same artery outlines the internal and external elastic lamina and better delineates the thick layer of intimal fibrosis that is present on the luminal side of the internal elastic lamina. Note also the hyperplastic endothelial cells.

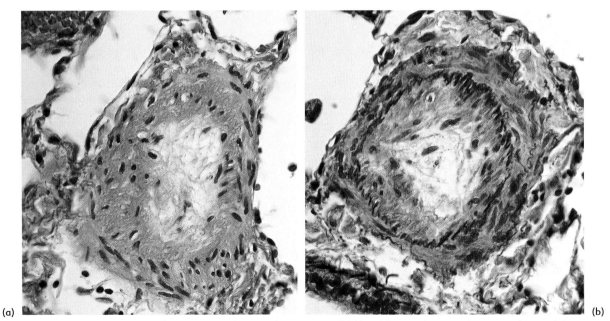

(a)   (b)

Figure 13–4 Marked intimal fibrosis in severe pulmonary hypertension. (a) H and E-stained section showing occlusion of the artery lumen by fibrosis. Note also the medial hypertrophy. **(b)** Elastic tissue stain of the same section better demarcates the intimal fibrosis obliterating the lumen. Note also the thickened media with increased numbers of nuclei.

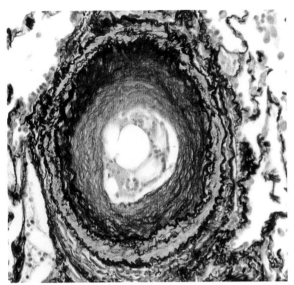

Figure 13–5 Concentric laminar fibrosis in severe pulmonary hypertension. Elastic tissue stain shows a prominent lamellar or onion-skin appearance to the intimal fibrosis that narrows the lumen of an artery.

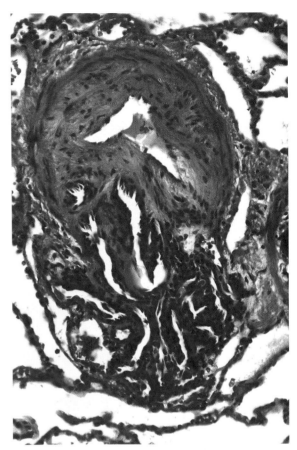

Figure 13–6 Plexiform lesion in severe pulmonary hypertension. Note the complex, interlacing, slit-like channels emanating from a muscular artery. The artery also shows intimal and medial hypertrophy.

Controversy exists about the origin of the cells lining the plexiform lesions. By electron microscopy, these cells show features of smooth muscle, myofibroblasts, or the so-called vasoformative reserve cells.[13,21] By immunohistochemistry, some studies have shown staining of the component cells for smooth muscle actin and vimentin, thus also suggesting myofibroblast origin.[28] Others, however, have demonstrated staining for endothelial markers, including factor VIII-related antigen and vascular endothelial growth factor receptor, thus indicating their derivation from endothelium.[5,22]

Traditionally, the pathogenesis of plexiform lesions has been related to vascular necrosis and secondary thrombosis with organization and recanalization.[13,14,21] More recent data, however, suggest that abnormal endothelial proliferation may be the primary abnormality.[15,23] Loss of transforming growth factor beta (TGFβ) signaling is thought to contribute to the abnormal endothelial cell proliferation in some cases.[51]

Various forms of dilatation lesions often accompany the plexiform lesions. These include the vein-like branches of hypertrophied muscular arteries, which consist of thin-walled dilated vessels arising from a muscular pulmonary artery that is proximal to an area of occlusion. These branches have a single elastic lamina, and so much of the media may disappear that, unless particular attention is paid to the anatomic location of these vessels and their origin from an artery,

they may be mistaken for pulmonary veins. A more common dilatation lesion is the *angiomatoid lesion*, which appears to be an exaggerated form of vein-like branches in which a discrete conglomeration of thin-walled, blood-filled vessels is found adjacent to a muscular pulmonary artery (Fig. 13–8). In practice, angiomatoid lesions and their variants are almost always found together with plexiform lesions. Hemosiderin-laden alveolar macrophages may accumulate in adjacent airspaces. The iron presumably results from the rupture of dilated small vessels.

Fibrinoid necrosis and *necrotizing arteritis* are uncommon features seen in muscular pulmonary arteries in the most severe forms of pulmonary hypertension. Early lesions are characterized by the deposition of glassy-appearing, brightly eosinophilic fibrinoid material in the vessel walls.[12] Electron microscopic studies indicate that actual necrosis of smooth

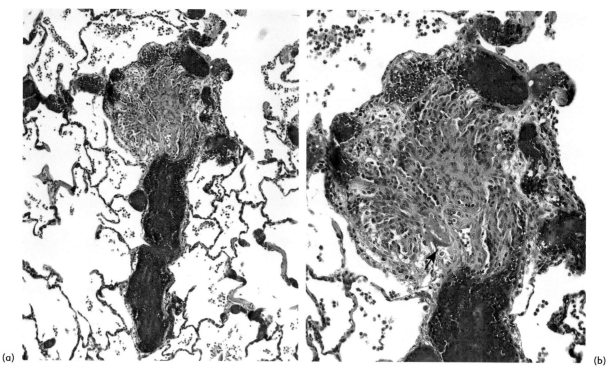

(a)

(b)

Figure 13–7 Plexiform lesion in severe pulmonary hypertension. (a) Low magnification view showing cellular lesion with adjacent dilated and congested thin-walled vessels. **(b)** Higher magnification of the plexiform lesion showing the cellular proliferation surrounding slit-like spaces. Fibrin disposition is seen focally as well (arrow).

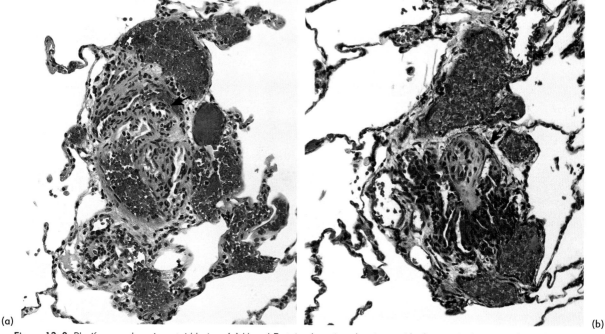

(a)

(b)

Figure 13–8 Plexiform and angiomatoid lesion. **(a)** H and E-stained section showing residual artery in the center (arrow) surrounded by and partially replaced by proliferative slit-like vascular spaces. In this case, there is also a proliferation of thin-walled congested vessels on the periphery that comprise the angiomatoid lesion. **(b)** Elastic tissue staining showing outlines of residual artery in the center (arrow).

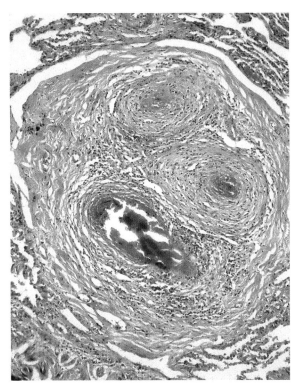

Figure 13–9 Vasculitis in severe pulmonary hypertension. This vessel is altered by severe chronic inflammation and fibrosis. There is also fibrinoid necrosis in the intima in areas.

muscle is rare in these early lesions. The fibrin that produces the characteristic light microscopic appearance lies between intact smooth muscle cells and appears to be forced into the medial layer from intraluminal thrombi. Thrombosis and necrosis of the arteries occur later, and a transmural infiltrate of polymorphonuclear leukocytes and occasional eosinophils eventually develops (Fig. 13–9). Older lesions show nodular masses of granulation tissue in and around the wall of the destroyed vessels. These nodules may represent old plexiform lesions.

Grading of Pulmonary Hypertension

Heath and Edwards devised a six-tiered grading system for pulmonary hypertension that was based on vascular changes observed in congenital left-to-right cardiac shunts (Table 13–3).[12,16,19,20,24,25,33] It was initially introduced to assess the potential reversibility of hypertensive vascular changes following surgical correction of congenital heart defects, and it retains limited usefulness in this regard. Its application to the primary forms of pulmonary hypertension has been questioned, however, since the morphologic grade of severity correlates poorly either with specific hemodynamic indices of severity or with clinical parameters such as response to therapy and prognosis.[46] Also, it implies an orderly progression of changes from grade I to grade VI, and it is not clear that the progression occurs, and, if so, whether it is related to severity or duration of the hypertension. Although this grading system is no longer widely utilized, evaluation of some of its features can provide an overall assessment of severity that may be helpful. Knowledge of its features is also beneficial for the pathologist, because it emphasizes the wide spectrum of vascular changes that can be encountered in pulmonary hypertension, and it describes the early subtle changes that may occur in the absence of more obvious plexiform lesions.

Primary Pulmonary Hypertension

The terminology used for idiopathic pulmonary hypertension has been confusing because a variety of different names have been applied, as summarized in Table 13–4.[33,47] The term primary pulmonary hypertension

Table 13–3	Heath and Edwards[12] Grading of Pulmonary Hypertension	
	Heath and Edwards Grades	**Clinicopathologic Correlation**
Grade I	Medial hypertrophy of small arteries and muscularization of arterioles	Mild to moderate hypertension (usually reversible)
Grade II	Medial hypertrophy plus intimal proliferation in small arteries	
Grade III	Medial hypertrophy, intimal proliferation plus intimal concentric laminar fibrosis	Severe hypertension (usually irreversible)
Grade IV	As in Grades I–III, plus plexiform lesions	
Grade V	Plexiform and angiomatoid lesions become prominent; hemosiderin deposition present	
Grade VI	All of the above, plus necrotizing arteritis	

Table 13–4   *Classification Schemes for Idiopathic Pulmonary Hypertension*

Wagenvoort[56]	Pietra et al[18,47]	Burke et al[33]	WHO, 1998[2,7]
Primary plexiform arteriopathy	Primary pulmonary arteriopathy • With plexiform lesions • With intimal fibrosis and medial hypertrophy • With isolated medial hypertrophy • With isolated arteritis	Arterial pulmonary hypertension • Plexiform type • Primary medial/intimal type	Primary pulmonary hypertension (sporadic/familial)
Thrombotic arteriopathy	• With thrombotic lesions	• Thrombotic type	Thromboembolic pulmonary hypertension (proximal artery/distal artery)
Pulmonary venoocclusive disease	Pulmonary occlusive venopathy Pulmonary microvasculopathy	Venous pulmonary hypertension • Pulmonary venoocclusive disease • Capillary hemangiomatosis	Pulmonary venoocclusive disease Pulmonary capillary hemangiomatosis

classically included primary plexiform arteriopathy, thrombotic arteriopathy, and pulmonary venoocclusive disease (PVOD),[31,42,56] whereas the current WHO classification (see Table 13–2) restricts its use to pulmonary arterial hypertension of unknown etiology (primary plexiform arteriopathy in the older terminology).[2,7] Both thrombotic arteriopathy and PVOD are considered to be separate from primary pulmonary hypertension in the WHO classification. More recently, the term idiopathic pulmonary arterial hypertension was advocated to replace primary pulmonary hypertension, although it seems unnecessarily cumbersome.[2]

Clinical Features

Primary pulmonary hypertension affects women about twice as often as men, and the mean age of onset is 36 years.[40,47,49,54] Approximately 6% of cases are familial. A mutation in the coding region of the gene for bone morphogenetic protein receptor 2 (BMPR2), a member of the TGFβ superfamily, has been demonstrated in half of the familial cases and about one-quarter of sporadic cases.[7,54] Exertional dyspnea is the most common presenting complaint, and fatigue, dizziness, and syncope are also frequent findings. Mortality is high, with current 5-year survival rates of 25–50%.[41] Right heart failure or sudden death is the usual cause of death. Treatment options include anticoagulants, calcium channel blockers, prostacyclin,

and lung transplantation, and recent reports have documented significantly improved survival in some patients.[2,41,53,54]

Pathologic Features

Microscopically, the entire spectrum of pathologic changes enumerated by the Heath and Edwards' grading system is found in primary pulmonary hypertension, and the findings are identical to those seen in other cases of severe pulmonary arterial hypertension.[14,33–35] Plexiform lesions are usually a prominent component, but in some cases they are absent and concentric laminar intimal fibrosis or medial hypertrophy are the main manifestations.[35,47] The paucity or absence of plexiform lesions may be explained in some cases by the fact that biopsy was performed early in the disease, before the plexiform lesions developed. Alternatively, plexiform lesions may be focal and patchy, and their absence in a biopsy specimen may reflect inadequate sampling. There is some evidence that the plexiform lesions in primary hypertension occur in more distal (intraacinar) arteries than the plexiform lesions of secondary forms of pulmonary arterial hypertension.[14] The adventitia of arteries is often thickened. Changes have also been documented in veins, including both intimal and adventitial thickening.[35] An additional common finding is evidence of recent and remote thrombosis in small arteries, including organizing thrombi, eccentric intimal fibrosis, and intravascular fibrous septa consistent with recanalized thrombi.[31,34,47,48,50,57] This finding has caused some investigators to question the rationale for separating the primary and thrombotic types of pulmonary hypertension (see further on).[44] Small thrombi, however, are common in well-documented secondary forms of pulmonary arterial hypertension and appear to correlate with patient age, occurring more often in adults than in children. The thrombi, therefore, are considered secondary phenomena in cases of primary pulmonary hypertension, rather than being important in pathogenesis. Furthermore, there are differences in the pathologic features and in the clinical manifestations and prognosis (see later on) of primary and thrombotic pulmonary hypertension, a fact that argues for maintaining these two entities as separate diseases.[57]

Pathogenesis

The pathogenesis of primary pulmonary hypertension is thought to be related to a combination of vaso-constriction due to an imbalance of vascular effectors, and abnormal proliferation of myofibroblasts and/or endothelial cells.[34,38,39,55] Whether patients with this disorder have inherently hyperreactive pulmonary arteries is an unresolved question.[40] Progesterone receptors, but not estrogen receptors, have been identified immunohistochemically within myofibroblasts of the vascular lesions, and their presence suggests a pathogenetic role for hormonal factors.[30] Evidence of monoclonality has been demonstrated in endothelial cells in plexiform lesions from primary but not secondary pulmonary hypertension.[15] Some authors consider primary pulmonary hypertension to represent an angioproliferative disorder possibly related to defective apoptosis.[23] Association with human herpesvirus 8 (HHV8) has been noted in some cases,[36] but not in others.[43] Evidence of tissue oxidative stress has been demonstrated in some.[32] Angiopoietin-1 may have a role in vascular smooth muscle hyperplasia in both primary and secondary forms of pulmonary hypertension.[37]

Pulmonary Arterial Hypertension Due to Cardiac Anomalies

Increased pulmonary blood flow is an important cause of pulmonary arterial hypertension and results from a number of cardiac anomalies with left-to-right shunts, especially ventricular and atrial septal defects and patent ductus arteriosus. Most of the vascular alterations related to cardiac shunts are similar regardless

of whether the shunt occurs proximal or distal to the tricuspid valve, and the Heath and Edwards' grading system is useful for assessing the severity of the morphologic changes.[12,58,60,63–65,71,72] The grade I changes may differ slightly, however, depending on the location of the shunt. Although the typical grade I change of medial hypertrophy is seen with post-tricuspid shunts, the earliest change related to pre-tricuspid shunts consists of intimal cell proliferation. As hypertension progresses, medial hypertrophy occurs and similar grade II through grade VI changes occur in both types of shunt, although severe hypertension (grades IV–VI) is unusual in pre-tricuspid lesions. The presence of longitudinally arranged smooth muscle bundles has also been noted in small arteries and arterioles in some cases.[69] This change, however, more commonly is a manifestation of alveolar hypoxia (see later on).

Lung biopsies are sometimes performed to assess the potential reversibility of pulmonary hypertension due to cardiac shunts before corrective surgery is undertaken, and the Heath–Edwards' grading system is usually a reliable predictor of reversibility.[1,12,58,61,62,63,66,68,70,73,74] When there are widespread lesions corresponding to grades IV to VI, the vascular resistance is irreversibly high, and corrective surgery will not improve pulmonary blood flow. The presence of extensive concentric laminar intimal fibrosis (grade III) usually also indicates fixed pulmonary vascular resistance, although individual exceptions do occur. It is important that both the extent and the severity of vascular lesions be considered when reversibility is evaluated. Other features also have predictive value in assessing reversibility. Fibrous obliteration of small pulmonary arteries with secondary medial atrophy in more peripheral arteries appears to correlate with irreversibility in some, but not all, patients.[73,74] In young children less than 2 years old, the extension of smooth muscle into arterioles is a more reliable indicator of severe hypertension than the Heath and Edwards' grading system.[19,20,74] Measurement of the ratio of the number of small arteries to alveoli is also helpful in evaluating hypertension in young children, since fixed pulmonary vascular resistance is often accompanied by a reduction in the number of arteries as compared to the number of alveoli.[10,59,60,62,67]

Miscellaneous Causes of Pulmonary Arterial Hypertension

Hepatic disease (usually cirrhosis) and extrahepatic causes of portal hypertension have both been associated with evidence of severe pulmonary hypertension, including plexiform lesions.[76,78,83,87,89,90,93,94,102,106] The cause of pulmonary hypertension in these cases is unknown, but occult thromboemboli from the portal venous system, portal-to-pulmonary vein anastomoses, and acquired pulmonary arteriovenous shunts have all been implicated. The presence of portocaval shunting, either surgical or spontaneous, appears to be a significant risk factor.[83] It has also been suggested that vasoactive substances produced in, or not properly inactivated by, the liver may cause pulmonary vasoconstriction.[78]

An association has been noted between *HIV infection* and pulmonary hypertension.[79,81,86,91,92,97–99] Most cases are idiopathic, although rare examples have been attributed to thromboembolic pulmonary hypertension and PVOD.[92] Germline mutations in BMPR2 have not been identified.[97] Vascular injury related to an immune reaction to the virus has been postulated in the etiology.[86] Stimulation and proliferation of endothelium due to viral-induced cytokine release has also been postulated.[92] The histologic changes in affected patients include a spectrum from moderate to severe pulmonary hypertension with the frequent presence of plexiform lesions.

A small number of therapeutic *drugs* (see Chapter 4), including prostaglandin E,[84] certain anorexigens (most recently fenfluramine derivatives),[75,77,96,101] and mitomycin,[118] have been associated with production of the clinical and histologic features of pulmonary hypertension, and similar changes have been noted following *L-tryptophan* ingestion.[85,105] A delayed onset of severe, plexiform pulmonary hypertension has been reported in some patients with *toxic oil syndrome* (see Chapter 2).[82] This syndrome was described following ingestion of tainted olive oil (rapeseed oil) in Spain in 1981. The vascular changes are thought to be related to direct endothelial injury by components of the ingested oil. Changes of mild to moderate pulmonary hypertension with medial hypertrophy of arteries has also been described in *cocaine* users and following chronic inhalation of *methamphetamine*.[95,103]

Collagen vascular diseases, especially scleroderma,[104] systemic lupus erythematosus,[100] and mixed connective tissue disease[80,88] (see Chapter 7), may be associated with pulmonary hypertension. While the hypertension is related in some cases to interstitial fibrosis with destruction of the capillary bed, it is often out of proportion to the interstitial fibrosis, and sometimes it is an isolated finding in the absence of interstitial lung disease.

Persistent Pulmonary Hypertension of the Newborn

Persistent pulmonary hypertension in the newborn (*persistent fetal circulation*) is another idiopathic form of pulmonary hypertension, but it is not considered a subtype of primary pulmonary hypertension.[60,107,108] Infants with this condition manifest respiratory distress and cyanosis related to failure of the decrease in pulmonary vascular resistance that normally occurs following birth. Cases are often associated with other conditions, including asphyxia, meconium aspiration, congenital pneumonia, sepsis, diaphragmatic hernia, and cardiac anomalies, although isolated examples also occur. Mortality is high, and most cases are encountered by the pathologist in autopsy rather than biopsy specimens. Muscularization of arterioles is the main pathologic finding.[60]

Pulmonary Venoocclusive Disease

PVOD is a rare form of pulmonary hypertension, characterized by obstruction of the small intrapulmonary veins. There is a wide age range of onset, from infancy to the seventh decade.[109,119,126] Approximately one-third of cases occur in children. The sex distribution is equal in children, while there is a slight male preponderance in adults.[110,123,129] Familial cases have been reported and a mutation in BMPR2 was noted in one case.[124,128] Some cases appear to be related to drug toxicity (see Chapter 4), especially to chemotherapeutic agents such as BCNU, bleomycin, and mitomycin,[118] and rare cases have followed bone marrow transplantation.[127,130] Rare examples have also been described in association with unilateral congenital absence of the pulmonary artery[117] and with a unilateral hyperlucent lung.[122]

Patients usually present with increasing dyspnea, and some give a history of an antecedent flu-like illness.[113,114,119] Hemoptysis may be a prominent manifestation. The chest radiographs often show a characteristic combination of enlarged pulmonary arteries and evidence of venous congestion (Kerley's lines and pleural effusions) without dilatation of the left atrium or large pulmonary veins. Intralobular septal thickening and diffuse or mosaic ground glass opacities are common on computed tomography (CT) examinations.[114,119] The demonstration of an elevated pulmonary artery wedge pressure may be helpful in diagnosing PVOD, but normal values can occur.[110] The

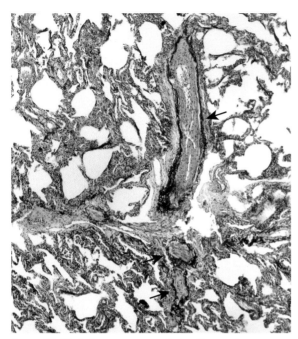

Figure 13–10 Pulmonary venoocclusive disease. Low magnification of elastic tissue stain showing veins (arrows) within an interlobular septum that are almost totally occluded by fibrosis.

prognosis is poor. Most patients die within 2 years of diagnosis, although prolonged survival has been reported rarely.[125]

The histologic findings in PVOD are characterized by a combination of chronic congestive changes, mild to moderate pulmonary hypertension, and obstruction of small veins. The single most important diagnostic feature is narrowing or occlusion of the small veins by eccentric or concentric intimal fibrosis (Fig. 13–10).[109,110,112,113,116,120,126,129] This feature is best appreciated with elastic tissue stains, which both identify the vessel as venous rather than arterial (since veins contain one elastic lamina rather than two), and distinguish fibrosed veins from background septal fibrosis (Fig. 13–11). Involvement of veins is often patchy, and a spectrum of normal to occluded veins may be seen. Dilatation of accompanying lymphatic spaces is common. The muscular pulmonary arteries usually show medial hypertrophy, but more severe hypertensive changes, such as concentric laminar intimal fibrosis and plexiform lesions, are generally not features. Arterial thrombi thought to be secondary to the venous congestion may occur but usually are not prominent.[115,129] Small infarcts are commonly found

adjacent to interlobular septa containing occluded veins (so-called *venous infarcts*) (Fig. 13–12). Hemosiderin deposition may be prominent within alveoli, and may be so striking that an alveolar hemorrhage syndrome (see Chapter 6) is considered in the differential diagnosis. In such cases, vascular elastic fibers may become coated with iron and calcium and elicit a foreign body granulomatous reaction (so-called *endogenous pneumoconiosis*, see Chapter 6).[121] The latter reaction is a nonspecific finding that can be seen in any example of longstanding alveolar hemorrhage regardless of cause. Alveolar septa usually show nonspecific thickening, a change that commonly occurs in any form of chronic venous congestion.

The cause of PVOD is unknown, although venous thrombosis is thought to be the inciting event for the development of intimal fibrous obliteration. A role has been postulated for a variety of potential pulmonary insults leading to thrombosis, including infection and immune complexes.[111,119,127]

The differential diagnosis of PVOD includes narrowing or obstruction of major pulmonary veins, idiopathic pulmonary hemosiderosis, and primary and thrombotic pulmonary hypertension. Obstruction to major pulmonary veins (see text following) can cause parenchymal changes similar to PVOD, except that arterialization of venules is often present and luminal fibrosis of veins may not be as prominent.[146] Clinical evaluation of the mediastinum and heart to exclude major venous obstruction (either in the mediastinum or because of cardiac anomalies such as mitral stenosis, for example) is recommended before diagnosing PVOD. Idiopathic pulmonary hemosiderosis (see Chapter 6) differs in that it is not associated with either medial hypertrophy of arteries (pulmonary hypertension) or fibrous obliteration of venules. Although so-called endogenous pneumoconiosis may also occur in idiopathic pulmonary hemosiderosis, it is a nonspecific manifestation of chronic alveolar hemorrhage due to any cause, and, thus, by itself, has no specific diagnostic implication.[121] The differentiation of PVOD from primary and thrombotic pulmonary hypertension (see further on) is somewhat easier, since significant venous occlusion is not a feature of either of these two disorders.

Pulmonary Capillary Hemangiomatosis

Capillary hemangiomatosis is another extremely rare cause of pulmonary hypertension. It is characterized by a proliferation of small vascular spaces that produces

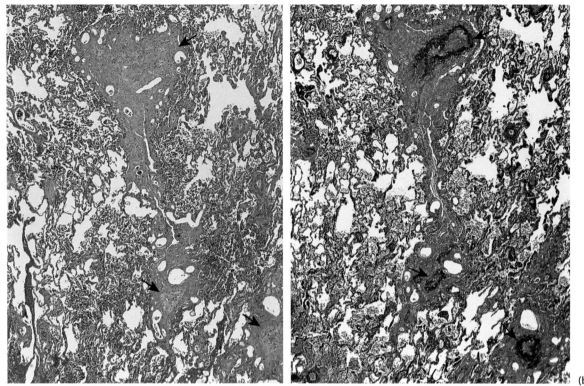

(a)
(b)

Figure 13–11 Pulmonary venoocclusive disease. (a) Low magnification showing patchy areas of parenchymal fibrosis. Remnants of occluded veins can be seen in the H and E-stained section (arrows), but they are better highlighted in an elastic tissue stain (**b**, arrows).

hypertension by surrounding and compressing intrapulmonary venules. Persons over a wide age range are affected, although most are between 20 and 40 years old.[131–133,135] Cases have been reported in infants and children, and a familial association has been described.[140,141] Most patients present with dyspnea, and, as in PVOD, hemoptysis occasionally occurs. Bilateral interstitial infiltrates are usually seen radiographically, and pleural effusions are sometimes present.[131] The prognosis is poor, with median survival of about 3 years. Treatment with recombinant interferon has been beneficial in a few cases, while lung transplantation has been undertaken in others.[131,133,135,144] Response to doxycycline, an angiogenesis inhibitor, was reported in one case.[136] In contrast to other forms of pulmonary hypertension, treatment with prostacyclin appears to be contraindicated.[131]

Histologically, capillary hemangiomatosis is characterized by a proliferation of thin-walled capillary-sized vascular channels within the interstitium (Figs 13–13 and 13–14).[133,135,138,142,143,145] Variable degrees of atypia may be seen in the component endothelial cells

(Fig. 13–15). The process is patchy and occurs within alveolar septa as well as around bronchioles and venules. The aberrant vascular spaces are often packed with erythrocytes, and hemosiderin and fresh blood may be found within adjacent airspaces. The changes may superficially resemble chronic passive congestion, but appreciation of the patchy nature of the process and the presence of large numbers of abnormal vascular spaces should suggest the correct diagnosis. Examination of alveolar septa in non-atelectatic areas helps, since no more than one row of capillaries is present between the alveolar epithelial layers in normal or congested lung, while two or more rows are present in areas of capillary hemangiomatosis.[137] Interestingly, some reported cases have occurred in patients with chronic congestive heart failure, an observation that suggests a role for chronic congestion in the pathogenesis.[134,139] In addition to the above findings, medium-sized arteries show intimal thickening and medial hypertrophy indicative of mild to moderate pulmonary hypertension. Sometimes, the lumens of venules are occluded by fibrosis as occurs in PVOD. This finding is thought to reflect thrombosis

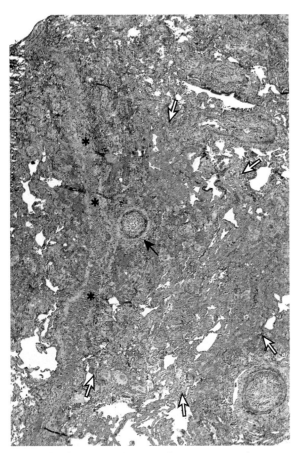

Figure 13–12 **Venous infarct in pulmonary venoocclusive disease.** A small hemorrhagic infarct (open arrows) is seen adjacent to an interlobular septum (asterisks). Note the occluded vein (black arrow) adjacent to the septum.

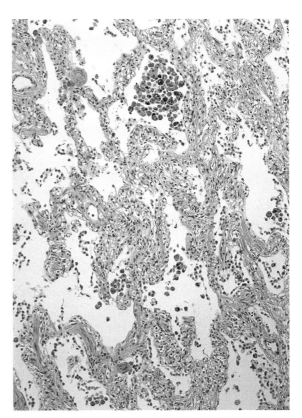

Figure 13–13 Low magnification view of capillary hemangiomatosis showing uniformly thickened alveolar septa along with intraalveolar hemosiderin-filled macrophages.

related to luminal narrowing by the perivenular capillary proliferation. It may cause initial consideration of PVOD in the diagnosis, but appreciation of the increased numbers of capillary-like spaces within the alveolar septa and elsewhere in the interstitium should indicate the correct diagnosis.

Pulmonary Venous Hypertension Due to Cardiac Abnormality

Mitral stenosis is a classical cause of pulmonary venous congestion with secondary pulmonary hypertension.[146,148] Similar findings can also occur with left atrial myxoma or aortic stenosis.[152] Histologic abnormalities are found in both arteries and veins. Mild (Heath and Edwards grade I to II) hypertensive arterial changes are characteristic. Plexiform lesions do not occur. Pulmonary veins show medial hypertrophy and

often evidence of 'arterialization'. In the latter lesion, the randomly distributed peripheral elastic fibrils of the venous wall condense, so that there are distinct internal and external elastic laminae. Fibrous intimal thickening similar to that seen in PVOD can also occur.[146] Dilated lymphatics are seen in the interlobular septa. Hemosiderin-filled macrophages are usually present in alveolar spaces, and alveolar septal thickening may be prominent. Features of so-called endogenous pneumoconiosis (see previous sections) are often present. Hemosiderin deposition may be so extensive, in fact, that clinically and pathologically the changes mimic an alveolar hemorrhage syndrome (see Chapter 6).

Pulmonary Venous Hypertension Due to Obstruction of Major Pulmonary Veins

Chronic narrowing or occlusion of major pulmonary veins within the mediastinum can cause secondary pulmonary hypertension related to venous congestion.[146,152,153] This process is most commonly encountered in cases of *fibrosing (sclerosing) mediastinitis* (see Chapter 15)[147,149]

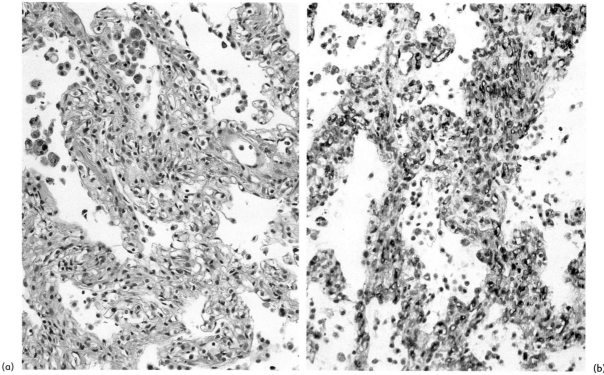

(a)

(b)

Figure 13–14 Capillary hemangiomatosis. (a) Higher magnification view of same case seen in Figure 13–13. Note the large numbers of thin-walled capillary-like spaces that thicken the alveolar septa. Hemosiderin-filled macrophages are present in adjacent alveolar spaces. **(b)** Immunohistochemical stain for CD34 outlines the large number of capillary-like spaces in alveolar septa.

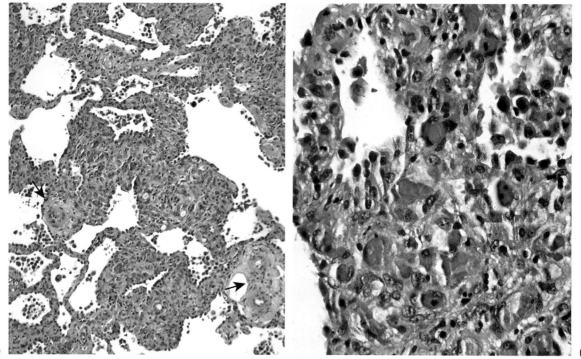

(a)

(b)

Figure 13–15 Cytologic atypia in capillary hemangiomatosis. (a) Low magnification view shows marked thickening of alveolar septa. Numerous capillary-like spaces can be appreciated even at this low magnification. Note also the medial hypertrophy in small arteries (arrows). **(b)** Higher magnification showing the enlarged nuclei and prominent nucleoli in some of the cells lining the capillary-like spaces.

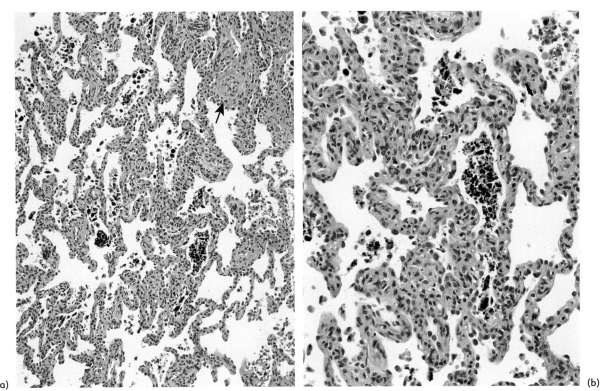

Figure 13–16 Pulmonary venous hypertension. (a) Low magnification view showing uniform-appearing alveolar septal thickening and intraalveolar hemosiderin-filled macrophages. A small artery at the top right (arrow) shows intimal and medial hypertrophy. This patient had occlusion of major pulmonary veins due to sarcoidosis. **(b)** Higher magnification view showing the mildly thickened alveolar septa with capillary congestion but no significant inflammation. Note the accompanying intraalveolar hemosiderin-filled macrophages.

or slowly growing mediastinal *neoplasms*. Rare examples of pulmonary vein atresia or stenosis have also been described.[150,151] The pathologic changes are identical to those occurring in mitral stenosis and other cardiac abnormalities causing venous congestion (see previous section) and include mild to moderate pulmonary hypertension (Heath and Edwards grades I and II), medial hypertrophy and arterialization of veins, hemosiderosis, and alveolar septal thickening (Fig. 13–16). Pulmonary infarction related to extrapulmonary venous obstruction has also been reported.[149] These venous infarcts are similar to those occurring in PVOD (see previous section) and are usually tiny and patchy and located near interlobular septa.

Pulmonary Hypertension Due to Lung Disease

Pulmonary hypertension is a common accompanying feature of diffuse interstitial fibrosis and honeycombing,

and it also occurs in emphysema and chronic bronchitis.[17,155,157,158,161,162] In these cases, the combined effects of hypoxia (see text following) and obliteration or distortion of the distal vascular bed play a role in producing the hypertension. Histologically, there is medial hypertrophy of muscular pulmonary arteries associated with the development of longitudinal intimal smooth muscle proliferation (Fig. 13–17).

Rarely, congenital pulmonary anomalies are associated with pulmonary hypertension. *Congenital alveolar capillary dysplasia* is a developmental disorder characterized by a striking paucity of alveolar wall capillaries and the presence of displaced or 'misaligned' veins accompanying pulmonary arteries.[154,156,160] This lesion causes pulmonary hypertension in neonates. Wagenvoort[159] has reported another structural anomaly that occurs in older patients with otherwise unexplained pulmonary hypertension. That disorder is characterized by focal, possibly congenital, defects in the media of pulmonary arteries.

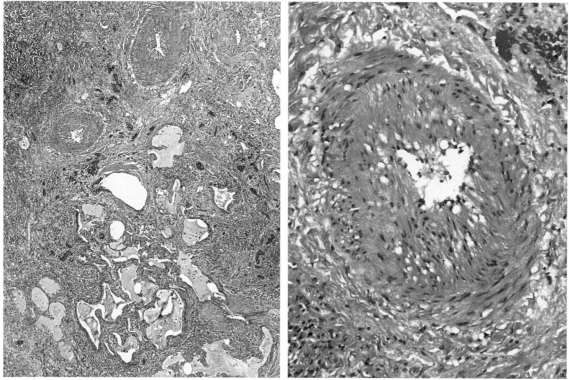

(a)

(b)

Figure 13–17 Pulmonary hypertension in usual interstitial pneumonia. (a) Low magnification view showing thick-walled arteries adjacent to an area of honeycomb change. (b) Higher magnification view of an artery showing both intimal and medial hypertrophy.

Pulmonary Hypertension Due to Alveolar Hypoxia

Hypoxia is a very potent stimulus to pulmonary vasoconstriction, and vascular changes may be seen in the lungs of high-altitude dwellers, patients with chronic obstructive pulmonary disease (bronchitis and emphysema), and obese patients with alveolar hypoventilation (sleep apnea syndrome).[155,157,158–164] Other factors in addition to hypoxia contribute to vascular changes in patients with chronic bronchitis and emphysema, as noted earlier, including loss of pulmonary vasculature and mechanical distortion of arteries.[161,162] Histologically, pulmonary hypertension related to hypoxia is characterized by medial hypertrophy of small arteries and extension of muscle into pulmonary arterioles. In addition, longitudinal bundles of smooth muscle appear in the intima of small muscular arteries. Medial hypertrophy may be seen in veins as well.[165,166] Interestingly, not all high-altitude dwellers develop these changes, thus indicating a role for individual (possibly genetic) predisposition.[164] Additional findings in obese patients with sleep apnea include hemosiderosis

and, rarely, capillary proliferation resembling pulmonary capillary hemangiomatosis.[163]

Pulmonary Hypertension Due to Chronic Thrombotic and/or Embolic Disease

Pulmonary hypertension can result from mechanical obstruction of small pulmonary arteries due to multiple, small pulmonary emboli or thrombi, or it can be associated with chronic thromboembolic occlusion of the main pulmonary artery. Emboli of substances other than clots also can cause pulmonary hypertension, and include foreign material injected intravenously by drug addicts (*drug abuser's lung*, see later on) or iatrogenically through intravenous infusions,[187] tumor emboli, and parasites such as schistosomes.

Chronic Thromboembolic Occlusion of Main Pulmonary Arteries

Chronic thromboembolism of the main pulmonary arteries is a rare occurrence that paradoxically may be associated with pulmonary hypertension (Fig. 13–18).[168,169,171–173,174] Many patients have an

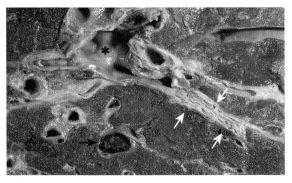

(a)

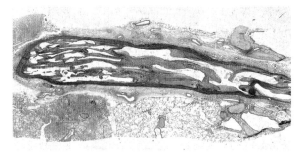

(b)

Figure 13-18 Thromboembolic occlusion of main pulmonary artery. (a) A branch of the main pulmonary artery (white arrows) is seen to be occluded by a web-like array of fibrosis, the typical gross appearance of recanalized remote thrombi. The proximal main artery (asterisk) is thick walled and contains focal atherosclerotic plaques. A recent thrombus (black arrow) is present in another artery. **(b)** Elastic tissue stain of the same portion of artery seen in Figure 13-18(a), showing the presence of multiple lumens characteristic of old, recanalized thrombi.

underlying predisposing condition such as tuberculosis or other chronic destructive lung disease, cardiac disease, especially mitral stenosis, or peripheral venous disease, although some have no underlying disease. A history of deep leg vein thrombosis is common, as is a history of previous pulmonary embolism.[168] Coagulation abnormalities and hematologic disorders are documented in a few individuals. The usual presenting complaint is progressive dyspnea, and there may be associated hemoptysis and signs of right heart failure. In patients with underlying lung disease, the thrombi are usually found on the side of greatest lung destruction, while in patients with no underlying disease, both right and left sides are affected equally.[173] Perfusion scans typically show reduced or absent blood flow to the affected areas, although angiography usually demonstrates more extensive and often bilateral

arterial occlusion.[167] Anticardiolipin antibodies are present in about 10% of patients.[169]

A lung biopsy may be undertaken in some patients, since the clinical presentation often mimics primary pulmonary hypertension. In such cases, the entire morphologic spectrum of pulmonary hypertensive changes ranging from mild to severe has been described.[172,173] Importantly, plexiform lesions may occur, and the changes may be identical to primary pulmonary hypertension. Surgical removal of the thrombus is associated with improved survival, even, surprisingly, in patients with plexiform lesions.[172] Thus, the distinction of this form of pulmonary hypertension from primary pulmonary hypertension is important and may require angiography.

The pathogenesis of pulmonary hypertension in thrombotic occlusion of main pulmonary arteries is thought to be related to the occurrence of multiple small thromboemboli distal to the main artery occlusion, perhaps related to recurrent fragmentation of the main thrombus. Certain cytokines may be important as well.[170]

Thrombotic/Thromboembolic Pulmonary Hypertension

Pulmonary hypertension can occur following obstruction of the distal arterial bed by thrombi or thromboemboli in the absence of thrombosis of a proximal major artery. This form of pulmonary hypertension was previously termed *thrombotic arteriopathy*, and it was included in the category of primary pulmonary hypertension in older classification schemes. Some patients have a history of peripheral venous disease or other evidence of recurrent, small pulmonary emboli, although more often patients present with an insidious onset of dyspnea without a history suggestive of emboli.[175,176] In such individuals, in situ thrombosis of the small arteries, rather than embolization, is thought to be the cause. This group can be difficult to distinguish clinically, and sometimes pathologically, from patients with primary pulmonary hypertension. There is no gender preference in thrombotic pulmonary hypertension, however, in contrast to a female preponderance in primary pulmonary hypertension.[47] Additionally, the prognosis may be slightly better for patients with thrombotic hypertension than for patients with primary pulmonary hypertension.[47] Anticoagulant therapy has been used, but there is little evidence that it is beneficial.[45]

The histologic hallmark of thrombotic pulmonary hypertension is the presence of widespread small artery thrombosis combined with the changes of moderate pulmonary hypertension.[29,177] Eccentric patches of intimal fibrosis in small pulmonary arteries are characteristic and are thought to represent remnants of organized thrombi (Fig. 13–19). Although occasionally the intimal fibrosis is circumferential rather than eccentric, the concentric laminar pattern characteristic of primary pulmonary hypertension is absent. Findings indicative of recanalized thrombi are also common, including multiple lumens, intravascular fibrous septa, and web formation (Fig. 13–20). Less often, recent fibrin thrombi, with or without organization, can be found (Fig. 13–21). Medial hypertrophy accompanies other changes, but features indicative of more severe pulmonary hypertension (plexiform lesions and intimal concentric laminar fibrosis) are absent.

Since small thrombi in various stages of organization are commonly found in primary pulmonary hypertension, some investigators have questioned whether thrombotic and primary forms of hypertension are separate entities or represent a spectrum of a single disease.[44] We agree with Wagenvoort and Mulder,[57] who point out that small thrombi are common in all forms of pulmonary hypertension (and in autopsy populations in general) and thus most likely represent incidental findings in primary hypertension rather than a characteristic or pathogenetic feature. In order to diagnose thrombotic hypertension, therefore, widespread,

rather than focal, evidence of small vessel thrombi should be present and should be the predominant finding. Additionally, changes indicative of severe pulmonary hypertension (plexiform lesions and concentric laminar intimal fibrosis) should be absent.

Drug Abuser's Lung (Talc Granulomatosis)

Emboli of foreign material, such as talc, cellulose, or other substances, may cause pulmonary hypertension in drug addicts who repeatedly inject oral medications intravenously. The foreign substances are insoluble filler materials used by pharmaceutical companies in the routine preparation of oral medications.[182,184-186] Histologically, medial hypertrophy of muscular pulmonary arteries (grade I, mild pulmonary hypertension) is usually found and is accompanied by evidence of thrombosis and recanalization.[182,186] Rarely, more severe hypertensive changes, including plexiform lesions, may be found. The diagnostic histologic feature is the presence of multiple foreign body granulomas containing exogenous particles, some of which are doubly refractile (Fig. 13–22). These granulomas occur in the lumina and walls of muscular pulmonary arteries, in perivascular connective tissue, and in alveolar septa.[178,182-186] The review by Tomashefski and Hirsch[184] illustrates the different appearances of various inert fillers that have been found within these lesions. Identification of these particles often suggests

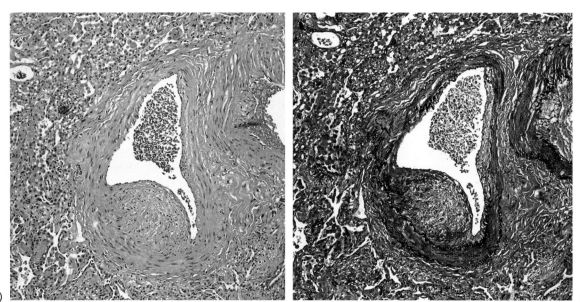

(a) (b)

Figure 13–19 Thrombotic pulmonary hypertension. (a) Small pulmonary artery showing eccentric intimal fibrosis that is indicative of an old thrombus. **(b)** Elastic tissue stain highlights the presence of the eccentric intimal fibrosis.

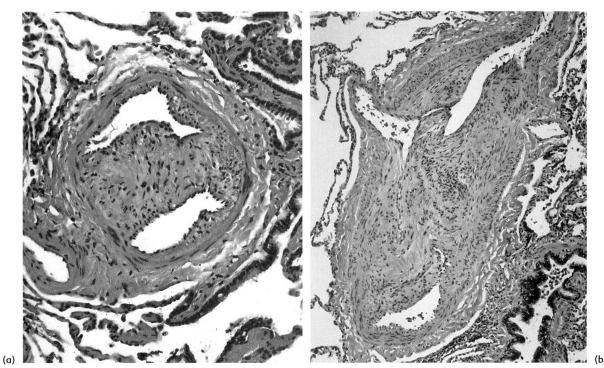

(a)   (b)

Figure 13–20 Thrombotic pulmonary hypertension. (a) A recanalized thrombus is characterized in this artery by a single 'web' that divides the lumen into two equal parts. **(b)** Multiple lumens indicative of old thrombi/thromboemboli are seen in this artery.

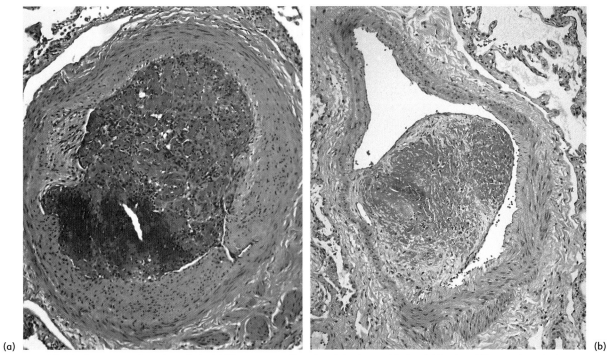

(a)   (b)

Figure 13–21 Organizing thromboemboli. (a) This artery is dilated and the lumen filled with blood and fibrin within which fibroblasts and granulation tissue are present. **(b)** In this example of an organizing thrombus, spindle-shaped fibroblasts can be seen surrounding residual central fibrin. Much of the thrombus has been replaced, and eventually the remnant will resemble the eccentric intimal fibrosis shown in Figure 13–19.

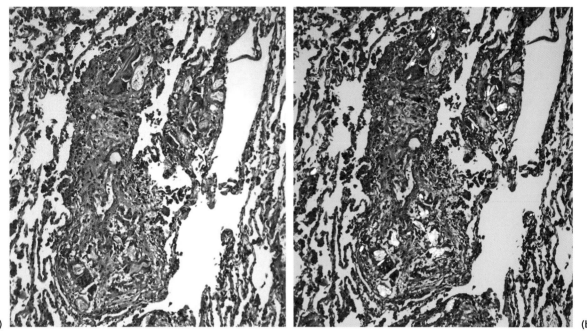

(a)   (b)

Figure 13–22 Intravenous drug abuser's lung. (a) H and E-stained slide showing foreign body granulomas in the interstitium around a small artery. (b) Under partially polarized light, large polarizable sheet-like crystals of talc are seen within foreign body giant cells.

the type of oral drug that was being injected. For example, the 6- to 23-μm-long, doubly refractile spicules of talc are found in methylphenidate (Ritalin) and methadone; starch granules resembling Maltese crosses in polarized light are found in barbiturates; large (up to 250 μm), pale gray, PAS-positive particles of microcrystalline cellulose are found in pentazocine (Talwin); and large, deeply basophilic, coral-like particles of crospovidone are found in hydromorphone (Fig. 13–23).[179,184,186] Another pathologic finding in drug abuser's lung is an acute and chronic inflammatory cell infiltrate, often containing eosinophils, within the alveolar septa.[182] Septic emboli from right-sided endocarditis may complicate the microscopic picture, and mycotic pulmonary artery aneurysms are also a complication.[243,244] Fungal or mycobacterial infections occasionally occur and should be suspected if necrosis is present within the granulomas.

Clinically, patients with drug abuser's lung present with increasing dyspnea. The chest radiograph may be normal or may show the vascular and cardiac changes associated with pulmonary hypertension.[182] In some cases, a diffuse, fine micronodular pattern has been reported. Ultimately, in rare cases, a lesion resembling progressive massive fibrosis (see Chapter 5) may develop.[180,181]

Tumor Emboli

Multiple small tumor emboli are uncommon causes of pulmonary hypertension.[187–199] They may occur in the absence of lung parenchymal metastasis, and the clinical manifestations in such cases may mimic primary pulmonary hypertension.[190,191,194–198] Adenocarcinomas, especially from the stomach, breast, lung, and ovary, are the most common tumors causing pulmonary hypertension, although others have been reported, including hepatocellular carcinoma, transitional cell carcinoma, and osteosarcoma, for example.[188,191,194–198]

OTHER DISORDERS OF THE PULMONARY VASCULATURE

Pulmonary Emboli

Thromboemboli are the most common cause of mechanical occlusion of the pulmonary vasculature. Most emboli arise in the deep veins of the lower extremities, although pelvic veins, renal veins, veins of the upper extremities and the right cardiac chamber are occasional sources.[205,213] If the pulmonary circulation is otherwise intact and the bronchial arterial system is adequate, pulmonary infarction (see text

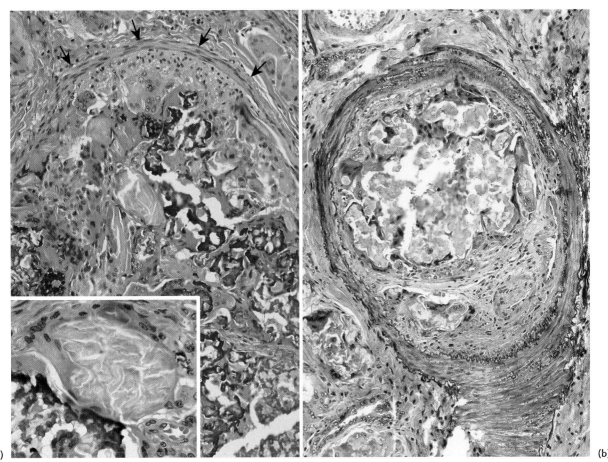

(a) (b)

Figure 13–23 Intravenous drug abuser's lung. Intravascular location of foreign material is illustrated in both H and E **(a)** (a portion of vascular media is seen at top, arrows) and elastic tissue stains **(b)**. The inset is a higher magnification showing the typical sheet-like appearance of a talc crystal. Also note the amorphous, coral-like basophilic material that fits with provolidine, a filler used in certain drugs.

following) rarely occurs, although small areas of hemorrhage or atelectasis may be seen.[203,213,221,223] As previously discussed, pulmonary hypertension can develop with chronic thromboemboli affecting either major pulmonary arteries or a large proportion of the distal arterial tree. More commonly, however, the thromboemboli are isolated events.

The histologic features of thromboemboli are indistinguishable from those of in situ thrombi, and they vary according to the age of the lesion.[223] *Acute thromboemboli* are composed of a mixture of blood, fibrin, platelets, and neutrophils, often arranged in alternating linear zones that correspond to the grossly visible *lines of Zahn*. The affected artery is usually dilated and thin walled. After 2 to 3 days the thrombus begins to undergo organization, with the ingrowth of fibroblasts and capillaries from the vessel wall (Fig. 13–24).

This process progresses over several weeks until the thrombus is completely replaced by fibrosis and variable numbers of small, capillary-sized vascular spaces (*organized thrombus*). *Recanalization* may occur by means of enlargement of one or more of the capillary-sized vessels within the organized thrombus. Eventually, all that remains is one or more fibrous *bands* (imparting the appearance of multiple lumens) or *webs* within the lumen (see Fig. 13–18). The latter lesions are common incidental autopsy findings indicative of thromboemboli occurring in the remote past.

Septic thromboemboli also can originate from the deep veins of the leg or the pelvic veins, or they may emanate from right-sided endocarditis. Lung abscesses (see Chapter 16) or infected infarcts are complications.[211]

Emboli of multiple other substances have been described. For example, emboli of *fat, bile, cotton fiber,*

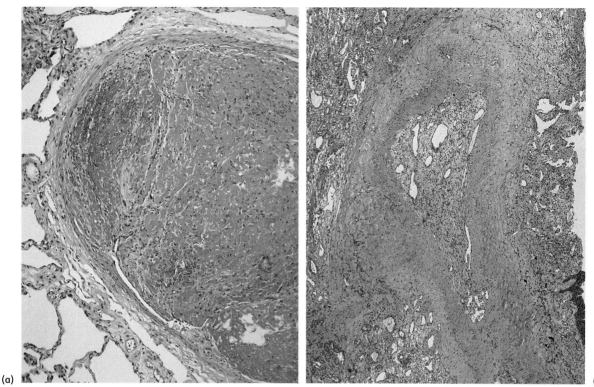

(a) (b)

Figure 13–24 (a) Low magnification of an organizing pulmonary embolus. Note the dilated thin-walled artery, the lumen of which is almost entirely occluded. Some blood is present but most of the material is fibrin admixed with fibroblasts. (b) This embolus is older and has undergone organization and recanalization. Note the almost complete occlusion of the artery lumen and the multiple small vascular spaces.

or *cardiac catheter material* have been found in patients subjected to invasive diagnostic or therapeutic procedures.[200,204,208,209,215,217,219,222] *Bone marrow* emboli are common autopsy findings, usually following resuscitative measures, and they are also occasionally present in open lung biopsy specimens (see Chapter 1), presumably related to rib manipulation during surgery. Emboli of foreign material occur in intravenous drug users (*drug abuser's lung* or *talc granulomatosis*) and of ova or parasites in certain *parasitic diseases*. The latter types of emboli may result in pulmonary hypertension and have been discussed in earlier sections. *Silicone emboli* are a rare complication of silicone fluid injection for breast augmentation, and have also been reported following illicit subcutaneous injection in other situations.[201,202,218] Acute pneumonitis, alveolar hemorrhage, and diffuse alveolar damage may accompany the emboli, and a fatal outcome is common. *Amniotic fluid embolism* occurs rarely in postpartum women and is characterized by systemic collapse and respiratory failure immediately after delivery.[207,216,224] The diagnostic

pathologic changes are usually encountered only at autopsy and consist of squames, lanugo hair, intestinal mucin (meconium), and fat droplets within the pulmonary arteries. Alcian blue and oil red O staining helps to demonstrate the meconium and fat droplets, while immunohistochemical staining for cytokeratin may help identify the squames.[206] Use of an antibody that reacts against meconium and an amniotic fluid-derived glycoprotein has also been described.[210] Squames may be demonstrable in pulmonary arterial blood samples by cytologic means.[212]

Pulmonary Infarcts

Pulmonary infarcts are not ordinarily excised, but, occasionally, clinically unsuspected examples that present as unresolving infiltrates or nodular opacities may be biopsied.[214] Histologically these lesions are characterized by central bland necrosis, often containing shadows, or 'ghosts', of alveolar septa (Fig. 13–25). There is variable associated hemorrhage, and often a

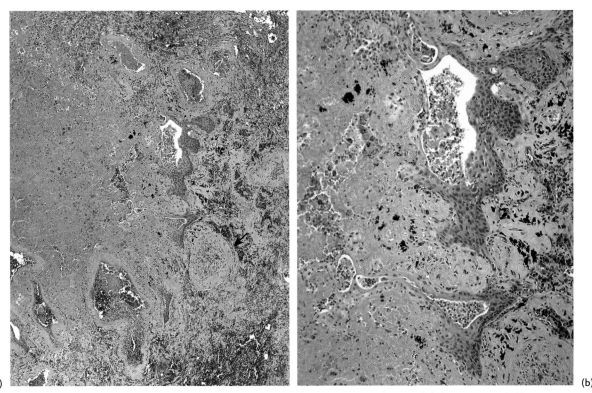

(a)

(b)

Figure 13–25 Pulmonary infarct. (a) Low magnification showing the necrotic parenchyma at left that is surrounded by squamous metaplasia, hemorrhage, and fibrosis on the right. An occluded artery containing an organized thrombus (arrow) is also present. **(b)** Higher magnification highlights the squamous metaplasia at the periphery of the infarct.

rim of active fibroblasts surrounds the necrotic center. Significant inflammation is not a feature. Recent or organizing thrombi or various types of emboli (see previous section) may be found in the adjacent pulmonary arteries. Squamous metaplasia and atypical alveolar cell proliferation are commonly seen around the periphery of the infarct and should not be misinterpreted as carcinoma. The natural history of pulmonary infarcts usually involves the eventual formation of a fibrous scar. Cavitation occurs in occasional cases,[211] and, in infants, peripheral lung cysts may result from infarcts (see Chapter 14).[220]

As noted in earlier sections, thromboemboli alone (in the absence of cardiac failure, shock, or underlying, chronic lung disease) rarely cause pulmonary infarction, because the lung possesses a dual blood supply. Therefore, when infarcts are encountered on lung biopsy specimens, causes other than uncomplicated thromboemboli should be considered. In our experience, pulmonary venous obstruction is a major cause, whether due to obstruction of major pulmonary veins in the mediastinum, as in fibrosing mediastinitis (see

Chapter 15) or tumor, for example, or due to obstruction of the small intrapulmonary veins (as in PVOD, see previous section). Infarcts related to pulmonary venous obstruction (so-called venous infarcts) tend to be small and irregular in shape and are located near interlobular septa.

Pulmonary Arteriovenous Malformations

Most pulmonary arteriovenous (AV) malformations or fistulae are congenital in origin, although acquired lesions related to infection,[231,232] neoplasm,[225] or trauma[235] have also been reported.[229] The congenital fistulae may be solitary or multiple,[225,228,236] and they are commonly associated with *Osler–Weber–Rendu disease (hereditary hemorrhagic telangiectasia)*.[227,228,237] The fistulae generally appear as discrete multilocular cystic lesions.

Dyspnea, cyanosis, and hemoptysis are common presenting complaints, while some patients are asymptomatic.[228,229] Digital clubbing is often present. Cerebral emboli and brain abscess are important complications. A bruit frequently is heard over the site of the fistula. The diagnosis is usually established by angiography, although suggestive changes may be found on chest CT examination.[233,238] The use of contrast echocardiography has also been advocated, and, when combined with chest radiographs, may obviate the need for other studies.[227] The current treatment of symptomatic lesions is embolotherapy, and surgery is usually not necessary.

Microscopically, the AV fistulae consist of multiple, anastomosing, small and large vascular channels with an irregularly thickened wall. Many AV fistulae abut the visceral pleura, which becomes thickened where it overlies the malformation. The blood supply is usually from a pulmonary artery, but a systemic blood supply has occasionally been reported.[226,230,234]

Pulmonary Artery Aneurysms

Pulmonary artery aneurysms occur most frequently in association with congenital or acquired cardiovascular diseases that produce pulmonary hypertension, but they may also arise on the basis of infection, trauma, atherosclerosis, metabolic defects, Behçet's disease, or collagen vascular disease.[239–241,243,245–247] Mycotic aneurysms have been reported in association with intravenous drug abuse.[243,244] Dissection, rupture, or pulmonary emboli may be fatal complications.[242]

REFERENCES

General Features of Pulmonary Hypertension

1. Aiello VD, Gutierrez PS, Chaves MJF, et al: Morphology of the internal elastic lamina in arteries from pulmonary hypertensive patients: A confocal laser microscopy study. Mod Pathol 16:411, 2003.
2. American College of Chest Physicians: Diagnosis and management of pulmonary arterial hypertension: ACCP evidence-based clinical practice guidelines. Chest 126(Suppl), 2004.
3. Berger RMF, Geiger, R, Hess J, et al: Altered arterial expression patterns of inducible and endothelial nitric oxide synthase in pulmonary plexogenic arteriopathy caused by congenital heart disease. Am J Respir Crit Care Med 163:1493, 2001.
4. Cool CD, Kennedy D, Voelkel NF, Tuder RM: Pathogenesis and evolution of plexiform lesions in pulmonary hypertension associated with scleroderma and human immunodeficiency virus infection. Hum Pathol 28:434, 1997.
5. Cool CD, Stewart JS, Werahera P, et al: Three-dimensional reconstruction of pulmonary arteries in plexiform pulmonary hypertension using cell-specific markers. Am J Pathol 155:411, 1999.
6. Deffebach ME, Charan NB, Lakshminarayan S, Butter J: The bronchial circulation. Small, but a vital attribute of the lung. Am Rev Respir Dis 135:463, 1987.
7. Farber HW, Loscalzo J: Pulmonary arterial hypertension. N Engl J Med 351:1655, 2004.
8. Fernie JM, Lamb D: A new method for quantitating the medial component of pulmonary arteries: The measurements. Arch Pathol Lab Med 109:156, 1985.
9. Gosrey J, Heath D, Smith P, et al: Pulmonary endocrine cells in pulmonary arterial disease. Arch Pathol Lab Med 113:337, 1989.
10. Haworth SG: Pulmonary vascular disease in different types of congenital heart disease. Implications for interpretation of lung biopsy findings in early childhood. Br Heart J 52:557, 1984.
11. Haworth SG, Hislop AA: Pulmonary vascular development: Normal values of peripheral vascular structure. Am J Cardiol 52:578, 1983.
12. Heath D, Edwards JE: The pathology of hypertensive pulmonary vascular disease. A description of six grades of structural changes in the pulmonary arteries with special reference to congenital cardiac septal defects. Circulation 18:533, 1958.
13. Heath D, Smith P, Gosney J: Ultrastructure of early plexogenic pulmonary arteriopathy. Histopathology 12:41, 1988.
14. Jamison BM, Michel RP: Different distribution of plexiform lesions in primary and secondary pulmonary hypertension. Hum Pathol 26:987, 1995.
15. Lee S-D, Shoyer KR, Markham NE, et al: Monoclonal endothelial cell proliferation is present in primary but not secondary pulmonary hypertension. J Clin Invest 101:927, 1998.
16. Meyrick B, Reid L: Pulmonary hypertension. Anatomic and physiologic correlates. Clin Chest Med 4:199, 1983.
17. Moore GW, Smith RRL, Hutchins GM: Pulmonary artery atherosclerosis. Correlation with systemic atherosclerosis and hypertensive pulmonary vascular disease. Arch Pathol Lab Med 106:378, 1982.
18. Pietra GG, Capron F, Steward S, et al: Pathologic assessment of vasculopathies in pulmonary hypertension. J Am Coll Cardiol 43:255, 2004.
19. Rabinovitch M, Haworth SG, Castaneda AR, et al: Lung biopsy in congenital heart disease: A morphometric approach to pulmonary vascular disease. Circulation 58:1107, 1978.
20. Rabinovitch M, Haworth S, Vance Z, et al: Early pulmonary vascular changes in congenital heart disease studied in biopsy tissue. Hum Pathol 11:499, 1980.
21. Smith P, Heath D: Electron microscopy of the plexiform lesion. Thorax 34:177, 1979.
22. Tuder RM, Groves B, Badesch D, Voelkel NF: Exuberant endothelial cell growth and elements of inflammation are present in plexiform lesions of pulmonary hypertension. Am J Pathol 144:275, 1994.
23. Voelkel NF, Cool CC: Pathology of pulmonary hypertension. Cardiol Clin 22:343, 2004.
24. Wagenvoort CA: Lung biopsy specimens in the

evaluation of pulmonary vascular disease. Chest 77:615, 1980.

25. Wagenvoort CA: Grading of pulmonary vascular lesions – a reappraisal. Histopathology 5:595, 1981.

26. Warnock ML, Kunmann A: Changes with age in muscular pulmonary arteries. Arch Pathol Lab Med 101:175, 1977.

27. Yamaki S, Wagenvoort CA: Plexogenic pulmonary arteriopathy: Significance of medial thickness with respect to advanced pulmonary vascular lesions. Am J Pathol 105:70, 1981.

28. Yi ES, Kim H, Hyekyung A, et al: Distribution of obstructive intimal lesions and their cellular phenotypes in chronic pulmonary hypertension. A morphometric and immunohistochemical study. Am J Respir Crit Care Med 162:1577, 2000.

Primary Pulmonary Hypertension

29. Anderson EG, Simon G, Reid L: Primary and thromboembolic pulmonary hypertension: A quantitative pathological study. J Pathol 110:273, 1973.

30. Barberis MCP, Veronese S, Bauer D, et al: Immunocytochemical detection of progesterone receptors. A study in a patient with primary pulmonary hypertension. Chest 107:869, 1995.

31. Bjornsson J, Edwards WD: Primary pulmonary hypertension: A histopathologic study of 80 cases. Mayo Clin Proc 60:16, 1985.

32. Bowers R, Cool C, Murphy RC, et al: Oxidative stress in severe pulmonary hypertension. Am J Respir Crit Care Med. 169:764, 2004.

33. Burke AP, Farb A, Virmani R: The pathology of primary pulmonary hypertension. Mod Pathol 4:269, 1991.

34. Caslin AW, Heath D, Madden B, et al: The histopathology of 36 cases of plexogenic pulmonary arteriopathy. Histopathology 16:9, 1990.

35. Chazova I, Loyd JE, Zhdanov VS, et al: Pulmonary artery adventitial changes and venous involvement in primary pulmonary hypertension. Am J Pathol 146:389, 1995.

36. Cool CD, Rai PR, Yeager ME, et al: Expression of human herpesvirus 8 in primary pulmonary hypertension. N Engl J Med 349:1113, 2003.

37. Du L, Sullivan CC, Chu D, et al: Signaling molecules in nonfamilial pulmonary hypertension. N Engl J Med 348:500, 2003.

38. Giaid A, Yanagisawa M, Langleben D, et al: Expression of endothelin-1 in the lungs of patients with pulmonary hypertension. N Engl J Med 328:1732, 1993.

39. Heath D, Smith P, Gosney J, et al: The pathology of the early and late stages of primary pulmonary hypertension. Br Heart J 58:204, 1987.

40. Hughes JD, Rubin LJ: Primary pulmonary hypertension. An analysis of 28 cases and a review of the literature. Medicine (Baltimore) 65:56, 1986.

41. Humbert M, Sitbon O, Simonneau G: Treatment of pulmonary arterial hypertension. N Engl J Med 351:1425, 2004.

42. Kay JM, Heath D: Pathologic study of unexplained pulmonary hypertension. Semin Respir Med 7:180, 1985.

43. Laney AS, DeMarco T, Peters JS, et al: Kaposi sarcoma-associated herpesvirus and primary and secondary pulmonary hypertension. Chest 127:762, 2005.

44. Loyd JE, Atkinson JB, Pietra GG, et al: Heterogeneity of pathologic lesions in familial primary pulmonary hypertension. Am Rev Respir Dis 138:952, 1988.

45. Nicod P, Moser KM: Primary pulmonary hypertension. The risk and benefit of lung biopsy. Circulation 80:1486, 1989.

46. Palevsky HI, Schloo BL, Pietra GG, et al: Primary pulmonary hypertension. Vascular structure, morphometry, and responsiveness to vasodilator agents. Circulation 80:1207, 1989.

47. Pietra GG, Edwards WD, Kay JM, et al: Histopathology of primary pulmonary hypertension. A qualitative and quantitative study of pulmonary blood vessels from 58 patients in the National Heart, Lung, and Blood Institute, Primary Pulmonary Hypertension Registry. Circulation 80:1198, 1989.

48. Pietra GG, Ruttner JR: Specificity of pulmonary vascular lesions in primary pulmonary hypertension. A reappraisal. Respiration 52:81, 1987.

49. Rich S, Dantzker DR, Ayres SM, et al: Primary pulmonary hypertension. A national prospective study. Ann Intern Med 107:216, 1987.

50. Rich S, Pietra GG, Kieras K, et al: Primary pulmonary hypertension: Radiographic and scintigraphic patterns of histologic subtypes. Ann Intern Med 105:499, 1986.

51. Richter A, Yeager ME, Zaiman A, et al: Impaired transforming growth factor-β signaling in idiopathic pulmonary arterial hypertension. Am J Respir Crit Care Med 170:1340, 2004.

52. Rubin LJ: Primary pulmonary hypertension. ACCP consensus statement. Chest 104:236, 1993.

53. Rubin LJ: Primary pulmonary hypertension. N Engl J Med 336:111, 1997.

54. Runo JR, Loyd JE: Primary pulmonary hypertension. Lancet 361:1533, 2003.

55. Smith P, Heath D, Yacoub M, et al: The ultrastructure of plexogenic pulmonary arteriopathy. J Pathol 160:111, 1990.

56. Wagenvoort CA: Primary pulmonary hypertension: A pathologic study of the lung vessels in 156 clinically diagnosed cases. Circulation 42:1163, 1970.

57. Wagenvoort CA, Mulder PGH: Thrombotic lesions in primary plexogenic arteriopathy. Similar pathogenesis or complication? Chest 103:844, 1993.

Pulmonary Arterial Hypertension Due to Cardiac Anomalies

58. Fried R, Falkovsky F, Newburger J, et al: Pulmonary artery changes in patients with ventricular septal defects and severe pulmonary hypertension. Pediatr Cardiol 7:147, 1986.

59. Haworth SG: Pulmonary vascular bed in children with complete atrioventricular septal defect: Relation between

structural and hemodynamic abnormalities. Am J Cardiol 57:833, 1980.

60. Haworth SG: Primary and secondary pulmonary hypertension in childhood: A clinicopathologic reappraisal. Curr Top Pathol 73:92, 1983.

61. Haworth SG: Pulmonary vascular disease in ventricular septal defect: Structural and functional correlations in lung biopsies from 85 patients, with outcome of intracardiac repair. J Pathol 152:157, 1987.

62. Haworth SG, Reid L: A morphometric study of regional variation in lung structure in infants with pulmonary hypertension and congenital cardiac defect. A justification of lung biopsy. Br Heart J 40:825, 1978.

63. Hoffman JIE, Rudolph AM, Heymann MA: Pulmonary vascular disease with congenital heart lesions: Pathologic features and causes. Circulation 64:873, 1981.

64. Meyrick B, Reid L: Ultrastructural findings in lung biopsy material from children with congenital heart defects. Am J Pathol 101:527, 1980.

65. Rabinovitch M, Bothwell T, Hayakawa BN, et al: Pulmonary artery endothelial abnormalities in patients with congenital heart defects and pulmonary hypertension. A correlation of light with scanning electron microscopy and transmission electron microscopy. Lab Invest 55:632, 1986.

66. Rabinovitch M, Keane JF, Norwood WI, et al: Vascular structure in lung tissue obtained at biopsy correlated with pulmonary hemodynamic findings after repair of congenital heart defects. Circulation 69:655, 1984.

67. Takahashi T, Wagenvoort CA: Density of muscularized arteries in the lung. Its role in congenital heart disease and its clinical significance. Arch Pathol Lab Med 107:23, 1983.

68. Wagenvoort CA: Open lung biopsies in congenital heart disease for evaluation of pulmonary vascular disease. Predictive value with regard to corrective operability. Histopathology 9:417, 1985.

69. Wagenvoort CA, Keutel J, Mooi WG, Wagenvoort N: Longitudinal smooth muscle in pulmonary arteries. Occurrence in congenital heart disease. Virchows Arch A Pathol Anat Histopathol 404:265, 1984.

70. Wagenvoort CA, Wagenvoort N, Draulans-Noe Y: Reversibility of plexogenic pulmonary arteriopathy following banding of the pulmonary artery. J Thorac Cardiovasc Surg 87:876, 1984.

71. Yaginuma G, Mohri H, Takahashi T: Distribution of arterial lesions and collateral pathways in the pulmonary hypertension of congenital heart disease: A computer aided reconstruction study. Thorax 45:586, 1990.

72. Yamaki S, Horiuchi T, Miura M, et al: Pulmonary vascular disease in secundum atrial septal defect with pulmonary hypertension. Chest 89:694, 1986.

73. Yamaki S, Kumate M, Yonesaka S, et al: Lung biopsy diagnosis of operative indication in secundum atrial septal defect with severe pulmonary vascular disease. Chest 126:1042, 2004.

74. Yamaki S, Mohri H, Haneda K, et al: Indications for surgery based on lung biopsy in cases of ventricular septal defect and/or patent ductus arteriosus with severe pulmonary hypertension. Chest 96:31, 1989.

Miscellaneous Causes of Pulmonary Arterial Hypertension

75. Abenhaim L, Moride Y, Brenot F, et al: Appetite suppressant drugs and the risk of primary pulmonary hypertension. N Engl J Med 335:609, 1996.

76. Bower JS, Pantzker DR, Naylor B: Idiopathic pulmonary hypertension associated with nodular pulmonary infiltrates and portal venous thrombosis. Chest 78:111, 1980.

77. Brenot F, Hervé P, Petipretz, P, et al: Primary pulmonary hypertension and fenfluramine use. Br Heart J 70:537, 1993.

78. Cohen MD, Rubin LJ, Taylor WE, Cuthbert JA: Primary pulmonary hypertension: An unusual case associated with extrahepatic portal hypertension. Hepatology 3:588, 1983.

79. Coplan NL, Shimony RY, Ioachim HL, et al: Primary pulmonary hypertension associated with human immunodeficiency viral infection. Am J Med 89:96, 1990.

80. Friedman DM, Mitnick HJ, Danilowicz D: Recovery from pulmonary hypertension in an adolescent with mixed connective tissue disease. Ann Rheum Dis 51:1001, 1992.

81. Goldsmith GH Jr, Baily RG, Brettler DB, et al: Primary pulmonary hypertension in patients with classic hemophilia. Ann Intern Med 108:797, 1988.

82. Gomez-Sanchez MA, Mestre de Juan MJ, Gomez-Pajuelo C, et al: Pulmonary hypertension due to toxic oil syndrome. A clinicopathologic study. Chest 95:325, 1989.

83. Hadengue A, Benhayoun MK, Lebrec D, Benhamou J-P: Pulmonary hypertension complicating portal hypertension: Prevalence and relation to splanchnic hemodynamics. Gastroenterology 100:520, 1991.

84. Heffelfinger S, Hawkins EP, Nihill M, Langston C: Pulmonary vascular changes associated with prolonged prostaglandin E_1 treatment. Pediatr Pathol 7:165, 1987.

85. Herrick MK, Chang Y, Horoupian DS, et al: L-tryptophan and the eosinophilia-myalgia syndrome: Pathologic findings in eight patients. Hum Pathol 22:12, 1991.

86. Jacques C, Richmond G, Tierney L, et al: Primary pulmonary hypertension and human immunodeficiency virus infection in a non-hemophiliac man. Hum Pathol 23:191, 1992.

87. Keren G, Boichis H, Zwas TS, Frand M: Pulmonary arteriovenous fistulae in hepatic cirrhosis. Arch Dis Child 58:302, 1983.

88. Martyn JB, Wong MJ, Huang SHK: Pulmonary and neuromuscular complications of mixed connective tissue disease: A report and review of the literature. J Rheumatol 15:703, 1988.

89. Matsubara O, Nakamura T, Uehara T, Kasuga T:

Histometrical investigation of the pulmonary artery in severe hepatic disease. J Pathol 143:31, 1984.

90. McDonnell PJ, Toye PA, Hutchins GM: Primary pulmonary hypertension and cirrhosis: Are they related? Am Rev Respir Dis 127:437, 1983.

91. Mehta NJ, Khan IA, Mehta RN, Sepkowitz DA: HIV-related pulmonary hypertension. Analytic review of 131 cases. Chest 118:1133, 2000.

92. Mesa RA, Edell ES, Dunn WF, Edwards WD: Human immunodeficiency virus infection and pulmonary hypertension: Two new cases and a review of 86 reported cases. Mayo Clin Proc 73:37, 1998.

93. Molden D, Abraham JL: Pulmonary hypertension. Its association with hepatic cirrhosis and iron accumulation. Arch Pathol Lab Med 106:328, 1982.

94. Morrison EB, Gaffney FA, Eigenbrodt EH, et al: Severe pulmonary hypertension associated with macronodular (postnecrotic) cirrhosis and autoimmune phenomena. Am J Med 69:513, 1980.

95. Murray RJ, Smialek JE, Golle M, Albin RJ: Pulmonary artery medial hypertrophy in cocaine users without foreign particle microembolization. Chest 96:1050, 1989.

96. Nall KC, Rubin LJ, Lipskind S, Sennesh JD: Reversible pulmonary hypertension associated with anorexigen use. Am J Med 91:97, 1991.

97. Nunes H, Humbert M, Sitbon O, et al: Prognostic factors for survival in human immunodeficiency virus-associated pulmonary arterial hypertension. Am J Respir Crit Care Med 167:1433, 2003.

98. Opravil M, Pechère, Speich R, et al: HIV-associated primary pulmonary hypertension. A case control study. Am J Respir Crit Care Med 155:990, 1997.

99. Polos PG, Wolfe D, Harley RA, et al: Pulmonary hypertension and human immunodeficiency virus infection. Two reports and a review of the literature. Chest 101:474, 1992.

100. Quismorio FP Jr, Sharma O, Koss M, et al: Immunopathologic and clinical studies in pulmonary hypertension associated with systemic lupus erythematosus. Semin Arthritis Rheum 13:349, 1984.

101. Rich S, Rubin L, Walker AM, et al: Anorexigens and pulmonary hypertension in the United States. Results from the surveillance of North American pulmonary hypertension. Chest 117:870, 2000.

102. Ruttner JR, Bartschi JP, Niedermann R, et al: Plexogenic pulmonary arteriopathy and liver cirrhosis. Thorax 35:133, 1980.

103. Schaiberger PH, Kennedy TC, Miller FC: Pulmonary hypertension associated with long term inhalation of "crack" methamphetamine. Chest 104:614, 1993.

104. Stupi AM, Steen VD, Owens GR, et al: Pulmonary hypertension in the crest syndrome variant of systemic sclerosis. Arthritis Rheum 29:515, 1986.

105. Tazelaar HD, Myers JL, Drage CW, et al: Pulmonary disease associated with L-tryptophan-induced eosinophilic myalgia syndrome. Clinical and pathologic features. Chest 97:1032, 1990.

106. Yutani C, Imakita M, Ishibashi-Ueda H, et al: Nodular regenerative hyperplasia of the liver associated with primary pulmonary hypertension. Hum Pathol 19:726, 1988.

Persistent Hypertension of Newborn

107. Morin FC, Stenmark KR: Persistent pulmonary hypertension of the newborn. Am J Respir Crit Care Med 151:2010, 1995.

108. Murphy J, Rabinovitch M, Goldstein J, et al: The structural basis of persistent pulmonary hypertension of the newborn infant. J Pediatr 98:962, 1981.

Pulmonary Venoocclusive Disease

109. Cagle P, Langston C: Pulmonary veno-occlusive disease as a cause of sudden infant death. Arch Pathol Lab Med 108:338, 1984.

110. Carrington CB, Liebow AA: Pulmonary veno-occlusive disease. Hum Pathol 1:322, 1970.

111. Corrin B, Spencer H, Turner-Warwick M, et al: Pulmonary venoocclusion – an immune complex disease? Virchows Arch A Pathol Anat Histol 364:81, 1974.

112. Daroca PM Jr, Mansfield RE, Ichinose H: Pulmonary veno-occlusive disease: Report of a case with pseudoangiomatous features. Am J Surg Pathol 1:349, 1977.

113. Hasleton PS, Ironside JW, Whittaker JS, et al: Pulmonary veno-occlusive disease. A report of four cases. Histopathology 10:933, 1986.

114. Holcomb BW, Loyd JE, Ely EW, et al: Pulmonary veno-occlusive disease. A case series and new observations. Chest 118:1671, 2000.

115. Katz DS, Scalzetti EM, Katzenstein A-LA, Kohman LJ: Pulmonary veno-occlusive disease presenting with thrombosis of pulmonary arteries. Thorax 50:699, 1995.

116. Kay JM, De Sa DJ, Mancer JFK: Ultrastructure of lung in pulmonary veno-occlusive disease. Hum Pathol 14:45, 1983.

117. Lang I, Kurmets R, Mlczoch J, et al: Pulmonary veno-occlusive disease in a patient with unilateral absence of right pulmonary artery. Chest 93:1307, 1988.

118. Lombard CM, Churg A, Winokur S: Pulmonary veno-occlusive disease following therapy for malignant neoplasms. Chest 92:871, 1987.

119. Mandel J, Mark EJ, Hales CA: Pulmonary veno-occlusive disease. Am J Respir Crit Care Med 162:1964, 2000.

120. Paakko P, Sutinen S, Remes M, et al: A case of pulmonary vascular occlusive disease: Comparison of post-mortem radiography and histology. Histopathology 9:253, 1985.

121. Pai U, McMahon J, Tomashefski JF Jr: Mineralizing pulmonary elastosis in chronic cardiac failure: "Endogenous pneumoconiosis" revisited. Am J Clin Pathol 101:22, 1994.

122. Pajewski M, Reif R, Manor H, et al: Pulmonary veno-occlusive disease in unilateral hypertransradiant lung. Thorax 36:397, 1981.

123. Palevsky HI, Pietra GG, Fishman AP: Pulmonary veno-occlusive disease and its response to vasodilator agents. Am Rev Respir Dis 142:426, 1990.

124. Runo JR, Vnencak-Jones CL, Prince M, et al: Pulmonary veno-occlusive disease caused by an inherited mutation in bone morphogenetic protein receptor II. Am J Respir Crit Care Med 167:889, 2003.

125. Salzman GA, Rosa UW: Prolonged survival in pulmonary veno-occlusive disease treated with nifedipine. Chest 95:1154, 1989.

126. Stoler MH, Anderson VM, Stuard ID: A case of pulmonary veno-occlusive disease in infancy. Arch Pathol Lab Med 106:645, 1982.

127. Troussard X, Bernaudin JF, Cordonnier C, et al: Pulmonary veno-occlusive disease after bone marrow transplantation. Thorax 39:956, 1984.

128. Voordes CG, Kuipers JRG, Elema JN: Familial pulmonary veno-occlusive disease: A case report. Thorax 32:763, 1977.

129. Wagenvoort CA, Wagenvoort P, Takahashi T: Pulmonary veno-occlusive disease: Involvement of pulmonary arteries and review of the literature. Hum Pathol 16:1033, 1985.

130. Williams LM, Fussell S, Veith RW, et al: Pulmonary veno-occlusive disease in an adult following bone marrow transplantation: Case report and review of the literature. Chest 109:1388, 1996.

Capillary Hemangiomatosis

131. Almagro P, Julia J, Sanjaume M, et al: Pulmonary capillary hemangiomatosis associated with primary pulmonary hypertension; report of 2 new cases and review of 35 cases from the literature. Medicine (Baltimore) 81:417, 2002.

132. Domingo C, Encabo B, Roig J, et al: Pulmonary capillary hemangiomatosis: Report of a case and review of the literature. Respiration 59:178, 1992.

133. Eltorky MA, Headley AS, Winer-Muram H, et al: Pulmonary capillary hemangiomatosis: A clinicopathologic review. Ann Thorac Surg 57:772, 1994.

134. Erbersdobler A, Niendorf A: Multifocal distribution of pulmonary capillary haemangiomatosis. Histopathology 49:88, 2002.

135. Faber CN, Yousem SA, Dauber JH, et al: Pulmonary capillary hemangiomatosis. A report of three cases and a review of the literature. Am Rev Respir Dis 140:808, 1989.

136. Ginns LC, Roberts DH, Mark EJ, et al: Pulmonary capillary hemangiomatosis with atypical endotheliomatosis. Successful antiangiogenic therapy with doxycycline. Chest 124:2017, 2003.

137. Havlik DM, Massie LW, Williams WL, Crooks LA: Pulmonary capillary hemangiomatosis-like foci. An autopsy study of 8 cases. Am J Clin Pathol 113:655, 2000.

138. Heath D, Reid R: Invasive pulmonary haemangiomatosis. Br J Dis Chest 79:284, 1985.

139. Jing X, Yokoi T, Nakamura Y, et al: Pulmonary capillary hemangiomatosis. A unique feature of congestive vasculopathy associated with hypertrophic cardiomyopathy. Arch Pathol Lab Med. 122:94, 1998.

140. Langleben D, Heneghan JM, Batten AP, et al: Familial pulmonary capillary hemangiomatosis resulting in primary pulmonary hypertension. Ann Intern Med 109:106, 1988.

141. Oviedo A, Abramson LP, Worthington R, et al: Congenital pulmonary capillary hemangiomatosis: Report of two cases and review of the literature. Pediatr Pulmonol 36:253, 2003.

142. Pycock CJ, Thomas AJ, Marshall AJ, Scarratt W: Capillary haemangiomatosis: A rare cause of pulmonary hypertension. Respir Med 88:153, 1994.

143. Tron V, Magee F, Wright JL, et al: Pulmonary capillary hemangiomatosis. Hum Pathol 17:1144, 1986.

144. White CW, Sondheimer HM, Crouch EC, et al: Treatment of pulmonary hemangiomatosis with recombinant interferon alfa-2a. N Engl J Med 320:1197, 1989.

145. Whittaker JS, Pickering CAC, Heath D, Smith P: Pulmonary capillary haemangiomatosis. Diagn Histopathol 6:77, 1983.

Other Causes of Pulmonary Venous Hypertension

146. Chazova I, Robbins I, Loyd J, et al: Venous and arterial changes in pulmonary veno-occlusive disease, mitral stenosis and fibrosing mediastinitis. Eur Respir J 15:116, 2000.

147. Espinosa RE, Edwards WD, Rosenow EC, Schaff HV: Idiopathic pulmonary hilar fibrosis: An unusual cause of pulmonary hypertension. Mayo Clin Proc 68:778, 1993.

148. Hutchins GM, Ostrow PT: The pathogenesis of the two forms of hypertensive pulmonary vascular disease. Am Heart J 92:797, 1976.

149. Katzenstein A-LA, Mazur MT: Pulmonary infarct: An unusual manifestation of fibrosing mediastinitis. Chest 77:521, 1980.

150. Kelley KM, Cheatham JP, Kugler JD, et al: Postnatal atresia of extraparenchymal pulmonary veins, fulminant necrotizing pulmonary arteritis and elevated circulatory immune complexes. J Am Coll Cardiol 9:1043, 1987.

151. Presbitero P, Bull C, Macartney FJ: Stenosis of pulmonary veins with ventricular septal defect. A cause of premature pulmonary hypertension in infancy. Br Heart J 49:600, 1983.

152. Wagenvoort CA: Pathology of congestive pulmonary hypertension. Prog Respir Res 9:195, 1975.

153. Wagenvoort CA, Wagenvoort N: Smooth muscle content and pulmonary arterial media in pulmonary venous hypertension compared with other forms of pulmonary hypertension. Chest 81:581, 1982.

Pulmonary Hypertension Due to Lung Disease

154. Cullinane C, Cox PN, Silver MM: Persistent pulmonary hypertension of the newborn due to alveolar capillary dysplasia. Pediatr Pathol 12:499, 1992.

155. Fernie JM, McLean A, Lamb D: Significant intimal abnormalities in muscular pulmonary arteries of patients with early obstructive lung disease. J Clin Pathol 41:730, 1988.

156. Janney CG, Askin FB, Kuhn CK III: Congenital alveolar capillary dysplasia – an unusual cause of respiratory distress in the newborn. Am J Clin Pathol 76:722, 1981.

157. Kessler R, Faller M, Weitzenblum E, et al: "Natural history" of pulmonary hypertension in a series of 131 patients with chronic obstructive lung disease. Am J Respir Crit Care Med 164:219, 2001.

158. Magee F, Wright JL, Wiggs BR, et al: Pulmonary vascular structure and function in chronic obstructive pulmonary disease. Thorax 43:183, 1988.

159. Wagenvoort, CA: Medial defects of lung vessels: A new cause of pulmonary hypertension. Hum Pathol 17:722, 1986.

160. Wagenvoort CA: Misalignment of lung vessels: A syndrome causing persistent neonatal pulmonary hypertension. Hum Pathol 17:727, 1986.

161. Wilkinson M, Landhorne CA, Heath D, et al: A pathophysiological study of 10 cases of hypoxic cor pulmonale. Q J Med 66:65, 1988.

162. Wright JL, Lawson L, Pare PD, et al: The structure and function of the pulmonary vasculature in mild chronic obstructive pulmonary disease. The effect of oxygen and exercise. Am Rev Respir Dis 128:702, 1983.

Pulmonary Hypertension Due to Alveolar Hypoxia

163. Ahmed Q, Chung-Park M, Tomashefski JF: Cardiopulmonary pathology in patients with sleep apnea/obesity hypoventilation syndrome. Hum Pathol 28:264, 1997.

164. Heath D, Williams D, Rios-Dalenz J, et al: Small pulmonary arterial vessels of Aymara Indians from the Bolivian Andes. Histopathology 16:565, 1990.

165. Wagenvoort CA, Wagenvoort N: Pulmonary venous changes in chronic hypoxia. Virchows Arch A Pathol Anat Histol 372:51, 1976.

166. Wagenvoort CA, Wagenvoort N: Pulmonary veins in high-altitude residents: A morphometric study. Thorax 37:931, 1982.

Chronic Thromboembolic Occlusion of Main Pulmonary Arteries

167. Auger WR, Fedullo PF, Moser KM, et al: Chronic major-vessel thromboembolic pulmonary artery obstruction: Appearance at angiography. Radiology 182:393, 1992.

168. Blauwet LA, Edwards WD, Tazelaar HD, et al: Surgical pathology of pulmonary thromboendarterectomy: A study of 54 cases from 1990 to 2001. Hum Pathol 34:1290, 2003.

169. Fedullo PF, Auger WR, Kerr KM, Rubin LJ: Chronic thromboembolic pulmonary hypertension. N Engl J Med 345:1465, 2001.

170. Kimura H, Okada O, Tanabe N, et al: Plasma monocyte chemoattractant protein-1 and pulmonary vascular resistance in chronic thromboembolic pulmonary hypertension. Am J Resp Crit Care Med 164:319, 2001.

171. Moser KM, Auger WA, Fedullo PF: Chronic major vessel thromboembolic pulmonary hypertension. Circulation 81:1735, 1990.

172. Moser KM, Bloor CM: Pulmonary vascular lesions occurring in patients with chronic major vessel thromboembolic pulmonary hypertension. Chest 103:685, 1993.

173. Presti B, Berthrong M, Sherwin RM: Chronic thrombosis of major pulmonary arteries. Hum Pathol 21:601, 1990.

174. Shuck J, Walder J, Kam T, Thomas H: Chronic persistent pulmonary embolism. Report of three cases. Am J Med 69:790, 1980.

Thrombotic Pulmonary Hypertension

175. D'Alonzo GE, Bower JS, Dantzker DR: Differentiation of patients with primary and thromboembolic pulmonary hypertension. Chest 85:457, 1984.

176. Rich S, Levitsky S, Brundage BH: Pulmonary hypertension from chronic pulmonary thromboembolism. Ann Intern Med 108:425, 1988.

177. Wagenvoort CA: Lung biopsies in the differential diagnosis of thromboembolic versus primary pulmonary hypertension. Prog Respir Res 13:16, 1980.

Drug Abuser's Lung

178. Farber HW, Fairman RP, Glausner FL: Talc granulomatosis: Laboratory findings similar to sarcoidosis. Am Rev Respir Dis 125:258, 1982.

179. Ganesan S, Felo J, Saldana M, et al: Embolized crospovidone (poly[N-vinyl-2-pyrrolidone]) in the lungs of intravenous drug users. Mod Pathol 16:286, 2003.

180. Padley SPG, Adler BD, Staples CA, et al: Pulmonary talcosis: CT findings in three cases. Radiology 186:125, 1993.

181. Pare JP, Cote G, Fraser RS: Long-term follow-up of drug abusers with intravenous talcosis. Am Rev Respir Dis 139:233, 1989.

182. Pare JP, Fraser RG, Hogg JC, et al: Pulmonary "mainline" granulomatosis: Talcosis of intravenous methadone abuse. Medicine (Baltimore) 58:229, 1979.

183. Siegel H: Human pulmonary pathology associated with narcotic and other addictive drugs. Hum Pathol 3:55, 1972.

184. Tomashefski JR Jr, Hirsch CS: The pulmonary vascular lesions of intravenous drug abuse. Hum Pathol 11:133, 1980.

185. Tomashefski JR Jr, Hirsch CS, Jolly PN: Microcrystalline cellulose pulmonary embolism and granulomatosis. A complication of illicit intravenous injections of pentazocine tablets. Arch Pathol Lab Med 105:89, 1981.

186. Zeltner TB, Nussbaumer U, Rudin O, Zimmerman A: Unusual pulmonary vascular lesions after intravenous injections of microcrystalline cellulose. A complication of pentazocine tablet abuse. Virchows Arch A Pathol Anat Histol 395:207, 1982.

Pulmonary Hypertension Due to Tumor and Other Emboli

187. Bowen JH, Woodard BH, Barton TK, et al: Infantile pulmonary hypertension associated with foreign body vasculitis. Am J Clin Pathol 75:609, 1981.

188. Brisbane JU, Howell DA, Bonkowsky HL: Pulmonary hypertension as a presentation of hepatocarcinoma. Report of a case and brief review of the literature. Am J Med 68:466, 1980.

189. Chakeres DW, Spiegel PK: Fatal pulmonary hypertension secondary to intravascular metastatic tumor emboli. AJR Am J Roentgenol 139:997, 1982.

190. Fanta CH, Compton CC: Microscopic tumour emboli to the lungs: A hidden cause of dyspnea and pulmonary hypertension. Thorax 43:794, 1980.

191. Fitzpatrick TM, Covelli HD, Tenholder MF: The acute and insidious onset of pulmonary metastatic transitional cell carcinoma. Chest 99:498, 1991.

192. Kupari M, Laitinen L, Kekali P, Luomanmaki K: Cor pulmonale due to tumor cell embolization. Report of a case and brief review of the literature. Acta Med Scand 210:507, 1981.

193. Schriner RW, Ryu JH, Edwards WD: Microscopic pulmonary tumor embolism causing subacute cor pulmonale: A difficult antemortem diagnosis. Mayo Clin Proc 66:143, 1991.

194. Soares FA, Landell GAM, de Oliveira JAM: Pulmonary tumor embolism to alveolar septal capillaries: A prospective study of 12 cases. Arch Pathol Lab Med 115:127, 1991.

195. Soares FA, Landell GAM, de Oliveira JAM: A prospective study of the morphological aspects of tumor involvement of the pulmonary vessels. Pathology 24:150, 1992.

196. Veinot JP, Ford SE, Price RG: Subacute cor pulmonale due to tumor embolization. Arch Pathol Lab Med 116:131, 1992.

197. von Herbay A, Illes A, Waldherr R, Otto HF: Pulmonary tumor thrombotic microangiopathy with pulmonary hypertension. Cancer 66:587, 1990.

198. Wakasa K, Sakurai M, Uchida A, et al: Massive pulmonary tumor emboli in osteosarcoma: Occult and fatal complication. Cancer 66:583, 1990.

199. Willett IR, Sutherland RC, O'Rourke MK, Dudley FJ: Pulmonary hypertension complicating hepatocellular carcinoma. Gastroenterology 87:1180, 1984.

Pulmonary Emboli and Infarcts

200. Balogh K: Pulmonary bile emboli. Sequelae of iatrogenic trauma. Arch Pathol Lab Med 108:814, 1984.

201. Chen YM, Lu C-C, Perng RP: Silicone fluid-induced pulmonary embolism. Am Rev Respir Dis 147:1299, 1993.

202. Chung KY, Se HK, Kwon H, et al: Clinicopathologic review of pulmonary silicone embolism with special emphasis on the resultant histologic diversity in the lung – a review of five cases. Yonsei Med J 43:152, 2002.

203. Dalen JE, Haffajee CI, Alpert JS, et al: Pulmonary embolism, pulmonary hemorrhage and pulmonary infarction. N Engl J Med 296:1431, 1977.

204. Dimmick JE, Bove KE, McAdams AJ, et al: Fiber embolization – a hazard of cardiac surgery and catheterization. N Engl J Med 292:685, 1975.

205. Dorfman GS, Cronan JJ, Tupper TB, et al: Occult pulmonary embolism: A common occurrence in deep venous thrombosis. AJR Am J Roentgenol 148:263, 1987.

206. Garland IWC, Thompson WP: Diagnosis of amniotic fluid embolism using an antiserum to keratin. J Clin Pathol 36:625, 1983.

207. Hardin L, Fox LS, O'Quinn AG: Amniotic fluid embolism. South Med J 84:1046, 1991.

208. Hulman G, Levene M: Intralipid microemboli. Arch Dis Child 61:702, 1986.

209. Kitchell CC, Balogh K: Pulmonary lipid emboli in association with long-term hyperalimentation. Hum Pathol 17:83, 1986.

210. Kobayashi H, Ooi H, Hayakawa H, et al: Histological diagnosis of amniotic fluid embolism by monoclonal antibody TKH-2 that recognizes NeuAc α 2-6GalNAc epitope. Hum Pathol 28:428, 1997.

211. Libby LS, King TE, LaForce FM, Schwarz MI: Pulmonary cavitation following pulmonary infarction. Medicine (Baltimore) 64:342, 1985.

212. Masson RG, Ruggiere J: Pulmonary microvascular cytology. A new diagnostic application of the pulmonary artery catheter. Chest 88:908, 1985.

213. Moser KM: Venous thromboembolism. Am Rev Respir Dis 141:235, 1990.

214. Parambil JG, Savci CD, Tazelaar HD, Ryu JH: Causes and presenting features of pulmonary infarctions in 43 cases identified by surgical lung biopsy. Chest 127:1178, 2005.

215. Pastore L, Kessler S: Pulmonary fat embolization in the immunocompromised patient. Its relationship to steroid medication. Am J Surg Pathol 6:315, 1982.

216. Price TP, Baker VV, Cefalo RC: Amniotic fluid embolism. Three case reports with a review of the literature. Obstet Gynecol Surv 40:462, 1985.

217. Rosen JM, Braman SS, Hassan FM, Teplitz C: Nontraumatic fat embolization. A rare cause of new pulmonary infiltrates in an immunocompromised patient. Am Rev Respir Dis 134:805, 1986.

218. Schmid A, Tzur A, Leshko L, Krieger BP: Silicone embolism syndrome. A case report, review of the literature, and comparison with fat embolism syndrome. Chest 127:2276, 2005.

219. Schulman RJ, Langston C, Schanler RJ: Pulmonary vascular lipid deposition after administration of intravenous fat to infants. Pediatrics 79:99, 1987.

220. Stocker JT, McGill LC, Orsini EN: Post-infarction peripheral cysts of the lung in pediatric patients: A possible cause of idiopathic spontaneous pneumothorax. Pediatr Pulmonol 1:7, 1985.

221. Tsao M-S, Schraufnagel D, Wang N-S: Pathogenesis of pulmonary infarction. Am J Med 72:599, 1982.

222. Vogler C, Sotelo-Avila C, Lagunoff D, et al: Aluminum-containing emboli in infants treated with extracorporeal membrane oxygenation. N Engl J Med 319:75, 1988.

223. Wagenvoort CA: Pathology of pulmonary thromboembolism. Chest 107:10S, 1995.

224. Ziadlourad F, Conklin KA: Amniotic fluid embolism. Semin Anesth 6:171, 1987.

Pulmonary Arteriovenous Malformations

225. Burke CM, Safai C, Nelson DP, Raffin TA: Pulmonary arteriovenous malformation: A critical update. Am Rev Respir Dis 134:334, 1986.

226. Chin RCJ, Herba MJ, Viloria J, Mulder DS: Thoracopulmonary hypogenesis with systemic artery-pulmonary vessel fistulae: Report of a case. Ann Thorac Surg 31:360, 1981.

227. Cottin V, Plauchu H, Bayle J-Y, et al: Pulmonary arteriovenous malformations in patients with hereditary hemorrhagic telangiectasia. Am J Respir Crit Care Med. 169:994, 2004.

228. Dines DE, Seward JB, Bernatz PC: Pulmonary arteriovenous fistulas. Mayo Clin Proc 58:176, 1983.

229. Gossage JR, Kanj G: Pulmonary arteriovenous malformations. A state of the art review. Am J Respir Crit Care Med 158:643, 1998.

230. Hearne SF, Burbank MK: Internal mammary artery-to-pulmonary artery fistulas. Case report and review of the literature. Circulation 62:1131, 1980.

231. Knoepfli HJ, Friedl B: Systemic-to-pulmonary artery fistula following actinomycosis. Chest 67:494, 1975.

232. Lundell C, Finch E: Arteriovenous fistulas originating from Rasmussen aneurysm. AJR Am J Roentgenol 140:687, 1983.

233. Remy J, Remy-Jardin M, Wattinne L, Deffontaines C: Pulmonary arteriovenous malformations: Evaluation with CT of the chest before and after treatment. Radiology 182:809, 1992.

234. Robinson LA, Sabiston DC Jr: Syndrome of congenital internal mammary-to-pulmonary arteriovenous fistula associated with mitral valve prolapse. Arch Surg 116:1265, 1981.

235. Symbas PN, Goldman M, Erbesfeld MH, et al: Pulmonary arteriovenous fistula, pulmonary artery aneurysm, and other vascular changes of the lung from penetrating trauma. Ann Surg 191:366, 1980.

236. Taylor GA: Pulmonary arteriovenous malformation: An uncommon cause for cyanosis in the newborn. Pediatr Radiol 13:339, 1983.

237. Trell E, Johansson BW, Linell F, et al: Familial pulmonary hypertension and multiple abnormalities of large systemic arteries in Osler's disease. Am J Med 53:50, 1972.

238. White RI Jr, Michell SE, Barth KH, et al: Angioarchitecture of pulmonary arteriovenous malformations: An important consideration before embolotherapy. AJR Am J Roentgenol 140:681, 1983.

Pulmonary Artery Aneurysms

239. Barrter T, Irwin RS, Nash G: Aneurysms of the pulmonary arteries. Chest 94:1065, 1988.

240. Butto F, Lucas RV Jr, Edwards JE: Pulmonary arterial aneurysm. A pathologic study of five cases. Chest 91:237, 1987.

241. Coffey MJ, Fantone J III, Stirling MC, Lynch JP III: Pseudoaneurysm of pulmonary artery in mucormycosis. Radiographic characteristics and management. Am Rev Respir Dis 145:1487, 1992.

242. Inayama Y, Nakatani Y, Kitamura H: Pulmonary artery dissection in patients without underlying pulmonary hypertension. Histopathology 38:435, 2001.

243. Navarro C, Dickinson PCT, Koondlapoodi P, Hagstrom JWC: Mycotic aneurysms of the pulmonary arteries in intravenous drug addicts. Report of three cases and review of the literature. Am J Med 76:1124, 1984.

244. San Dretto MA, Scanlon GT: Multiple mycotic pulmonary artery aneurysms secondary to intravenous drug abuse. AJR Am J Roentgenol 142:89, 1984.

245. Steurer J, Jenni R, Medici TC, et al: Dissecting aneurysm of the pulmonary artery with pulmonary hypertension. Am Rev Respir Dis 142:1219, 1990.

246. Stricker H, Malinverni R: Multiple, large aneurysms of pulmonary arteries in Behçet's disease. Clinical remission and radiologic resolution after corticosteroid therapy. Arch Intern Med 149:925, 1989.

247. Symbas PN, Goldman M, Erbesfeld MH, et al: Pulmonary arteriovenous fistula, pulmonary artery aneurysm, and other vascular changes of the lung from penetrating trauma. Ann Surg 191:366, 1980.

PEDIATRIC DISORDERS

This chapter reviews the pulmonary conditions occurring primarily in infants and children that are likely to be encountered by the surgical pathologist. Congenital malformations comprise the main entities, while a few lesions are acquired in the neonatal period.[1–7] Interstitial lung disease occurring in childhood is also reviewed, with emphasis on those lesions that differ from adult diseases. Conditions that are seen mainly in autopsy specimens are not discussed but can be found in other reviews.[1,2,4,6]

PULMONARY SEQUESTRATION

Pulmonary sequestration is defined as a mass of abnormal pulmonary tissue that lacks communication with the tracheobronchial tree through normally located bronchi and receives its blood supply from one or more anomalous systemic arteries.[1–3,35] Intralobar sequestrations occur within the visceral pleural lining of a pulmonary lobe, and extralobar sequestrations are found outside of this pleural investment. Both types of sequestration most commonly occur on the left side. Either type rarely may have a connection to the esophagus or stomach,[16,20,24,32,40] and congestive heart failure related to arteriovenous shunting has been associated with both. In a small number of cases, intralobar and extralobar sequestration have occurred together. The two forms of sequestration are discussed separately because there are important differences in the clinical, anatomic, and histologic features of each (Table 14–1).

Intralobar Sequestration

Intralobar sequestrations are found within the substance of the lung, and are usually (90% of cases) located in a lower lobe. About 60% involve the left side in the posterior basal segment. Bilateral lesions have been reported rarely.[11,33] The blood supply is usually provided by one or more elastic systemic arteries arising from the thoracic aorta, but origin of the vascular supply

Table 14-1 Contrasting Features of Intralobar and Extralobar Sequestrations*

	Intralobar	Extralobar
Age at diagnosis	50% >20 years	60% <1 year
Sex distribution	M:F = 1:1	M:F = 3–4:1
Relation to lung	Within	Separate (outside of visceral pleura)
Side affected	Left, 60%	Left, 90%
Venous drainage	Pulmonary	Systemic or portal
Associated anomalies	Rare	Present in 50% (pectus excavatum, diaphragmatic defects, cardiovascular malformations)
Pathogenesis	Acquired or congenital	Congenital

*Adapted from references 1–3, 35.

from beneath the diaphragm (aorta or celiac axis) is not uncommon. Generally, there is vascular drainage to the pulmonary venous system of the affected lobe, although systemic venous drainage may occur.[3,8,39]

Clinical Features

Many cases of intralobar sequestration occur in children, but at least one-half of patients are over 20 years of age at the time of diagnosis.[3,26,35,37] The incidence is equal in both sexes. Symptomatic patients present with recurrent pulmonary infection, cough, or chest pain. Up to one-third of patients are asymptomatic, and the sequestration is discovered on a routine chest film. Radiographically, the lesion may appear as a discrete mass, an inhomogeneous density, or one or more cysts with an air–fluid level. Bronchography generally fails to fill the sequestration. There is usually displacement of the adjacent bronchi by the lesion but no reduction in the number of segmental branches to the involved lobe. Angiography reveals the abnormal vascular supply and is especially useful for identifying cases in which there is an infradiaphragmatic origin of the vascular pedicle.

Gross and Histologic Features

In most cases of intralobar sequestration, the operative specimen is an entire pulmonary lobe, although segmental resections have been performed. The sequestration usually appears grossly as an ill-defined, poorly circumscribed firm area in the parenchyma, with a variable cystic component (Fig. 14–1). The solid

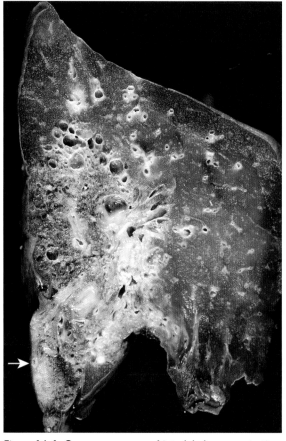

Figure 14–1 Gross appearance of intralobular sequestration. A mixture of solid and cystic areas that are poorly demarcated from adjacent lung is seen in this example. The feeding systemic artery is seen at lower left (arrow).

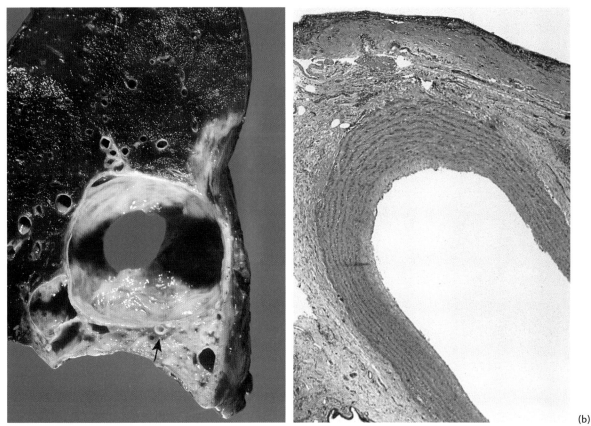

Figure 14–2 Cystic degeneration in intralobar sequestration. (a) This example is composed almost entirely of a large cyst with some residual inflamed and fibrotic parenchyma at the bottom. The systemic artery is seen beneath the cyst (arrow). **(b)** Low magnification microscopic view showing the systemic artery containing multiple elastic layers in the media. It is present adjacent to the cyst cavity.

portion varies from yellow to white depending on the proportion of inflammation and fibrosis. Cysts are usually small but may be the predominant finding in some cases (Fig. 14–2). The arterial supply forms a separate pedicle or hilus distinct from the normal bronchovascular structures and is easily recognized by its large size and thick wall. In older patients, the anomalous systemic artery is often markedly atherosclerotic. Dissection of the bronchi along probes (see Chapter 1) is helpful in demonstrating the lack of relationship of the sequestered area to the normal tracheobronchial tree.

The pathologic features of intralobar sequestration vary with the patient's age.[30,35] Because of the lack of communication with the normal tracheobronchial tree, the natural history of the disorder is one of continued accumulation of secretions accompanied by acute and chronic inflammation and infection. In younger children, the microscopic pattern is essentially that of normal distal lung parenchyma containing large, irregularly distributed, elastic arteries and their muscular branches. In these cases, a preoperative or specimen bronchogram or dissection of the bronchial tree along probes is necessary to confirm that the tissue is a true sequestration rather than a segment of otherwise normal lung supplied by systemic arteries.[15,18,25,44]

In older patients, the sequestration shows the effects of recurrent infection and obstructive pneumonia (Fig. 14–3). There are usually dense infiltrates of lymphocytes, plasma cells, and fibroblasts. Lipid-filled macrophages and giant cells are often prominent. Scarring may be so extensive that very little recognizable lung parenchyma remains and the end result may be a large multilocular cyst. Skeletal muscle fibers are sometimes found (so-called *rhabdomyomatous dysplasia*) (Fig. 14–4), although they are more common

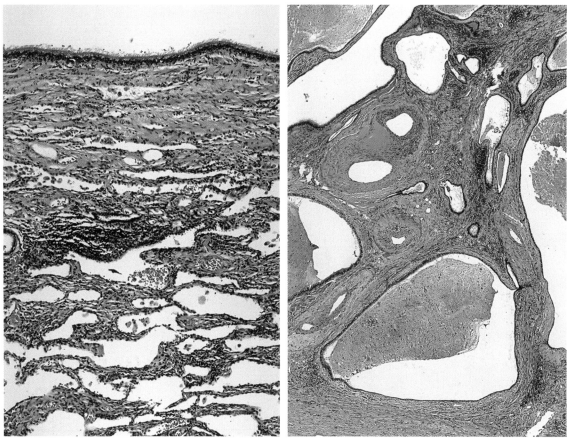

(a)   (b)

Figure 14-3 Microscopic findings in intralobar sequestration. Same case as in Figure 14-2. **(a)** Fibrosis and chronic inflammation are prominent in the interstitium adjacent to the cyst. **(b)** In this area there is destruction of parenchyma by scarring that surrounds residual bronchioles and altered airspaces. Note the medial and intimal hyperplasia in the arteries (center) that is indicative of pulmonary hypertension.

in extralobar sequestrations (see further on).[17] Vascular changes of pulmonary hypertension may be seen, including intimal and medial hypertrophy and even plexiform lesions, and are likely related to the systemic blood supply.[38] The main feeding systemic artery is usually identifiable by its size as well as the presence of multiple elastic layers in the media (see Fig. 14-2b).

Although large patent connections between classic intralobar sequestrations and the normal tracheobronchial tree are excluded by definition, some investigators have been able to demonstrate small areas of communication between the sequestered area and normal lung parenchyma.[1,2] Whether these communications precede or follow the inflammatory process is not clear, but their presence helps to explain the appearance of air–fluid levels in some sequestrations. They may also be one route of access for infectious agents.[42]

Extralobar Sequestration

Extralobar sequestration (accessory lung, Rokitansky's lobe) is separate from the lung, but has its own pleural investment. It occurs on the left side in over 90% of cases and usually appears in the lower hemithorax.[3,20,35] There are variations, including upper thoracic, paraesophageal, mediastinal, or paracardiac locations, and, in some cases, the lesion has occurred within substance of or below the diaphragm, including the retroperitoneum.[23,43] The blood supply generally is from anomalous systemic arteries, but, in contrast to intralobar sequestrations, venous drainage is usually through the systemic or portal venous system. The vascular routes may vary and include a blood supply from the pulmonary artery, venous drainage through the pulmonary system, or both. There is a frequent

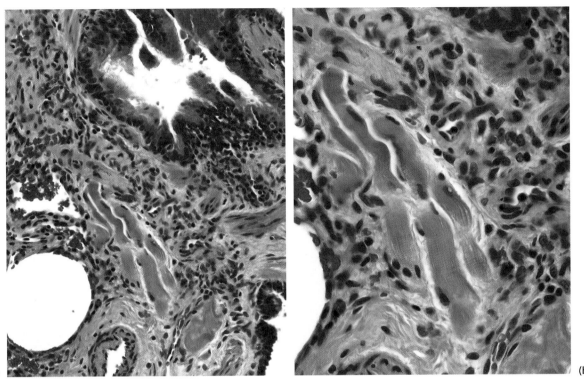

(a)

(b)

Figure 14–4 Skeletal muscle fibers in intralobar sequestration. (a) Low magnification showing skeletal muscle fibers in the interstitium between a bronchiole and its accompanying artery. (b) Higher magnification view showing the characteristic cross-striations. Skeletal muscle is found more commonly in extralobar than intralobar sequestration.

association with other congenital anomalies, especially ipsilateral congenital diaphragmatic defects, which occur in over half of the cases.[3,35] Funnel chest (pectus excavatum) is another associated anomaly,[3] and cardiovascular anomalies such as patent ductus arteriosus and ventricular septal defect occur less often.[26]

Clinical Features

The majority (60%) of extralobar sequestrations are found in children under 1 year of age, but the lesion occurs in older children and in adults as well.[3,35,37] There is a marked preponderance of cases in males. Extralobar sequestrations frequently are discovered incidentally during repair of a posterior diaphragmatic defect. A small number of the lesions are found on chest radiographs taken routinely or for some unrelated problem. Other patients are symptomatic as a result of recurrent infection. Radiographically, an extrapulmonary, intrathoracic radiodense mass is characteristic.[23] Because of the occasional mediastinal or hilar location of this anomaly, symptoms are sometimes due to bronchial obstruction with resultant congenital lobar

overinflation (see text following) or to compression of the normal pulmonary parenchyma.[22,43] Rarely, extralobar sequestrations may be associated with a large ipsilateral pleural effusion with mediastinal shift and ipsilateral pulmonary hypoplasia.[27] Massive hemothorax was the presenting manifestation in one adult.[9] Infarction of sequestrations has been reported.[29,35] Communication with the esophagus or stomach may be present and can lead to the development of air–fluid levels.[16,20,24,32]

Pathologic Features

Grossly, the extralobar sequestration is usually a spongy pyramidal mass of tissue with a complete pleural investment. The microscopic features depend on the patient's age. In young children, the lesion is composed either of histologically normal lung or of immature or dysplastic pulmonary parenchyma with minimal inflammation.[3,35] The last-mentioned feature is characterized by absent or reduced numbers of cartilaginous bronchi and an irregular proliferation of bronchiole-like structures resembling a congenital adenomatoid malformation (Fig. 14–5, see further on).[14,91] Striated

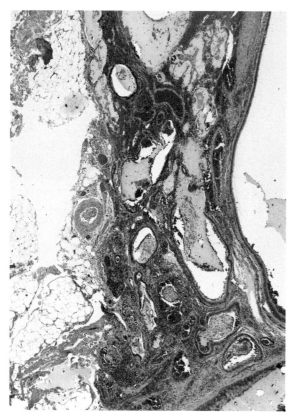

Figure 14–5 Extralobar sequestration. Low magnification view showing altered lung parenchyma adjacent to adipose tissue (left). This example was found near the adrenal gland.

muscle cells have been noted in some cases.[17] Septal interstitial edema and dilated lymphatics may be prominent in either microscopic pattern. In older patients, accumulation of secretions and recurrent infection may produce a multicystic lesion with chronically inflamed fibrotic stroma.

Pathogenesis of Sequestration

There is general agreement that extralobar sequestrations represent true congenital malformations that develop from an accessory lung bud arising from the primitive foregut.[1–3,12,20,35] By this theory, formation of the accessory bud occurs late in pulmonary organogenesis. The original communication to the foregut generally involutes, although occasionally it may persist as a patent connection to the esophagus or stomach. The systemic arterial supply is more difficult to explain, but it may represent the persistence of embryonic splanchnic plexus connections to the primitive foregut.

Controversy exists regarding the origin of intralobar sequestrations.[4] Some authors consider them to represent congenital anomalies analogous to extralobar sequestrations, the difference being that in intralobar sequestrations the accessory lung bud develops before the pleura is delineated.[30] Other authors, however, believe that the lesion is acquired postnatally and the systemic arterial supply develops secondary to chronic inflammation.[21,35] By this theory, chronic or recurrent infection in the lower lobe destroys the normal bronchial and pulmonary vascular connections and produces enlargement of small systemic arterial branches that are normally present in the inferior pulmonary ligament.[36] Some evidence exists in support of both mechanisms, and it may be that different cases have differing pathogenesis.[41]

Other Anomalies Related to Sequestration

The theory of abnormal lung bud origin suggests that pulmonary sequestrations may represent part of a spectrum of abnormalities ranging from bronchogenic or enteric-lined mediastinal or intrapulmonary cysts to sequestrations containing a central bronchial diverticulum and, ultimately, to complicated lesions communicating with the esophagus or stomach.[12,20,22,24] The term *bronchopulmonary foregut malformation*[20] has been suggested to encompass sequestration and all lesions with a connection to the upper gastrointestinal tract.

The *scimitar syndrome*, like sequestration, is characterized by a systemic vascular supply and absent bronchus. It derives its name from the radiographic picture produced by an anomalous vein that drains the right lung and enters the inferior vena cava.[19,39] The right lung is often smaller than the left and may have only a single lobe. In addition, the bronchus to the right upper lobe may be small or absent. The pulmonary artery is reduced in caliber, and an anomalous systemic arterial supply to the lower lobe occurs frequently. Dextroposition of the heart and congenital cardiac defects, especially atrial septal defect, are often present. Patients with this anomaly may be remarkably asymptomatic, but some present with either pulmonary hypertension[19] or repeated respiratory infection that may lead to resection of the abnormal lung. Venolobar syndrome is another term that has been utilized to encompass this syndrome and related entities.[13,31]

Total sequestration is a term that refers to a complex anomaly in which the lung is sequestered because the mainstem bronchus to the affected side originates from the esophagus instead of from the normal tracheobronchial tree.[3,10,28] The arterial supply may be either systemic or pulmonary in origin.

BRONCHOGENIC CYSTS

Bronchogenic, or bronchial, cysts usually occur in the subcarinal area or middle mediastinum, but they may be found in the lungs as well as below the diaphragm.[45,46,48-51] Similar lesions have also been noted in the subcutaneous tissue of the thorax.[47,52] Bronchogenic cysts presumably represent supernumerary lung buds from the primitive foregut, but, in contrast to sequestrations, they only rarely contain distal lung parenchyma.

Radiographically, most bronchogenic cysts in the mediastinum appear as homogeneous water-density masses with smooth margins. In the lung, air–fluid levels may be present, suggesting small communications with the surrounding parenchyma.[48] Cases are often detected incidentally on a chest radiograph taken for other reasons, although, in some instances, infection, rupture of the cyst, or compression of the normal tracheobronchial tree may lead to diagnosis. It is possible that some reported intrapulmonary bronchogenic cysts may actually represent type 1 congenital cystic adenomatoid malformations (see later on).

Pathologic Features

Microscopically, the cysts are usually lined by ciliated columnar epithelium with variable acute and chronic inflammation.[48,49,51] Areas of ulceration are common. The wall generally contains smooth muscle, cartilage, and bronchial glands, although multiple tissue sections may be needed in order to demonstrate these features. The cyst may be filled with clear or turbid and serous or viscous fluid, depending on the presence or absence of infection.

Differential Diagnosis

The differential diagnosis of bronchogenic cysts includes lung abscess (see Chapter 16), enteric cyst, esophageal cyst, and cystic teratoma. Since infection and inflammation may lead to squamous metaplasia in both the lining of a bronchogenic cyst and the inner wall of an abscess, the most reliable feature in distinguishing these two lesions is the frequent communication of multiple bronchi with the lumen of an abscess. In contrast to bronchogenic cysts, enteric cysts appear in the posterior mediastinum and are lined

by gastric epithelium. These lesions, which also arise as accessory buds or outpouchings of the foregut, may be associated with vertebral malformations.[48-50] In the area of the esophagus, bronchogenic cysts must also be separated from esophageal cysts. The latter can be recognized by a squamous epithelial lining and a double layer of muscle in a wall without cartilage.[48,49] Esophageal cysts probably do not represent abnormal foregut buds but apparently result from the persistence of vacuoles that form in the solid tube stage of the primitive esophagus and that, in normal development, coalesce longitudinally to form the esophageal lumen.[48] Adult cystic teratomas are usually found in the anterior mediastinum, although they rarely occur in the lung. They differ from bronchogenic cysts in that they are often multilocular and histologically show evidence of ectodermal and other endodermal derivatives, in addition to bronchial tissue.

MALFORMATIONS OF THE TRACHEOBRONCHIAL TREE

Bronchial anomalies and abnormalities of lobation are probably the most common congenital malformations of the lung.[3,66] Many of these lesions are anatomic curiosities, but some are of interest to the surgical pathologist. Certain abnormalities of the tracheobronchial tree are regularly associated with the asplenia syndrome and related cardiac defects.[3,65,66]

Displaced and Supernumerary Bronchi

Abnormally placed bronchi may be *displaced* and supply their usual pulmonary segment from an ectopic origin, or they may be *supernumerary*.[3,63,66,70] The tracheal bronchus[3,54] usually arises proximal to the carina and may supply either the apical segment or the entire upper lobe of either lung. The right tracheal bronchus may be supernumerary or displaced, but the less common left tracheal bronchus is described only as a displaced airway. Bilateral tracheal bronchi are rare.[59] In many cases, the tracheal bronchus is asymptomatic, but recurrent pneumonia and respiratory distress have been described in some patients. Associated tracheal stenosis may be present as well.[66,71,75] A supernumerary right tracheal bronchus with accessory lung tissue has been reported.[1,2] The anomalous origin of the anterior segmental bronchus of the right upper lobe from the middle lobe bronchus is a rare finding.[3,74] The accessory cardiac bronchus arises from the medial wall of the bronchus intermedius and forms a long or short diverticulum that supplies an accessory segment of lung. Recurrent pulmonary infection and hemoptysis, presumably a result of poor drainage, have been reported in patients with that anomaly.[3,72] The bridging bronchus[57,62] is a unique abnormality in which the bronchial supply of a portion of the right lung arises from the left mainstem bronchus.

Congenital Stenosis

Congenital stenosis of a mainstem bronchus is a rarely reported entity. In one case, a conical segment of bronchus with a small lumen and hypoplastic cartilage was found.[58] Atelectasis is the predominant clinical feature, in contrast to overinflation or focal mucoid impaction that results from stenosis or atresia of a segmental bronchus (see Regional Pulmonary Overinflation, later on).

Congenital Bronchiectasis

Congenital bronchiectasis is a disputed entity. Many cases may, in fact, be postinfectious in origin.[73] True congenital cases (also known as *tracheobronchomalacia*) likely are due to diffuse cartilage deficiency or immaturity, and in a strict sense should not be classified as bronchiectasis (see Chapter 16).[3,53,64] The few patients reported have had collapsible, ectatic bronchi with distal air trapping. Whether or not this lesion is the same as tracheobronchomegaly (Mounier–Kuhn syndrome)[1-3] is not clear, although that disorder involves larger airways than does congenital bronchiectasis. Similar changes have been reported in infants with bronchopulmonary dysplasia and other complications of hyaline membrane disease and likely are acquired rather than congenital.[61,64,76,77]

Fistulas

Tracheoesophageal or bronchoesophageal fistulas can occur with or without associated esophageal atresia.[3,56,69,78] Diagnostic tissue is not usually examined by the surgical pathologist, but cartilage abnormalities and squamous metaplasia have been described in autopsy studies.[78] Several cases of congenital tracheobiliary or bronchobiliary fistula have been reported.[60,67,68] The fistulous tract originates near the carina, and patients may produce yellow- or green-stained sputum. An apparently congenital bronchopleurocutaneous fistula has also been reported.[55]

CONGENITAL CYSTIC ADENOMATOID MALFORMATION

The congenital cystic adenomatoid malformation (CCAM) is seen most commonly in the lungs of infants and has features of both immaturity and malformation of the small airways and distal lung parenchyma.[1,2,4,86,96,105] Some authors prefer the term *congenital pulmonary airway malformation (CPAM)*.[5,104] Many lesions described in the past as congenital cystic disease, bronchiolectasis, and a variety of related names probably were adenomatoid malformations.[3,81,96,105] Most CCAMs occur in two distinct clinical settings: in a stillborn or extremely ill premature infant with anasarca or in a newborn infant who rapidly develops respiratory distress that is related to an expanding mass in one hemithorax. Less often, the lesion is seen in older children, and a few cases have been reported in adults.[80,90,93]

The radiographic appearance of CCAM is variable.[7] There may be a homogeneous mass, multiple air- or fluid-filled cysts, or a single or dominant radiolucent area.[96,105] Spontaneous pneumothorax is an unusual presenting feature.[89] The respiratory distress produced by the adenomatoid malformation is usually related either to tissue bulk or to air trapping within the lesion. In both instances, there is compression of the underlying normal lung parenchyma and even mediastinal shift. Circulatory symptoms occur because the mass obstructs the vena cava and interferes with venous return to the heart, producing anasarca. This fetal edema, and perhaps also the overproduction of lung fluid by the malformation, may contribute to the maternal hydramnios that is frequently seen as an obstetric complication.[105] The lesion may be diagnosed by antenatal ultrasound examination.[95,101,102] Elevation of maternal serum alpha fetoprotein (AFP) is sometimes an associated feature.[100]

Most CCAMs communicate with the normal tracheobronchial tree,[105] and air trapping presumably results from the usual lack of cartilaginous bronchi within the lesion. In some instances, however, there may be atresia of bronchi leading to the lesion.[83,97]

Pathologic Classification

CCAM is classified into five types based on gross and histologic features (Table 14–2).[4,5,85,88,94,104,105] This classification is useful both to emphasize the spectrum of pathologic findings in CCAM, and also to highlight

Type	Gross Appearance	Microscopic Appearance
0	Solid	Bronchial-like structures, abundant cartilage
1	Large, multilocular cysts 3–10 cm	Broad fibrous septa, mucigenic cells, focal cartilage in 5–10%
2	Small, uniform cysts <2 cm	Irregular proliferation of bronchiolar-like structures, may contain striated muscle
3	Solid, bulky lesion; cysts <0.2 cm	Irregular curved channels and small spaces lined by cuboidal epithelium
4	Large cysts, up to 7 cm, in peripheral lung	Thin-walled cysts lined by type 1 pneumocytes and low columnar epithelium, hypercellular stroma

Table 14–2 Congenital Adenomatoid Malformation*

*Adapted from references 4, 96, 104, 105.

certain associations among individual types. In our experience, however, some lesions may combine features of several types, and it can be difficult to pigeon-hole individual cases into a single subtype. Also, the classification may not be applicable to CCAMs occurring in immature lungs, a situation encountered following prenatal intrauterine surgery or in abortuses.[85] The utility of this classification system has been questioned by others as well, and some suggest lumping Types 1, 2, and 3 into a single category.[98,99]

Type 1 lesions are the most common, accounting for over half the cases.[94,102] Grossly, they are composed of one or more large cysts ranging from 3 to 10 cm in diameter (Fig. 14–6). Microscopically, there are fibrous septa lined by pseudostratified, ciliated columnar or cuboidal cells. Cartilaginous plates may be present focally in 5–10% of cases. In the more solid areas between the large cysts there are scattered bronchiole-like structures that differ from true bronchioles in that they are irregularly sized and shaped and they are not accompanied by an artery as would be expected in normal bronchioles (Fig. 14–7). Plump, mucus-filled cells may occur in clusters and are found in up to one-half of cases (Fig. 14–8). Histochemically, these cells resemble the goblet cells found in bronchial or intestinal mucous glands.[87] Morphologic features of adenocarcinoma, usually the bronchoalveolar variant, have been reported in association with Type 1 CCAM, but metastatic spread is extremely rare.[94,102]

Type 2 lesions are the second most common variant and are characterized grossly by multiple, evenly spaced cysts that are usually less than 2 cm in diameter (Fig. 14–9). They may be associated with other congenital anomalies, including renal agenesis, diaphragmatic hernia, cardiovascular anomalies, and extralobar sequestration.[92,96,105,106] Histologically, they are characterized by uniformly distributed small cysts lined by cuboidal to ciliated columnar epithelium that superficially resemble ectatic bronchioles, except that they are too numerous and, as in Type 1 lesions, are distributed randomly without an accompanying pulmonary artery

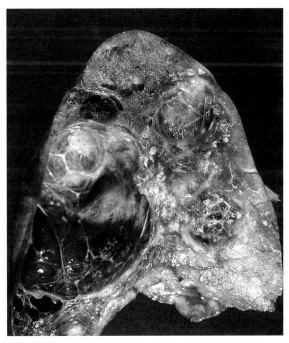

Figure 14–6 Gross appearance of Type 1 CCAM, showing large cysts replacing lung parenchyma.

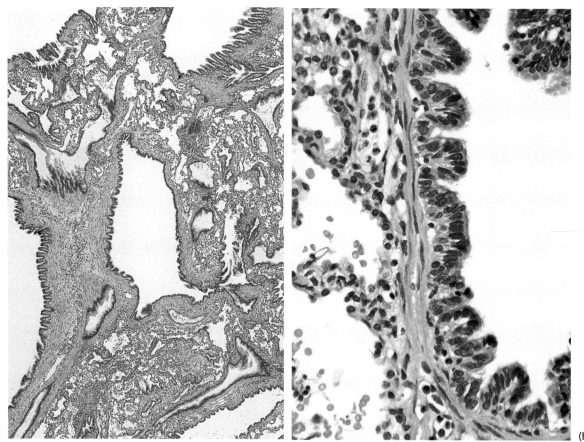

(a) (b)

Figure 14–7 Type 1 CCAM. (a) Low magnification photomicrograph showing cystic spaces lined by bronchiolar epithelium. Numerous smaller bronchiole-like structures are present among alveoli. They differ from normal bronchioles in that they are not accompanied by arteries. **(b)** Higher magnification showing the bronchiolar-type epithelial lining of the cysts. Smooth muscle is also present around the cyst in this example.

branch (Fig. 14–10). Striated muscle may be present in the septa or adjacent to the cysts.[17]

Type 3 CCAMs are uncommon. They occur almost exclusively in males and are usually associated with maternal polyhydramnios. Babies with this lesion are often stillborn or develop severe respiratory distress. They are characterized grossly by a firm or spongy mass of tissue in which macroscopic cysts are not readily found (Fig. 14–11). Microscopically, curved channels or microscopic cysts lined by cuboidal to low columnar epithelium are seen (Fig. 14–12). By both light and electron microscopy, this epithelium resembles that seen in late-intrauterine fetal lung. Bronchial structures are not present.

Type 0 and Type 4 CCAMs were added more recently to the original three types of CCAM and are extremely rare.[4] *Type 0* is felt to be a malformation of the proximal tracheobronchial tree and was previously termed *acinar dysplasia* or *agenesis*. It is incompatible with life and is often associated with cardiovascular, renal, and other abnormalities. Grossly, the lungs are small, firm, and granular appearing on cut section. Histologically, it is characterized by the presence of bronchial-like structures lined by respiratory epithelium and containing smooth muscle, glands, and cartilage in the walls. This variant may include previously described examples of Type 2 lesions containing unusually prominent cartilage formation.[81,96] *Type 4* CCAM is considered to represent a malformation of the distal acinus and is characterized by thin-walled cysts in the peripheral lung that are lined by type 1 alveolar pneumocytes and low cuboidal cells. Hypercellular stroma may sometimes be present, and the lesion may be difficult to distinguish from pleuropulmonary blastoma.[94] Tension

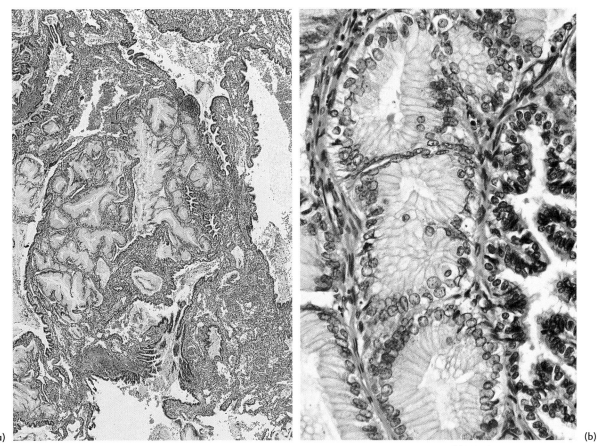

Figure 14–8 Mucigenic cells in CCAM. (a) Low magnification showing goblet-like cells in a Type 1 CCAM. **(b)** Higher magnification showing the bland-appearing goblet-like cells containing abundant apical mucin and basally located nuclei.

pneumothorax occurs in some infants, and is unique to this form of CCAM.

Pathogenesis

The pathogenesis of CCAM is unknown, but is thought to be related to defective lung development.[84,98] The absence of cartilage in most cases suggests that there is an embryologic insult before the sixteenth week of intrauterine life, by which time the cartilaginous bronchi are formed.[105] Other histologic aspects of the lesion suggest that there may be a focal overgrowth of bronchioles with the suppression of alveolar development.[96] There is also some evidence that the changes may occur secondary to bronchial atresia and other congenital and acquired lung lesions.[91,97] The variability in gross and microscopic appearance and a peripheral rim of more normal lung in most cases suggest that the lesion has some ability to undergo maturation.

CONGENITAL PULMONARY OVERINFLATION (EMPHYSEMA)

The term 'congenital pulmonary overinflation' denotes two entities (Table 14–3): (1) congenital lobar overinflation, in which an entire pulmonary lobe is overexpanded and compresses the remaining pulmonary parenchyma, and (2) regional or segmental pulmonary overinflation, in which a small segment of the lung is hyperinflated. There is no tissue destruction in the distal lung in either of these conditions, and, therefore, the term 'emphysema' is not strictly correct (see Chapter 16). Similar changes can sometimes develop postnatally (*acquired* lobar overinflation) and they are also briefly reviewed in this section.

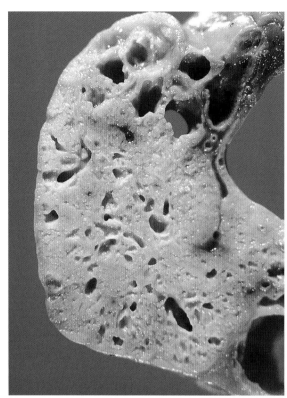

Figure 14–9 Gross appearance of a Type 2 CCAM, showing small, relatively uniform cysts.

Congenital Lobar Overinflation

Clinical Features

Congenital lobar overinflation involves hyperinflation, usually of an upper or middle lobe of the lung. Lower lobe involvement is distinctly uncommon.[2,3,119] The condition most frequently occurs in the newborn period, and 95% of cases develop before the infant is 6 months of age. Rare familial cases have also been reported.[126] Patients usually present with dyspnea, and the chest radiograph shows an enlarging lucent area in one hemithorax with compression of the ipsilateral and contralateral lung parenchyma.[112,119,124] The radiographic diagnosis may be complicated early in the course of the disease by the retention of fluid that is normally present before birth in the affected lobe. In these cases, the initial radiographic appearance is of a homogeneous density. As the lung fluid is absorbed, the characteristic lucent area appears.

Histopathologic Features

Grossly, the affected lobe appears overinflated and retains its shape after excision (Fig. 14–13). Gentle insufflation

Table 14–3 Classification and Etiology of Congenital Pulmonary Overinflation

Congenital Lobar Overinflation
  Obstructive (partial bronchial obstruction)
    Extrinsic: pulmonary vessels, intrathoracic masses
      (cysts, lymph nodes, neoplasms), rotation of the
      lung pedicle
    Intrinsic: cartilage abnormalities, mucosal flaps or
      fibrous webs (congenital or acquired), mucous
      plugs
  Nonobstructive
    Polyalveolar lobe
    Hypoplastic lobe with emphysema
  Unknown

Regional (Focal, Segmental) Overinflation
  Bronchial atresia
  Displaced tracheal bronchus

of the specimen with formalin through the bronchi will preserve the gross features of the lesion. Microscopically, the distal airspaces show enlargement (overinflation) only. Interstitial or bronchial inflammation has been described, but both are unusual, and their presence suggests a complicating infection.[3,119]

Causes

There are numerous causes of congenital lobar overinflation, as listed in Table 14–3, and the relative frequency with which these various lesions are found will depend to a great degree on the interest and determination with which a search is conducted. In nearly half the reported cases, however, a cause is not identified. Most cases are related to bronchial obstruction, which can be due to either intrinsic or extrinsic abnormalities. It should be remembered that the obstruction is partial rather than complete, since complete obstruction results in atelectasis rather than hyperinflation.[120]

Extrinsic bronchial obstruction may result from dilated pulmonary vessels, as in patent ductus arteriosus, total anomalous venous return, and other cardiac defects that cause increased pulmonary bloodflow.[119,122,123,125] Mediastinal masses, such as bronchogenic cysts,[127] extralobar sequestrations,[113] an azygous lobe,[110] enlarged hilar lymph nodes, and neoplasms may also cause bronchial compression. A case due to rotation of the lung pedicle has been reported.[111]

Intrinsic bronchial obstruction is most often related to focal deficiencies of bronchial cartilage.[2,3,119,121] It is

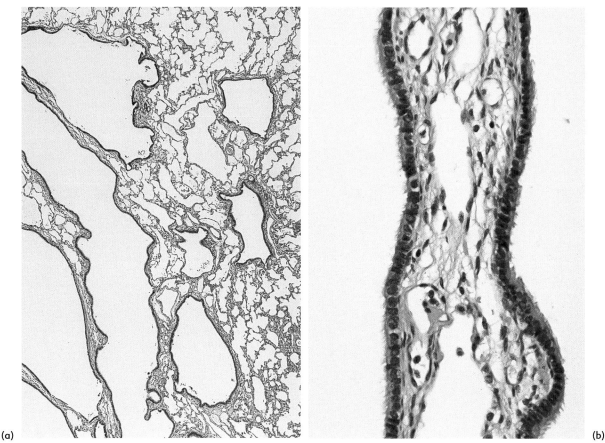

(a)   (b)

Figure 14–10 Type 2 CCAM. (a) Low magnification photomicrograph showing multiple bronchiole-like structures scattered within alveolated parenchyma. Note the lack of accompanying arteries. **(b)** Higher magnification showing the ciliated respiratory epithelium lining the small cysts.

thought that the abnormal bronchi collapse during expiration, leading to distal air trapping and lobar overinflation. Partial stenosis of the bronchus to the overinflated lobe has also been reported, owing either to congenital fibrous bands or webs or to bulky, abnormally shaped cartilaginous rings.[119] Mucous plugs and congenital mucosal flaps have been noted as well.[119]

Rarely, nonobstructive causes of lobar overinflation have been identified.[2,3] Several investigators have described a polyalveolar lobe in which the number of alveoli is increased, and the alveolar spaces become overinflated.[111,118] The lesion has most often involved the left upper lobe. Although the total alveolar number was determined in early reported cases, the use of *radial alveolar counts* is more practical for the surgical pathologist. In a radial alveolar count, the number of alveoli transected by a perpendicular line drawn from a respiratory bronchiole to the nearest connective tissue septum or pleural surface is recorded. Counts

vary with the patient's age, but they should range from five to seven alveoli for infants at birth to 1 year of age.[1,2,4] The pathogenesis of the polyalveolar lobe is not known. The clinical and experimental data, however, have suggested that intrauterine bronchial obstruction may lead to excessive alveolar proliferation.

Another form of nonobstructive overinflation is the hypoplastic lobe with emphysema,[109] in which an affected lung, lobe, or segment has a reduced number of airways and alveoli. The airspaces that are present are markedly increased in size.

Therapy

The therapy for lobar overinflation usually involves lobectomy, although conservative, nonsurgical management has been successful in cases without severe respiratory embarrassment or mediastinal shift.[108,112,117] Follow-up lung function studies have shown evidence of similar mild residual airflow obstruction regardless

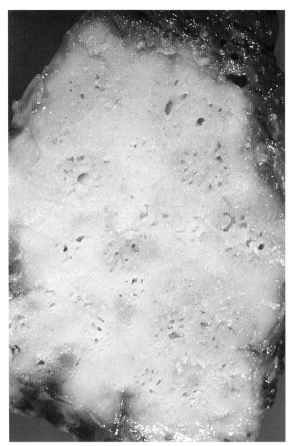

Figure 14–11 Type 3 CCAM. Gross appearance is characterized by solid parenchyma with only minute cysts. A rim of normal lung is seen at top.

of whether patients were treated conservatively or by surgery.[114]

Regional Pulmonary Overinflation

Regional overinflation of the lung may be caused by segmental bronchial atresia or, rarely, by the displaced type of tracheal bronchus (see Table 14–3). Segmental bronchial atresia is found in older children and young adults and characteristically affects the apical portion of the left upper lobe.[129–131] The chest radiograph shows hyperlucency in the affected area and often reveals a dense shadow near the hilum. On gross examination, there is atresia of the segmental bronchus with no communication to the mainstem bronchus. Dissection of the bronchi along probes (see Chapter 1) or specimen bronchography is essential to demonstrate the atretic segment. A large, mucus-filled bronchocele may be found distal to the atretic segment and explains the hilar

shadow. In the distal lung parenchyma, the alveoli are overexpanded and the small airways may contain mucous plugs. The pathogenesis of this lesion is unknown; abnormal branching of a bronchial bud during embryogenesis and segmental loss of the bronchial artery supply have been suggested as factors. It is possible also that the lesion is acquired as a result of infection or aspiration. The air supply of the overinflated area is presumed to be via collateral ventilation through the pores of Kohn from the surrounding normal segments.

In one reported case, regional overinflation of the lung was described in a right upper lobe supplied by a displaced tracheal bronchus.[128] The cause of the overinflation in that case was not clear.

Acquired Lobar Overinflation

Acquired lobar overinflation is one complication of longstanding bronchopulmonary dysplasia (see text following).[107,115,116] In contrast to congenital lobar over-inflation, the middle and lower lobes, rather than the upper lobes, are primarily affected. In some cases, intrinsic bronchial obstruction related to intraluminal granulation tissue can be identified. The location and histologic appearance suggest that this lesion results from trauma caused by suctioning. More often, however, an obstructing intrabronchial lesion cannot be found, and the changes are thought to be due to localized bronchomalacia.[107]

CONGENITAL PULMONARY LYMPHANGIECTASIS

Congenital pulmonary lymphangiectasis is characterized by prominent dilatation of the septal and subpleural lymphatic channels of the lung. It can be divided into three main categories: (1) primary, (2) secondary, and (3) generalized.[132–139]

Primary pulmonary lymphangiectasis is an almost uniformly fatal developmental defect that is related to an apparent failure of the pulmonary lymphatics to communicate with the systemic lymph channels.[2,3,133,134,138] Affected infants die of respiratory distress shortly after birth. This lesion occurs rarely and can be diagnosed only if cardiovascular or systemic lymphatic abnormalities are not present (see text following). Wagenaar et al[141] have described a peculiar form of primary lymphangiectasis that apparently was limited to focal involvement of the lung, mediastinum, or both. These patients were asymptomatic young adults who had

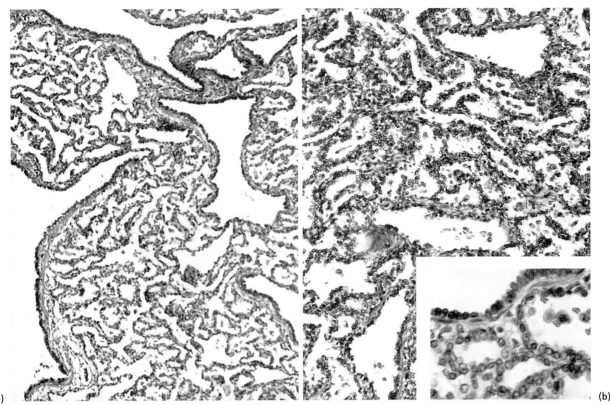

(a)
(b)

Figure 14–12 Type 3 CCAM. (a) Low magnification showing dilated, irregularly branching structures next to smaller structures resembling primitive airspaces. **(b)** Higher magnification view showing low cuboidal epithelium lining spaces. Inset is a higher magnification of the lining epithelium.

localized cystic lesions that were discovered on a routine chest radiograph.

Secondary pulmonary lymphangiectasis is associated with cardiovascular anomalies, most frequently, total anomalous pulmonary venous return,[2,3,133] but it has been noted with other lesions, including atresia of the common pulmonary veins.[135] It is thought that obstruction of the pulmonary venous flow may cause lymphangiectasis in some cases by producing interstitial edema. According to this theory, the large lymphatic channels normally present in fetal life persist in an attempt to clear the edema fluid from the lung.[135] This mechanism does not explain all cases, however, since some have not had associated venous obstruction.[132,133]

Generalized lymphangiectasis involves the lung as part of a systemic abnormality with lymphangiomas and occasionally hemangiomas in the bones, viscera, and soft tissue.[137,139,140] Pleural effusion and chylothorax are frequently present, and there may be a diffuse mediastinal or abdominal lymphangioma. In some cases, the intestines and spleen have shown lymphangiectasis as

well. These cases may be more appropriately classified as *diffuse pulmonary lymphangiomatosis* (see further on), since they are characterized by lymphatic proliferation as well as dilatation.

Pathologic Features

The pathologic features of primary and secondary lymphangiectasis are identical. Grossly, the markedly dilated lymphatics impart a firm, bosselated appearance to the lung. Microscopically, dilated, endothelial-lined spaces are seen in the bronchovascular connective tissue, along the interlobular septa and in the pleura (Fig. 14–14). Although the dilated lymphatic channels may initially resemble other cystic lesions, the presence of a distinct endothelial lining distinguishes them from the epithelium-lined spaces of adenomatoid malformation and the air cysts of pulmonary interstitial emphysema (Fig. 14–15). Immunohistochemical staining for CD34 can facilitate identification of lymphatic endothelium in difficult cases.

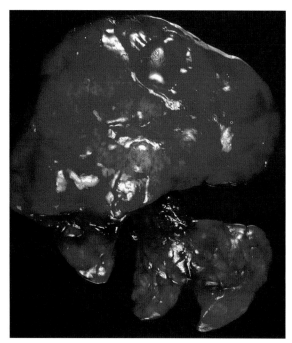

Figure 14–13 Congenital lobar overinflation. The left upper lobe (top) is markedly overinflated compared to the normally expanded lingula (bottom). The lobes were excised from a 1-month-old infant who developed dyspnea and was found to have a lucent area in the left upper lobe and a mediastinal shift. The cause was not identified in this case.

PULMONARY INTERSTITIAL EMPHYSEMA

Pulmonary interstitial emphysema is an acquired lesion in which air dissects out of the alveolar spaces and accumulates within the loose connective tissue of the interlobular septa, the subpleural region, and the bronchovascular bundles.[2,124,142,143,148,154] Some of the air appears to be within the lymphatic spaces as well.[150,152,153] Interstitial emphysema occurs in both *diffuse* and *localized* forms.[2,142,150,153] The diffuse form involves both lungs and usually occurs in infants with hyaline membrane disease who are treated with mechanical ventilation. Other cases involve neonates with meconium aspiration or pulmonary hypoplasia. Many of these patients also develop pneumothorax, dissection of air into the mediastinum, or both.

In the localized form, which occurs predominantly in infants receiving mechanical ventilation, interstitial emphysema is confined to one or two lobes of a lung. Clinically, patients present with an enlarging cystic mass that causes respiratory distress by compression of the adjacent lung parenchyma.[2,142,144,150,152,154] This form of the lesion clinically may mimic lobar overinflation or congenital adenomatoid malformation (see earlier sections).

Formerly, the therapy for localized pulmonary interstitial emphysema involved lobectomy. Selective bronchial intubation of the more normal lung, bypassing and decompressing the affected lobe, has been successful in preventing the need for surgery.[2,146]

Pathologic Features

On gross examination, the lung in both forms of interstitial emphysema shows irregular, clear cystic spaces in the interlobular septa and following the branching pattern of the bronchovascular bundles (Fig. 14–16). In severe cases, the cysts may expand and destroy the parenchyma, so that their relationship to the septa or bronchovascular bundles is no longer apparent (Fig. 14–16b). Microscopically, these cysts appear as round or oval empty spaces in the connective tissue of the interlobular septa and surrounding bronchi and pulmonary arteries (Fig. 14–17). The interstitial air may dissect so extensively around the bronchi or vessels that they appear as isolated structures in the center of a cyst. Usually, the air-filled spaces have no apparent lining, but, occasionally, a giant cell reaction resembling that seen in pneumatosis intestinalis is found (Fig. 14–17b).

Localized interstitial emphysema is distinguishable from CCAM (see earlier section) because in interstitial emphysema there are areas of normal lung between the cysts and the cysts lack an epithelial lining. In contrast, adenomatoid malformation is composed of abnormally arranged lung components in which the cysts are lined by bronchiolar or prominent cuboidal epithelium and, occasionally, by mucinous goblet cells. Congenital lymphangiectasis (see earlier section) differs from interstitial emphysema in that the cystic spaces possess an endothelial lining. In difficult cases, immunohistochemical markers of endothelial cells such as CD31, CD34 or factor VIII should clarify the issue.

MISCELLANEOUS LUNG CYSTS

Posttraumatic cysts have been described in the lung. Microscopic examination of one such case demonstrated a lining composed of granulation tissue.[149] Postinfarction lung cysts have been described in neonates, infants, and children with a variety of underlying

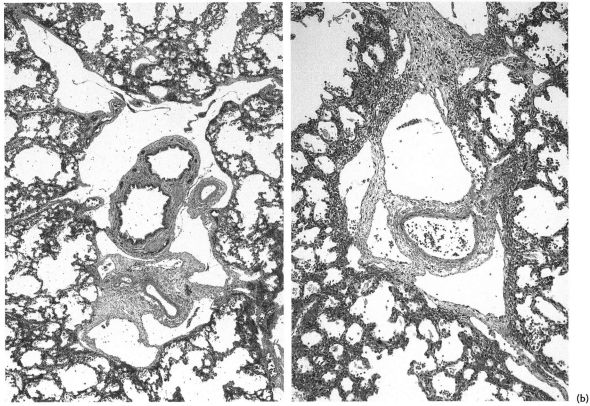

Figure 14–14 Lymphangiectasis. (a) Low magnification view showing the dilated lymphatic spaces in the bronchovascular connective tissue. **(b)** Dilated lymphatic spaces surrounding a vein in an interlobular septum.

disorders.[151] The cysts are formed from subpleural areas of lung destruction and fibrosis, and a thrombosed pulmonary artery is often associated with the affected area. Similar lesions have been described in infants with Down syndrome, especially when associated with cardiac anomalies.[145] Pneumatoceles are solitary or multiple thin-walled parenchymal cysts of debated etiology. Parenchymal necrosis and bronchial obstruction are likely important in their pathogenesis.[147]

INTERSTITIAL LUNG DISEASE IN CHILDREN

Children may be affected by many of the same interstitial lung diseases that occur in adults, but it is clear that diseases unique to children also occur, and some adult interstitial lung diseases do not affect children.[166] Infections are the most common, but chronic noninfectious conditions occasionally also occur. These conditions are most prevalent in patients under the age of 2 years and there is a slight male predominance.

Involvement of siblings by a similar disease occurs in almost 10%, and consanguinity of parents is found in about 7%.[166] The following discussion concentrates on interstitial pneumonias, many of which have unique features in childhood. Conditions encountered only at autopsy, such as hyaline membrane disease, are reviewed elsewhere.[6]

Interstitial Pneumonias

A variety of noninfectious interstitial pneumonias have been reported in children, and a familial occurrence has been noted in some.[166,180,200] Lymphoid interstitial pneumonia (LIP, see Chapter 9) and hypersensitivity pneumonia (extrinsic allergic alveolitis, see Chapter 6) are the most common noninfectious pneumonias encountered in children, and they are histologically identical to adult versions. LIP is usually associated with underlying connective tissue diseases, such as juvenile rheumatoid arthritis, for example, or with immunodeficiency, especially HIV infection, although it can occur as an isolated lesion.[165,171,172,178,182,185,188] The presence

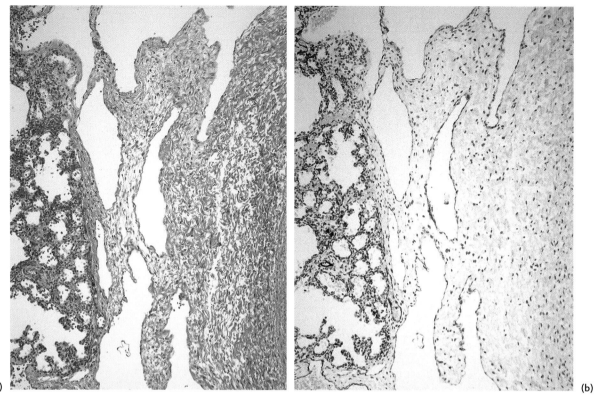

(a)   (b)

Figure 14–15 Higher magnification of dilated lymphatic spaces in lymphangiectasis. A thin endothelial lining can be appreciated along the lymphatic spaces in routine stains **(a)**, but are better appreciated in immunohistochemical stains for the endothelial marker CD34 **(b)**.

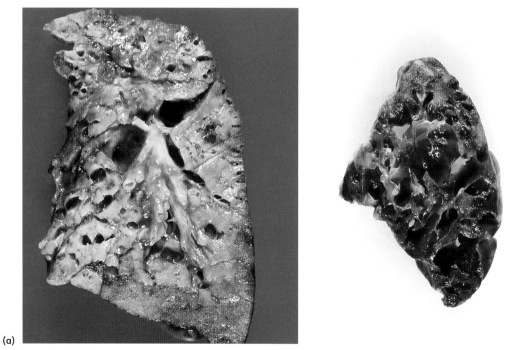

(a)   (b)

Figure 14–16 Pulmonary interstitial emphysema. (a) In this example, air-filled spaces are seen along the bronchovascular tree and extending into distal parenchyma. **(b)** Multiple air-filled spaces almost completely replace the parenchyma in this lobe removed from a 5-week-old infant who was receiving mechanical ventilation for hyaline membrane disease. (Case courtesy of Dr John Blair, St. Louis.)

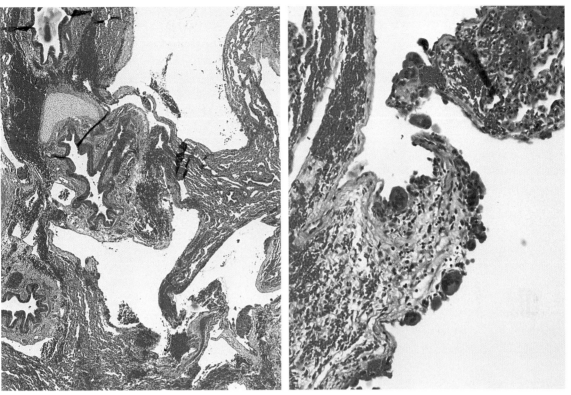

(a)

(b)

Figure 14–17 Pulmonary interstitial emphysema. (a) Low magnification showing irregular, dilated spaces surrounding a bronchovascular bundle. (b) Higher magnification showing foreign body giant cells arranged along the cyst wall in areas.

of LIP in an HIV-infected child is a diagnostic criterion of AIDS. Most cases of hypersensitivity pneumonia in children are caused by chronic exposure to birds.[171]

Usual interstitial pneumonia (UIP) and desquamative interstitial pneumonia (DIP) (see Chapter 3) have been reported occasionally in children,[183,195,198,200,202] although there is a controversy as to whether veritable examples occur in this age group. A critical review of the reported cases suggests that most, if not all, represent another form of interstitial pneumonia. We have not seen a provable case of UIP in a child, and we believe that if the diagnostic criteria for UIP as outlined in Chapter 3 are followed (i.e. a temporally variegated chronic interstitial pneumonia with alternating zones of interstitial inflammation, collagen deposition, fibroblast foci, honeycomb change, and normal lung), most reported cases will be reclassified as another disease. Likewise, the temporally uniform, mild interstitial pneumonia associated with diffusely increased numbers of alveolar macrophages that is typical of DIP is rare in children. As in adults, however, care must be taken not to overdiagnose as DIP a DIP-like reaction (the

focal or patchy accumulation of alveolar macrophages in an area of stiffened lung) that occasionally occurs in children. In our experience, most idiopathic interstitial pneumonias in children represent examples of so-called nonspecific interstitial pneumonia (see Chapter 3).[179] This lesion is a temporally uniform, inflammatory, and fibrotic interstitial process that differs pathologically from both UIP and DIP and is associated with a relatively good prognosis.

Acute lung injury can occur in childhood as in adulthood, and diffuse alveolar damage (DAD, see Chapter 2) is the characteristic pathologic finding in both situations. This lesion usually follows an identifiable pulmonary insult such as sepsis or intrauterine or perinatal asphyxia, for example, while, rarely, the cause is unknown (so-called Hamman–Rich disease or acute interstitial pneumonia).[164,181,192,193] In either situation, respiratory failure rapidly develops, and the prognosis is poor. Pathologically, hyaline membranes are seen early in the course of the lesion, while interstitial fibroblast proliferation and alveolar pneumocyte hyperplasia are prominent in later stages.

Bronchopulmonary Dysplasia

Bronchopulmonary dysplasia (BPD) represents the spectrum of pathologic changes resulting from oxygen and ventilator therapy used in treating respiratory failure in newborn infants, and it is an important cause of chronic lung disease in infants.[190] In most cases, hyaline membrane disease (idiopathic respiratory distress syndrome) is the underlying cause of the initial respiratory failure. The pathogenesis is thought to be related to a combination of the effects of oxygen toxicity and barotrauma imposed on immature lungs. A possible role for altered surfactant proteins has also been postulated.[167]

The diagnosis of BPD is usually established on the basis of clinical findings, including a history of positive pressure ventilation during the first 2 weeks of life, characteristic radiographic changes, and respiratory compromise that requires supplemental oxygen therapy for more than 28 days. Most cases of BPD are encountered by the pathologist at autopsy, although occasionally a baby with continued chronic lung disease that clinically seems out of proportion to the initial injury will undergo biopsy late in the course of disease.

The pathologic features of BPD have changed significantly since its description in 1967 due to advancements in mechanical ventilation, the widespread use of surfactant therapy, and younger gestational age of affected babies.[177] Early cases were characterized by hyaline membranes and bronchial ulceration acutely, and by interstitial fibrosis and squamous metaplasia of bronchial epithelium later on.[155–158,162,170,184,191,199] A 'healed' stage characterized by interstitial fibrosis that may be patchy and separated by emphysematous changes was noted in infants after several months (Fig. 14–18).[199] Bronchiolar abnormalities are inconspicuous or absent in this stage.

The current use of surfactant has decreased the oxygen tensions and ventilatory pressures needed to support oxygenation and it is thus postulated that there is less injury to the pulmonary acini, although the injury is more diffuse. While mild to moderate alveolar

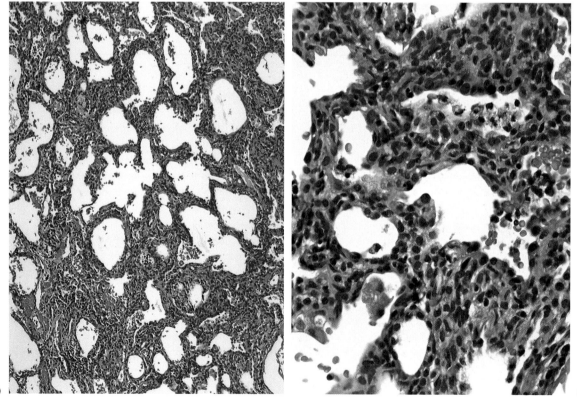

(a) (b)

Figure 14–18 Bronchopulmonary dysplasia. (a) Low magnification showing prominent uniform-appearing alveolar septal thickening. **(b)** Higher magnification showing interstitial fibrosis characterized by fibroblasts and myofibroblasts thickening the alveolar septa.

septal fibrosis is still seen in some infants, the main finding is an apparent arrest in acinar development that can be documented by measuring radial alveolar counts and mean linear intercepts.[176] Disrupted alveolar vascular development and impaired expression of angiogenic growth factors have been noted as well.[160]

Chronic Pneumonitis of Infancy and Related Entities

Chronic pneumonitis of infancy (CPI) is a rare and unique form of interstitial pneumonia that affects infants and young children.[180] In the past, cases may have been misdiagnosed as UIP, fibrosing alveolitis, DIP, and pulmonary alveolar proteinosis.[159,168,173,174,183,186,187,189,195,200,202] A few cases likely have also been included under the designation of *cellular interstitial pneumonitis*.[196]

Reported cases have involved full-term infants who appear healthy at birth. A few cases are familial.[173,180,200]

The onset occurs several weeks to months following birth and is characterized by dyspnea, cough, and failure to thrive. Some cases are likely related to surfactant protein deficiencies.[187,189] Pathologically, there is a distinct mixture of interstitial and airspace abnormalities (Fig. 14–19). The alveolar septa are thickened by mesenchymal cells that resemble myofibroblasts, combined with marked alveolar pneumocyte hyperplasia, but there is only minimal inflammation. Increased numbers of macrophages are seen within alveolar spaces, and there is also focal accumulation of granular eosinophilic debris within alveolar spaces that superficially resembles pulmonary alveolar proteinosis (see Chapter 15) (Fig. 14–20a). Sometimes, cholesterol clefts are present along with the alveolar macrophages (Fig. 14–20b). The prognosis is not good, with continued severe chronic lung disease and eventual death in most.

A different interstitial process, termed *pulmonary interstitial glycogenolysis*,[163] has been described, in

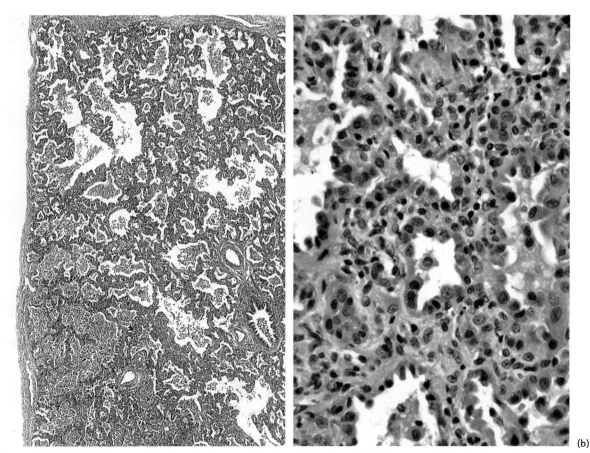

(a)　　　　　　　　　　　　　　　　　　　　　　　　(b)

Figure 14–19 CPI. (a) Low magnification showing a combination of alveolar septal thickening and intraalveolar exudates. **(b)** Higher magnification view showing interstitial mesenchymal cells and prominent alveolar pneumocyte hyperplasia causing the alveolar septal thickening. Minimal inflammation is seen.

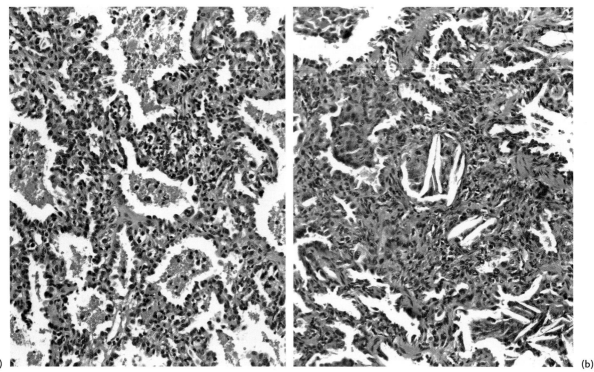

(a)   (b)

Figure 14–20 CPI. (a) Pulmonary alveolar proteinosis-like areas in CPI. Note the granular eosinophilic material within alveolar spaces. **(b)** Cholesterol clefts are seen in alveolar spaces along with alveolar macrophages in this example.

which glycogen-containing mesenchymal cells are present within alveolar septa. It occurs mainly in premature infants, with an onset usually within the first few days of birth. Mechanical ventilation was used in most. Histologically, there is mild interstitial fibrosis similar to that seen in healed BPD, except for the demonstration of glycogen. Most reported infants have recovered, and most were treated with steroids.

Persistent Tachypnea of Infancy

Persistent tachypnea of infancy is a recently described entity occurring in the first year of life.[169] The reported infants were full term and presented with symptoms of interstitial lung disease. High-resolution computed tomography scans showed mild peribronchial thickening and patchy ground glass opacities. The prognosis was good, with no deaths reported and eventual improvement over time.

Microscopically, mildly increased airway smooth muscle was described along with increased numbers of intraalveolar macrophages. Additionally, there were increased numbers of clear cells in distal airways that stained positively with immunohistochemical stains for bombesin. The lesion may be related to so-called chronic idiopathic bronchiolitis of infancy, except that increased numbers of neuroendocrine cells have not been noted in the latter entity.[175]

Diffuse Pulmonary Lymphangiomatosis

Diffuse pulmonary lymphangiomatosis is a rare cause of interstitial lung disease that occurs predominantly in young children, although young adults are sometimes affected as well.[161,197,201] Dyspnea or wheezing is the usual presenting complaint, and bilateral interstitial infiltrates are seen radiographically. Chylous pleural or pericardial effusions are common complications, and there may be involvement of extrapulmonary organs. The disease is usually slowly progressive, although patients may survive for many years.

The pathologic features are characterized by a proliferation of thin-walled lymphatic channels which sometimes contain smooth muscle in their walls (Fig. 14–21).[194,197,201] They are present within the bronchovascular bundles, the interlobular septa, and the pleura – locations where lymphatic spaces are normally found – and they are recognized by being

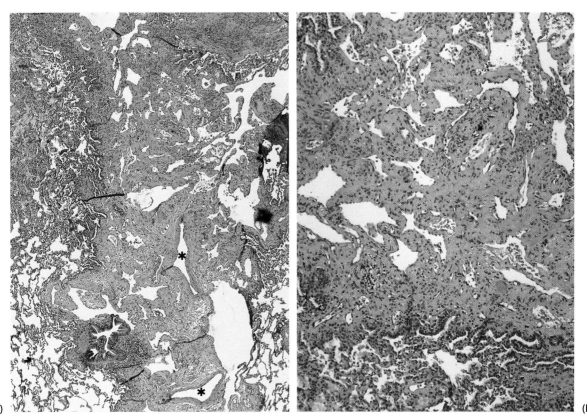

Figure 14–21 Lymphangiomatosis. (a) Low magnification view showing a proliferation of lymphatic spaces that extends along and widens the bronchovascular connective tissue. The normal pulmonary artery branches are marked by an asterisk. **(b)** Higher magnification illustrating the numerous irregular lymphatic spaces within the thickened bronchovascular connective tissue.

often dilated and irregular in shape and more numerous than normal. In some instances, an associated finding in the dilated lymphatic spaces is the presence of clusters of bland, spindle-shaped cells intermingled with hemosiderin granules. These proliferative foci likely result from organization of prior hemorrhage. Their appearance may initially suggest Kaposi's sarcoma, but they are focal, and recognition of large numbers of abnormal lymphatic spaces should indicate the correct diagnosis.

Diffuse lymphangiomatosis needs to be distinguished from lymphangiectasis and from lymphangiomyomatosis (LAM). Lymphangiectasis (see earlier section) is characterized by lymphatic dilatation but not proliferation. It is a developmental anomaly that usually occurs in infants and may be associated with cardiovascular abnormalities. Some cases of lymphangiomatosis, however, may have been incorrectly included under the term generalized lymphangiectasis.[134,137,139] LAM (see Chapter 15) is a proliferative, smooth muscle process that occurs mainly in women of reproductive age. It is characterized by random proliferation of bland-appearing smooth muscle bundles within the pulmonary interstitium. Although the lymphatic spaces may be secondarily dilated, they are not increased in number.

REFERENCES

General

1. Askin FB: Respiratory tract disorders in the fetus and neonate. In: Wigglesworth JS, Singer DB, eds: *Textbook of Fetal and Perinatal Pathology*, 2nd ed, Boston, Blackwell Scientific,1998, pp 555–592.

2. Askin FB, Langston C, Rosenberg HS, Bernstein J: Pulmonary disease. *Perspectives in Pediatric Pathology*, Vol. 18, Basel, Karger, 1995.

3. Landing BH, Dixon LG: Congenital malformations and genetic disorders of the respiratory tract (larynx, trachea, bronchi and lungs). Am Rev Respir Dis 120:151, 1979.

4. Stocker JT: Congenital and developmental diseases. In: Dail DH, Hammar SP, eds: *Pulmonary Pathology*, 2nd ed, New York, Springer-Verlag, 1994, pp 155–190.

5. Stocker JT: The respiratory tract. In: Stocker JT, Dehner LP, eds: *Pediatric Pathology*, Philadelphia, Lippincott Williams & Williams, 2001, pp 445–517.

6. Stocker JT, Dehner LP: Acquired neonatal and pediatric disease, In: Dail DH, Hammar SP, eds: *Pulmonary Pathology*, 2nd ed, New York, Springer-Verlag, 1994, pp 191–254.

7. Winters WD, Effmann EL: Congenital masses of the lung: Prenatal and postnatal imaging evaluation. J Thorac Imaging 16:196, 2001.

Pulmonary Sequestration and Related Anomalies

8. Alivizatos P, Cheatle T, de Laval M, Stark J: Pulmonary sequestration complicated by anomalies of pulmonary venous return. J Pediatr Surg 20:76, 1986.

9. Avishai V, Dolev E, Weissberg D, et al: Extralobar sequestration presenting as massive hemothorax. Chest 109:843, 1996.

10. Bates M: Total unilateral pulmonary sequestration. Thorax 23:311, 1968.

11. Cerruti MM, Marmolejos F, Cacciarelli T: Bilateral intralobar pulmonary sequestration with horseshoe lung. Ann Thorac Surg 55:509, 1993.

12. Clements BS, Warner JO: Pulmonary sequestration and related congenital bronchopulmonary vascular malformations: Nomenclature and classification based on anatomical and embryological considerations. Thorax 42:401, 1987.

13. Clements BS, Warner JO: The crossover lung segment: Congenital malformation associated with a variant of scimitar syndrome. Thorax 42:417, 1987.

14. Conran RM, Stocker JT: Extralobar sequestration with frequently associated congenital cystic adenomatoid malformation, type 2: Report of 50 cases. Pediatr Dev Pathol 2:454, 1999.

15. Ernst SMPG, Bruschke AVG: An aberrant systemic artery to the right lung with normal pulmonary tissue. Chest 60:606, 1971.

16. Flye MW, Izant RJ: Extralobar pulmonary sequestration with esophageal communication and complete duplication of the colon. Surgery 71:744, 1972.

17. Fraggetta F, Davenport M, Magro G, et al: Striated muscle cells in non-neoplastic lung tissue: A clinicopathologic study. Hum Pathol 31:1477, 2000.

18. Gay BB Jr, Atkinson GO Jr, Ball TI, et al: Pediatric case of the day. Case 1. Systemic arterial supply to normal pulmonary parenchyma. AJR Am J Roentgenol 140:1016, 1983.

19. Haworth SG, Sauer U, Bühlmeyer K: Pulmonary hypertension in scimitar syndrome in infancy. Br Heart J 50:182, 1983.

20. Heithoff KB, Sane SM, Williams HJ, et al: Bronchopulmonary foregut malformations. A unifying etiological concept. AJR Am J Roentgenol 126:46, 1976.

21. Holder PD, Langston C: Intralobar pulmonary sequestration (a nonentity?). Pediatr Pulmonol 2:147, 1986.

22. Hruban RH, Shumway SJ, Orel SB, et al: Congenital bronchopulmonary foregut malformations. Intralobar and extralobar pulmonary sequestrations communicating with the foregut. Am J Clin Pathol 91:403, 1989.

23. Lager DJ, Kuper KA, Haake GK: Subdiaphragmatic extralobar pulmonary sequestration. Arch Pathol Lab Med 115:536, 1991.

24. Leithiser RE Jr, Capitanio MA, Macpherson RI, Wood BP: "Communicating" bronchopulmonary foregut malformations. AJR Am J Roentgenol 146:227, 1986.

25. Litwin SB, Plauth WH Jr, Nadas AS: Anomalous systemic arterial supply to the lung causing pulmonary artery hypertension. N Engl J Med 283:1098, 1970.

26. Louie HW, Martin SM, Mulder DG: Pulmonary sequestration: 17-year experience at UCLA. Am Surg 59:801, 1993.

27. Lucaya J, Carcia-Conesa JA, Bernado L: Pulmonary sequestration associated with unilateral pulmonary hypoplasia and massive pleural effusion. A case report and review of the literature. Pediatr Radiol 14:228, 1984.

28. Masaoka A, Maeda M, Monden M, et al: Total lung ectoplasia with systemic arterial supply. Ann Thorac Surg 27:76, 1979.

29. Maull KI, McElvein RB: Infarcted extralobar pulmonary sequestration. Chest 68:98, 1975.

30. Nicolette LA, Kosloske AM, Bartow SA, Murphy S: Intralobar pulmonary sequestration: A clinical and pathological spectrum. J Pediatr Surg 28:802, 1993.

31. Partridge JB, Osborne JM, Slaughter RE: Scimitar et cetera – the dysmorphic right lung. Clin Radiol 39:11, 1988.

32. Rodgers BM, Harman PK, Johnson AM: Bronchopulmonary foregut malformations. The spectrum of anomalies. Ann Surg 203:517, 1986.

33. Roe JP, Mack JW, Shirley JH: Bilateral pulmonary sequestrations. J Thorac Cardiovasc Surg 80:8, 1980.

34. Shuman RL, Libby G, Riker J: Pulmonary sequestration with aneurysmal anomalous systemic artery. Vasc Surg 17:183, 1983.

35. Stocker JT: Sequestrations of the lung. Semin Diagn Pathol 3:106, 1986.

36. Stocker JT, Malczak HT: A study of pulmonary ligament arteries. Relationship to intralobar pulmonary sequestration. Chest 86:611, 1984.

37. Sugio K, Kaneko S, Yokoyama H, et al: Pulmonary sequestration in older child and in adults. Int Surg 77:102, 1992.

38. Tandon M, Warnock ML: Plexogenic angiopathy in pulmonary intralobar sequestrations: Pathogenetic mechanisms. Hum Pathol 24:263, 1993.

39. Thilenius OG, Ruschaput DG, Replogle RL, et al: Spectrum of pulmonary sequestration: Association with anomalous pulmonary venous drainage in infants. Pediatr Cardiol 4:97, 1983.

40. Thornhill BA, Cho KC, Morehouse HT: Gastric duplication associated with pulmonary sequestration:

CT manifestations. AJR Am J Roentgenol 138:1168, 1982.

41. Tomashefski JF, Wen P, Giampoli E, et al: Pulmonary intralobar sequestration in a patient with cystic fibrosis. Hum Pathol 28:1436, 1997.

42. Uppal MS, Kohman LJ, Katzenstein A-LA: Mycetoma within an intralobar sequestration. Evidence supporting acquired origin for this pulmonary anomaly. Chest 103:1627, 1993.

43. Werthammer JW, Hatten HP Jr, Blake WB Jr: Upper thoracic extralobar pulmonary sequestration presenting with respiratory distress in a newborn. Pediatr Radiol 9:116, 1980.

44. Yabek SM, Burstein J, Berman W Jr, Dillon T: Aberrant systemic arterial supply to the left lung with congestive heart failure. Chest 80:636, 1981.

Bronchogenic Cysts

45. Amendola BS, Shirazi KK, Brooks J, et al: Transdiaphragmatic bronchopulmonary foregut anomaly: "Dumbbell bronchogenic cyst." AJR Am J Roentgenol 138:1165, 1982.

46. Coselli MP, de Ipolyi P, Bloss RS, et al: Bronchogenic cysts above and below the diaphragm: Report of eight cases. Ann Thorac Surg 44:491, 1987.

47. Dubois P, Belanger R, Wellington JL: Bronchogenic cyst presenting as a supraclavicular mass. Can J Surg 24:530, 1981.

48. Reed JC, Sobonya RE: Morphologic analysis of foregut cysts in the thorax. Am J Roentgenol Radium Ther Nucl Med 120:851, 1974.

49. Salyer DC, Salyer WR, Eggleston JC: Benign developmental cysts of the mediastinum. Arch Pathol Lab Med 101:136, 1977.

50. Snyder ME, Luck SR, Hernandez R, et al: Diagnostic dilemmas of mediastinal cysts. J Pediatr Surg 20:810, 1985.

51. St-Georges R, Deslauriers J, Duranceau A, et al: Clinical spectrum of bronchogenic cysts of the mediastinum and lung in the adult. Ann Thorac Surg 52:6, 1991.

52. Van der Putte SCJ, Toonstra J: Cutaneous "bronchogenic" cyst. J Cutan Pathol 12:404, 1985.

Congenital Abnormalities of the Bronchial Tree

53. Agosti E, deFilippi G, Fior R, et al: Generalized familial bronchomalacia. Acta Paediatr Scand 63:616, 1974.

54. Barat M, Konrad HR: Tracheal bronchus. Am J Otolaryngol 8:118, 1987.

55. Bashour T, Kabbami S, Cheng TO: Congenital bronchopleurocutaneous fistula. Chest 79:489, 1981.

56. Benson JE, Olsen MM, Fletcher BD: A spectrum of bronchopulmonary anomalies associated with tracheoesophageal malformations. Pediatr Radiol 15:377, 1985.

57. Bertucci GM, Dickman PS, Lachman RS, et al: Bridging bronchus and posterior left pulmonary artery: A unique association. Pediatr Pathol 7:637, 1987.

58. Chang N, Hertzler JH, Gregg RH, et al: Congenital stenosis of the right mainstem bronchus. Pediatrics 41:739, 1968.

59. Cope R, Campbell JR, Wall M: Bilateral tracheal bronchi. J Pediatr Surg 21:443, 1986.

60. de Carvalho CRR, Barbas CSV, de Moraes Goncalves Guarnieri RM, et al: Congenital bronchobiliary fistula: First case in an adult. Thorax 43:792, 1988.

61. Engle WA, Cohen MD, McAlister WH, Griscom MT: Neonatal tracheobronchomegaly. Am J Perinatol 4:81, 1987.

62. Gonzales-Crussi F, Padilla L-M, Miller JK, et al: "Bridging bronchus." A previously undescribed airway anomaly. Am J Dis Child 130:1015, 1976.

63. Hosker HSR, Clague HW, Morrett GN: Ectopic right upper lobe bronchus as a cause of breathlessness. Thorax 42:473, 1987.

64. Jacobs IN, Wetmore RF, Tom LWC, et al: Tracheobronchomalacia in children. Arch Otolaryngol Head Neck Surg 120:154, 1994.

65. Landing BH: Syndromes of congenital heart disease with tracheobronchial anomalies. Am J Roentgenol Radium Ther Nucl Med 123:679, 1975.

66. Landing BH, Wells TR: Tracheobronchial anomalies in children. Perspect Pediatr Pathol 1:1, 1973.

67. Lavasseur P, Navajas M: Congenital tracheobiliary fistula. Ann Thorac Surg 44:318, 1987.

68. Lindahl H, Nyman R: Congenital bronchobiliary fistula successfully treated at the age of three days. J Pediatr Surg 21:734, 1986.

69. Loyer EM: Case of the season: Congenital left bronchoesophageal fistula. Semin Roentgenol 21:169, 1986.

70. Maesen FPV, Santana B, Lamers J, Brekel B: A supernumerary bronchus of the right upper lobe. Eur J Respir Dis 64:473, 1983.

71. Maisel RH, Fried MP, Swain R, et al: Anomalous tracheal bronchus with tracheal hypoplasia. Arch Otolaryngol 100:69, 1974.

72. Mangiulea VG, Stinghe RV: The accessory cardiac bronchus. Bronchologic aspect and review of the literature. Chest 54:433, 1968.

73. Mitchell RE, Bury RG: Congenital bronchiectasis due to deficiency of bronchial cartilage (Williams-Campbell syndrome). A case report. J Pediatr 87:230, 1975.

74. Odell J: Anomalous origin of the anterior segmental bronchus of the right upper lobe. Thorax 35:213, 1980.

75. Siegel MJ, Shackleford GD, Francis RS, et al: Tracheal bronchus. Radiology 130:353, 1979.

76. Smith KP, Cavett CM: Segmental bronchomalacia: Successful surgical correction in an infant. J Pediatr Surg 20:240, 1985.

77. Sotomayor JL, Godinez RI, Borden S, Wilmott RW: Large-airway collapse due to acquired tracheobronchomalacia in infancy. Am J Dis Child 140:367, 1986.

78. Wailoo M, Emory J: The trachea in children with tracheo-esophageal fistula. Histopathology 3:329, 1979.

Congenital Cystic Adenomatoid Malformation

79. Alt B, Shikes RH, Stanford RE, Silverberg SG: Ultrastructure of congenital cystic adenomatoid of the lung. Ultrastruct Pathol 3:217, 1982.

80. Avitabile AM, Greco MA, Hulnick DH, Feiner HD: Congenital cystic adenomatoid malformation of the lung in adults. Am J Surg Pathol 8:193, 1984.

81. Bale PM: Congenital cystic malformation of the lung. A form of congenital bronchiolar ("adenomatoid") malformation. Am J Clin Pathol 71:411, 1979.

82. Benning TL, Godwin JD, Roggli VL, Askin FB: Cartilaginous variant of congenital adenomatoid malformation of the lung. Chest 92:514, 1987.

83. Cachia R, Sobonya RE: Congenital cystic adenomatoid malformation of the lung with bronchial atresia. Hum Pathol 12:947, 1981.

84. Cangiarella J, Greco A, Askin F, et al: Congenital cystic adenomatoid malformation of the lung: Insights into the pathogenesis utilizing quantitative analysis of vascular marker CD34 (QBEND-10) and cell proliferation marker MIB-1. Mod Pathol 8:913, 1995.

85. Cha I, Adzick NS, Harrison MR, Finkbeiner WE: Fetal congenital cystic adenomatoid malformations of the lung: A clinicopathologic study of eleven cases. Am J Surg Pathol 21:537, 1997.

86. Cloutier MM, Schaeffer DA, Hight D: Congenital cystic adenomatoid malformation. Chest 103:761, 1993.

87. Deroca PJ Jr: Mucogenic cells of congenital adenomatoid malformation of lung. Arch Pathol Lab Med 103:258, 1979.

88. Fisher JE, Nelson SJ, Allen JE, Holzman RS: Congenital cystic adenomatoid malformation of lung. A unique variant. Am J Dis Child 136:1071, 1982.

89. Gaisie G, Oh KS: Spontaneous pneumothorax in cystic adenomatoid malformation. Pediatr Radiol 13:281, 1983.

90. Hulnick DH, Naidich DP, McCauley DI, et al: Late presentation of congenital cystic adenomatoid malformation of the lung. Radiology 151:569, 1984.

91. Imai Y, Mark EJ: Cystic adenomatoid change is common to various forms of cystic lung diseases of children: A clinicopathologic analysis of 10 cases with emphasis on tracing the bronchial tree. Arch Pathol Lab Med 126:934, 2002.

92. Krous HF, Harper PE, Perlman M: Congenital cystic adenomatoid malformation in bilateral renal agenesis. Its mitigation of Potter's syndrome. Arch Pathol Lab Med 104:368, 1980.

93. Luján M, Bosque M, Mirapeix RM, et al: Late-onset congenital cystic adenomatoid malformation of the lung. Respiration 69:148, 2002.

94. MacSweeney F, Papagiannopoulos K, Goldstraw P, et al: An assessment of the expanded classification of congenital cystic adenomatoid malformations and their relationship to malignant transformation. Am J Surg Pathol 27:1139, 2003.

95. Mendoza A, Wolf P, Edwards DK, et al: Prenatal ultrasonographic diagnosis of congenital adenomatoid malformation of the lung. Correlation with pathology and implication for pregnancy management. Arch Pathol Lab Med 110:402, 1986.

96. Miller RK, Sieber WK, Yunis EJ: Congenital adenomatoid malformation of the lung. A report of 17 cases and review of the literature. Pathol Annu 15(Pt 1):387, 1980.

97. Moerman P, Fryns J-P, Vandenberghe K, et al: Pathogenesis of congenital cystic adenomatoid malformation of the lung. Histopathology 21:315, 1992.

98. Morotti RA, Cangiarella J, Gutierrez MC, et al: Congenital cystic adenomatoid malformation of the lung (CCAM): Evaluation of the cellular components. Hum Pathol 30:618, 1999.

99. Morotti RA, Gutierrez MC, Askin F, et al: Expression of thyroid transcription factor-1 in congenital cystic adenomatoid malformation of the lung. Pediatr Dev Pathol 3:455, 2000.

100. Petit P, Bossens M, Thomas D, et al: Type III congenital cystic adenomatoid malformation of the lung: Another cause of elevated alpha fetoprotein? Clin Genet 32:172, 1987.

101. Roelofsen J, Oostendorp R, Volovics A, Hoogland H: Prenatal diagnosis and fetal outcome of cystic adenomatoid malformation of the lung: Case report and historical survey. Ultrasound Obstet Gynecol 4:78, 1994.

102. Saltzman DH, Adzick NS, Benacerraf BR: Fetal cystic adenomatoid malformation of the lung: Apparent improvement in utero. Obstet Gynecol 71:1000, 1989.

103. Stacher E, Ullmann R, Halbwedl I, et al: Atypical goblet cell hyperplasia in congenital cystic adenomatoid malformation as a possible preneoplasia for pulmonary adenocarcinoma in childhood: A genetic analysis. Hum Pathol 35:565, 2004.

104. Stocker JT: Congenital pulmonary airway malformation – a new name for and an expanded classification of congenital cystic adenomatoid malformation of the lung. Histopathology 41:424, 2002.

105. Stocker JT, Madewell JF, Drake RM: Congenital cystic adenomatoid malformation of the lung. Classification, and morphologic spectrum. Hum Pathol 8:155, 1977.

106. Wilson SK, Moore GW, Hutchins G: Congenital cystic adenomatoid malformation of the lung associated with abdominal musculature deficiency (prune belly). Pediatrics 62:421, 1978.

Congenital Lobar Overinflation

107. Azizkhan RG, Grimmer DL, Askin FB, et al: Acquired lobar emphysema (overinflation): Clinical and pathological evaluation of infants requiring lobectomy. J Pediatr Surg 27:1145, 1992.

108. Glenski JA, Thibeault DW, Hall FK, et al: Selective bronchial intubation in infants with lobar emphysema: Indications, complications, and long-term outcome. Am J Perinatol 3:149, 1986.

109. Henderson R, Hislop A, Reid L: New pathological findings in emphysema of childhood: 3. Unilateral

congenital emphysema with hypoplasia and compensatory emphysema of contralateral lung. Thorax 26:195, 1971.

110. Hill RC, Mantese V, Spock A, Wolfe WG: Management of an unusual case of congenital lobar emphysema. Pediatr Pulmonol 5:252, 1988.

111. Hislop A, Reid L: New pathological findings in emphysema of childhood: 2. Overinflation of a normal lobe. Thorax 26:190, 1971.

112. Kennedy CD, Habibi P, Matthew DJ, Gordon I: Lobar emphysema: Long-term imaging follow-up. Radiology 180:189, 1991.

113. Knudson RJ, Lindgren I, Gaensler EA: Accessory lung (or extrapulmonary sequestration) as a cause of lobar emphysema. Med Thorac 23:52, 1966.

114. McBride JT, Wohl MEB, Strieder DJ, et al: Lung growth and airway function after lobectomy in infancy for congenital lobar emphysema. J Clin Invest 66:962, 1980.

115. Miller KE, Edwards DK, Hilton S, et al: Acquired lobar emphysema in premature infants with bronchopulmonary dysplasia: An iatrogenic disease? Radiology 138:589, 1981.

116. Miller RW, Woo P, Kellman RK, Slagle TS: Tracheobronchial abnormalities in infants with bronchopulmonary dysplasia. J Pediatr 111:779, 1987.

117. Morgan WJ, Lemen RJ, Rojas R: Acute worsening of congenital lobar emphysema and subsequent spontaneous improvement. Pediatrics 71:844, 1983.

118. Munnell ER, Lambird PA, Austin RL: Polyalveolar lobe causing lobar emphysema of infancy. Ann Thorac Surg 16:624, 1973.

119. Murray GF: Congenital lobar emphysema. Surg Gynecol Obstet 124:611, 1967.

120. Nagaraj HS, Shott R, Fellows R, Yacoub U: Recurrent lobar atelectasis due to acquired bronchial stenosis in neonates. J Pediatr Surg 15:411, 1980.

121. Powell HC, Elliott ML: Congenital lobar emphysema. Virchows Arch A Pathol Anat Histol 374:197, 1977.

122. Rabinovitch M, Grady S, David I, et al: Compression of intrapulmonary bronchi by abnormally branching pulmonary arteries associated with absent pulmonary valves. Am J Cardiol 50:804, 1982.

123. Stanger P, Lucas RV Jr, Edwards JE: Anatomic factors causing respiratory distress in acyanotic congenital cardiac disease: Special reference to bronchial obstruction. Pediatrics 43:760, 1969.

124. Stocker JT, Drake RM, Madewell JE: Cystic and congenital lung disease in the newborn. Perspect Pediatr Pathol 4:93, 1978.

125. Sulayman R, Thilenius O, Replogle R, Arcilla RA: Unilateral emphysema in total anomalous pulmonary venous return. J Pediatr 87:433, 1975.

126. Wall MA, Eisenberg JD, Campbell JR: Congenital lobar emphysema in a mother and daughter. Pediatrics 70:131, 1982.

127. Weichert RF III, Lindsey ES, Pearce LW, Waring WW: Bronchogenic cyst with unilateral obstructive emphysema. J Thorac Cardiovasc Surg 59:287, 1970.

Regional Pulmonary Overinflation

128. Iancu T, Boyanover Y, Eilam N, et al: Infantile sublobar emphysema and tracheal bronchus. Acta Paediatr Scand 64:551, 1975.

129. Jederlinic PJ, Sicilian LS, Baigelman W, Gaensler EA: Congenital bronchial atresia. A report of 4 cases and a review of the literature. Medicine (Baltimore) 66:73, 1987.

130. Talner LB, Gmelich JT, Liebow AA, et al: The syndrome of bronchial mucocele and regional hyperinflation of the lung. Am J Roentgenol Radium Nucl Med 110:675, 1970.

131. Williams LE, Murray GF, Wilcox BR: Congenital atresia of the bronchus. J Thorac Cardiovasc Surg 68:957, 1974.

Pulmonary Lymphangiectasis

132. Esterly JR, Oppenheimer EH: Lymphangiectasis and other pulmonary lesions in the asplenia syndrome. Arch Pathol 90:553, 1970.

133. France NE, Brown RJK: Congenital pulmonary lymphangiectasis: Report of 11 examples with special reference to cardiovascular findings. Arch Dis Child 46:528, 1971.

134. Gardner TW, Domm AC, Brock CB, Pruitt AW: Congenital pulmonary lymphangiectasis. A case complicated by chylothorax. Clin Pediatr 22:75, 1983.

135. Hawker RE, Celermajer JM, Gengos DC, et al: Common pulmonary vein atresia. Premortem diagnosis in two infants. Circulation 46:368, 1972.

136. Hernandez RJ, Stein AM, Rosenthal A: Pulmonary lymphangiectasis in Noonan syndrome. AJR Am J Roentgenol 134:75, 1980.

137. Moerman P, Vandenberghe K, Devlieger H, et al: Congenital pulmonary lymphangiectasis with chylothorax: A heterogeneous lymphatic vessel abnormality. Am J Med Genet 47:54, 1993.

138. Shannon MP, Grantmyre EB, Reid WD, Wotherspoon AS: Congenital pulmonary lymphangiectasis. Report of two cases. Pediatr Radiol 2:235, 1974.

139. Sindel LJ, Blackburn WR, Brogdon BG, Harris RO III: Progressive pulmonary lymphangiectasis. Pediatr Pulmonol 10:57, 1991.

140. Smeltzer DM, Stickler GB, Fleming RE: Primary lymphatic dysplasia in children. Chylothorax, chylous ascites, and generalized lymphatic dysplasia. Eur J Pediatr 145:286, 1986.

141. Wagenaar SS, Swierenga J, Wagenvoort CA: Late presentation of primary pulmonary lymphangiectasis. Thorax 33:791, 1978.

Interstitial Emphysema and Miscellaneous Cystic Lesions

142. Askin FB: Pulmonary interstitial air and pneumothorax in the neonate. In: Stocker JT, ed: *Pediatric Pulmonary Disease*, New York, Hemisphere Publishing, 1989, pp 165–174.

143. Boothroyd AE, Barson AJ: Pulmonary interstitial emphysema – a radiological and pathological correlation. Pediatr Radiol 18:194, 1988.

144. Ivey HH, Kattwinkel J, Alford BA: Subvisceral pleural air in neonates with respiratory distress. Am J Dis Child 135:544, 1981.

145. Joshi VV, Kasznica J, Ali Khan MA, et al: Cystic lung disease in Down's syndrome. A report of two cases. Pediatr Pathol 5:79, 1986.

146. Levine DH, Trump DS, Waterkotte G: Unilateral pulmonary interstitial emphysema. A surgical approach to treatment. Pediatrics 68:510, 1981.

147. Quigley MJ, Fraser RS: Pulmonary pneumatocele: Pathology and pathogenesis. AJR Am J Roentgenol 150:1275, 1988.

148. Schneider JR, St. Cyr JS, Thompson TR, et al: The changing spectrum of cystic pulmonary lesions requiring surgical resection in infants. J Thorac Cardiovasc Surg 89:332, 1985.

149. Shirakusa T, Araki Y, Tsutsui M, et al: Traumatic lung pseudocyst. Thorax 42:516, 1987.

150. Smith TH, Currarino G, Rutledge JC: Spontaneous occurrence of localized pulmonary interstitial and endolymphatic emphysema in infancy. Pediatr Radiol 14:142, 1984.

151. Stocker JT: Post-infarction peripheral cysts of the lung in pediatric patients: A possible cause of idiopathic spontaneous pneumothorax. Pediatr Pulmonol 1:7, 1985.

152. Stocker JT, Madewell JE: Persistent interstitial pulmonary emphysema: Another complication of the respiratory distress syndrome. Pediatrics 59:847, 1977.

153. Wood BP, Anderson VM, Mauk JE, Merritt TA: Pulmonary lymphatic air: Locating "pulmonary interstitial emphysema" of the premature infant. AJR Am J Roentgenol 138:809, 1982.

154. Zimmerman H: Progressive interstitial pulmonary lobar emphysema. Eur J Pediatr 138:258, 1982.

Interstitial Lung Diseases

155. Anderson WR: Bronchopulmonary dysplasia: A correlative study by light, scanning, and transmission electron microscopy. Ultrastruct Pathol 14:221, 1990.

156. Anderson W, Strickland M: Pulmonary complications of oxygen therapy in the neonate. Postmortem study of bronchopulmonary dysplasia with emphasis on fibroproliferative obliterative bronchitis and bronchiolitis. Arch Pathol 91:506, 1971.

157. Anderson W, Strickland M, Tsai S, Haglin J: Light microscopic and ultrastructural study of the adverse effects of oxygen therapy on the neonate lung. Am J Pathol 73:327, 1973.

158. Banerjee CK, Girling DJ, Wigglesworth JS: Pulmonary fibroplasia in newborn babies treated with oxygen and artificial ventilation. Arch Dis Child 47:509, 1972.

159. Bellon G, Ninet J, Louis D, et al: Heart-lung transplantation in a 16 month-old infant. Chest 102:299, 1992.

160. Bhatt AJ, Pryhuber GS, Huyck H, et al: Disrupted pulmonary vasculature and decreased vascular endothelial growth factor, Flt-1, and TIE-2 in human infants dying with bronchopulmonary dysplasia. Am J Respir Crit Care Med 164:1971, 2001.

161. Bhatti MAK, Ferrante JW, Gielchinsky I, Norman JC: Pleuropulmonary and skeletal lymphangiomatosis with chylothorax and chylopericardium. Ann Thorac Surg 40:398, 1986.

162. Bonikos D, Bensch K, Northway W Jr, Edwards D: Bronchopulmonary dysplasia: The pulmonary pathologic sequel of necrotizing bronchiolitis and pulmonary fibrosis. Hum Pathol 7:643, 1976.

163. Canakis A-M, Cutz E, Manson D, O'Brodovich H: Pulmonary interstitial glycogenosis: A new variant of neonatal interstitial lung disease. Am J Respir Crit Care Med 165:1557, 2002.

164. Chou P, Blei ED, Sherr-Schwarz S, et al: Pulmonary changes following extracorporeal membrane oxygenation: Autopsy study of 23 cases. Hum Pathol 24:405, 1993.

165. Church J, Isaacs H, Saxon A, et al: Lymphoid interstitial pneumonitis and hypogammaglobulinemia in children. Am Rev Respir Dis 124:491, 1981.

166. Clement A, Allen J, Corrin B, et al: Task force on chronic interstitial lung disease in immunocompetent children. Eur Respir J 24:886, 2004.

167. Coalson JJ, King RJ, Yang F, et al: SP-A deficiency in primate model of bronchopulmonary dysplasia with infection. In situ mRNA and immunostains. Am J Respir Crit Care Med 151:854, 1995.

168. Coleman M, Dehner LP, Sibley RK, et al: Pulmonary alveolar proteinosis: An uncommon cause of chronic neonatal respiratory distress. Am Rev Respir Dis 121:583, 1980.

169. Deterding RR, Fan LL, Morton R, et al: Persistent tachypnea of infancy (PTI) – a new entity. Pediatr Pulmonol 23:72, 2001.

170. Erickson AM, de la Monte SM, Moore GW, Hutchins GM: The progression of morphologic changes in bronchopulmonary dysplasia. Am J Pathol 127:474, 1987.

171. Fan LL, Langston C: Chronic interstitial lung disease in children. State of the art review. Pediatr Pulmonol 16:184, 1993.

172. Fan LL, Mullen ALW, Brugman SM, Inscore SC, Parks DP, White CW: Clinical spectrum of chronic interstitial lung disease in children. J Pediatr 121:867, 1992.

173. Farrell P, Gilbert EF, Zimmerman JJ, et al: Familial lung disease associated with proliferation and desquamation of type II pneumonocytes. Am J Dis Child 140:262, 1986.

174. Fisher M, Roggli V, Merten D, et al: Coexisting endogenous lipoid pneumonia, cholesterol granulomas, and pulmonary alveolar proteinosis in a pediatric population: A clinical, radiographic, and pathologic correlation. Pediatr Pathol 12:365, 1992.

175. Hull J, Chow CW, Robertson CF: Chronic idiopathic bronchiolitis of infancy. Arch Dis Child 77:512, 1997.

176. Husain AN, Siddiqui NH, Stocker JT: Pathology of arrested acinar development in postsurfactant

bronchopulmonary dysplasia. Hum Pathol 29:710, 1998.

177. Jobe AH, Bancalari E: Bronchopulmonary dysplasia. Am J Respir Crit Care Med 163:1723, 2001.

178. Joshi VV, Oleske JM, Minnefor AB, et al: Pathological pulmonary findings in children with AIDS. Hum Pathol 16:241, 1985.

179. Katzenstein A-LA, Fiorelli RF: Nonspecific interstitial pneumonia/fibrosis. Histologic features and clinical significance. Am J Surg Pathol 18:136, 1994.

180. Katzenstein A-LA, Gordon LP, Oliphant M, Swender PT: Chronic pneumonitis of infancy. A unique form of interstitial lung disease occurring in early childhood. Am J Surg Pathol 19:439, 1995.

181. Katzenstein A-LA, Myers JL, Mazur MT: Acute interstitial pneumonia. A clinicopathologic, ultrastructural, and cell kinetic study. Am J Surg Pathol 10:256, 1986.

182. Koss MN: Pulmonary lymphoproliferative disorders. In: Churg A, Katzenstein A, eds: *The Lung: Current Concepts*, Baltimore, Williams and Wilkins, 1993, pp 145–194.

183. Mak H, Moser RL, Hallett JS, Robotham JL: Usual interstitial pneumonia in infancy. Clinical and pathologic evolution. Chest 82:124, 1982.

184. Margraf LR, Tomashefski JF Jr, Bruce MC, Dahms BB: Morphometric analysis of the lung in bronchopulmonary dysplasia. Am Rev Respir Dis 143:391, 1991.

185. Marolda J, Pace B, Bonforte RJ, et al: Pulmonary manifestations of HIV infection in children. Pediatr Pulmonol 10:231, 1991.

186. McDonald JW, Roggli VL, Bradford WD: Coexisting endogenous and exogenous lipoid pneumonia and pulmonary alveolar proteinosis in a patient with neurodevelopmental disease. Pediatr Pathol 14:505, 1994.

187. Mildenberger E, deMello DE, Lin Z, et al: Focal congenital alveolar proteinosis associated with abnormal surfactant protein B messenger RNA. Chest 119:645, 2001.

188. Moran CA, Suster S, Pavlova Z, et al: The spectrum of pathological changes in the lung in children with the acquired immunodeficiency syndrome: An autopsy study of 36 cases. Hum Pathol 25:877, 1994.

189. Nogee LM, deMello DE, Dehner LP, Colten HR: Deficiency of pulmonary surfactant protein B in congenital alveolar proteinosis. N Engl J Med 328:406, 1993.

190. Northway WH Jr: Bronchopulmonary dysplasia: Twenty-five years later. Pediatrics 89:969, 1992.

191. Northway WH Jr, Rosan RC, Porter DY: Pulmonary disease following respiratory therapy of hyaline-membrane disease. Bronchopulmonary dysplasia. N Engl J Med 276:357, 1967.

192. Olsen J, Colby T, Elliott C: Hamman-Rich syndrome revisited. Mayo Clin Proc 65:1538, 1990.

193. Pfenninger J, Tschaeppeler H, Wagner BP, et al: The paradox of adult respiratory distress syndrome in neonates. Pediatr Pulmonol 10:18, 1991.

194. Ramani P, Shah A: Lymphangiomatosis. Histologic and immunohistochemical analysis of four cases. Am J Surg Pathol 17:329, 1993.

195. Riedler J, Golser A, Huttegger I: Fibrosing alveolitis in an infant. Eur Respir J 5:359, 1992.

196. Schroeder SA, Shannon DC, Mark EJ: Cellular interstitial pneumonitis in infants. A clinicopathologic study. Chest 101:1065, 1992.

197. Shah AR, Dinwiddie R, Woolf D, et al: Generalized lymphangiomatosis and chylothorax in the pediatric age group. Pediatr Pulmonol 14:126, 1992.

198. Stillwell PC, Norris DG, O'Connell EJ, Rosenow EC III, Weiland LH, Harrison EG Jr: Desquamative interstitial pneumonitis in children. Chest 77:165, 1980.

199. Stocker JT: Pathologic features of long-standing "healed" bronchopulmonary dysplasia: A study of 28 3- to 40-month-old infants. Hum Pathol 17:943, 1986.

200. Tal A, Maor E, Bar-Ziv J, Gorodischer R: Fatal desquamative interstitial pneumonia in three infant siblings. J Pediatr 104:873, 1984.

201. Tazelaar HD, Kerr D, Yousem SA, et al: Diffuse pulmonary lymphangiomatosis. Hum Pathol 24:1313, 1993.

202. Wigger HJ, Berdon WE, Ores CN: Fatal desquamative interstitial pneumonia in an infant. Case report with transmission and scanning electron microscopical studies. Arch Pathol Lab Med 101:129, 1977.

MISCELLANEOUS I. SPECIFIC DISEASES OF UNCERTAIN ETIOLOGY

This chapter includes miscellaneous forms of infiltrative lung diseases that have specific clinical and pathologic features and usually require a lung biopsy for diagnosis.

PULMONARY ALVEOLAR PROTEINOSIS

Pulmonary alveolar proteinosis (PAP), first described in 1958 by Rosen et al,[32] is a rare and fascinating disease characterized by the accumulation of surfactant-like material within alveolar spaces. Other names have been proposed, including *pulmonary alveolar lipoproteinosis* and *pulmonary alveolar phospholipoproteinosis*, that more accurately portray the nature of the intraalveolar material[30,35] but are too cumbersome for routine use. The disease is divided into four categories as listed in Table 15–1. The *acquired* or *idiopathic* form is the most common, and it is discussed in detail in the following sections. *Secondary alveolar proteinosis* occurs in persons who have conditions or treatments associated with impaired macrophage function, including malignancies (especially hematologic, but also solid tumors), cytotoxic or immunosuppressive therapy, HIV infection, and the rare inherited disorder of amino acid transport, lysinuric protein intolerance.[2,29,30,32,33,36,39,48] *Dust-related alveolar proteinosis* is often included under the category of secondary alveolar proteinosis. It has been reported most commonly following high exposures to silica dust, as in sandblasters (see Chapter 5),

Table 15–1   Classification of Pulmonary Alveolar Proteinosis
Acquired (idiopathic, primary)
Secondary
Dust-related
Congenital

and occasional cases have been reported following aluminum, titanium, and fibrous insulation material exposures.[20,25,26,28,30,34] *Congenital alveolar proteinosis*, as the name implies, occurs in newborn and young infants, and some cases are familial.[9,22,24,42] It differs clinically, histologically, and pathogenetically from the other forms of alveolar proteinosis, however, and should be considered a different disease. Most cases are due to genetic abnormalities in surfactant proteins. Histologically, many fit with chronic pneumonitis of infancy (see Chapter 14) rather that PAP, and the prognosis is poor.

Clinical Features

Acquired PAP occurs most often in adults in the fourth to fifth decade and the mean age of onset is 39 years.[1,13,30,32,35,37,43] Cases have been reported in older children, although, as noted earlier, the disease reported in children younger than 1 year old probably represents a different entity. There is a male predominance. Rare familial cases have been reported.[24,45] Dyspnea and cough are the most common presenting complaints, while low-grade fever and streaky hemoptysis are encountered occasionally. A few patients are asymptomatic. Pulmonary function studies show restrictive defects. Elevated serum levels of lactate dehydrogenase (LDH), surfactant proteins A, B, and D, and KL-6, a mucin-like glycoprotein, are usually observed but are not specific.[15,40] Neutralizing IgG autoantibodies to granulocyte–macrophage colony-stimulating factor (GM-CSF) are present both in the serum and in broncho-alveolar lavage (BAL) fluid.[3,21] They are important both for diagnosis and for understanding pathogenesis (see further on).

Chest x-rays usually show bilateral symmetric airspace opacities with perihilar accentuation that may resemble pulmonary edema.[32,34] Less commonly, the lesions are patchy, asymmetric, and even unilateral,[30,32,34] and, rarely, interstitial opacities may occur.[8,27] Ground glass densities often associated with thickened interlobular septa that have characteristic polygonal shapes (so-called 'crazy paving') are typically seen on high-resolution computed tomography (HRCT) scans.[16,23] The radiographic findings often seem to be out of proportion to the patient's symptoms. The diagnosis is usually made from transbronchial or surgical lung biopsies, although sometimes cytologic specimens from sputum or BAL are diagnostic.[4,7,30,35]

Whole lung lavage is the usual therapy, and prognosis is good, with greater than 90% survival reported in recent years.[18,30,37,43] Lobar lavage with fiberoptic bronchoscopy has been utilized in some patients.[6] Spontaneous remission without therapy has also been reported.[46] Recently, therapy with GM-CSF has been used with beneficial results in some patients.[19,38,41,43]

Pathology

Grossly, the affected parenchyma is firm and yellow–tan. The fluid removed in lavage specimens has a characteristic opaque, milky appearance (Fig. 15–1). The striking histologic feature is the filling of the alveolar spaces with eosinophilic, amorphous to coarsely granular material (Figs 15–2 and 15–3). The intraalveolar material usually stains weakly positive with periodic acid–Schiff (PAS), and this stain helps emphasize the characteristic granularity (Fig. 15–4). Basophilic, rather than eosinophilic, staining has been reported in unfixed frozen-section preparations.[10] The intraalveolar material stains strongly with an antibody to surfactant apoprotein in acquired PAP, whereas staining is focal or absent in secondary alveolar proteinosis.[39] Vacuolated, foamy macrophages and ghost-like cell remnants may be prominent within the eosinophilic material, and needle-like, acicular spaces resulting from cholesterol deposition are also common. Hyperplastic, cuboidal, alveolar type 2 pneumocytes often line alveolar septa.

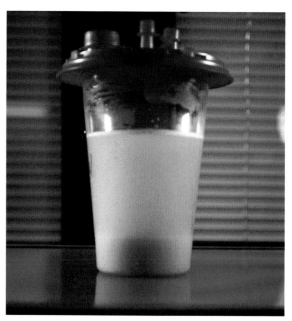

Figure 15–1 Gross photo of fluid removed during whole lung lavage from a patient with PAP. Note the characteristic milky appearance.

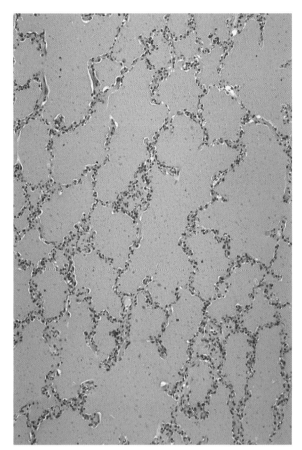

Figure 15–2 Low magnification view of PAP. The alveolar spaces are filled with eosinophilic material while the alveolar septa are nearly normal.

The interstitial architecture of the lung is usually not otherwise abnormal, although interstitial fibrosis may rarely accompany the other changes.[8,27]

Significant inflammation and parenchymal necrosis are not seen in uncomplicated cases, and their presence should suggest an associated infection. Nocardia infection is encountered with increased frequency in this disease, and infections due to other organisms, including various fungi and mycobacteria, have also been described.[31,32,47]

Electron microscopy of the intraalveolar material demonstrates numerous, concentrically laminated myelin figures and lamellar bodies that are similar to the cytoplasmic inclusions normally found in type 2 alveolar pneumocytes (Fig. 15–5).[12,17] These structures, along with lipid droplets, cellular debris, scattered macrophages, and unattached type 2 alveolar pneumocytes, are dispersed in an electron-dense granular material. Biochemical and immunologic studies on BAL fluid show the presence of surfactant phospholipids and proteins, including large amounts of surfactant proteins A and D.[11]

Differential Diagnosis

The differential diagnosis of PAP includes any disease characterized by intraalveolar accumulation of eosinophilic material. *Pulmonary edema* is an important lesion to be distinguished from PAP. The edema fluid differs from the intraalveolar material of PAP in that it appears homogeneous and lacks granularity, acicular spaces, and foam cells (Fig. 15–6). *Pneumocystis carinii pneumonia* also enters the differential diagnosis. Identification of the typical frothy or honeycomb exudate of pneumocystis (see Chapter 10) should facilitate the diagnosis, and, of course, a Gomori's methenamine silver (GMS) stain will demonstrate the organisms.

Changes resembling PAP can occasionally be encountered in parenchyma distal to *bronchial obstruction*.[44] The presence of numerous foamy macrophages along with a prominent inflammatory component, often with fibrosis, should indicate the correct diagnosis. The relationship to an obstructed bronchus is also usually obvious.

Etiology and Pathogenesis

Early theories postulated an overproduction of surfactant related to inhaled irritants, defective alveolar clearance mechanisms, or a combination of both in the pathogenesis of PAP.[2,30,31] It is now clear that the presence of neutralizing IgG antibodies to GM-CSF has a central role in etiology. These antibodies are found in serum and BAL fluid of all patients with PAP.[3,5,19,21,37,41,43] GM-CSF is a cytokine important in modulating macrophage function, and the presence of anti-GM-CSF antibodies causes a relative deficiency of GM-CSF with subsequent impairment of macrophage function and inability to appropriately clear the alveolar spaces.

LANGERHANS CELL HISTIOCYTOSIS (PULMONARY EOSINOPHILIC GRANULOMA)

Langerhans cell histiocytosis (also known as pulmonary eosinophilic granuloma) is a proliferative disorder of Langerhans histiocytes that belongs to the spectrum of disorders known as *histiocytosis-X* or *differentiated histiocytosis*.[69,76,97] Although pulmonary involvement is

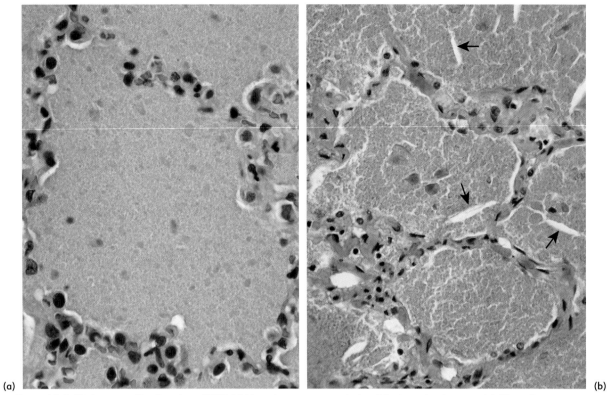

(a)   (b)

Figure 15–3 Higher magnification view of PAP. (a) Note the coarse granularity of the intraalveolar material. The adjacent alveolar septa contain mildly hyperplastic alveolar pneumocytes but are otherwise unremarkable. (b) Cholesterol clefts (arrows) are seen in this example of PAP. Note the prominent granularity in the background.

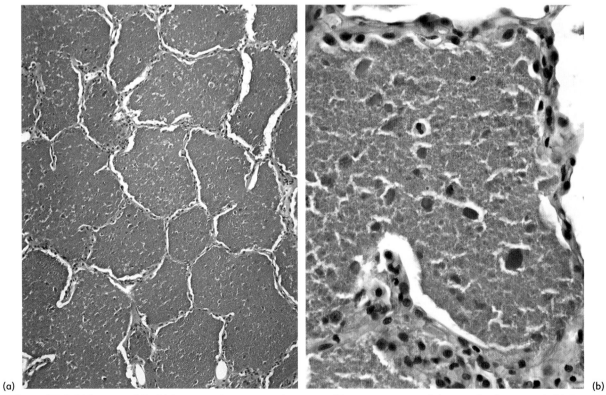

(a)   (b)

Figure 15–4 PAS stain in PAP. (a) Low magnification view showing weakly positive staining of the intraalveolar material. (b) At higher magnification, the PAS stain highlights the granularity of the intraalveolar material.

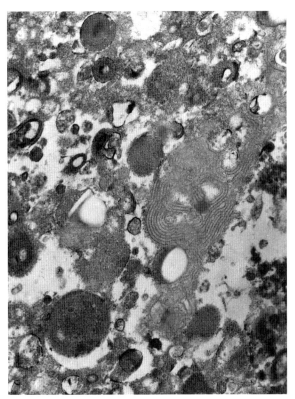

Figure 15–5 Electron micrograph of alveolar material in **PAP**. Note the concentric lamellated structures as well as the cellular debris.

common in all these diseases, the primary lesion known as 'pulmonary eosinophilic granuloma' or 'pulmonary Langerhans cell histiocytosis' is distinctly different and should be considered separately from the disseminated forms of histiocytosis. Currently, the term 'Langerhans cell histiocytosis' is preferred over 'eosinophilic granuloma' although the latter term has been used for many years. 'Eosinophilic granuloma' is a misnomer since the process is not truly granulomatous and eosinophils are not always present.

The pathogenesis of pulmonary Langerhans cell histiocytosis is uncertain, although there is some evidence that the characteristic proliferation of Langerhans cells represents an abnormal immune reaction, possibly directed at components in cigarette smoke.[93,102] Clonality has been demonstrated in extrapulmonary lesions,[101] but is not a consistent feature of lung lesions.[58,102]

Clinical Features

Pulmonary Langerhans cell histiocytosis occurs almost exclusively in cigarette smokers, including both current and ex-smokers.[57,66,90,95] Cough and dyspnea are common presenting complaints, but symptoms may be minimal or absent. Systemic manifestations such as fever, weight loss, and malaise occur occasionally, and spontaneous pneumothorax is the presenting manifestation in a few cases.[81] The peak incidence is in the fourth decade, with only rare cases reported in children.[84,85] The gender distribution varies from male predominance in earlier series to female predominance in more recent studies.[52,59,66,69,90,95-98] Restrictive defects and decreased diffusing capacity are often found on pulmonary function tests.[57] Extrapulmonary involvement is seen in about 15% of patients and includes bone, anterior pituitary (usually manifesting as diabetes insipidus), skin, or lymph node lesions.[66,80,84,90,95,97]

The radiographic features of Langerhans cell histiocytosis vary depending on the age of the lesion.[52,66,75,90] Early in the disease, the chest radiograph typically shows multiple, bilateral nodules averaging 0.5 to 1.0 cm in diameter that are most prominent in upper lung zones and often spare the lung bases. Solitary pulmonary nodules have been reported rarely,[64,90] and hilar adenopathy is uncommonly found.[53,66] An example of total lung collapse due to endobronchial obstruction by eosinophilic granuloma has also been reported.[85] In older lesions, the nodules may be replaced by small cysts, or, less commonly, honeycomb lung with interstitial fibrosis may develop.[88] Unlike the late stages of the chronic interstitial pneumonias, however, lung volumes in advanced pulmonary eosinophilic granuloma often remain normal or are increased. HRCT scans are helpful in that they emphasize the characteristic thin-walled cystic lesions in addition to small nodules and reticulations.[90,91]

The clinical course of Langerhans cell histiocytosis is variable. The median survival is 12–13 years, with 5- and 10-year survival rates of 74% and 64%, respectively.[59,66,88,90,95,98,99] About 15–20% of patients develop respiratory failure due to irreversible fibrosis, and a smaller proportion die of malignancies. Many recover completely, however, and the efficacy of any particular therapy is difficult to determine since the untreated disease may disappear spontaneously. Smoking cessation is advocated in all cases, and prednisone is usually used for severe disease.[97,98] Lung transplantation has been successful in treating some patients, although relapse in the transplanted lung has been reported.[62]

Association with Malignancy

Several studies have noted an association of pulmonary Langerhans cell histiocytosis with malignant

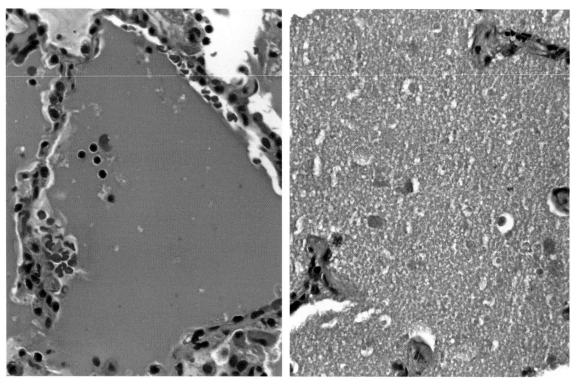

(a)   (b)

Figure 15–6 Contrasting appearance of pulmonary edema and PAP. (a) Pulmonary edema. Note the homogenous eosinophilic appearance to the edema fluid. **(b)** PAP. Note the distinct granularity of the intraalveolar material.

neoplasms.[56,59,60,74,77,83,89,94,97,98] Malignant lymphoma, especially Hodgkin's disease, is the most common associated neoplasm, although the Langerhans cell histiocytosis in these cases occurs more frequently in lymph nodes than in lung. Carcinomas, usually arising in the lung, but occasionally also from various extrapulmonary sites, have likewise been associated with Langerhans cell histiocytosis. The tumors can precede, occur concurrently, or follow the development of the disease. Whether or not there is a true relationship between Langerhans cell histiocytosis and malignancy is speculative. The development of lung carcinoma and Langerhans cell histiocytosis in the same patient may be explained partly by the association of both conditions with cigarette smoking. Additionally, the fact that patients with prior malignancy are often followed with frequent chest x-rays suggests that asymptomatic disease which ordinarily would remain undetected may be identified. This is not the entire explanation, however, at least for lymphomas, since lymph nodes are the organs most commonly involved by Langerhans cell histiocytosis in those diseases.

Histologic Features

The diagnostic histologic features of pulmonary Langerhans cell histiocytosis are listed in Table 15–2. Typically there are discrete, often nodular, interstitial lesions that are localized around bronchioles and separated by areas of normal lung (Fig. 15–7).[51,52,66,72,95] The nodules often assume a stellate shape due to extension of the interstitial infiltrate along alveolar septa, and adjacent airspaces may be enlarged (traction

---

Table 15–2 Diagnostic Histologic Features of Langerhans Cell Histiocytosis

- Nodular interstitial infiltrates of Langerhans cells (S-100, CD1a+)

- Peribronchiolar location, stellate shape

- Adjacent traction emphysema

- Respiratory bronchiolitis with intraalveolar macrophage accumulation (DIP-like reaction)

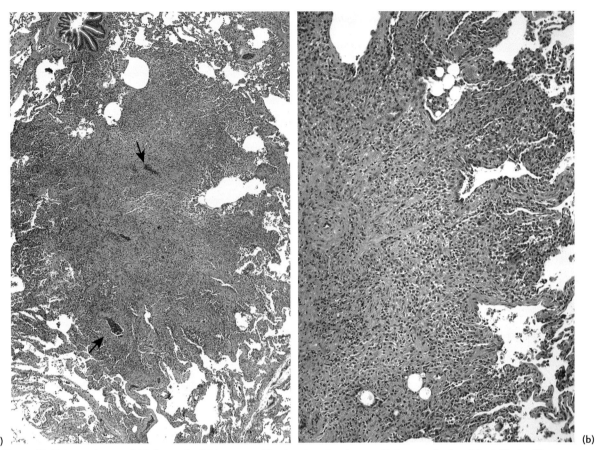

Figure 15–7 Langerhans cell histiocytosis. (a) Low magnification view showing a well-circumscribed nodular infiltrate. The bronchiolocentric location is inferred because the infiltrate is located adjacent to pulmonary arteries (arrows). **(b)** Higher magnification view illustrating extension of the cellular infiltrate along alveolar septa, imparting a stellate configuration. Note the central fibrosis.

emphysema) (Fig. 15–8). The cellular infiltrate comprising the nodules is composed of a mixture of histiocytes and variable numbers of eosinophils, plasma cells, and lymphocytes. Variable fibrosis may be found in the center of the nodules. Eosinophils are not necessary for the diagnosis, and they may be absent. Rather, the diagnosis depends on finding clusters of Langerhans cells within the infiltrate (Fig. 15–8b). These cells are large histiocytes containing bland, folded or indented nuclei, inconspicuous nucleoli, and abundant eosinophilic cytoplasm with indistinct cell borders. In active lesions, Langerhans cells are numerous and occur in small nests or sheets. Central areas of cystic change may be seen in cellular foci (Fig. 15–9). These cystic areas represent residual bronchiolar lumens rather than degenerative or necrotic foci, although they may cause the appearance of cavitation radiographically.[72]

In older lesions, fibrosis becomes prominent, and the diagnostic Langerhans cells may be scant (Fig. 15–10).

The fibrosis affects mainly peribronchiolar interstitium. Often a mixture of chronic inflammatory cells, pigmented histiocytes, and scattered eosinophils is present in the fibrotic areas, and entrapped alveoli lined by hyperplastic alveolar pneumocytes may be seen (Fig. 15–10b). Frequently, stellate- or starfish-shaped scars are found in peribronchiolar parenchyma that follow the original pattern of cellular infiltration along the interstitium (Fig. 15–11). Traction emphysema is characteristically present in adjacent alveoli, and is thought to be due to air trapping related to bronchiolar obstruction from the scarring. Multiple tissue sections may be necessary in such cases to demonstrate the presence of small, active lesions containing diagnostic Langerhans cells. The diagnosis of Langerhans cell histiocytosis, however, cannot be made in the absence of Langerhans cell clusters, although the presence of typical stellate-shaped scars in the correct clinical setting with typical HRCT findings can be considered

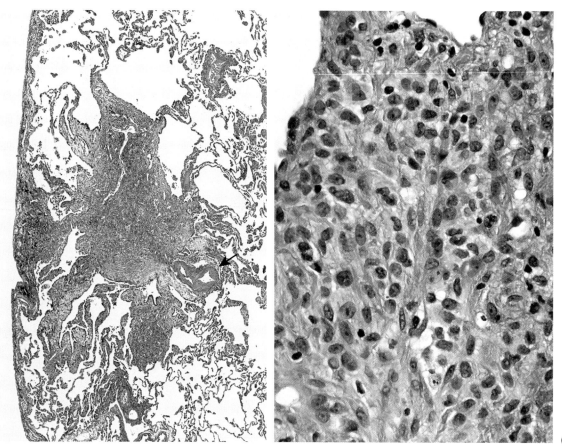

(a)
(b)

Figure 15–8 Langerhans cell histiocytosis. (a) Low magnification view showing the marked stellate or starfish shape to the typical infiltrate. The lesion is located next to a pulmonary artery (arrow), indicating that it has partially replaced a bronchiole. Note also the enlarged airspaces at the periphery (traction emphysema). **(b)** Higher magnification of the cellular infiltrate demonstrating sheets of Langerhans cells. These cells have bland-appearing folded and convoluted nuclei with abundant cytoplasm. Eosinophils are not numerous in this example.

consistent with the diagnosis. Elastic fiber degradation is thought to contribute to the eventual formation of end-stage lung that occurs in some cases.[67] Transforming growth factor β1 has been identified in alveolar pneumocytes and macrophages, while certain metallo-proteinases have been identified in Langerhans cells.[49,70]

In addition to the characteristic interstitial changes of Langerhans cell histiocytosis, evidence of respiratory bronchiolitis (see Chapters 3 and 16) is seen in most cases.[96] This lesion is a manifestation of cigarette smoking, and it occurs in Langerhans cell histiocytosis since patients either are or have been cigarette smokers. Respiratory bronchiolitis is characterized by the accumulation within bronchioles and peribronchiolar airspaces of macrophages containing light brown to golden yellow, coarsely granular cytoplasmic pigmenta-tion. The pigmented macrophages also can accumulate

more widely, often affecting alveolar spaces adjacent to the interstitial lesions of Langerhans cells histiocytosis, and, because of the similarity of such changes to desquamative interstitial pneumonia (DIP), they have been referred to as DIP-like reaction (Fig. 15–12).[87,95,96] As discussed in Chapter 3, this intraalveolar macro-phage accumulation can occur in cigarette smokers in any condition in which the lung is stiffened, including, in addition to Langerhans cell histiocytosis, the chronic interstitial pneumonias as well as localized areas of nonspecific interstitial fibrosis.

The pulmonary arteries in Langerhans cell histio-cytosis may show reactive intimal proliferation and a transmural infiltrate of eosinophils as well as chronic inflammatory cells.[57] The term 'vasculitis' has been used to describe this phenomenon,[51] but it is not appropriate, since the vascular infiltration is a passive

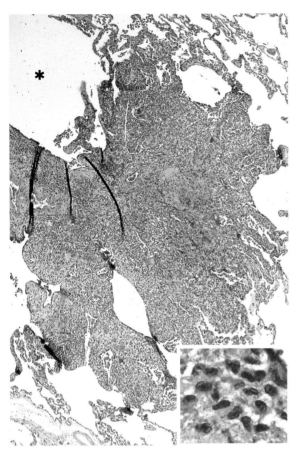

Figure 15–9 Langerhans cell histiocytosis. A cystic space (asterisk) that represents the residuum of a bronchiolar lumen is seen in the center of this infiltrate. Note the stellate shape of the infiltrate due to extension along alveolar septa. Inset is a high magnification showing the typical Langerhans cells that comprise the infiltrate.

phenomenon related to the contiguous parenchymal infiltrate rather than representing a primary event. Changes of pulmonary hypertension have also been described and correlate with clinical evidence of pulmonary hypertension. Some investigators postulate the presence of a small vessel vasculopathy independent of the characteristic Langerhans cell lesions.[63]

Immunohistochemistry and Electron Microscopy

Most cases of pulmonary Langerhans cell histiocytosis are readily diagnosed on hematoxylin and eosin (H and E)-stained sections.[95,100] Difficulty in diagnosis, however, may be encountered occasionally in small transbronchial biopsy specimens or in larger biopsies when

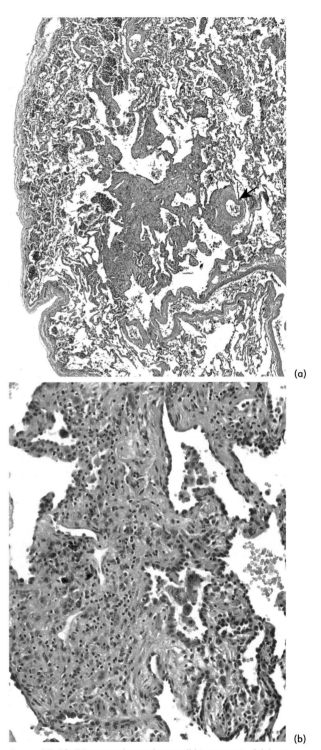

Figure 15–10 Fibrosis in Langerhans cell histiocytosis. (a) Low magnification view showing a bronchiolocentric area of scarring with a partially stellate shape. Note the adjacent pulmonary artery (arrow). **(b)** Higher magnification showing a mixture of chronic inflammatory cells and pigmented histiocytes in the scarred area. Note the entrapped alveoli lined by hyperplastic pneumocytes and the intraalveolar pigmented macrophages.

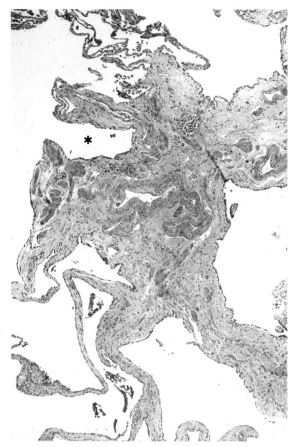

Figure 15–11 Interstitial scar in Langerhans cell histiocytosis. In this example of scarred eosinophilic granuloma, a stellate-shaped scar is seen around a bronchiole (asterisk) and is associated with prominent traction emphysema.

diagnostic areas are focal or artifactually distorted, and immunohistochemistry or electron microscopy can help to confirm the diagnosis.[71]

Immunohistochemistry has largely replaced electron microscopy as a diagnostic tool in Langerhans cell histiocytosis. Immunoperoxidase staining for S-100 protein or CD1a is the most widely used method for identifying Langerhans cells, and it works well on routine paraffin-embedded, formalin-fixed tissue.[54,55,61,65,82,92,93,100] In positive cases, clusters of strongly staining Langerhans cells are identifiable within the pulmonary interstitium as well as in adjacent alveoli (Fig. 15–13). It should be emphasized, however, that scattered Langerhans cells can be found in a variety of other inflammatory (and neoplastic) lung diseases, where they occur singly and are often associated with bronchioles.[68,73,100] Therefore, to confirm the diagnosis of Langerhans cell histiocytosis, these cells must be aggregated in clusters.

Positive staining has been demonstrated for fascin in Langerhans cell histiocytosis, but this staining is not as specific as S-100 or CD1a.[86]

By electron microscopy, characteristic rod- to racquet-shaped, pentalaminar inclusions, known as *Langerhans cell granules*, *Birbeck granules*, or *X bodies*, can be found within the cytoplasm of Langerhans cells (Fig. 15–14).[76] There are no firm ultrastructural criteria for separating Langerhans cells of Langerhans cell histiocytosis from those present in other conditions, although the former cells are said to contain more deeply indented nuclei and more granules.

Differential Diagnosis

The differential diagnosis of Langerhans cell histiocytosis depends on the stage of the disease. When active, cellular lesions containing numerous eosinophils are present, *eosinophilic pneumonia* (see Chapter 6) enters the differential diagnosis. Eosinophilic pneumonia differs in that the mixture of eosinophils and macrophages is present mainly within airspaces rather than the interstitium. Also, the changes lack a peribronchiolar distribution, and the macrophages have round nuclei rather than the folded nuclei of Langerhans cells. In difficult cases, immunohistochemical staining for S-100 antigen or CD1a will answer the question, since only Langerhans cells are positive.

When intraalveolar macrophage accumulation is prominent, the changes can be suggestive of *respiratory bronchiolitis interstitial lung disease (RBILD)/DIP* (see Chapter 3). Finding the characteristic interstitial Langerhans cell infiltrates indicates the correct diagnosis.

When fibrosis is prominent and cellularity is minimal, as in advanced Langerhans cell histiocytosis, the changes may be difficult to differentiate from *usual interstitial pneumonia* (UIP, see Chapter 3). The presence of discrete scars with stellate shape and surrounding traction emphysema occurring in a peribronchiolar distribution is not a feature of UIP. Also, the characteristic honeycomb change of UIP is not seen in Langerhans cell histiocytosis.

Pulmonary Langerhans cell histiocytosis also must be differentiated from *reactive eosinophilic pleuritis*, a lesion that occurs in patients with spontaneous pneumothorax due to various different causes, including underlying Langerhans cell histiocytosis (see Chapter 16).[50,78,79,95] This lesion consists of an infiltrate of eosinophils, macrophages, and mesothelial cells that is confined to the pleura. It appears to represent a nonspecific response to pleural injury. Perivascular

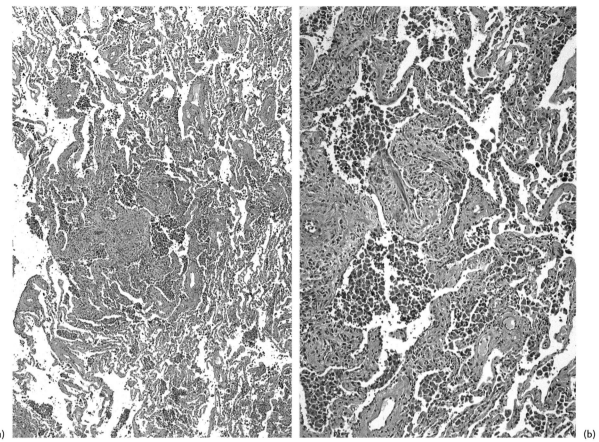

(a)   (b)

Figure 15–12 DIP-like reaction in Langerhans cell histiocytosis. (a) At low magnification the characteristic peribronchiolar stellate-shaped interstitial lesion (left of center) is nearly overshadowed by large numbers of intraalveolar macrophages. **(b)** A higher magnification view highlights the intraalveolar pigmented macrophages. Numerous Langerhans cells are present in the thickened interstitium in the center and at left.

eosinophil infiltrates in lung tissue resected for pneumothorax may accompany the reactive eosinophilic pleuritis.[78] Langerhans cells are not a part of this reaction, and the finding thus should not be confused with eosinophilic granuloma.

PULMONARY LYMPHANGIOMYOMATOSIS

Lymphangiomyomatosis (or lymphangioleiomyomatosis – LAM) is a rare disease occurring almost exclusively in women that is characterized by smooth muscle proliferation in the pulmonary interstitium.[114,118] The term 'lymphangiomyomatosis' should not be confused with *lymphangiomatosis*, an unrelated condition characterized by proliferation of lymphatic spaces (see Chapter 14). Extrapulmonary involvement can occur in LAM, especially of thoracic or abdominal lymph nodes or lymphatics.[137,155]

LAM is an important pulmonary manifestation in women with *tuberous sclerosis*, occurring in as many as 34–39%,[115,119,121,139,152] although most cases of LAM encountered on biopsy specimens are sporadic. Angiomyolipomas of the kidney, which are characteristic findings in tuberous sclerosis, are common both in sporadic LAM and in LAM associated with tuberous sclerosis.[109] Similar gene mutations as well as identical loss of heterozygosity on chromosome 16 have been demonstrated in pulmonary LAM cells and angiomyolipomas from patients with both sporadic LAM and LAM associated with tuberous sclerosis.[121,159] The genes responsible for tuberous sclerosis, *TSC1* and *TSC2*, act as tumor suppressor genes, and their presence in both sporadic LAM and tuberous sclerosis-associated LAM suggests a common pathogenesis for these two diseases.

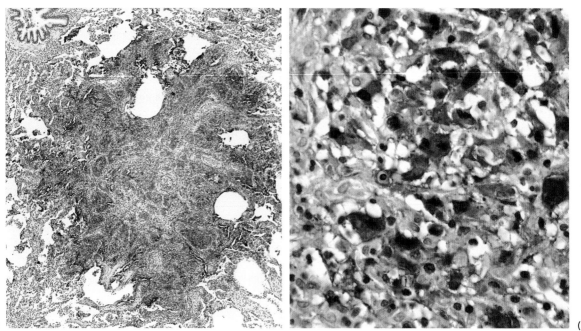

(a)

(b)

Figure 15–13 S-100 staining in Langerhans cell histiocytosis. (a) Low magnification view of S-100 stain showing marked positivity in a nodule of Langerhans cell histiocytosis. (b) Higher magnification view showing the typical nuclear and cytoplasmic staining of Langerhans cells.

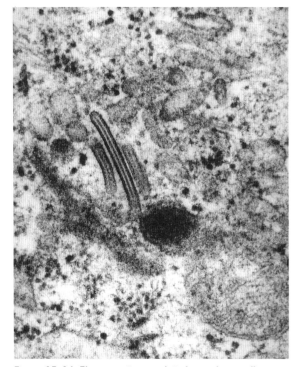

Figure 15–14 Electron micrograph in Langerhans cell histiocytosis, showing the characteristic pentalaminar rod-like Birbeck or Langerhans granules.

Clinical Features

Lymphangiomyomatosis occurs almost exclusively in women and there has been only a single well-documented example reported in a man.[105] Most cases occur during the reproductive years, with a mean age ranging from 32 to 36 years, although occasional cases have been reported in postmenopausal women.[106,114,116,118,131,147, 148,152,153,157] Patients usually present with progressive dyspnea, chylous pleural effusions, recurrent pneumothoraces, or a combination of these findings. Hemoptysis or blood-streaked sputum is occasionally found, and, in rare instances, massive pulmonary hemorrhage may occur. Pulmonary function tests usually show both restrictive and obstructive defects with decreased diffusing capacity and normal or increased total lung capacity.[119,152,157]

Chest radiographs show diffuse reticular interstitial opacities that occasionally appear nodular or resemble honeycomb changes.[103,114,118,131,141] Bullae, pleural effusions, and pneumothorax are frequently demonstrated as well. Lung volume often appears normal sized or slightly enlarged, despite the presence of diffuse interstitial infiltrates. This appearance differs from most other interstitial diseases (except Langerhans cell histiocytosis and sarcoidosis), where the lungs appear radiographically small. Numerous thin-walled cystic spaces are seen on HRCT scans and are considered highly suggestive of the diagnosis.[103,141,148,157]

The clinical course in LAM is variable but is usually characterized by slowly progressive disease, with reported 5- and 10-year survival rates of 78–91% and 40–79%, respectively.[131,134,153,156,157] Outcome can be correlated with the extent of parenchymal involvement by smooth muscle proliferation and cysts (so-called *LAM histologic score – LHS*).[134] Antiestrogenic hormonal therapy is usually advocated, and beneficial effects have been reported with both ovarian ablation and progesterone.[120,152,156,157] Lung transplantation has been successful in some cases, although recurrence has been reported in the allograft in a few cases.[110,111,129,142,149] Analysis of microsatellite markers in one case showed that recurrent LAM in the allograft was derived from the patient and contained the same *TSC* gene mutation as in the native LAM.[129]

Histologic Features

The light microscopic findings in LAM are characterized by a disorderly proliferation of benign-appearing smooth muscle bundles within the interstitium.[114,118] Although the prefix *lymphangio-* implies localization of the process to lymphatic spaces, the distribution is quite random. Delicate smooth muscle fibers can be found around bronchioles, in alveolar septa, around arteries, veins, and lymphatic spaces, and in the pleura (Fig. 15–15). The component smooth muscle cells are mostly spindle shaped with bland-appearing elongated nuclei, although some are round and epithelioid appearing, often containing clear cytoplasm. Type 2 pneumocyte hyperplasia frequently accompanies the smooth muscle proliferation.[135] A common, helpful microscopic feature is the presence of small air-filled cysts that contain smooth muscle bundles, at least focally, in their walls (Fig. 15–16). They are thought

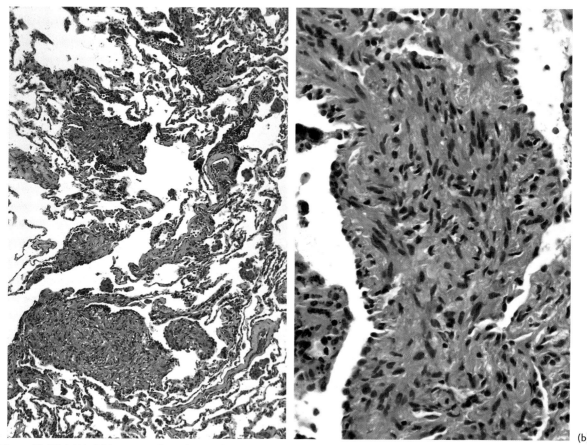

(a)   (b)

Figure 15–15 LAM. (a) Low magnification view showing scattered randomly dispersed areas of smooth muscle proliferation in the interstitium. **(b)** Higher magnification showing the uniform, bland-appearing spindle-shaped smooth muscle cells within an alveolar septum.

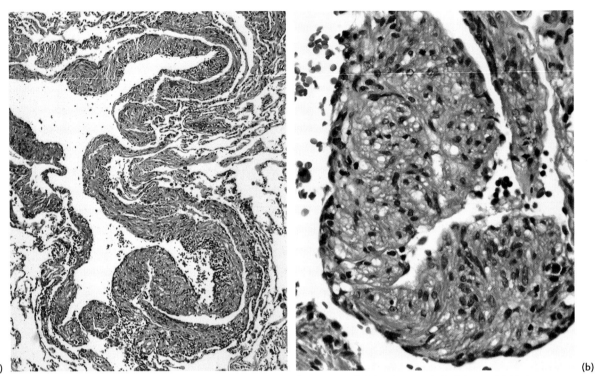

(a)   (b)

Figure 15–16 Cystic spaces in LAM. (a) Low magnification view showing a well-defined cyst with thick lining. **(b)** Higher magnification showing the characteristic smooth muscle lining of the cyst. In this example, many of the cells have an epithelioid rather than spindle cell configuration.

to result from air trapping secondary to bronchiolar narrowing from smooth muscle proliferation. There is also evidence that elastic fiber degradation in areas of smooth muscle proliferation may contribute to the cyst formation and a role for matrix metalloproteinases has been postulated.[122] Some cysts are located directly beneath the pleura, and rupture may cause pneumothorax (Fig. 15–17). Hemosiderin deposition due to occlusion of small veins by the process is common in longstanding cases, and it may be prominent (Fig. 15–18). In such cases, iron encrustation of vascular elastic tissue with a foreign body granulomatous reaction (so-called *endogenous pneumoconiosis*, see Chapter 6) may occur.[118] Occasionally, small aggregates of immature-appearing round to ovoid cells (thought to represent immature smooth muscle cells) are also found and have been termed *myoblastic foci*.[118] A proliferation of lymphatic spaces in and around LAM lesions has been demonstrated.[133]

The smooth muscle proliferation may also affect the lymphatics in the thorax and abdomen, transforming them into thick, cord-like structures or replacing the

parenchyma of adjacent lymph nodes.[118,155] Rupture of these lymphatic channels may lead to chylothorax.

Peculiar nodular proliferations of type 2 alveolar pneumocytes have been observed in LAM and are termed *micronodular pneumocyte hyperplasia (MNPH).*[118,125,140,145] They are found most often in patients with tuberous sclerosis and thus are considered a marker of that condition. They can occur, however, in cases of sporadic LAM, and rare examples have been reported unassociated with tuberous sclerosis or LAM. They are characterized by enlarged, often atypical alveolar pneumocytes lining thickened alveolar septa, and they average a few millimeters in greatest dimension (Fig. 15–19). The process is thought to represent a hamartomatous proliferation.

Immunohistochemistry and Electron Microscopy

The aberrant smooth muscle bundles of LAM usually stain for the melanoma-associated antigen HMB-45 in addition to smooth muscle actin, vimentin, and some-

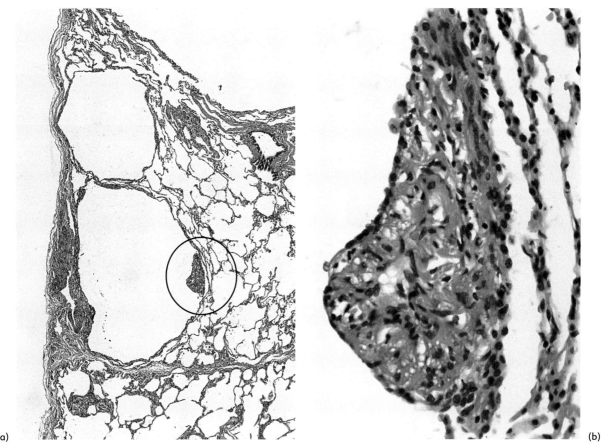

(a)   (b)

Figure 15–17 Cystic spaces in LAM. (a) At low magnification, thin-walled cysts are seen beneath the pleura in this example, and in areas their walls are thickened by nests of smooth muscle (left beneath the pleura and in circle). **(b)** Higher magnification from the circled area shows a small focus of bland-appearing smooth muscle in the cyst wall.

times desmin (Fig. 15–20).[112,116,127,137,138,144] Estrogen and progesterone receptor antigens have been identified in some, but not all, cases of LAM.[108,113,117,124,136,143] They appear to be present more often in patients without other associated features of tuberous sclerosis and are observed mainly in the epithelioid cells.[136]

Ultrastructural studies demonstrate smooth muscle features in the proliferating spindle cells.[107,128,144] Abundant cytoplasmic glycogen is a consistent feature, and distinct membrane-bound crystalloid structures have been noted in some cases.

Differential Diagnosis

The main lesions in the differential diagnosis of LAM include other conditions in which smooth muscle proliferation is prominent. *Benign metastasizing leiomyoma*, a rare condition thought to represent a metastatic, low-grade leiomyosarcoma from the uterus in most cases, is characterized by similar bland-appearing smooth muscle proliferation (Fig. 15–21).[123,154,158] The smooth muscle differs from that in LAM in that it is more likely to be nodular and contain entrapped alveolar epithelium. The distinction between these two diseases can be difficult in some cases, however, and staining for HMB-45 helps, since it is negative in benign metastasizing leiomyoma. The differentiation of these two entities is not crucial for patient management, since hormonal treatment is used for both and their prognosis is similar.

LAM needs to be distinguished from the smooth muscle hyperplasia that frequently occurs in the late stage of interstitial fibrosis, so-called *muscular cirrhosis* (see Fig. 3–5b).[130] This lesion is composed of thicker smooth muscle bundles in areas of honeycomb change that are arranged around or replace a bronchiole. Transitions from normal bronchiolar smooth muscle can often be seen, and background

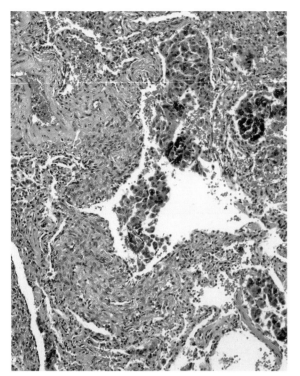

Figure 15–18 Hemosiderin deposition in LAM. In this example there are numerous hemosiderin-filled macrophages within the airspaces. Note a small cyst in the center that is lined by smooth muscle.

interstitial fibrosis is extensive. Occasionally, *smooth muscle hyperplasia* occurs around bronchioles in cases of chronic obstructive pulmonary disease or chronic bronchiolitis in the absence of parenchymal scarring. This lesion differs from LAM in that it only occurs where smooth muscle normally is found, and it is confined to peribronchiolar parenchyma. Again, in difficult cases, staining for HMB-45 should help, since non-LAM processes are negative.

When cysts are prominent, the changes may superficially resemble *emphysema*. The finding of aberrant smooth muscle bundles in the cyst walls, however, should indicate the correct diagnosis. The fact that emphysema is uncommon in young women is an important clue to look carefully for another cause of the cysts. The *alveolar hemorrhage syndromes* (see Chapter 6) may enter the differential diagnosis when hemosiderin deposition is prominent. Attention to the smooth muscle proliferation should clarify the issue in these diseases as well.

Another low-grade uterine lesion that can resemble LAM is metastatic *endometrial stromal sarcoma*, and

patients can present with lung lesions before a uterine primary is recognized.[104] The cells of this neoplasm appear more stellate shaped and have only scant cytoplasm. They are present within a delicate myxoid stroma with prominent vascularity. Immunohistochemical stains are strongly positive for CD110 and estrogen receptor protein, and they are negative for HMB-45.

PULMONARY ALVEOLAR MICROLITHIASIS

Pulmonary alveolar microlithiasis is a rare disorder that is characterized by the appearance of laminated calcospherites in the lung in the absence of any known abnormality of calcium metabolism. The disease appears in a sporadic, isolated form and as a familial condition, apparently transmitted by an autosomal recessive gene.[160,165,172,176] A disproportionate number of cases have been reported from Turkey.[173,176]

Clinical Features

The early clinical features of alveolar microlithiasis are minimal and nonspecific, and the majority of cases are diagnosed on the basis of an incidental or routine chest radiograph.[172,176] Patients usually present in their twenties and early thirties,[161,165,167,170–172,176] although cases have been reported in infants, children, and the elderly.[173,177] In the sporadic form of the disorder, there is a male prevalence, whereas in familial cases, females predominate in most series. The chest film shows distinct, diffusely scattered micronodular calcifications throughout the lung, with accentuation toward the bases. The appearance has been described as sand-like.[165,173] There is usually marked disparity between the paucity of symptoms and the striking radiographic picture.[165] Spontaneous pneumothorax has been noted in a few cases.

The clinical course of pulmonary alveolar microlithiasis is variable. Little or no progression occurs in some patients, whereas in others, interstitial fibrosis and cor pulmonale may develop.[165,167,169] There is no known effective therapy. Lung lavage has been attempted in a few patients, but has had no beneficial effect.[165–167] Disodium etidronate, a drug that inhibits hydroxyapatite metabolism, has also been used with minimal success.[166,171] Lung transplantation has been undertaken occasionally.[161,174]

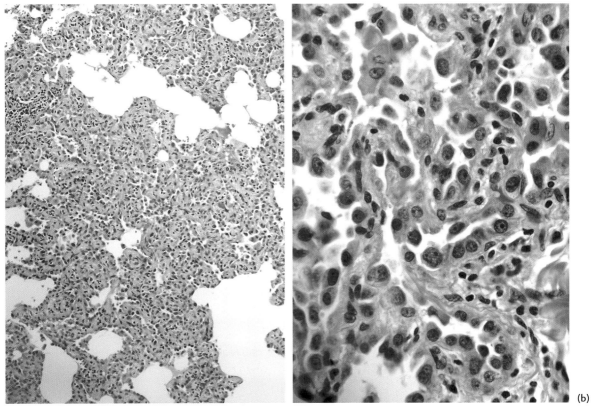

Figure 15–19 Multinodular pneumocyte hyperplasia in LAM. (a) Low magnification view showing a cellular nodular lesion.
(b) Higher magnification demonstrates that the lesion is composed of hyperplastic pneumocytes.

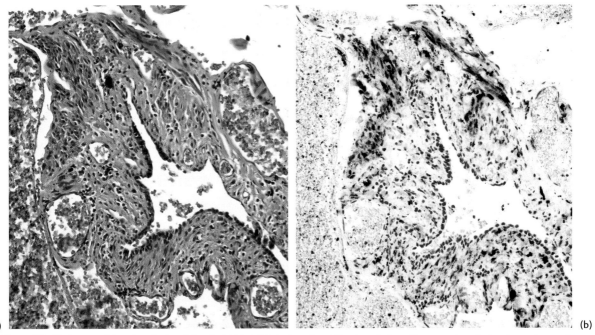

Figure 15–20 Immunohistochemical staining in LAM. (a) Subpleural cyst lined partly by collagen and partly by aberrant smooth
muscle (darker staining areas). (b) Prominent staining of smooth muscle cells in the cyst wall for HMB-45.

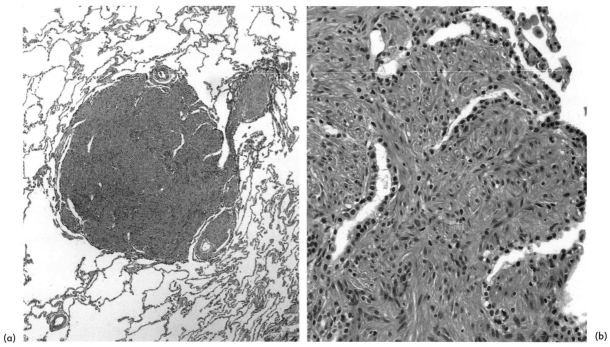

(a)   (b)

Figure 15–21 Benign metastasizing leiomyoma. (a) Low magnification showing a well-circumscribed nodular lesion. **(b)** At higher magnification the lesion is composed of bland-appearing spindle-shaped cells similar to the cells of LAM. One difference, in addition to the distinct nodularity, is the presence of entrapped alveoli lined by hyperplastic alveolar pneumocytes.

Pathologic Features

A distinct gritty sensation is noted grossly when sectioning the lung. Histologically, there is an intraalveolar and interstitial accumulation of concentrically laminated calcified bodies that also can be seen in the submucosa of bronchi and bronchioles (Fig. 15–22).[163,168,169] These calcospherites vary in size from several microns to a millimeter or more, and may appear either blue or pink in H and E stains, depending on whether or not decalcification is required for histologic preparations. Sometimes, in older lesions, ossification may be present on the periphery of the calcospherites. Calcospherites have been noted in extrapulmonary sites in a few cases, and they can be identified in sputum and BAL specimens.[172] Their presence in sputum preparations is not diagnostic of alveolar microlithiasis, however, since similar structures may be found in the sputum of patients with chronic obstructive lung disease.[175]

Several analytic techniques have demonstrated that the calcospherites are composed mainly of calcium and phosphorus, sometimes with small amounts of calcium carbonate and traces of silicon, magnesium, and iron.[169,172] There is some evidence that they represent a form of carboxyapatite, a close relative of hydroxyapatite.[160] The pathogenesis is unknown. A relationship has been postulated to inhalation of sand particles, but this exposure has been documented in only a few cases.[170,176]

Differential Diagnosis

Various other forms of *calcification* (see Chapter 16) enter the differential diagnosis of alveolar microlithiasis. They differ because they do not form calcospherites, and calcium is usually deposited in the interstitium rather than the airspaces. *Corpora amylacea* (see Chapter 1, Figs 1–8, 1–9) must be distinguished from calcospherites. These are large, round, eosinophilic structures that are common, incidental findings. They occur within alveolar spaces and do not contain calcium.[162] So-called *blue bodies* must also be distinguished from calcospherites (see Chapters 1 and 3, Figs 1–10, 3–13).[164] These structures are gray to basophilic, round forms, and they are smaller than most microliths, averaging 15 to 25 μm in size. They stain for calcium and iron at their periphery, and connective tissue mucin at their center. They occur mainly within alveolar macrophage cytoplasm and are nonspecific findings in any condition in which macrophages are numerous.

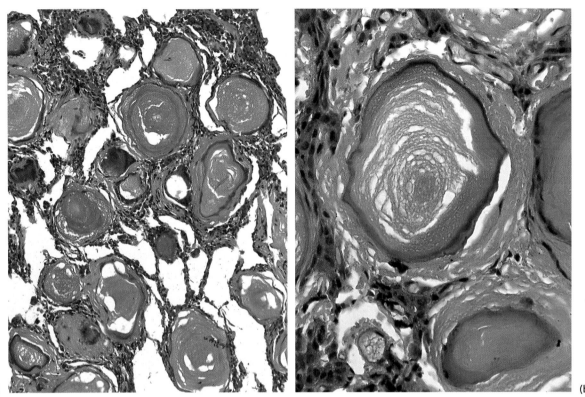

(a)   (b)

Figure 15–22 Pulmonary alveolar microlithiasis. (a) Varying-sized concentric laminated calcospherites are seen in both the airspaces and the interstitium. **(b)** Higher magnification showing the typical lamellated appearance of an interstitial calcospherite. (Photomicrographs courtesy of Dr Jeffrey Myers, Ann Arbor, Michigan.)

PULMONARY HYALINIZING GRANULOMA AND FIBROSING MEDIASTINITIS

Pulmonary hyalinizing granuloma and fibrosing media-stinitis are related disorders with identical pathologic features. The latter occurs in the mediastinum and hilar area, and it may extend focally into adjacent lung parenchyma. The term pulmonary hyalinizing granuloma is used when the process occurs within the lung parenchyma in the absence of contiguous mediastinal involvement. Both lesions are thought to represent abnormal immunologic reactions to previous granulomatous infections, mainly histoplasmosis and possibly also tuberculosis.[185,189,193,198,203] A few patients manifest both lesions concurrently,[185,207] and they also have been reported in association with other fibrosing lesions such as retroperitoneal fibrosis and orbital pseudotumor.[181,199,201]

Pulmonary Hyalinizing Granuloma

Pulmonary hyalinizing granuloma is a rare disorder characterized by slowly enlarging nodules in the pulmonary parenchyma that clinically may suggest metastatic carcinoma.[185,207]

Clinical Features

Pulmonary hyalinizing granuloma usually occurs in young or middle-aged adults.[179,185,207] Most patients present with mild or nonspecific symptoms, including cough, fatigue, fever, or pleuritic chest pain, although approximately one-quarter are asymptomatic. Laboratory studies have detected various autoimmune phenomena, including antinuclear antibody (ANA), rheumatoid factor, anti-smooth muscle antibody, and Coombs-positive hemolytic anemia. Circulating immune complexes have also been identified in some cases.[202,207] Multiple, bilateral nodular densities are the most common chest radiographic finding. Solitary lesions occur occasionally. When serial chest films are available, gradual enlargement of the lesions can often be demonstrated. The clinical course is usually benign, despite the increasing size of the nodules.

Histologic Features

Lung biopsy specimens in pulmonary hyalinizing granuloma show well-defined nodules in the lung parenchyma that are sharply demarcated from adjacent parenchyma (Fig. 15–23). They are composed of thick, relatively acellular, eosinophilic collagen bundles that have a characteristic lamellar arrangement, often forming whorls or storiform arrays (Fig. 15–24).[185,207] They are usually separated by a clear space in which variable numbers of lymphocytes and plasma cells are found. A perivascular inflammatory cell infiltrate is common, and a mild non-necrotizing vasculitis may be seen. The number of inflammatory cells tends to

be most prominent at the periphery of the lesion, and germinal centers may be found. Areas of ischemic necrosis, often containing karyorrhectic cellular debris, are common in the center. Discrete foci of calcification are usually not seen, although focal calcification of collagen bundles has been reported in a few cases.[207] Foreign body granulomas, and chondroid or osseous metaplasia are not features.

Differential Diagnosis

The main lesions in the differential diagnosis of pulmonary hyalinizing granuloma include *amyloid nodule* and involuting *plasma cell granuloma*. Amyloid nodules (see Chapter 7) are composed of globular eosinophilic material that lacks the distinct lamellar arrangement seen in pulmonary hyalinizing granuloma. Foci of calcification and ossification, and foreign body granulomas are common in amyloidosis but are usually absent in hyalinizing granulomas. An additional helpful feature is that amyloid deposits are frequently found in the pulmonary blood vessels surrounding the amyloid nodule. Of course, the Congo red stain should be positive in amyloidosis and negative in hyalinizing granuloma. Electron microscopy may help in difficult cases since it can easily distinguish the ultrastructural features of amyloid and collagen.[190] The contrasting features of hyalinizing granulomas and amyloid nodules are summarized in Table 15–3.

Although plasma cell granulomas (inflammatory myofibroblastic pseudotumor) may contain hyalinized areas, cellular foci composed of fibroblasts, plasma cells, lymphocytes, and other inflammatory cells are consis-

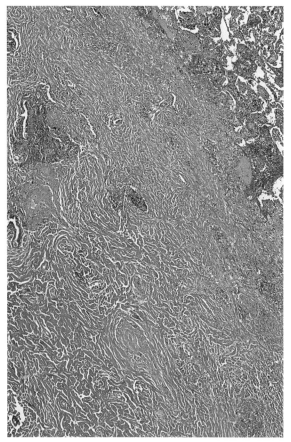

Figure 15–23 Low magnification view of pulmonary hyalinizing granuloma. The lesion is well demarcated from normal lung (top right). The characteristic dense collagen bundles can be appreciated even at this low magnification.

Table 15–3 Contrasting Features of Pulmonary Hyalinizing Granulomas and Amyloid Nodules

Pulmonary Hyalinizing Granulomas	Amyloid Nodules
Thick collagen bundles, lamellar arrangement	Amorphous, globular eosinophilic material
Calcification usually absent, occasional necrosis	Calcification and ossification common
Variable inflammatory cell infiltrate, most prominent at periphery, but no foreign body giant cells	Foreign body giant cell reaction common Amyloid in adjacent blood vessels Positive Congo red stain

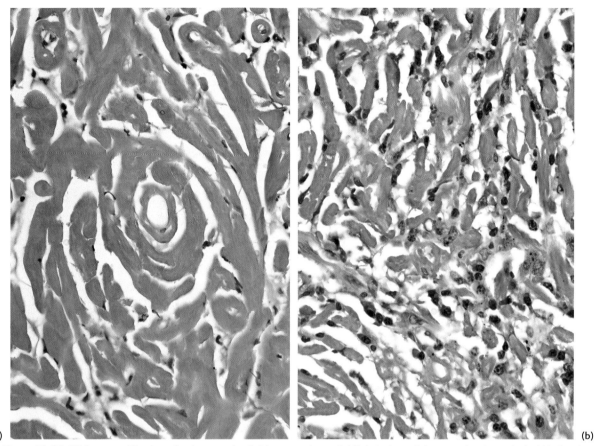

Figure 15–24 Higher magnification of pulmonary hyalinizing granuloma. (a) Relatively acellular area showing typical whirled and lamellated pattern of the collagen bundles. **(b)** Plasma cells are prominent between the collagen bundles in this area.

tently present.[196,200] Furthermore, these neoplasms are almost always solitary and frequently occur in children.

When necrosis is prominent, hyalinizing granulomas need to be distinguished from old, 'burned out' *infectious granulomas*.[206] These lesions are usually surrounded by a thin rim of collagen lamellae that are arranged concentrically around areas of central necrosis, in contrast to the wide area of more haphazardly arranged collagen bundles in hyalinizing granuloma. They often contain broad areas of calcification within the necrotic zones, and usually epithelioid histiocytes can be identified at least focally around the necrotic zones. In contrast, the necrosis in hyalinizing granulomas tends to be patchy and randomly distributed rather than being extensive and centrally located as in necrotizing granulomas, and calcification is usually absent or at least very focal. In questionable cases, special stains for organisms should be performed.

Fibrosing Mediastinitis

Fibrosing mediastinitis is a much more frequently reported condition than pulmonary hyalinizing granuloma.[182,187,189,191,193,198,200,203] It is a destructive and infiltrative fibrosing process involving the mediastinum and hilar areas. Some, but not all, cases surround and appear to develop from caseating granulomas (so-called *granulomatous mediastinitis*).[203] Evidence of prior histoplasmosis is present in most patients in the United States, while prior tuberculosis is more common in Europe.[198]

Clinical Features

Symptoms in fibrosing mediastinitis result from infiltration or compression of vital mediastinal or hilar structures by the dense fibrosis.[186,187,191,195,198,201,203] Cough, hemoptysis, and dyspnea are the most common presenting complaints.[194,201] There may be stridor, collapse of a lobe or entire lung, or distal obstructive pneumonia from narrowing or occlusion of the trachea or major bronchi. In rare instances, dysphagia occurs secondary to esophageal constriction. Compression and obstruction of systemic or pulmonary veins may occur with resultant superior vena cava syndrome, pulmonary venous obstruction, pulmonary hypertension, and even lung infarcts.[178,180,192,193,197] Significant occlusion of the pulmonary artery is rare, but it may cause right ventricular failure.[186,205]

The most common chest x-ray finding is a mediastinal mass or widening.[187,201,204] Calcification is often present and parenchymal lung masses occasionally accompany the other findings. Chest CT demonstrates an infiltrative soft tissue mass that encases or invades normal structures. Two radiographic manifestations on CT have been described: a focal pattern occurring in the majority of patients and a less common diffuse pattern.[201,204] The focal pattern is characterized by a mass that is frequently calcified and usually located in the right paratracheal or subcarinal region or occasionally in the hilum, while a diffusely infiltrating non-calcified mass involving multiple mediastinal compartments is seen in the diffuse pattern. The latter pattern may be related to other idiopathic fibrosing disorders such as retroperitoneal fibrosis rather than to histoplasmosis.

The clinical course is variable, with spontaneous remissions and exacerbations occurring. Prognosis depends on the location of the fibrosis and which mediastinal structures are involved. In one study, mortality rates approaching 30% were noted in patients with subcarinal or bilateral hilar involvement, while outcome was excellent with localized fibrosis.[193] Surgical intervention has been used in cases with airway or vascular compromise, but may be associated with significant mortality.[184,186,188,191] Some success has been reported with percutaneous stenting of vascular structures.[183] Beneficial results have also been reported in a few studies with antifungal agents, but there is no evidence that corticosteroids or other medical treatments are useful.[201]

Pathologic Features

Grossly, fibrosing mediastinitis appears as a mass of firm, white, fibrous tissue that surrounds and compresses mediastinal structures and may extend into the lung parenchyma (Fig. 15–25). Because of its solid consistency and infiltrative growth pattern, it may be mistaken clinically for a malignant tumor.

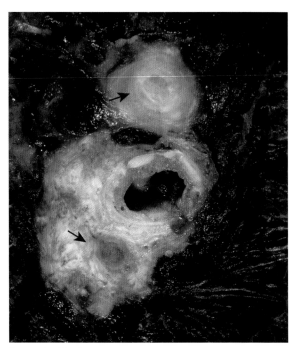

Figure 15–25 Gross appearance of sclerosing mediastinitis. In this example, the process has extended into the hilum, where it surrounds the bronchus and occludes the blood vessels (arrows). This patient underwent pneumonectomy because of a hilar mass that was suspicious for cancer.

The histologic appearance of fibrosing mediastinitis is identical to that of pulmonary hyalinizing granuloma and is characterized by dense bands of collagen often having a lamellar arrangement and separated by variable numbers of lymphocytes and plasma cells (Fig. 15–26).[182,187,189,193,198,201,205] The sclerotic process surrounds, infiltrates, and compresses blood vessels and nerves, and often extends into the lung (Fig. 15–27). Foci of calcification, necrosis, and metaplastic bone formation can sometimes be seen. Occasionally, remnants of necrotizing granulomas are seen within the dense fibrosis, and organisms, especially histoplasma, can sometimes be found in the necrotic granulomas. Organisms are not, however, found in the areas of fibrosis, and cultures are consistently negative.

Differential Diagnosis

Fibrosing mediastinitis needs to be distinguished from other fibrosing processes in the mediastinum, most commonly the fibrosis surrounding or associated with malignancies, especially Hodgkin's disease. The thick collagen bundles in a lamellated pattern would be

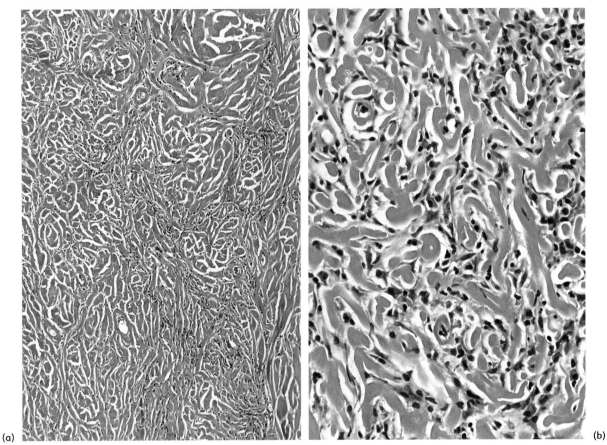

(a)   (b)

Figure 15–26 Sclerosing mediastinitis. (a) Low magnification view showing the typical thick, glassy-appearing collagen bundles often arranged in parallel. **(b)** Higher magnification showing moderate numbers of plasma cells between the collagen bundles.

unusual in this type of reactive fibrosis, but the adequacy of the biopsy should always be assessed and the surgeon urged to take tissue from the center, not the edge, of the lesion. When fibrosing mediastinitis involves the lung, the histologic appearance is indistinguishable from *pulmonary hyalinizing granuloma*, as already discussed. These two lesions often occur together, and their pathogenesis is similar.

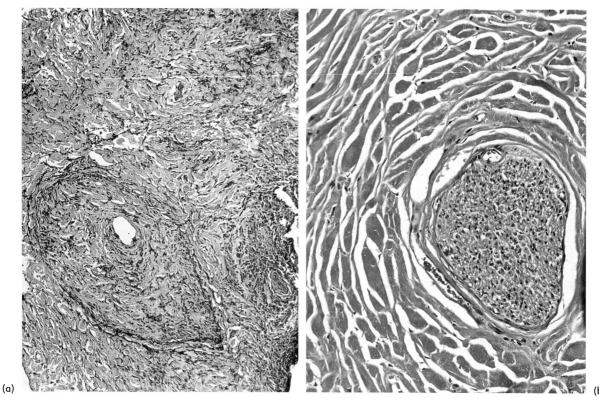

(a)   (b)

Figure 15–27 Infiltrative pattern in sclerosing mediastinitis. (a) Elastic tissue stain showing infiltration of a pulmonary vein by the fibrosing process with almost complete occlusion of its lumen. **(b)** Infiltration around a nerve by the fibrosing process.

REFERENCES

Pulmonary Alveolar Proteinosis

1. Asamoto H, Kitaichi M, Nishimura K, et al: Primary pulmonary alveolar proteinosis – clinical observation of 68 patients in Japan. Nihon Kyobu Shikkan Gakkai Zasshi 33:835, 1995.
2. Bedrossian CWM, Luna MA, Conklin RH, et al: Alveolar proteinosis as a consequence of immunosuppression. A hypothesis based on clinical and pathologic observations. Hum Pathol 71:527, 1980.
3. Bonfield TL, Russell D, Burgess S, et al: Autoantibodies against granulocyte macrophage colony-stimulating factor are diagnostic for pulmonary alveolar proteinosis. Am J Respir Cell Mol Biol 27:481, 2002.
4. Burkhalter A, Silverman JF, Hopkins MB III, Geisinger KR: Bronchoalveolar lavage cytology in pulmonary alveolar proteinosis. Am J Clin Pathol 106:504, 1996.
5. Carraway MS, Ghio AJ, Carter JD, Piantadosi CA: Detection of granulocyte-macrophage colony-stimulating factor in patients with pulmonary alveolar proteinosis. Am J Respir Crit Care Med 161:1294, 2000.
6. Cheng S-L, Chang H-T, Lau H-P, et al: Pulmonary alveolar proteinosis. Treatment by bronchofiberscopic lobar lavage. Chest 122:1480, 2002.
7. Chou CW, Lin FC, Tung SM, et al: Diagnosis of pulmonary alveolar proteinosis: Usefulness of Papanicolaou-stained smears of bronchoalveolar lavage fluid. Arch Intern Med 161:562, 2001.
8. Clague HW, Wallace AC, Morgan WKC: Pulmonary interstitial fibrosis associated with alveolar proteinosis. Thorax 38:865, 1983.
9. Coleman M, Dehner LP, Sibley RK, et al: Pulmonary alveolar proteinosis: An uncommon cause of chronic neonatal respiratory distress. Am Rev Respir Dis 121:583, 1980.
10. Corsello BP, Choi H: Basophilic staining in pulmonary alveolar proteinosis. Arch Pathol Lab Med 108:68, 1984.
11. Crouch E, Persson A, Chang D: Accumulation of surfactant protein D in human pulmonary alveolar proteinosis. Am J Pathol 142:241, 1993.
12. Gilmore LB, Talley FA, Hook GER: Classification and morphometric quantitation of insoluble materials from the lungs of patients with alveolar proteinosis. Am J Pathol 133:252, 1988.
13. Goldstein LS, Kavuru MS, Curtis-McCarthy P, Christie HA, Farver C, Stoller JK: Pulmonary alveolar proteinosis. Clinical features and outcomes. Chest 114:1357, 1998.
14. Hoffman RM, Dauber JH, Rogers RM: Improvement in alveolar macrophage migration after therapeutic whole

lung lavage in pulmonary alveolar proteinosis. Am Rev Respir Dis 139:1030, 1989.

15. Hoffman RM, Rogers RM: Serum and lavage lactate dehydrogenase isoenzymes in pulmonary alveolar proteinosis. Am Rev Respir Dis 143:42, 1991.

16. Holbert JM, Costello P, Li W, et al: CT features of pulmonary alveolar proteinosis. AJR Am J Roentgenol 176:1287, 2001.

17. Hook GER, Gilmore LB, Talley FA: Multilamellated structures from the lungs of patients with pulmonary alveolar proteinosis. Lab Invest 50:711, 1984.

18. Kariman K, Kylstra JA, Spock A: Pulmonary alveolar proteinosis: Prospective clinical experience in 23 patients for 15 years. Lung 162:223, 1984.

19. Kavuru MS, Sullivan EJ, Piccin R, Thomassen MJ, Stoller JK: Exogenous granulocyte-macrophage colony-stimulating factor administration for pulmonary alveolar proteinosis. Am J Respir Crit Care Med 161:1143, 2000.

20. Keller CA, Frost A, Cagle PT, Abraham JL: Pulmonary alveolar proteinosis in a painter with elevated pulmonary concentrations of titanium. Chest 108:277, 1995.

21. Kitamura T, Uchida K, Tanaka N, et al: Serological diagnosis of idiopathic pulmonary alveolar proteinosis. Am J Respir Crit Care Med 162:658, 2000.

22. Knight DP, Knight JA: Pulmonary alveolar proteinosis in the newborn. Arch Pathol Lab Med 109:529, 1985.

23. Lee K-N, Levin DL, Webb WR, et al: Pulmonary alveolar proteinosis. High-resolution CT, chest radiographic, and functional correlations. Chest 111:989, 1997.

24. Mahut B, Delacourt C, Scheinmann P, et al: Pulmonary alveolar proteinosis: Experience with eight pediatric cases and a review. Pediatrics 97:117, 1996.

25. McDonald JW, Alvarez F, Keller CA: Pulmonary alveolar proteinosis in association with household exposure to fibrous insulation material. Chest 117:1813, 2000.

26. McEuen DD, Abraham JL: Particulate concentrations in pulmonary alveolar proteinosis. Environ Res 17:334, 1978.

27. Miller PA, Ravin CE, Smith GJW, Osborne DRS: Pulmonary alveolar proteinosis with interstitial involvement. AJR Am J Roentgenol 137:1069, 1981.

28. Miller R, Churg A, Hutcheon M, Lam S: Pulmonary alveolar proteinosis and aluminum dust exposure. Am Rev Respir Dis 130:312, 1984.

29. Parto K, Kallajoki M, Aho H, Simell O: Pulmonary alveolar proteinosis and glomerulonephritis in lysinuric protein intolerance: Case reports and autopsy findings of four pediatric patients. Hum Pathol 25:400, 1994.

30. Prakash UBS, Barham SS, Carpenter HA, et al: Pulmonary alveolar phospholipoproteinosis: Experience with 34 cases and a review. Mayo Clin Proc 62:499, 1987.

31. Reyes JM, Putong PB: Association of pulmonary alveolar lipoproteinosis with mycobacterial infection. Am J Clin Pathol 74:478, 1980.

32. Rosen SH, Castleman B, Liebow AA, et al: Pulmonary alveolar proteinosis. N Engl J Med 258:1123, 1958.

33. Ruben FL, Talamo TS: Secondary pulmonary alveolar proteinosis occurring in two patients with acquired immunodeficiency syndrome. Am J Med 80:1187, 1986.

34. Rubin E, Weisbrod GL, Sanders DE: Pulmonary alveolar proteinosis. Relationship to silicosis and pulmonary infection. Radiology 135:35, 1980.

35. Rubinstein I, Mullen JBM, Hoffstein V: Morphologic diagnosis of idiopathic pulmonary alveolar lipoproteinosis – revisited. Arch Intern Med 148:813, 1988.

36. Schiller V, Aberle DR, Aberle AM: Pulmonary alveolar proteinosis: Occurrence with metastatic melanoma to lung. Chest 95:466, 1989.

37. Seymour JF, Presneill JJ. Pulmonary alveolar proteinosis: Progress in the first 44 years. Am J Respir Crit Care Med 166:215, 2002.

38. Seymour JF, Presneill JJ, Schoch OD, et al: Therapeutic efficacy of granulocyte-macrophage colony-stimulating factor in patients with idiopathic acquired alveolar proteinosis. Am J Respir Crit Care Med 163:524, 2001.

39. Singh G, Katyal SL, Bedrossian CWM, Rogers RM: Pulmonary alveolar proteinosis. Staining for surfactant apoprotein in alveolar proteinosis and in conditions simulating it. Chest 83:82, 1983.

40. Takahashi T, Munakata M, Suzuki I, Kawakami Y: Serum and bronchoalveolar fluid KL-6 levels in patients with pulmonary alveolar proteinosis. Am J Respir Crit Care Med 158:1294, 1998.

41. Tazawa R, Hamano E, Arai T, Ohta H, et al; Granulocyte-macrophage colony-stimulating factor and lung immunity in pulmonary alveolar proteinosis. Am J Respir Crit Care Med 171:1142, 2005.

42. Teja K, Cooper P, Squires J, Schnatterly P: Pulmonary alveolar proteinosis in four siblings. N Engl J Med 305:1390, 1981.

43. Trapnell BC, Whitsett JA, Nakata K: Pulmonary alveolar proteinosis. N Engl J Med 349:2527, 2003.

44. Verbeken EK, Demedts M, Vanwing J, et al: Pulmonary phospholipid accumulation distal to an obstructed bronchus. A morphologic study. Arch Pathol Lab Med 113:886, 1989.

45. Webster J Jr, Battifora H, Turey L, et al: Pulmonary alveolar proteinosis in two siblings with decreased immunoglobulin A. Am J Med 69:786, 1980.

46. Wilson DO, Rogers RM: Prolonged spontaneous remission in a patient with untreated pulmonary alveolar proteinosis. Am J Med 82:1014, 1987.

47. Witty LA, Tapson VF, Piantadosi CA: Isolation of mycobacteria in patients with pulmonary alveolar proteinosis. Medicine (Baltimore) 73:103, 1994.

48. Yousem SA: Alveolar lipoproteinosis in lung allograft recipients. Hum Pathol 28:1383, 1997.

Langerhans Cell Histiocytosis (Pulmonary Eosinophilic Granuloma)

49. Asakura S, Colby TV, Limper AH: Tissue localization of transforming growth factor-beta 1 in pulmonary eosinophilic granuloma. Am J Respir Crit Care Med 154:1525, 1996.

50. Askin FB, McCann BG, Kuhn C: Reactive eosinophilic pleuritis. A lesion to be distinguished from eosinophilic granuloma. Arch Pathol Lab Med 101:187, 1977.
51. Auld D: Pathology of eosinophilic granuloma of the lung. Arch Pathol 62:113, 1957.
52. Basset F, Corrin B, Spencer H, et al: Pulmonary histiocytosis-X. Am Rev Respir Dis 118:811, 1978.
53. Brambilla E, Fontaine E, Pison CM, et al: Pulmonary histiocytosis X with mediastinal lymph node involvement. Am Rev Respir Dis 142:1216, 1990.
54. Cagle PT, Mattioli CA, Truong LD, Greenberg SD: Immunohistochemical diagnosis of pulmonary eosinophilic granuloma on lung biopsy. Chest 94:1133, 1988.
55. Chollet S, Soler P, Dournovo P, et al: Diagnosis of pulmonary histiocytosis X by immunodetection of Langerhans cells in bronchoalveolar lavage fluid. Am J Pathol 115:225, 1984.
56. Coli A, Bigotti G, Ferrone S: Histiocytosis X arising in Hodgkin's disease: Immunophenotypic characterization with a panel of monoclonal antibodies. Virchows Arch A Pathol Anat Histopathol 418:369, 1991.
57. Crausman RS, Jennings CA, Tuder RM, et al: Pulmonary histiocytosis X: Pulmonary function and exercise pathophysiology. Am J Respir Crit Care Med 153:426, 1996.
58. Dacic S, Trusky C, Bakker A, et al: Genotypic analysis of pulmonary Langerhans cell histiocytosis. Hum Pathol 34:1345, 2003.
59. Delobbe A, Durieu J, Duhamel A, et al: Determinants of survival in pulmonary Langerhans' cell granulomatosis (histiocytosis X). Eur Respir J 9:2002, 1996.
60. Egeler RM, Neglia JP, Puccetti DM, et al: Association of Langerhans cell histiocytosis with malignant neoplasms. Cancer 71:865, 1993.
61. Emile J-F, Wechsler J, Brousse N, et al: Langerhans' cell histiocytosis. Definitive diagnosis with the use of monoclonal antibody O10 on routinely paraffin-embedded samples. Am J Surg Pathol 19:636, 1995.
62. Etienne B, Bertocchi M, Gamondes J-P, et al: Relapsing pulmonary Langerhans cell histiocytosis after lung transplantation. Am J Respir Crit Care Med 157:288, 1998.
63. Fartoukh M, Humbert M, Capron F, et al: Severe pulmonary hypertension in histiocytosis X. Am J Respir Crit Care Med 161:216, 2000.
64. Fichtenbaum CJ, Kleinman GM, Haddad RG: Eosinophilic granuloma of the lung presenting as a solitary pulmonary nodule. Thorax 45:905, 1991.
65. Flint A, Lloyd RV, Colby TV, Wilson BW: Pulmonary histiocytosis X. Immunoperoxidase staining for HLA-DR antigen and S100 protein. Arch Pathol Lab Med 110:930, 1986.
66. Friedman PJ, Liebow AA, Sokoloff J: Eosinophilic granuloma of lung. Clinical aspects of primary pulmonary histiocytosis in the adult. Medicine (Baltimore) 60:385, 1981.
67. Fukuda Y, Basset F, Soler P, Ferrans VJ, Masugi Y, Crystal RG: Intraluminal fibrosis and elastic fiber degradation lead to lung remodeling in pulmonary Langerhans cell granulomatosis (histiocytosis X). Am J Pathol 137:415, 1990.
68. Hammar S, Bockus D, Remington F, Bartha M: The widespread distribution of Langerhans cells in pathologic tissues: An ultrastructural and immunohistochemical study. Hum Pathol 17:894, 1986.
69. Hance AJ, Cadranel J, Soler P, Basset F: Pulmonary and extrapulmonary Langerhans' cell granulomatosis (histiocytosis X). Semin Respir Med 9:349, 1988.
70. Hayashi T, Rush WL, Travis WD, Liotta LA, Stetler-Stevenson WG, Ferrans VJ: Immunohistochemical study of matrix metalloproteinases and their tissue inhibitors in pulmonary Langerhans' cell granulomatosis. Arch Pathol Lab Med 121:930, 1997.
71. Housini I, Tomashefski JF Jr, Cohen A, et al: Transbronchial biopsy in patients with pulmonary eosinophilic granuloma. Comparison with findings on open lung biopsy. Arch Pathol Lab Med 118:523, 1994.
72. Kambouchner M, Basset F, Marchal J, et al: Three-dimensional characterization of pathologic lesions in pulmonary Langerhans cell histiocytosis. Am J Respir Crit Care Med 166:1483, 2002.
73. Kawanami O, Basset F, Ferrans VJ, et al: Pulmonary Langerhans' cells in patients with fibrotic lung disorders. Lab Invest 44:227, 1981.
74. Kjeldsberg CR, Kim H: Eosinophilic granuloma as an incidental finding in malignant lymphoma. Arch Pathol Lab Med 104:137, 1980.
75. Lacronique J, Roth C, Battesti J-P, et al: Chest radiological features of pulmonary histiocytosis X: A report based on 50 adult cases. Thorax 37:104, 1982.
76. Lieberman PH, Jones CR, Steinman RM, et al: Langerhans cell (eosinophilic) granulomatosis. A clinicopathologic study encompassing 50 years. Am J Surg Pathol 20:519, 1996.
77. Lombard CM, Medeiros LJ, Colby TV: Pulmonary histiocytosis X and carcinoma. Arch Pathol Lab Med 111:339, 1987.
78. Luna E, Tomashefski JF Jr, Brown D, et al: Reactive eosinophilic pulmonary vascular infiltration in patients with spontaneous pneumothorax. Am J Surg Pathol 18:195, 1994.
79. McDonnell TJ, Crouch EC, Gonzalez JG: Reactive eosinophilic pleuritis. A sequela of pneumothorax in pulmonary eosinophilic granuloma. Am J Clin Pathol 91:107, 1989.
80. Meier B, Rhyner K, Medici TC, Kistler G: Eosinophilic granuloma of the skeleton with involvement of the lung: A report of three cases. Eur J Respir Dis 64:551, 1983.
81. Mendez JL, Nadrous HF, Vassalo R, et al: Pneumothorax in pulmonary Langerhans cell histiocytosis. Chest 125:1028, 2004.
82. Mierau GW, Favara BE: S-100 protein immunohisto-chemistry and electron microscopy in the diagnosis of

Langerhans cell proliferative disorders: A comparative assessment. Ultrastruct Pathol 10:303, 1986.

83. Neumann MP, Frizzera G: The coexistence of Langerhans' cell granulomatosis and malignant lymphoma may take different forms: Report of seven cases with a review of the literature. Hum Pathol 17:1060, 1986.

84. Nondahl SR, Finlay JL, Farrell PM, et al: A case report and literature review of "primary" pulmonary histiocytosis-X of childhood. Med Pediatr Oncol 14:57, 1986.

85. O'Donnell AE, Tsou E, Awh C, et al: Endobronchial eosinophilic granuloma: A rare cause of total lung atelectasis. Am Rev Respir Dis 136:1478, 1987.

86. Pinkus GS, Lones MA, Matsumura F, et al: Langerhans cell histiocytosis. Immunohistochemical expression of fascin, a dendritic cell marker. Am J Clin Pathol 118:335, 2002.

87. Pomeranz SJ, Proto AV: Histiocytosis X. Unusual-confusing features of eosinophilic granuloma. Chest 89:88, 1986.

88. Powers MA, Askin FB, Cresson DH: Pulmonary eosinophilic granuloma: 25-year follow-up. Am Rev Respir Dis 129:503, 1984.

89. Sadoun D, Vaylet F, Valeyre D, et al: Bronchogenic carcinoma in patients with pulmonary histiocytosis X. Chest 101:1610, 1992.

90. Schönfeld N, Frank W, Wenig S, et al: Clinical and radiologic features, lung function and therapeutic results in pulmonary histiocytosis X. Respiration 60:38, 1993.

91. Soler P, Bergeron A, Kambouchner M, et al: Is high-resolution computed tomography a reliable tool to predict the histopathological activity of pulmonary Langerhans cell histiocytosis? Am J Respir Crit Care Med 162:264, 2000.

92. Soler P, Chollet S, Jacque C, et al: Immunocytochemical characterization of pulmonary histiocytosis X cells in lung biopsies. Am J Pathol 118:439, 1985.

93. Tazi A, Bonay M, Grandsaigne M, et al: Surface phenotype of Langerhans cells and lymphocytes in granulomatous lesions from patients with pulmonary histiocytosis X. Am Rev Respir Dis 147:1531, 1993.

94. Tomashefski JF Jr, Khiyami A, Kleinerman J: Neoplasms associated with pulmonary eosinophilic granuloma. Arch Pathol Lab Med 115:499, 1991.

95. Travis WD, Borok Z, Roum JH, et al: Pulmonary Langerhans cell granulomatosis (histiocytosis X). A clinicopathologic study of 48 cases. Am J Surg Pathol 17:971, 1993.

96. Vassallo R, Jensen EA, Colby TV, et al: The overlap between respiratory bronchiolitis and desquamative interstitial pneumonia in pulmonary Langerhans cell histiocytosis. High-resolution CT, histologic and functional correlations. Chest 124:1199, 2003.

97. Vassallo R, Ryu JH, Colby TV, et al: Pulmonary Langerhans'-cell histiocytosis. N Engl J Med 342:1969, 2000.

98. Vassallo R, Ryu JH, Schroeder DR, et al: Clinical outcomes of pulmonary Langerhans'-cell histiocytosis in adults. N Engl J Med 346:484, 2002.

99. Von Essen S, West W, Sitorius M, Rennard SI: Complete resolution of roentgenographic changes in a patient with pulmonary histiocytosis X. Chest 98:765, 1990.

100. Webber D, Tron V, Askin F, Churg A: S-100 staining in the diagnosis of eosinophilic granuloma of lung. Am J Clin Pathol 84:447, 1985.

101. Willman CL, Busque L, Griffith BB, et al: Langerhans'-cell histiocytosis (histiocytosis X) – a clonal proliferative disease. N Engl J Med 331:154, 1994.

102. Yousem SA, Colby TV, Chen Y-Y, et al: Pulmonary Langerhans' cell histiocytosis. Molecular analysis of clonality. Am J Surg Pathol 25:630, 2001.

Pulmonary Lymphangiomyomatosis
103. Aberle DR, Hansell DM, Brown K, Tashkin DP: Lymphangiomyomatosis: CT, chest radiographic, and functional correlations. Radiology 176:381, 1990.

104. Aubry M-C, Myers JL, Colby TV, et al: Endometrial stromal sarcoma metastatic to the lung: A detailed analysis of 16 patients. Am J Surg Pathol 26:440, 2002.

105. Aubry M-C, Myers JL, Ryu JH, et al: Pulmonary lymphangioleiomyomatosis in a man. Am J Respir Crit Care Med 162:749, 2000.

106. Baldi S, Papotti M, Valente ML, et al: Pulmonary lymphangioleiomyomatosis in postmenopausal women: Report of two cases and review of the literature. Eur Respir J 7:1013, 1994.

107. Basset F, Soler P, Marsac J, et al: Pulmonary lymphangiomyomatosis. Three new cases studied with electron microscopy. Cancer 38:2357, 1976.

108. Berger U, Khaghani A, Pomerance A, Yacoub MH, Coombes RC: Pulmonary lymphangioleiomyomatosis and steroid receptors. An immunocytochemical study. Am J Clin Pathol 93:609, 1990.

109. Bernstein SM, Newell JD Jr, Adamczyk D, et al: How common are renal angiomyolipomas in patients with pulmonary lymphangiomyomatosis? Am J Respir Crit Care Med 152:2138, 1995.

110. Bittman I, Dose TB, Müller C, et al: Lymphangioleiomyomatosis: Recurrence after single lung transplantation. Hum Pathol 26:1420, 1997.

111. Boehler A, Speich R, Russo EW, Weder W: Lung transplantation for lymphangioleiomyomatosis. N Engl J Med 335:1275, 1996.

112. Bonetti F, Chiodera PL, Pea M, et al: Transbronchial biopsy in lymphangiomyomatosis of the lung. HMB45 for diagnosis. Am J Surg Pathol 17:1092, 1993.

113. Brentani MM, Carvalho CRR, Saldiva PH, et al: Steroid receptors in pulmonary lymphangiomyomatosis. Chest 85:96, 1984.

114. Carrington CB, Cugell DW, Gaensler EA, et al: Lymphangiomyomatosis. Physiologic-pathologic-radiologic correlations. Am Rev Respir Dis 116:977, 1977.

115. Castro M, Shepherd CW, Gomez MR, et al: Pulmonary tuberous sclerosis. Chest 107:189, 1995.

116. Chu SC, Horiba K, Usuki J, et al: Comprehensive evaluation of 35 patients with lymphangio-leiomyomatosis. Chest 115:1041, 1999.

117. Colley MH, Geppert E, Franklin WA: Immunohistochemical detection of steroid receptors in a case of pulmonary lymphangioleiomyomatosis. Am J Surg Pathol 13:803, 1989.

118. Corrin B, Liebow AA, Friedman PJ: Pulmonary lymphangiomyomatosis. A review. Am J Pathol 79:347, 1975.

119. Crausman RS, Jennings CA, Mortenson RL, et al: Lymphangioleiomyomatosis: The pathophysiology of diminished exercise capacity. Am J Respir Crit Care Med 153:1368, 1996.

120. Eliasson AH, Phillips YY, Tenholder MF: Treatment of lymphangioleiomyomatosis. A meta-analysis. Chest 196:1352, 1989.

121. Franz DN, Brody A, Meyer C, et al: Mutational and radiographic analysis of pulmonary disease consistent with lymphangioleiomyomatosis and micronodular pneumocyte hyperplasia in women with tuberous sclerosis. Am J Respir Crit Care Med 164:661, 2001.

122. Fukuda Y, Kawamoto M, Yamamoto A, et al: Role of elastic fiber degradation in emphysema-like lesions of pulmonary lymphangiomyomatosis. Hum Pathol 21:1252, 1990.

123. Gal AA, Brooks JSJ, Pietra GG: Leiomyomatous neoplasms of the lung: A clinical, histologic, and immunohistochemical study. Mod Pathol 2:209, 1989.

124. Graham ML II, Spelsberg TC, Dines DE, et al: Pulmonary lymphangiomyomatosis: With particular reference to steroid-receptor assay studies and pathologic correlation. Mayo Clin Proc 59:3, 1984.

125. Guinee D, Singh R, Azumi N, et al: Multifocal micronodular pneumocyte hyperplasia: A distinctive pulmonary manifestation of tuberous sclerosis. Mod Pathol 8:902, 1995.

126. Hayashi T, Fleming MV, Stetler-Stevenson WG, et al: Immunohistochemical study of matrix metalloproteinases (MMPs) and their tissue inhibitors (TIMPs) in pulmonary lymphangioleiomyomatosis (LAM). Hum Pathol 28:1071, 1997.

127. Hoon V, Thung SN, Kaneko M, Unger PD: HMB-45 reactivity in renal angiomyolipoma and lymphangioleiomyomatosis. Arch Pathol Lab Med 118:732, 1994.

128. Kane PB, Lane BP, Cordice JWV, et al: Ultrastructure of the proliferating cells in pulmonary lymphangio-myomatosis. Arch Pathol Lab Med 102:618, 1978.

129. Karbowniczek M, Astrinidis A, Balsara BR, et al: Recurrent lymphangiomyomatosis after transplantation. Genetic analyses reveal a metastatic mechanism. Am J Respir Crit Care Med 167:976, 2003.

130. Kay JM, Kahana LM, Rihal C: Diffuse smooth muscle proliferation of the lungs with severe pulmonary hypertension. Hum Pathol 27:969, 1996.

131. Kitaichi M, Nishimura K, Itoh H, Izumi T: Pulmonary lymphangioleiomyomatosis: A report of 46 patients including a clinicopathologic study of prognostic factors. Am J Respir Crit Care Med 151:527, 1995.

132. Kumaki F, Takeda K, Yu Z-X, et al: Expression of human telomerase reverse transcriptase in lymphangioleio-myomatosis. Am J Respir Crit Care Med 166:187, 2002.

133. Kumasaka T, Seyama K, Mitani K, et al: Lymphangio-genesis in lymphangioleiomyomatosis. Its implication in the progression of lymphangioleiomyomatosis. Am J Surg Pathol 28:1007, 2004.

134. Matsui K, Beasley MB, Nelson WK, et al: Prognostic significance of pulmonary lymphangioleiomyomatosis histologic score. Am J Surg Pathol 25:479, 2001.

135. Matsui K, Riemenschneider WK, Hilbert SL, et al: Hyperplasia of type II pneumocytes in pulmonary lymphangioleiomyomatosis. Immunohistochemical and electron microscopic study. Arch Pathol Lab Med 124:1642, 2000.

136. Matsui K, Takeda K, Yu Z-X, et al: Downregulation of estrogen and progesterone receptors in the abnormal smooth muscle cells in pulmonary lymphangioleio-myomatosis following therapy. An immunohistochemical study. Am J Respir Crit Care Med 161:1002, 2000.

137. Matsui K, Tatsuguchi A, Valencia J, et al: Extrapulmonary lymphangioleiomyomatosis (LAM): Clinicopathologic features in 22 cases. Hum Pathol 31:1242, 2000.

138. Matsumoto Y, Horiba K, Usuki J, et al: Markers of cell proliferation and expression of melanosomal antigen in lymphangioleiomyomatosis. Am J Respir Cell Mol Biol 21:327, 1999.

139. Moss J, Avila NA, Barnes PM, et al: Prevalence and clinical characteristics of lymphangioleiomyomatosis (LAM) in patients with tuberous sclerosis complex. Am J Respir Crit Care Med 163:669, 2001.

140. Muir TE, Leslie KO, Popper H, et al: Micronodular pneumocyte hyperplasia. Am J Surg Pathol 22:465, 1998.

141. Muller NL, Chiles C, Kullnig P: Pulmonary lymphangio-myomatosis: Correlation of CT with radiographic and functional findings. Radiology 175:335, 1990.

142. O'Brien JD, Lium JH, Parosa JF, et al: Lymphangiomyomatosis in the allograft after single-lung transplantation. Am J Respir Crit Care Med 151:2033, 1995.

143. Ohori NP, Yousem SA, Sonmez-Alpan E, Colby TV: Estrogen and progesterone receptors in lymphangioleiomyomatosis, epithelioid hemangioendothelioma, and sclerosing hemangioma of the lung. Am J Clin Pathol 96:529, 1991.

144. Peyrol S, Gindre D, Cordier JF, Loire R, Grimaud JA: Characterization of the smooth muscle cell infiltrate and associated connective tissue matrix of lymphangiomyomatosis. Immunohistochemical and ultrastructural study of two cases. J Pathol 168:387, 1992.

145. Popper HH, Juettner-Smolle FM, Pongratz MG: Micronodular hyperplasia of type II pneumocytes – a

new lung lesion associated with tuberous sclerosis. Histopathology 18:347, 1990.

146. Rappaport DC, Weisbrod GL, Herman SJ, Chamberlain DW: Pulmonary lymphangioleiomyomatosis. High-resolution CT findings in four cases. AJR Am J Roentgenol 152:961, 1989.

147. Ryu JH, Doerr CH, Fisher SD, et al: Chylothorax in lymphangioleiomyomatosis. Chest 123:623, 2003.

148. Sinclair W, Wright JL, Churg A: Lymphangioleiomyomatosis presenting in a postmenopausal woman. Thorax 40:475, 1985.

149. Sleiman C, Mal H, Jebrak G, et al: Pulmonary lymphangiomyomatosis treated by single lung transplantation. Am Rev Respir Dis 145:964, 1992.

150. Sobonya RE, Quan SF, Fleishman JS: Pulmonary lymphangioleiomyomatosis: Quantitative analysis of lesions producing airflow limitation. Hum Pathol 16:1122, 1985.

151. Sullivan EJ: Lymphangioleiomyomatosis. A review. Chest 114:1689, 1998.

152. Taveira-DaSilva AM, Hedin C, Stylianou MP, et al: Reversible airflow obstruction, proliferation of abnormal smooth muscle cells, and impairment of gas exchange as predictors of outcome in lymphangioleiomyomatosis. Am J Respir Crit Care Med 164:1072, 2001.

153. Taylor JR, Ryu J, Colby TV, Raffin TA: Lymphangioleiomyomatosis. Clinical course in 32 patients. N Engl J Med 323:1254, 1990.

154. Tietze L, Gunther K, Horbe A, et al: Benign metastasizing leiomyoma: A cytogenetically balanced but clonal disease. Hum Pathol 31:126, 2000.

155. Torres VE, Bjornsson J, King BF, et al: Extrapulmonary lymphangioleiomyomatosis and lymphangiomatous cysts in tuberous sclerosis complex. Mayo Clin Proc 70:641, 1995.

156. Urban T, Kuttenn F, Gompel A, Marsac J, Lacronique J: Pulmonary lymphangiomyomatosis. Follow-up and long-term outcome with antiestrogen therapy: A report of eight cases. Chest 102:472, 1992.

157. Urban T, Lazor R, Lacronique J, et al: Pulmonary lymphangioleiomyomatosis: A study of 69 patients. Medicine (Baltimore) 78:321, 1999.

158. Wolff M, Kaye G, Silva F: Pulmonary metastases (with admixed epithelial elements) from smooth muscle neoplasms. Report of nine cases including three males. Am J Surg Pathol 3:325, 1979.

159. Yu J, Astrinidis A, Henske EP: Chromosome 16 loss of heterozygosity in tuberous sclerosis and sporadic lymphangiomyomatosis. Am J Respir Crit Care Med 164:1537, 2001.

Pulmonary Alveolar Microlithiasis

160. Barnard NJ, Crocker PR, Blainey AD, et al: Pulmonary alveolar microlithiasis. A new analytical approach. Histopathology 11:639, 1987.

161. Castellana G, Lamorgese V: Pulmonary alveolar microlithiasis. World cases and review of the literature. Respiration 70:549, 2003.

162. Dobashi M, Yuda F, Narabayashi M, et al: Histopathological study of corpora amylacea pulmonum. Histol Histopathol 4:153, 1989.

163. Hawass ND, Noah MS: Pulmonary alveolar microlithiasis. Eur J Respir Dis 69:1, 1986.

164. Koss MN, Johnson FB, Hochholzer L: Pulmonary blue bodies. Hum Pathol 12:258, 1981.

165. Lauta VM: Pulmonary alveolar microlithiasis: An overview of clinical and pathological features together with possible therapies. Respir Med 10:1081, 2003.

166. Mariotta S, Guidi L, Mattia P, et al: Pulmonary microlithiasis. Report of two cases. Respiration 64:165, 1997.

167. Mascie-Taylor BH, Wardman AG, Madden CA, Page RL: A case of alveolar microlithiasis: Observation over 22 years and recovery of material by lavage. Thorax 40:952, 1985.

168. Miro JM, Moreno A, Coca A, et al: Pulmonary alveolar microlithiasis with an unusual radiological pattern. Br J Dis Chest 76:91, 1982.

169. Moran CA, Hochholtzer L, Hasleton PS, et al: Pulmonary alveolar microlithiasis. A clinicopathologic and chemical analysis of seven cases. Arch Pathol Lab Med 121:607, 1997.

170. Nouh MS: Is the desert lung syndrome (nonoccupational pneumoconiosis) a variant of pulmonary alveolar microlithiasis? Report of 4 cases with review of the literature. Respiration 55:122, 1989.

171. Pavlov JS, Ivkosic A, Glavina-Durdov M, et al: Pulmonary alveolar microlithiasis in childhood: Clinical and radiological follow-up. Pediatr Pulmonol 34:384, 2002.

172. Prakash UBS, Barham SS, Rosenow EC III, et al: Pulmonary alveolar microlithiasis. A review including ultrastructural and pulmonary function studies. Mayo Clin Proc 58:290, 1983.

173. Senyigit A, Yaramis A, Gurkan F, et al: Pulmonary alveolar microlithiasis: A rare familial inheritance with report of six cases in a family. Contribution of six new cases to number of case results in Turkey. Respiration 68:204, 2001.

174. Stamatis G, Zerkowski H-R, Doetsch N, et al: Sequential bilateral lung transplantation for pulmonary alveolar microlithiasis. Ann Thorac Surg 56:972, 1993.

175. Tao L-C: Microliths in sputum specimens and their relationship to pulmonary alveolar microlithiasis. Am J Clin Pathol 19:482, 1978.

176. Ucan ES, Keyf AI, Aydilek R, et al: Pulmonary alveolar microlithiasis: Review of Turkish reports. Thorax 48:171, 1993.

177. Voile E, Kaufmann HJ: Pulmonary alveolar microlithiasis in pediatric patients – review of the world literature and two new observations. Pediatr Radiol 17:439, 1987.

Pulmonary Hyalinizing Granuloma and Sclerosing Mediastinitis

178. Berry DF, Buccigrossi D, Peabody J, et al: Pulmonary vascular occlusion and fibrosing mediastinitis. Chest 89:296, 1986.

179. Chalaoui J, Gregoire P, Sylvestre J, et al: Pulmonary hyalinizing granuloma: A cause of pulmonary nodules. Radiology 152:23, 1984.

180. Chazova I, Robbins I, Loyd J, et al: Venous and arterial changes in pulmonary veno-occlusive disease, mitral stenosis and fibrosing mediastinitis. Eur Respir J 15:116, 2000.

181. Dent RG, Godden DJ, Stovin PGI, Stark JE: Pulmonary hyalinising granuloma in association with retroperitoneal fibrosis. Thorax 38:955, 1983.

182. Dines DE, Payne WS, Bernatz PE, et al: Mediastinal granuloma and fibrosing mediastinitis. Chest 75:320, 1979.

183. Doyle TP, Loyd JE, Robbins IM: Percutaneous pulmonary artery and vein stenting. A novel treatment for mediastinal fibrosis. Am J Respir Crit Care Med 164:657, 2001.

184. Dunn EJ, Ulicny KS Jr, Wright CB, Gottesman L: Surgical implications of sclerosing mediastinitis. A report of six cases and review of the literature. Chest 97:338, 1990.

185. Engleman P, Liebow AA, Gmelich J, et al: Pulmonary hyalinizing granuloma. Am Rev Respir Dis 115:997, 1977.

186. Espinosa RE, Edwards WD, Rosenow EC III, Schaff HV: Idiopathic pulmonary hilar fibrosis: An unusual cause of pulmonary hypertension. Mayo Clin Proc 68:778, 1993.

187. Flieder DB, Suster S, Moran CA: Idiopathic fibroinflammatory (fibrosing/sclerosing) lesions of the mediastinum: A study of 30 cases with emphasis on morphologic heterogeneity. Mod Pathol 12:257, 1999.

188. Garrett HE Jr, Roper CL: Surgical intervention in histoplasmosis. Ann Thorac Surg 42:711, 1986.

189. Goodwin RA, Nickell JA, DesPrez RM: Mediastinal fibrosis complicating healed airway histoplasmosis and tuberculosis. Medicine (Baltimore) 51:227, 1972.

190. Guccion JG, Rohatgi PK, Saini N: Pulmonary hyalinizing granuloma. Electron microscopic and immunologic studies. Chest 85:571, 1984.

191. Kalweit G, Huwer H, Straub U, Gams E: Mediastinal compression syndromes due to idiopathic fibrosing mediastinitis – report of three cases and review of the literature. Thorac Cardiovasc Surg 44:105, 1996.

192. Katzenstein A-LA, Mazur MT: Pulmonary infarct. An unusual manifestation of fibrosing mediastinitis. Chest 77:521, 1980.

193. Loyd JE, Tillman BF, Atkinson JB, DesPrez RM: Mediastinal fibrosis complicating histoplasmosis. Medicine (Baltimore) 67:295, 1988.

194. Manali ED, Saas CP, Krizmanich G, Mehta AC: Endobronchial findings of fibrosing mediastinitis. Respir Care 48:1038, 2003.

195. Mathisen DJ, Grillo HC: Clinical manifestations of mediastinal fibrosis and histoplasmosis. Ann Thorac Surg 54:1053, 1992.

196. Matsubara O, Tan-Liu NS, Kenney RM, Mark E: Inflammatory pseudotumors of the lung: Progression from organizing pneumonia to fibrous histiocytoma or to plasma cell granuloma in 32 cases. Hum Pathol 19:807, 1988.

197. Mendelson EB, Mintzer RA, Hidvegi DF: Venoocclusive pulmonary infarct: An unusual complication of fibrosing mediastinitis. AJR Am J Roentgenol 141:175, 1983.

198. Mole TM, Glover J, Sheppard MN: Sclerosing mediastinitis: A report of 18 cases. Thorax 50:280, 1995.

199. Morgan AD, Loughridge LW, Calve RV: Combined mediastinal and retroperitoneal fibrosis. Lancet 1:67, 1966.

200. Pettinato G, Manivel JC, DeRosa N, Dehner LP: Inflammatory myofibroblastic tumor (plasma cell granuloma). Clinicopathologic study of 20 cases with immunohistochemical and ultrastructural observations. Am J Clin Pathol 94:538, 1990.

201. Rossi SE, McAdams HP, Rosado-de-Christenson ML, et al: Fibrosing mediastinitis. Radiographics 21:737, 2001.

202. Schlosnagle DC, Check IJ, Sewell CW, et al: Immunologic abnormalities in two patients with pulmonary hyalinizing granuloma. Am J Clin Pathol 78:231, 1982.

203. Schowengerdt CG, Suyemoto R, Main FB: Granulomatous and fibrous mediatinitis. A review and analysis of 180 cases. J Thorac Cardiovasc Surg 57:365, 1969.

204. Sherrick AD, Brown LR, Harms GF, Myers JL: The radiographic findings of fibrosing mediastinitis. Chest 106:484, 1994.

205. Sobrinho-Simoes M, Vaz Saleiro J, Wagenvoort C: Mediastinal and hilar fibrosis. Histopathology 5:53, 1981.

206. Ulbright TM, Katzenstein A-LA: Solitary necrotizing granulomas of the lung. Differentiating features and etiology. Am J Surg Pathol 4:13, 1980.

207. Yousem SA, Hochholzer L: Pulmonary hyalinizing granuloma. Am J Clin Pathol 87:1, 1987.

16

MISCELLANEOUS
II. NONSPECIFIC INFLAMMATORY
AND DESTRUCTIVE DISEASES

This chapter discusses the various nonspecific inflammatory or destructive lesions that may be encountered in lung biopsy or lobectomy specimens.

MISCELLANEOUS PNEUMONIAS

Aspiration Pneumonia

Aspiration of gastric contents into the lung causes varying manifestations depending on the amount and type of material aspirated and the time course of the aspiration. The classic form of aspiration pneumonia that is commonly encountered by pathologists is a necrotizing acute bronchopneumonia in which there are foreign body granulomas to exogenous (usually vegetable) material. The process centers around bronchioles, which are often destroyed and replaced by acute inflammation and necrosis (Fig. 16–1). Multinucleated giant cells are usually a striking feature in the surrounding infiltrate. In the early stages, aspirated vegetable matter is easily recognized because of a thick, golden-yellow, refractile cell wall. Sometimes skeletal muscle fragments are seen, and irregularly shaped brown pigmented structures can be found. Later on, the aspirated material loses its structure and appears as eosinophilic, amorphous structures surrounded by foreign body giant cells. The process can undergo organization and may superficially resemble bronchiolitis obliterans–organizing pneumonia (Fig. 16–2). Aspiration pneumonia is a common incidental finding at autopsy in severely debilitated patients dying of other causes. It is occasionally seen in biopsy specimens as well, although it is easy to overlook if the characteristic foreign body giant cell reaction is not recognized.[21,27a]

Massive aspiration of gastric acid produces a pattern of diffuse alveolar damage (DAD, see Chapter 2) associated with intraalveolar hemorrhage, pulmonary edema, and

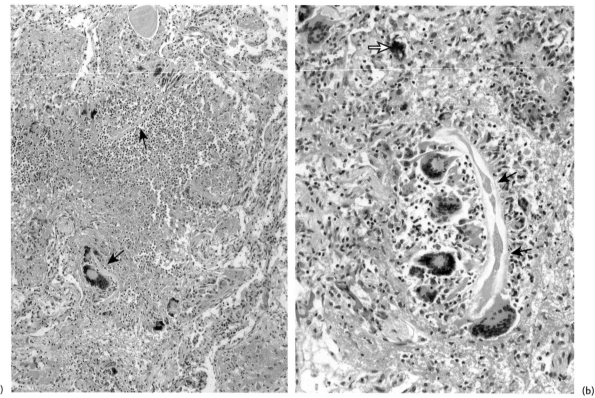

(a)   (b)

Figure 16–1 Acute aspiration pneumonia. (a) Low magnification view showing replacement of a bronchiole by acute inflammation and necrosis surrounded by a prominent foreign body giant cell reaction. Aspirated material (arrows) can be appreciated even at this low magnification. **(b)** Higher magnification showing degenerated vegetable matter (black arrows) surrounded by foreign body giant cells. Note also the darkly pigmented amorphous material at top center (open arrow).

necrosis of alveolar lining cells.[14,20] This acute syndrome (*Mendelson's syndrome*) has a significant mortality, especially when complicated by bacterial superinfection. It is usually observed only in autopsy specimens.

There is considerable controversy whether *chronic aspiration of gastric acid*, as occurs in patients with gastroesophageal reflux, esophageal diverticula, or hiatal hernias, for example, causes significant lung disease.[1,4,28,29,31,37] A relationship seems to exist between gastroesophageal reflux and asthma and possibly also other airway lesions such as chronic bronchitis or bronchiectasis. Good evidence linking chronic aspiration with inflammatory or fibrotic parenchymal lesions does not exist, however.

Cytologic examination of sputum, tracheal aspirate, and bronchoalveolar lavage (BAL) specimens has been used, especially in pediatric, but also in adult, populations, to diagnose gastroesophageal reflux and chronic aspiration of gastric contents.[11–13,29] Sudan black or oil red O stains are used to identify lipid-filled macrophages,

and the relative number of these cells is quantitated. Although large numbers of lipid-filled macrophages appear to correlate with the presence of aspiration, this finding is by no means specific, since lipid-filled macrophages can be seen in a wide variety of parenchymal disease.[23] Their absence, however, may be used as evidence against aspiration.

Exogenous Lipid Pneumonia

Lipid pneumonia of exogenous origin is related to the chronic aspiration of mineral oil or a related substance into the distal lung.[8,17–19,25] Most patients are chronic users of mineral oil laxatives or oily nose drops, and there are often associated neurologic or other disorders predisposing to chronic aspiration.[8,18] Other less common causes of lipid pneumonia have been reported, including industrial inhalation of burning fats,[30] the use of tobacco moistened with mineral oil and Vaseline,[27] ingestion of shark liver oil (squalene),[2] inhalation of

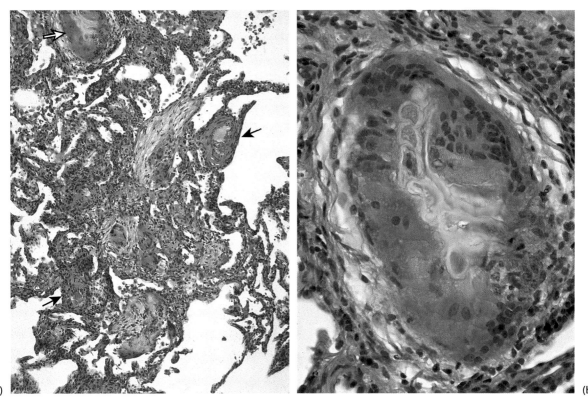

(a)

(b)

Figure 16–2 Organizing aspiration pneumonia. (a) Intraluminal fibrosis and chronic inflammation have replaced a bronchiole, and the process resembles bronchiolitis obliterans–organizing pneumonia (BOOP) except for the presence of multinucleated giant cells. The fact that the reaction involves parenchyma adjacent to pulmonary arteries (black arrows) indicates a bronchiolar location. **(b)** Higher magnification view of multinucleated giant cell seen in top left of Fig. 16–2a (open arrow). Note the remnant of vegetable matter in the center.

spray lubricant (WD-40) used as a liniment for sore muscles and joints,[16] use of lip gloss,[5] and intravenous injection of lipoid material (olive oil).[7]

Patients often are asymptomatic and are diagnosed during evaluation of an abnormal chest radiograph. Basilar infiltrates or an intrapulmonary mass lesion resembling a neoplasm are the most common radiographic findings.[8,25] The clinical course of patients with exogenous lipid pneumonia is usually benign after the use of the offending oil ceases.[18,24] Fibrosis may develop, however, if aspiration continues.

Histologically, exogenous lipid pneumonia is characterized by the presence within alveolar spaces and the interstitium of numerous macrophages containing large, clear cytoplasmic vacuoles (Fig. 16–3). Multinucleated foreign body giant cells are often seen surrounding lipid droplets, and there may be an associated chronic interstitial pneumonia (Fig. 16–4). Interstitial fibrosis may be prominent in longstanding cases. Special stains for acid-fast bacteria should be examined

routinely, since nontuberculous mycobacterial infection may occasionally complicate this lesion.[17,19] The demonstration of mineral oil by fat stains or chromatography may help in diagnosing difficult cases but is usually not necessary.[19] Examination of BAL specimens may suggest the diagnosis in some cases.[24]

The main lesion in the differential diagnosis of exogenous lipid pneumonia is the much more common *endogenous lipid pneumonia (postobstructive, golden, or cholesterol pneumonia)* that occurs distal to major airway obstruction.[9,35] In this lesion, macrophages also accumulate within the alveolar spaces and to a lesser extent within the interstitium, but they contain foamy or finely vacuolated cytoplasm rather than the large vacuoles characteristic of exogenous lipid pneumonia (Fig. 16–5). They may degenerate, with the liberation of cholesterol and other lipids and the formation of cholesterol clefts. The foamy macrophages may be multinucleated, but foreign body-type giant cells surrounding large lipid droplets are not seen.

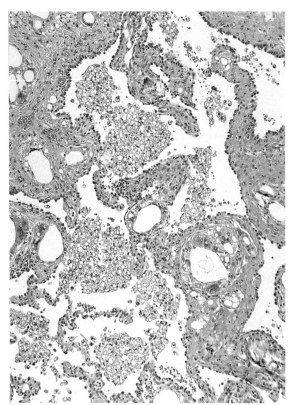

Figure 16–3 Exogenous lipid pneumonia. Low magnification showing vacuolated macrophages filling alveolar spaces and interstitium.

Middle Lobe Syndrome

Middle lobe syndrome is a clinical term that refers to persistent or recurring atelectasis or opacification of the middle lobe or lingula.[6,22,26,32–34,36] The condition occurs in both children and adults, and lobectomy is frequently undertaken for treatment.[3] The etiology is varied and includes bronchiectasis, bronchial obstruction (both intrinsic and extrinsic), and recurrent infection.[6,22,32] Some cases are a manifestation of allergic bronchopulmonary aspergillosis (see Chapter 6), and endobronchial silicosis has been implicated rarely.[10,15] Although bronchial compression by enlarged (often granulomatous) lymph nodes was a major cause in the past, poor clearance of secretions inherent to this anatomic location may be a more important cause.[32]

The most common pathologic finding in lobectomy specimens is bronchiectasis and it is usually accompanied by inflammation in adjacent bronchioles and surrounding parenchyma.[22] Secondary changes such as organizing pneumonia, atelectasis, and abscess

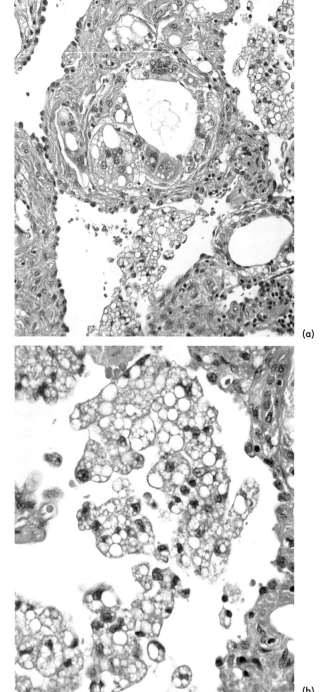

(a)

(b)

Figure 16–4 Higher magnification of exogenous lipid pneumonia. Interstitial foreign body giant cell reaction to lipid vacuoles is seen in **(a)**, and intraalveolar lipid filled macrophages are present in **(b)**. Note the large vacuoles within the macrophages in contrast to the foamy appearance to the cytoplasm that is characteristic of endogenous lipid pneumonia (compare with Fig. 16–5).

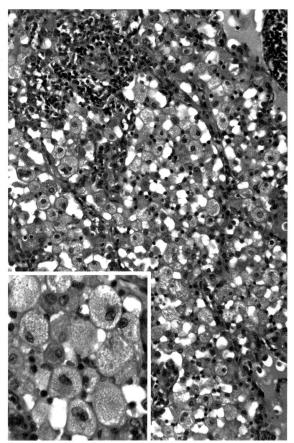

Figure 16–5 Endogenous lipid (postobstructive) pneumonia. Low magnification shows the filling of alveolar spaces by large numbers of macrophages containing foamy-appearing cytoplasm. Note the background chronic inflammation. Inset is a higher magnification showing numerous tiny cytoplasmic vacuoles that impart a foamy appearance to the macrophages.

formation are frequent. Granulomatous inflammation, both necrotizing and non-necrotizing, may also be found, and *Mycobacterium avium* complex (MAC) is frequently isolated.[22,32] MAC infections of the middle lobe have a propensity for elderly women and may be related to the voluntary suppression of cough in this patient population (*Lady Windermere syndrome*).[32]

LUNG ABSCESS

A lung abscess is a localized suppurative, destructive process in the pulmonary parenchyma. Three general categories, which are based on etiology, are recognized:[38] (1) aspiration, (2) postpneumonic, and (3) secondary. *Aspiration lung abscesses* result from the aspiration of infected oropharyngeal debris, vomitus, or other particulates. Many of the patients with this lesion are debilitated, have poor dental hygiene, or have some neurologic or mechanical interference with swallowing. The bacterial content of this type of lesion characteristically includes anaerobic organisms.[38–40] Most aspiration lung abscesses are located in the posterior segment of the right upper lobe or the superior segment of either lower lobe, depending on the patient's position during aspiration.[38,41] *Postpneumonic lung abscesses* usually result from a prior necrotizing bacterial bronchopneumonia. Staphylococcal or klebsiella organisms are often responsible, but a wide variety of other pathogens can also cause this complication.[38–43] *Secondary lung abscesses* usually occur distal to bronchial obstruction but can also result from superinfection of a pulmonary infarct, from septic pulmonary emboli, or from hematogenous dissemination of infection in other sites.[42] In rare instances, infection of a preexisting bronchial cyst or related abnormality or of a pulmonary bulla can lead to abscess formation.[38]

Clinical Features

Generally, aspiration and secondary lung abscesses are more common in adults, whereas children are more likely to develop the postinfectious variety. However, each type of abscess has been reported in all age groups.[38–42,44] Drainage and treatment with antimicrobials are usually adequate therapy.[39,40] Occasionally, however, a lung abscess is resected either for therapeutic purposes or in an attempt to define the nature of a cavitary lung lesion. Massive hemoptysis due to bleeding into an abscess also may lead to resection.

Pathologic Features

The gross appearance of an abscess depends on its age (Fig. 16–6). In the early stages, it is filled with yellow, purulent, necrotic debris and is surrounded by a firm rim. As the lesion heals, much of the debris is expectorated or is cleared by inflammatory cells, and there may eventually be an empty cavity lined by a smooth fibrous wall. Communication with one or more bronchi is usually present. This feature can be demonstrated by dissection of the bronchial tree, and the probe technique described in Chapter 1 is useful. Microscopically, the abscess contains necrotic debris and acute inflammatory cells. Bacteria or other organisms can often be identified by special stains. Early in the

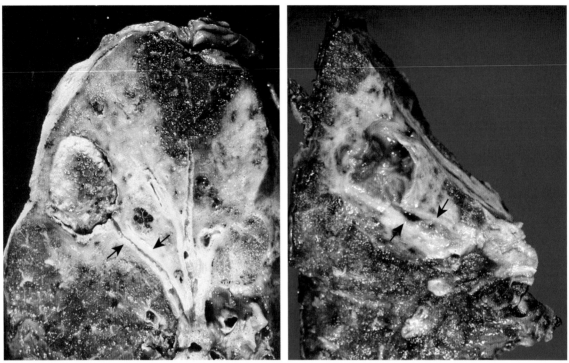

(a) (b)

Figure 16–6 Lung abscess. (a) Acute abscess containing necrotic inflammatory debris. The abscess is surrounded by a thick rim of organizing pneumonia. Note the continuity with a bronchus (arrows). **(b)** The inflammatory exudate has been cleared from the center of this abscess. It is surrounded by dense fibrosis. This abscess also communicates with a bronchus (arrows).

process, it is surrounded by acute and chronic inflammatory cells and granulation tissue. Later, the wall becomes fibrotic and may acquire a squamous or columnar epithelial lining. Continuity with an adjacent bronchus may be demonstrable, and organizing pneumonia is often prominent in the surrounding alveolated parenchyma.

A healed abscess cavity, especially if it has acquired an epithelial lining, should not be confused with a congenital cyst. Features that favor an abscess cavity over a cyst include communication with one or more bronchi and the presence of surrounding organizing pneumonia.

NON-NEOPLASTIC MASSES

A variety of inflammatory and reactive processes may produce localized nodular opacities or masses that radiographically mimic neoplasms. *Bronchiolitis obliterans–organizing pneumonia (BOOP)* or *cryptogenic organizing pneumonia (COP)* is probably the most common and is reviewed in detail in Chapter 2. *Round*

atelectasis is another example of this phenomenon.[52] In this condition, a collapsed area of lung assumes a round or ovoid appearance under a thickened, fibrotic pleura. Most patients have a history of asbestos exposure, although the disorder can result from any type of pleural inflammatory reaction with resultant fibrosis.[46,48,51,53] The lesion is sometimes excised because of the clinical suspicion of malignancy, but surgery may be avoidable if the characteristic radiographic features are recognized.[53] Pathologically, the main finding is marked pleural fibrosis with invagination of thickened pleura into the subjacent lung parenchyma (Fig. 16–7).[45,50] Nonspecific fibrosis, atelectasis, and patchy organizing pneumonia are common in the adjacent lung. Occasionally, acute bacterial pneumonia may also produce a nodular lesion in the lung parenchyma. This *round pneumonia* is more common in children than in adults.[47]

Sometimes, inflammatory and fibrotic masses are encountered that cannot be classified as BOOP, round atelectasis, or related entities. Such lesions usually have a central scar surrounded by a rim of chronic inflammation. Lymphoid follicles containing germinal

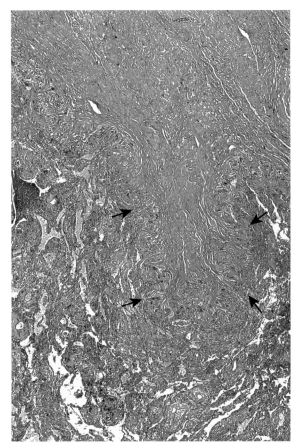

Figure 16–7 Round atelectasis. There is the characteristic invagination of thickened, fibrotic pleura into the underlying lung parenchyma (arrows). Note the adjacent lung atelectasis.

centers are often prominent in the inflammatory cell infiltrate, and foci of BOOP may be present in the adjacent lung. These lesions likely represent the residuum of a prior necrotizing bronchopneumonia and are best classified as *inflammatory pseudotumor*.[49] This lesion has overlapping histologic findings with nodular lymphoid hyperplasia and is discussed in more detail in Chapter 9.

Subpleural scars, also known as *pulmonary apical caps*, are common autopsy findings, especially in the lung apices. Occasionally, however, they are found on chest radiographs and excised because of the clinical suspicion of malignancy.[54] They are composed of dense collagen deposition with variable associated elastosis. Scattered foci of calcification or metaplastic ossification may be seen (Fig. 16–8). The pathogenesis is thought to be related either to chronic ischemia or to a prior infectious process.

DISORDERS OF THE LARGE AIRWAYS

This section includes a discussion of the disorders involving the cartilaginous bronchi. Cystic fibrosis is also briefly discussed, since its major pathologic manifestation is bronchiectasis.

Bronchiectasis

Bronchiectasis is a chronic disorder characterized by permanent dilatation of bronchi accompanied by inflammatory changes in their walls and in adjacent lung parenchyma.[55] The pathogenesis is related to recurrent inflammation of the bronchial walls combined with fibrosis in the surrounding parenchyma. The resultant traction on weakened walls leads to eventual irreversible dilatation. Bronchiectasis is generally divided into *postobstructive* and *postinflammatory (nonobstructive)* forms. *Congenital bronchiectasis (tracheobronchomalacia)* is a rare disorder that results from bronchial flaccidity related to deficient cartilage rings in the airways (see Chapter 14).[61] Thin-walled, generalized bronchiectatic cysts occur, and chest radiographs show hyperinflation. It differs from ordinary bronchiectasis in etiology and pathogenesis, and in a strict sense should be considered a separate entity.

Postinflammatory or Nonobstructive Bronchiectasis

Most cases of bronchiectasis are of the postinflammatory (nonobstructive) type and presumably are related to prior episodes of pneumonia.[56,63] Certain preexisting conditions may be associated with this form of bronchiectasis, including various types of immunodeficiency, cystic fibrosis (see further on), ciliary dyskinesia (see further on), and inflammatory bowel disease (see Chapter 7), for example. Allergic bronchopulmonary aspergillosis can cause an unusual proximal bronchiectasis (see Chapter 6). Rarely, reactions to inhaled toxic fumes or gastric aspiration may result in bronchiectasis.[58,63] An etiology is not identifiable in about one-half of patients.[63]

Postinflammatory bronchiectasis may be localized or widespread. Localized disease most commonly involves the basal segments of the lower lobes, the right middle lobe, and the lingula, and most cases can be related to an episode of pneumonia, often occurring many years previously.[62] Widespread bronchiectasis occurs almost exclusively in patients with underlying predisposing diseases.

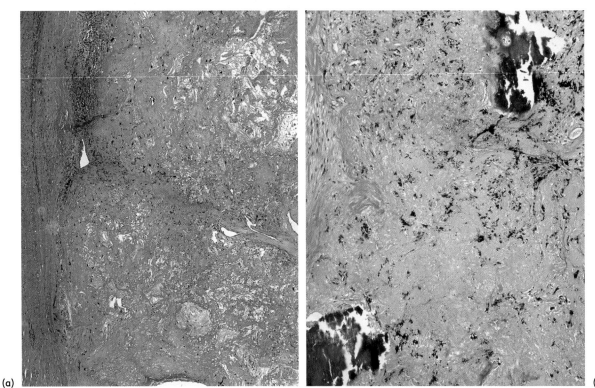

(a)   (b)

Figure 16–8 Pulmonary apical cap. (a) Low magnification showing replacement of subpleural lung parenchyma by fibrosis and elastosis. The pleura is on the left. **(b)** Higher magnification showing collagen deposition, elastosis, pigment deposition, and foci of calcification and ossification.

The most common clinical manifestations of bronchiectasis include productive cough, hemoptysis, and recurrent fevers. Most patients are in their mid fifties at the time of diagnosis, although symptoms are often present for many years prior to the diagnosis.[62] A younger age at onset is seen in patients with inherited diseases such as cystic fibrosis (see text following). High-resolution computed tomography (HRCT) examination is the diagnostic modality of choice, although routine chest radiographs are almost always abnormal.[55,59,60,65] Most patients are treated with conservative, nonsurgical therapy, but resection may be performed in cases with severely affected lobes.[55,64] Massive hemoptysis that is related to submucosal granulation tissue in bronchiectatic airways or to erosion of a bronchial artery may sometimes necessitate emergency surgery.[55,57]

Postobstructive Bronchiectasis

Postobstructive bronchiectasis results from any cause of longstanding bronchial obstruction, including a slow-growing neoplasm, foreign body, external compression, or, rarely, bronchial webs or atresia (see Chapter 14). It follows the branching pattern of the obstructed bronchus and can occur in any area of the lung. Infection and inflammation in the distal lung may cause changes that are irreversible, even after the obstruction is relieved.

Pathologic Features

Grossly, the dilated bronchi in bronchiectasis extend almost to the pleural surface and are often filled with mucopurulent material and surrounded by scarring (Fig. 16–9).[59,205] There may be an exaggerated transverse ridging and trabeculation of the bronchial mucosa caused by hypertrophy of the underlying circular smooth muscle. Small pockets, or 'pits', representing dilated bronchial mucous gland ducts may be seen in the wall of the affected bronchi. Saccular, cylindrical, or varicose forms of bronchiectasis have been described, but this morphologic classification has little value other than for radiographic–pathologic correlation. Postobstructive bronchiectasis differs only in that the cause of the obstruction is visible in the proximal bronchus (Fig. 16–10).

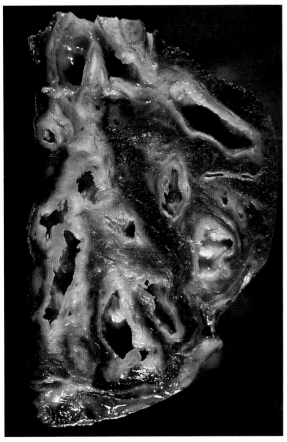

Figure 16–9 Postinflammatory bronchiectasis. Note the dilated bronchi that extend to the pleural surface.

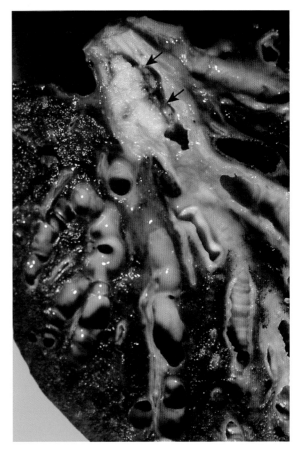

Figure 16–10 Postobstructive bronchiectasis. The dilated bronchi contain a purulent exudate and extend almost to the pleural surface. Note the proximal obstruction by squamous cell carcinoma (arrows).

Microscopically, the submucosa of the dilated bronchus is chronically inflamed and lymphoid aggregates with germinal centers may be present.[56] Granulation tissue is often prominent and the bronchial arteries are commonly hypertrophied. Acute and organizing pneumonia routinely occurs in the adjacent alveolated parenchyma. Small carcinoid tumorlets (see Chapter 1) often are seen surrounding the chronically inflamed and dilated bronchi and they may replace damaged or scarred bronchioles in the distal parenchyma.

All lobes resected for bronchiectasis should be carefully examined to detect the presence of tumors, foreign bodies, or other causes of bronchial obstruction, as well as to identify the sources of bleeding in patients whose lobes were removed because of hemoptysis. Dissection of the bronchi along probes (see Chapter 1) is a helpful technique for demonstrating mucosal abnormalities or obstructed areas.

Cystic Fibrosis

Cystic fibrosis is a genetically transmitted autosomal recessive disease manifested by multiple systemic problems.[69,70] Mutations in the cystic fibrosis transmembrane conductance regulator (*CFTR*) gene have been shown to be etiologic.[69] Most cases are diagnosed in infancy or early childhood, although rarely the disease is not recognized until adulthood.[70,78] The major pulmonary problems are related to recurrent infection, and the mucoid strains of *Pseudomonas aeruginosa* or *Staphylococcus aureus* are the most common causative organisms. Specimens are usually encountered by the pathologist only at autopsy, although occasionally a lobe is resected for severe bronchiectasis.

The main pathologic manifestation in older children and adults is widespread bronchiectasis, and there are no specific histologic features that separate the bronchiectasis of cystic fibrosis from that due to other causes.[66,71,73,74] Several investigators have shown an age-related progression of changes, from bronchitis and bronchiolitis with mucous plugging in infants to bronchiectasis with squamous metaplasia in older patients.[66,75–77] Interstitial pneumonia may accompany the other changes,[81] and pneumothorax is an occasional complication in adults.[79,80] Fungal colonization or localized infection is identified in about 15% of patients at autopsy, although invasive, disseminated infection is less common.[67,74] Ultrastructurally, nonspecific ciliary and basement membrane abnormalities can be found in bronchial mucosa.[68,72]

Intrinsic Obstructive Lesions of Bronchi

Neoplasms are probably the most common cause of intrinsic intrabronchial obstruction, but there are also a number of less common, non-neoplastic causes. *Broncholithiasis* results from old calcified granulomas in hilar or peribronchial lymph nodes that erode into an adjacent bronchus, producing a *broncholith*.[84–86,88,90] The broncholith may partially or completely occlude the bronchus, with the development of postobstructive pneumonia and eventually bronchiectasis. Hemoptysis may also occur. Sometimes, bronchial biopsies are undertaken. In addition to fragments of calcified tissue, dense, acute and chronic inflammation with granulation tissue is usually seen in the bronchial wall.[84]

Rare examples of bronchial obstruction or narrowing due to *inflammatory polyps* have been reported following smoke inhalation and foreign body aspiration as well as in asthmatics.[82,83,91] Most are composed of polypoid granulation tissue. Cases of fibrous obliteration of multiple bronchi (*bronchitis obliterans*) resulting in collapse of an entire lung have also been described.[87,89]

Inspissated mucus (mucoid impaction of bronchi, plastic bronchitis) is another cause of intrinsic bronchial obstruction, and it is discussed in Chapter 6.

Primary Ciliary Dyskinesia

Primary ciliary dyskinesia encompasses a group of diseases caused by abnormal cilia and characterized by recurrent pulmonary infection and associated upper respiratory tract disease.[92,93,95,103,116,118,124] There is evidence of autosomal recessive inheritance in some cases, and most male patients are infertile. The term encompasses, but is not limited to, *Kartagener's triad* of bronchiectasis, sinusitis, and situs inversus. *Immotile cilia syndrome* is another term that has been used for

these conditions, but it is not as accurate, since a spectrum of motility abnormalities occur, ranging from absent to nearly normal motility.[119,123] The prognosis for patients with primary ciliary dyskinesia is variable but may be reasonably good in the absence of cigarette smoking.[122,124] In some instances, the symptoms are most severe during childhood and partially remit during adult life.

Diagnosis

The diagnosis of primary ciliary dyskinesia is made by observation of ciliary motility and by electron microscopic examination of nasal or bronchial ciliated epithelium or of spermatozoa. The light microscopic appearance of the affected cilia is not recognizably abnormal. Measurement of nasal nitric oxide (NO) is a good screening test, since patients have consistently low values of nasal NO.[118]

A variety of ultrastructural defects in the cilia have been described.[92,94,95,101,103,106,111–113,115–118,126–130,134] Patients whose cilia lack dynein arms have been reported most often. Other defects, including the absence of radial spokes, absence of central microtubules, a deficiency of nexin links, abnormally long cilia, and the transposition of peripheral microtubules, have been described (Fig. 16–11). Peculiar cyst-like structures in ciliary shafts have been noted in a few cases.[131] In some cases, abnormalities of the basal ciliary apparatus may be the only ultrastructural disorder.[114] Rarely, no ultrastructural abnormalities are found, and, in such cases, measurements of ciliary orientation may show random orientation.[99,100,121,125]

Differential Diagnosis

It is important to remember that several nonspecific and potentially reversible ultrastructural abnormalities of cilia have been noted in a variety of chronic inflammatory diseases of the respiratory tract, including various infections, cystic fibrosis, and chronic bronchitis, although these disorders are not necessarily associated with abnormal ciliary motility.[93,96–98,100,102,108–111,126] Ciliary abnormalities are also associated with cigarette smoking.[133] The nonspecific abnormalities include compound cilia, abnormal microtubular arrangements, excess cytoplasmic matrix, and ruffled ciliary contours (Fig. 16–12). Ciliary disorientation also has been noted secondary to inflammation and is reversible following treatment of the inflammatory reaction.[120] Fox et al[105] found abnormal cilia in patients with retinitis pigmentosa, and, along with others, have commented

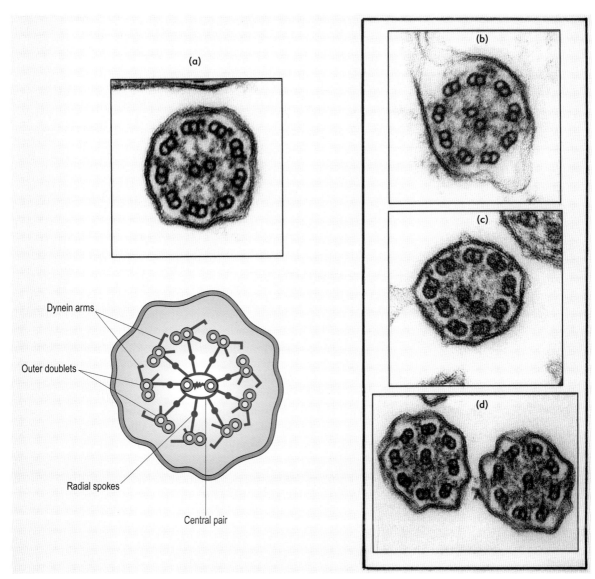

Figure 16–11 Ultrastructural abnormalities of cilia. (a) Normal cilium. The ultrastructural features are labeled in the accompanying drawing. Nine doublets surround a central pair of microtubules. Dynein arms join the peripheral doublets. Radial spokes run from the doublets toward the central pair. **(b)** Patient with Kartagener's syndrome. The dynein arms are absent. **(c)** Radial spoke defect. Compare with (a) and (b). This patient was one of three siblings with chronic respiratory disease and defective mucociliary clearance. **(d)** Transposition of microtubules. There are only eight peripheral doublets. The other peripheral pair of tubules has been transposed to the center of the cilium. The central pair is absent. Radial spokes are not uniformly present. (a) and (b), ×115,000; (c), ×122,000; (d), ×103,950. Patients (b) through (d) have immotile or poorly motile cilia. ((a) through (d) courtesy of Dr Jennifer Sturgess, Toronto, Ontario, Canada. (a) through (c) reproduced with permission from Sturgess JM, Chas J, Wong J, et al: Cilia with defective radial spokes: A cause of human respiratory disease. N Engl J Med 300:53, 1979.)

on the extreme difficulty that may be encountered in attempting to identify absolutely perfect cilia – even in normal controls.[104,126] In males, the examination of sperm rather than respiratory mucosa may be helpful, although, sometimes, different ultrastructural abnormalities are found in bronchial or nasal cilia and

spermatozoa, and motility at these two sites may also be different.[130,135]

Young's syndrome of obstructive azoospermia and chronic sinopulmonary infections may mimic primary ciliary dyskinesia clinically but is not associated with ciliary ultrastructural or motility abnormalities.[107]

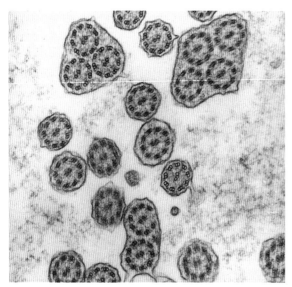

Figure 16-12 Nonspecific abnormalities of cilia. Compound cilia contain two, three, and four complete sets of microtubules with peripheral doublets and central pairs. These types of cilia can be found in patients with chronic bronchitis and are not in themselves diagnostic features of ciliary dyskinesia. ×38,200. (Courtesy of Dr Jennifer Sturgess, Toronto, Ontario, Canada.)

Pathogenetic Mechanisms

The structural abnormalities of the cilia are believed to cause abnormal motility leading to interference with the clearance and defense mechanisms of the upper and lower respiratory tract, thus predisposing affected individuals to recurrent infection. Since sperm are essentially modified cilia, immotile sperm and male infertility are components of the clinical picture. In individuals with normal ciliary ultrastructure, random ciliary orientation may decrease ciliary efficiency in mucociliary clearance because of disoriented beat direction.

SMALL AIRWAYS DISEASE

'Small airways disease' is a nonspecific, descriptive term used to denote various lesions that affect bronchioles having diameters less than 2 mm.[138,140] Patients with most forms of small airways disease share a common spectrum of clinical manifestations, including dyspnea, cough, obstructive pulmonary function defects, and overinflation on chest radiographs. The literature in this area is confusing since many studies combine under one category several pathologically distinct lesions, and terminology tends to be inconsistent.[136,137,139] Table 16-1 is a pathologic classification of small airways disease that attempts to clarify these issues. Abnormalities of small airways are also frequently found as one component of other diseases, such as emphysema, bronchitis, bronchiectasis, and asbestosis, for example. BOOP (see Chapter 2) is an additional lesion that involves small airways. It is not included in the category of primary small airways disease, however, since alveolar ducts and peribronchiolar alveoli are usually affected to the same extent as bronchioles.

Respiratory (Smokers') Bronchiolitis

Respiratory bronchiolitis (RB), also known as *smokers' bronchiolitis*, is by far the most common form of small airways disease encountered by the surgical pathologist.[142,144] It is seen in virtually all cigarette smokers

Table 16-1 Pathologic Classification of Small Airways Disease		
Small Airways Disease	Major Pathologic Manifestations	Cause of Clinical Symptoms?
Respiratory (smokers') bronchiolitis	Intraluminal pigmented macrophages	Rarely
Follicular bronchiolitis	Peribronchiolar lymphoid follicles and reactive germinal centers	Yes
Diffuse panbronchiolitis	Bronchiolar inflammation and foamy histiocytes in peribronchiolar interstitium	Yes
Cellular bronchiolitis	Acute and chronic bronchiolar inflammation	Yes
Constrictive bronchiolitis obliterans	Fibrous luminal obliteration and replacement by scars	Yes
Nonspecific chronic bronchiolitis	Bronchiolar smooth muscle hyperplasia, scant inflammation	Maybe

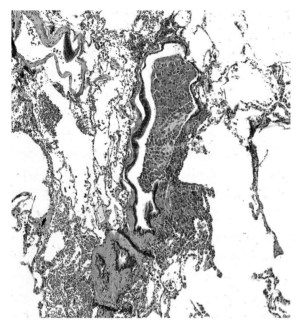

Figure 16–13 Respiratory bronchiolitis. Low magnification view showing the filling of a small bronchiole by lightly pigmented macrophages. Note that the changes are confined to the bronchiolar lumen and immediate peribronchiolar airspaces.

and can be present for many years after having stopped smoking.[142] It is usually an incidental pathologic finding of little significance. In rare cases (so-called *respiratory bronchiolitis interstitial lung disease, RBILD,* see Chapter 3), it causes clinical features of interstitial lung disease, including dyspnea and cough, along with mild restrictive defects on pulmonary function testing, and ground glass infiltrates radiographically.[143,145]

The histologic features of RB are characterized by the accumulation, within the lumens of distal bronchioles and adjacent alveolar ducts and spaces, of macrophages containing coarsely granular yellow–brown pigment in their cytoplasm (Fig. 16–13, and see Fig. 3–11).[142,144] The macrophages stain lightly with Prussian blue (Fig. 16–14a, and see Fig. 3–12). Ultrastructurally, they contain numerous lysosomes and phagolysosomes (Fig. 16–14b).[141,143] Needle-like inclusions representing aluminum silicates thought to be derived from cigarette smoke can be found within their cytoplasm.[141] There are no histologic features that distinguish RBILD from RB, and, therefore, the diagnosis of RBILD requires clinical evidence of interstitial lung disease. It should be remembered, however, that RB is a very common finding, while RBILD is rare.

Follicular Bronchiolitis

Follicular bronchiolitis is a rare small airways disorder characterized by a dense chronic inflammatory cell infiltrate containing prominent reactive germinal centers within bronchiole walls. There is usually associated luminal narrowing, and an intraluminal acute inflammatory cell exudate may be present. The clinical and pathologic findings are discussed in detail in Chapter 9 (see Fig. 9–2). The pathologic findings in follicular bronchiolitis may overlap with those of *lymphoid interstitial pneumonia* (LIP) and nonspecific reactive lymphoid hyperplasia (see Chapter 9). The diagnosis of LIP should be made only when the lymphoid infiltrate is truly diffuse, involving not only the peribronchiolar interstitium but also the alveolar septa between the affected bronchioles. Nonspecific lymphoid hyperplasia is diagnosed when scattered lymphoid follicles with germinal centers occur within interlobular septa and bronchovascular bundles, usually in association with other inflammatory conditions. Follicular bronchiolitis should be used only for cases in which the process is confined to peribronchiolar interstitium and other processes are absent or minimal.

Diffuse Panbronchiolitis

Diffuse panbronchiolitis is a distinct form of small airways disease that has been reported mainly from Japan, with only rare cases described in non-Japanese individuals.[147–153] An association has been demonstrated with HLA Bw54, which is found only in Japanese, Chinese, and Korean persons.[158] The disease occurs predominantly in men, with an average age of 50 years. Patients present with dyspnea and cough that is usually productive of purulent sputum. Chronic sinusitis is commonly present as well. Rales and rhonchi are found on physical examination, and chest radiographs demonstrate fine nodular opacities and hyperinflation.[156] Centrilobular nodules along with thickened bronchioles and air trapping are seen on HRCT scans.[150,156] Elevated cold agglutinins are often present. Pulmonary function tests show obstructive defects. The disease is usually slowly progressive, with 5- and 10-year survival rates of only 50% and 25%, respectively, in untreated patients.[150,156] Treatment with erythromycin significantly improves survival, with 90% 10-year survival reported.[154] Recurrence has been noted following lung transplantation.[148]

Pathologically, there is a cellular, chronic bronchiolitis characterized by a dense peribronchiolar infiltrate of

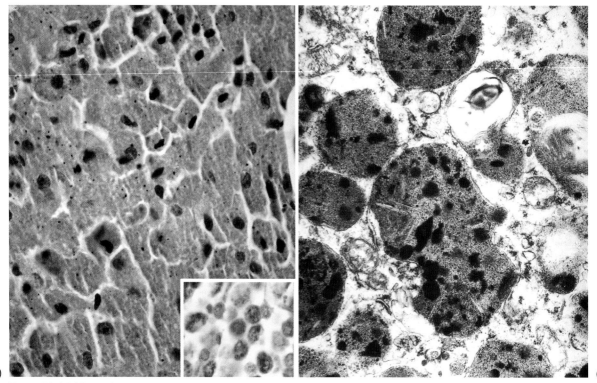

(a)   (b)

Figure 16–14 Macrophages in respiratory bronchiolitis. (a) High magnification showing coarsely granular yellow–brown cytoplasmic pigmentation. Inset is a Prussian blue iron stain. Note the uneven staining characteristics. **(b)** Electron micrograph of macrophage cytoplasm showing phagolysosomes containing characteristic needle-like inclusions.

lymphocytes and plasma cells that is sometimes accompanied by an acute inflammatory cell intraluminal exudate (Fig. 16–15).[152,157] Increased numbers of dendritic cells have been noted by immunohistochemistry.[159] The distinct finding, however, is the accumulation of foamy histiocytes within the inflammatory cell infiltrate that extends into the adjacent interstitium (Fig. 16–16). In the early stage, the lumens of affected bronchioles are narrowed, while, in the late stage, secondary ectasia occurs in the proximal terminal bronchioles.[146,155] A similarity has been noted between diffuse panbronchiolitis and the bronchiolitis associated with human T-cell lymphotropic virus type 1 (HTLV-1), and some authors suggest that diffuse panbronchiolitis may be a manifestation of HTLV-1 infection.[154]

The interstitial accumulation of foamy histiocytes, while highly characteristic of panbronchiolitis, is not unique to this condition, since similar changes can occur uncommonly in association with other diseases such as cystic fibrosis and bronchiectasis.[153] The diagnosis of panbronchiolitis, therefore, should be made only when clinical manifestations fit and when other conditions are absent.

Cellular Bronchiolitis

Cellular bronchiolitis is a term used to describe a type of bronchiolitis in which there is a prominent chronic and sometimes acute inflammatory cell infiltrate in the walls of small airways, often accompanied by an acute inflammatory cell intraluminal exudate (Fig. 16–17). It corresponds to some of the cases described by Macklem et al,[138] Kindt et al,[137] and Edwards et al[136] as *small airways disease*, *adult bronchiolitis*, and *chronic transmural bronchiolitis*, respectively. The clinical findings are similar to those observed in other forms of small airways disease, and most patients respond favorably to corticosteroid therapy. Whether this lesion predisposes to the eventual development of constrictive bronchiolitis obliterans (see later on) is not known.

This form of small airways disease differs from follicular bronchiolitis by its lack of germinal centers and from diffuse panbronchiolitis by its lack of foam cells. Similar bronchiolar inflammation can be associated with other conditions, including BOOP, constrictive bronchiolitis, bronchiectasis, and acute bronchopneumonia. The diagnosis of cellular bronchiolitis,

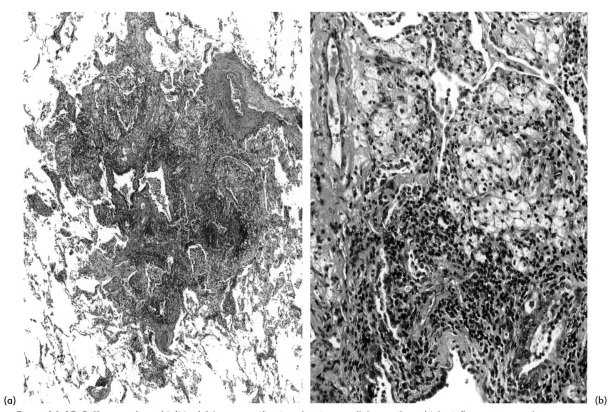

(a) (b)

Figure 16–15 Diffuse panbronchiolitis. (a) Low magnification showing a cellular, peribronchiolar inflammatory exudate. Numerous foam cells can be seen even at this low magnification. **(b)** Higher magnification showing the prominent component of foamy macrophages admixed with lymphocytes and plasma cells that surround the bronchiole.

however, pertains only to cases in which the bronchiolitis is the predominant finding. Infection should always be excluded clinically in the etiology.

Constrictive Bronchiolitis Obliterans

Constrictive bronchiolitis obliterans, also known as *obliterative bronchiolitis*, is an uncommon bronchiolar disease characterized by fibrous luminal narrowing of small airways, usually associated with obstructive pulmonary function defects and hyperinflation on chest radiographs. Terminology is confusing since the same lesion has been referred to as bronchiolitis obliterans, especially in the transplantation literature (see Chapter 6), and that term has also been used for cases of bronchiolitis obliterans–organizing pneumonia (BOOP). The latter lesion differs both pathologically and clinically, however, and it is recommended that the term bronchiolitis obliterans, if used at all, be restricted to those rare examples of BOOP lacking organizing pneumonia.

Constrictive bronchiolitis obliterans is most commonly encountered in lung allograft recipients and bone marrow transplant recipients, where it is considered a manifestation of chronic rejection and graft-versus-host disease, respectively (see Chapter 6), and it is only rarely encountered in other situations.[160,162,181,182] It has been described as a manifestation of drug toxicity, especially to gold and penicillamine,[167,177] and it can occur in patients with rheumatoid arthritis.[165] It is a rare complication following infections, especially adenovirus and mycoplasma.[170,179] Inhalation of certain organic compounds, as described in workers at a microwave popcorn factory who were exposed to volatile butter flavoring ingredients, can cause the lesion.[161,174] Toxic fume exposure, including ammonia, nitrogen dioxide, and certain isocyanates, has also been implicated in a few cases.[176] The lesion has been related to ingestion of juice from *Sauropus androgynus*, a vegetable cultivated primarily in Southeast Asia and used for weight reduction and blood pressure control.[163,164] Certain dermatologic conditions may be complicated by constrictive

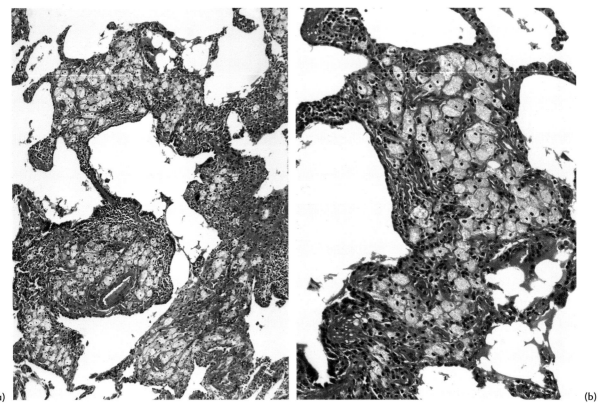

(a)   (b)

Figure 16–16 **Diffuse panbronchiolitis. (a)** In this lesion, the respiratory bronchiole (center) is mildly dilated and there is a striking surrounding infiltrate of foamy histiocytes, while other inflammatory cells are not numerous. **(b)** Higher magnification showing the interstitial foamy macrophages.

bronchiolitis obliterans, including paraneoplastic pemphigus, Stevens–Johnson syndrome, and toxic epidermal necrolysis.[171,175,178] Idiopathic cases also occur.[139,166,168,169,172,176,180]

Clinically, patients present with progressive dyspnea and cough.[139,170,172,176] Pulmonary function tests demonstrate airway obstruction with variable associated restrictive defects. Chest x-ray films show overinflation, usually without infiltrates, and HRCT examinations show air trapping, often associated with ground glass opacities and bronchial wall thickening. Rarely, only one lung is affected and appears small, hyperlucent, and hypovascular (*Swyer–James [Macleod's] syndrome*).[170,173,179] The prognosis is not good, with progressive disease in most patients that is unresponsive to corticosteroid or cytotoxic therapy. Many patients undergo lung transplantation.[164]

Histologically, constrictive bronchiolitis obliterans is characterized by peribronchiolar fibrosis that is associated with luminal narrowing and eventually replacement of bronchioles by small scars. In the early

stages, fibrosis is seen beneath the bronchiolar epithelium and it widens the ordinarily narrow space between epithelium and smooth muscle (Fig. 16–18).[139,172,176] The fibrosis often has a concentric, 'onion skin' pattern, and the epithelium is compressed (Fig. 16–19). Eventually, the lumen is entirely obliterated by the fibrosis and the bronchiole is identifiable only by the presence of smooth muscle bundles or discontinuous elastic tissue around a scar (Fig. 16–20). Fibrosis has also been described in the bronchiolar adventitium, but the presence in this location is not specific. The changes can be extremely subtle, especially when only tiny scars are widely scattered in otherwise normal parenchyma. In difficult cases, an elastic tissue stain can help by outlining the residual bronchiolar elastic tissue around the scars and by identifying the adjacent blood vessel as an artery (which normally is accompanied by a bronchiole) (Fig. 16–21).

Variable amounts of chronic inflammation may accompany the bronchiolar fibrosis. Some investigators include cases with bronchiolar narrowing due to

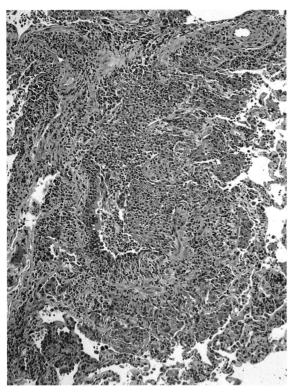

Figure 16–17 Cellular bronchiolitis. This bronchiole is infiltrated by acute and chronic inflammatory cells. The cells ulcerate the mucosa and narrow the lumen, which also contains a necrotic acute inflammatory cell exudate.

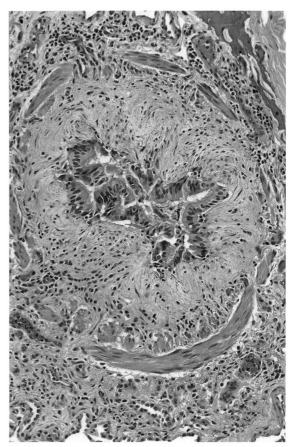

Figure 16–18 Constrictive bronchiolitis obliterans. A prominent layer of fibrosis with mild chronic inflammation is present between the bronchiolar epithelium and the smooth muscle, and there is luminal narrowing.

inflammation without significant fibrosis in the category of constrictive bronchiolitis obliterans.[176] There is no evidence, however, that this type of inflammatory bronchiolitis necessarily progresses to fibrotic luminal narrowing or even that all cases of constrictive bronchiolitis obliterans are preceded by inflammation. We prefer, therefore, to restrict the term constrictive bronchiolitis obliterans to cases characterized by periluminal fibrosis and use the more generic 'cellular bronchiolitis' or 'acute and chronic bronchiolitis' for the inflammatory lesion.

The main condition in the differential diagnosis of constrictive bronchiolitis obliterans is BOOP, and the differentiating features of these two lesions are outlined in Table 16–2. The fibrosis in BOOP occurs as a polypoid intraluminal excrescence, in contrast to the periepithelial concentric fibrosis in constrictive bronchiolitis obliterans, and the lumen in BOOP is thus not narrowed. Neither fibrosis of peribronchiolar airspaces nor adjacent chronic interstitial pneumonia that are characteristic of BOOP occur in constrictive bronchiolitis

obliterans. Clinically, obstructive defects are seen in constrictive bronchiolitis obliterans, in contrast to restrictive defects in BOOP, and there is overinflation radiographically rather than infiltrates.

Nonspecific Chronic Bronchiolitis

This form of small airways disease is characterized by smooth muscle hyperplasia in bronchiole walls, associated with mild luminal narrowing. An inflammatory cell infiltrate is scant, if present at all, and there may be accompanying goblet cell hyperplasia and intraluminal mucus accumulation. This lesion commonly accompanies a wide variety of other lung disorders, but occasionally it is encountered as the only abnormality on a lung biopsy specimen. In such cases, it is difficult to know whether the biopsy has failed to sample another more important lesion or whether this form

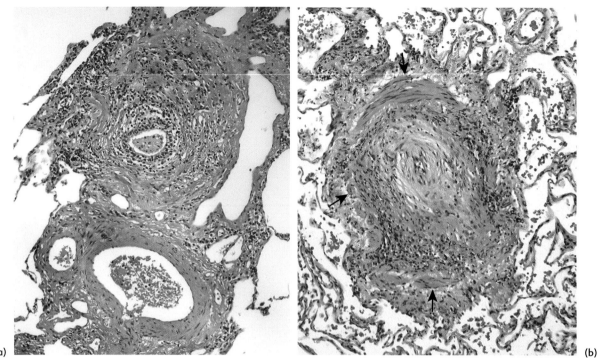

(a)   (b)

Figure 16–19 Constrictive bronchiolitis obliterans. In these more advanced examples there is prominent concentric fibrosis surrounding the bronchiole lumens. In **(a)**, the lumen is markedly narrowed, while in **(b)** it is almost completely obliterated. There is mild chronic inflammation as well. Note the residual bronchiole smooth muscle (arrows).

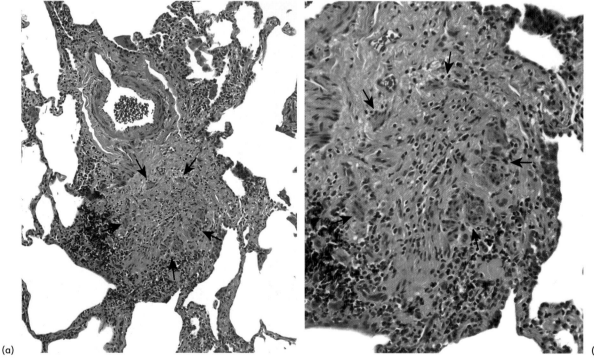

(a)   (b)

Figure 16–20 Constrictive bronchiolitis obliterans. (a) In this example, only a small scar remains adjacent to an artery in the location normally occupied by a bronchiole. Remnants of bronchiolar smooth muscle (arrows) can still be seen, however, and they are better illustrated at higher magnification **(b)**.

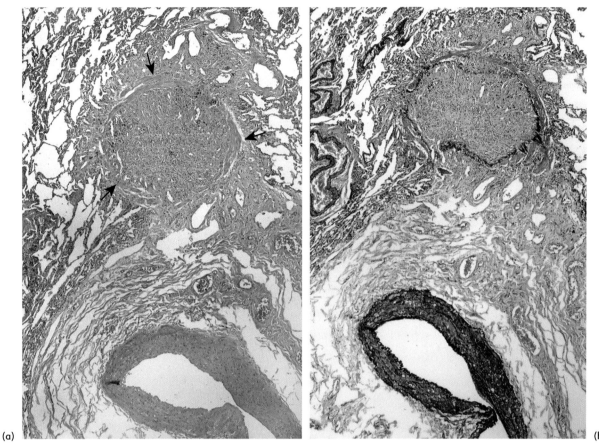

(a)
(b)

Figure 16–21 Constrictive bronchiolitis obliterans. (a) Low magnification view shows a small scar adjacent to a pulmonary artery. Note the residual bronchiolar smooth muscle surrounding the scar (arrows). **(b)** An elastic tissue stain outlines the residual bronchiolar elastic tissue (black) as well as the smooth muscle (red) that surrounds the scar. Note that the diameter of the scar is considerably less than that of the adjacent artery, confirming that the bronchiole has undergone 'constriction' in addition to obliteration.

Table 16–2   Contrasting Features of Constrictive Bronchiolitis Obliterans and BOOP

	CBO	BOOP
Clinical Features		
CXR/CT	Overinflation, air trapping	Airspace opacities
PFTs	Obstruction	Normal to mild restriction
Prognosis	Poor	Good
Pathologic Features		
Airway lesion	Concentric mural fibrosis	Intraluminal fibrous polyp
Luminal narrowing	Yes	No
Extension of fibrosis into adjacent airspaces	No	Usually
Intraalveolar foamy macrophages	No	Common
Associated interstitial pneumonia	No	Usually

Abbreviations: CBO = constrictive bronchiolitis obliterans; BOOP = bronchiolitis obliterans organizing pneumonia; CXR = chest x-ray; CT = computed tomography; PFT = pulmonary function test.

of small airways disease is causing significant clinical manifestations.

EMPHYSEMA

Pulmonary emphysema is defined as the abnormal, permanent enlargement of airspaces distal to the terminal bronchiole accompanied by destruction of their walls without obvious fibrosis.[184,186,203,207] Thus, it differs from congenital lobar overinflation ('emphysema', see Chapter 14), in which there is enlargement, but not destruction, of airspaces, and from interstitial emphysema (see Chapter 14), which involves interstitial and subpleural connective tissue.

Emphysema is classified into three types according to the portion of the pulmonary acinus that is predominantly affected.[84,203,205,207] (1) *Panacinar emphysema* involves the acinus uniformly, and it is most prominent in the lower lobes. It is the form usually associated with α_1-antitrypsin deficiency,[206] and it has also been described in young intravenous drug users.[190,202] (2) *Proximal acinar (centrilobular) emphysema* involves the respiratory bronchioles and surrounding airspaces (proximal acinus). It is the form usually associated with cigarette smoking and predominantly involves the upper lobes. Cases with overlapping features of these two forms of emphysema are common in advanced disease. (3) *Distal acinar (paraseptal) emphysema* involves the distal portion of the acinus, especially along the interlobular septa and beneath the pleura. Although it is associated with relatively few functional defects, it may cause bulla formation or spontaneous pneumothorax (see later on).[201] Focal airspace enlargement may occur around parenchymal scars and has previously been termed 'irregular emphysema', 'traction emphysema', or 'scar emphysema', but this lesion is not considered to represent true emphysema since there is no associated alveolar wall destruction.

The pathogenesis of emphysema has long been considered to be related to an imbalance in the protease–antiprotease system, with resultant tissue destruction.[184,193] An alternative hypothesis suggests that inflammation and subsequent repair may be pathogenetic.[207] It is possible that both mechanisms may be involved, and the different morphologic forms of emphysema might be explained by a difference in pathogenesis.[186,203,207]

The diagnosis of emphysema is usually based on clinical and radiographic evidence,[185,188] and morphologic studies are generally done on whole lungs

obtained at autopsy or on lobes resected for other reasons.[189,192,195, 200,205,207,208] The pathologic changes of emphysema, however, are commonly encountered in lung specimens excised for diagnosis of other lesions, and there are also a few situations in which portions of lung are resected because of emphysema or its complications.

Blebs and Bullae

Blebs

Blebs are defined as collections of air within the visceral pleura.[205] Thus, they are a form of interstitial emphysema, presumably resulting from the rupture of paraseptal, subpleural, or peribronchiolar alveoli, with dissection of air into adjacent connective tissue. They are commonly encountered in lung tissue resected from patients with *idiopathic spontaneous pneumothorax* and consist of spaces with surrounding fibrosis and varying amounts of inflammation and hemosiderin deposition.[201] Foreign body granulomas sometimes surround the interstitial air. The adjacent lung parenchyma often contains scattered interstitial scars, and a perivascular eosinophil infiltrate has been described in some cases.[196] The overlying pleura is commonly inflamed, and it may show the features of so-called *reactive eosinophilic pleuritis*.[183,198] This lesion is characterized by an inflammatory exudate containing a mixture of histiocytes, numerous eosinophils, and fibrin (Fig. 16–22). Multinucleated giant cells and hyperplastic mesothelial cells may be present as well. The appearance may superficially resemble pulmonary Langerhans cell histiocytosis (eosinophilic granuloma, see Chapter 15), but Langerhans cells are not identified by immunohistochemistry or electron microscopy, and the underlying lung in most patients shows no evidence of Langerhans cell histiocytosis. Reactive eosinophilic pleuritis may represent a reaction to prior chest tube placement used in treating the pneumothorax. It can, of course, occur in any condition associated with pneumothorax, including Langerhans cell histiocytosis.

Bullae

Bullae are large, air-filled spaces in the lung, and, by definition, are greater than 1 cm in diameter.[205] They may be associated with any of the various forms of emphysema, or, less commonly, they may occur as isolated lesions in an otherwise normal lung. An increased incidence of upper lobe bullae has been reported in intravenous drug abusers, and there is some evidence

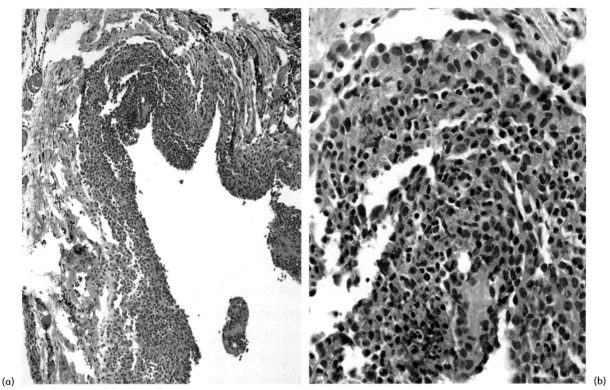

(a)   (b)

Figure 16–22 Reactive eosinophilic pleuritis. (a) Low magnification view showing a prominent cellular infiltrate over fibrotic pleura. Eosinophils can be appreciated even at this low magnification. (b) Higher magnification showing numerous eosinophils in a background of histiocytes and mesothelial cells.

that marijuana smoking is associated with bullae formation.[190,194,202] When bullae are prominent and bilateral with compression of the adjacent lung, the condition is referred to as *giant bullous emphysema*, or *vanishing lung syndrome*.[204] Many of these cases are related to underlying distal acinar emphysema, and bullectomy may significantly improve pulmonary function.[199,204]

Microscopically, bullae characteristically have thick fibrotic walls on the pleural surface, in which smooth muscle and large systemic (bronchial) arteries can be seen.[201] They may contain papillary-appearing fibrous strands that some workers have likened to placental villi (so-called *placental bullous lesion*, or *placental transmogrification of the lung*).[187,197,209] Rarely, fatty tissue (so-called *pulmonary lipomatosis*) is seen in the papillary tissue.[191]

PULMONARY CALCIFICATION AND OSSIFICATION

Pulmonary calcification and ossification constitute a group of disorders in which either calcium or metaplastic bone is deposited in the distal lung parenchyma.[214] In the majority of cases, these depositions are secondary to some underlying local or systemic disorder. In tracheobronchopathia osteoplastica, a rare disorder, the cause is unknown.

Pulmonary Calcification

Calcium deposition in the lungs occurs in two forms, *dystrophic* and *metastatic*.[214] In the *dystrophic* form, calcification occurs focally in areas of caseation, necrosis, or scarring, and it is usually of little, if any, functional significance. The calcified granulomas of tuberculosis or histoplasmosis and the calcified lesions of healed varicella pneumonia are characteristic examples.

Metastatic Calcification

In *metastatic* calcification, the process is usually diffuse and related to renal failure, especially in patients on long-term dialysis.[211,215,217,224,235] Some cases develop after renal transplantation.[213,219,228] Occasionally, other disorders of calcium and phosphorus metabolism may be found, including primary hyperparathyroidism and widespread destructive bone lesions (as in multiple myeloma or other malignancies).[221] In some instances, the therapy for hypercalcemia in these conditions may contribute to calcium deposition. Rare examples of metastatic calcification have been described, however, in patients with normal renal function, normal serum calcium and phosphate levels, and no underlying pulmonary disorder or malignancy.[210,213] Local tissue factors, such as hypoxia related to arterial thrombi, for example, may promote calcium deposition in some patients.[212]

Patients with metastatic calcification are usually asymptomatic, but a small number develop respiratory insufficiency.[213,215,228] The chest radiograph in such cases may show diffuse infiltrates or patterns that resemble pneumonia or even pulmonary edema.[217] In most cases, however, distinct calcific densities cannot be demonstrated on routine chest radiographs, although they may be detectable by more sophisticated methods, such as the dual-energy digital radiography technique.[235] Pulmonary function studies may show a restrictive defect with decreased diffusing capacity in advanced disease.

Microscopically, metastatic calcification is characterized by diffuse deposition of calcium within the alveolar septa and within the walls of blood vessels, bronchioles, and bronchi (Fig. 16–23).[212,215,219,221] Isolated deposition involving the bronchial tree without alveolar involvement has been reported rarely.[237] The calcium appears as finely granular, broad, linear basophilic deposits that have a particular affinity for elastic tissue. Sometimes, a foreign body giant cell reaction to the calcium can be found.[215] Interstitial fibrosis has been reported in some cases of metastatic calcification, and small foci of interstitial bone formation have been noted rarely as well.

Pulmonary Ossification

Pulmonary ossification may be focal or diffuse.[214] The *focal* lesion often is seen in association with dystrophic calcification in areas of prior scarring or necrosis, or it may occur in nodular amyloidosis (see Chapter 7). Some cases have been encountered in a background of organizing pneumonia.[229] The lesion consists of metaplastic bone formation with or without marrow elements.

Diffuse pulmonary ossification can predominantly affect either the airspaces or the interstitium. The airspace form is more common and usually results from pulmonary congestion, as in mitral valve disease. It consists of nodular masses of bone that are located

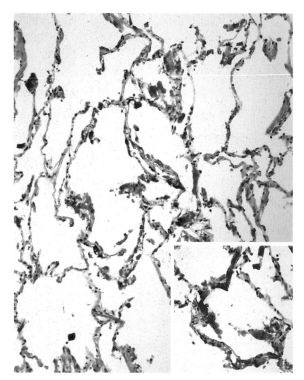

Figure 16–23 Metastatic calcification. Irregular basophilic calcified fragments are seen within the alveolar septa. Inset is a higher magnification of the calcium deposits.

predominantly within alveolar spaces,[231] and it is also termed *nodular pulmonary ossification*. Sometimes, similar nodular bony deposits are encountered in lung biopsy specimens with various other diseases and have no known significance. An interstitial form of diffuse pulmonary ossification, also known as *dendriform pulmonary ossification*, has been described less frequently, and the pathogenesis of this lesion is unclear.[216,218,220,223,225,226,230,231] It usually occurs in a background of interstitial fibrosis and is generally an incidental finding in biopsy or autopsy specimens. Characteristic branching bony deposits, often containing marrow elements, are present in the interstitium (Fig. 16–24). It is not associated with metastatic calcification.

Tracheobronchopathia Osteoplastica

This is a rare disorder that is characterized by the projection of multiple submucosal nodules of bone and cartilage into the lumen of the trachea and large airways.[222,234,238] Patients with this disease are usually middle-aged or elderly men. A familial occurrence

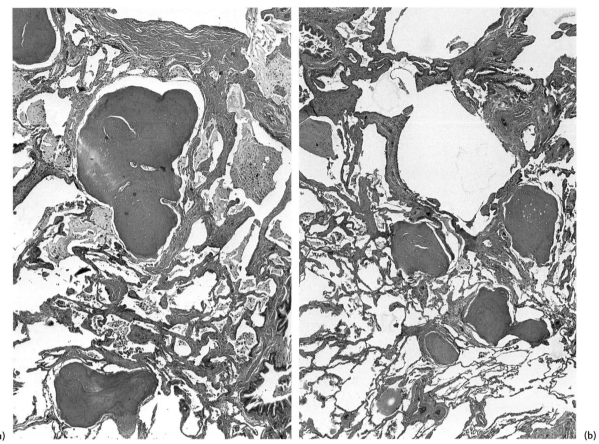

Figure 16–24 Pulmonary ossification. Metaplastic bone formation is present within both the interstitium and the airspaces in this example. Note the associated interstitial fibrosis in **(a)** and honeycomb change (top) in **(b)**.

has been noted rarely.[234] Symptoms include hoarseness, stridor, hemoptysis, and recurrent pulmonary infection.[238] Lobar collapse may occur, and the clinical impression is frequently that of neoplasia.[222] At bronchoscopy, typical hard, yellow–white, papilla-like formations are seen on the cartilaginous portion of the trachea or bronchi.[227] Histologically, the lesion is composed of nodules of bone and cartilage in the submucosa of the airway, superficial to the normal bronchial cartilage (Fig. 16–25).[210,233,236,238] An inflammatory infiltrate of lymphocytes and plasma cells often surrounds the nodules.

The pathogenesis of this disorder is unknown. An association with tracheobronchial amyloidosis has been suggested in the past, but most investigators maintain that the disease is a discrete entity. The lesion may represent an outgrowth or exostosis of normal tracheal rings.[232,233] Tracheobronchopathia osteoplastica should not be confused with the ossification that occurs within normally located tracheal and bronchial cartilage as a manifestation of aging. In this lesion, the cartilaginous rings maintain their normal size and position but contain central ossification.

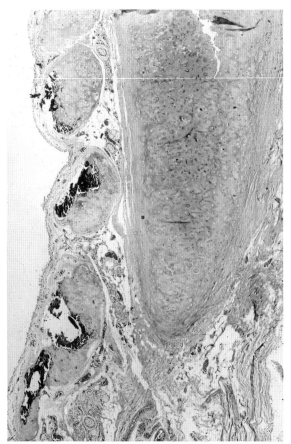

Figure 16–25 Tracheobronchopathia osteoplastica. Nodules of bone and cartilage are located in the submucosa superficial to the normal cartilage ring (right) of this large bronchus.

REFERENCES

Miscellaneous Pneumonias
1. Allen CJ, Newhouse MT: Gastroesophageal reflux and chronic respiratory disease. Am Rev Respir Dis 129:645, 1984.
2. Asnis DS, Saltzman HP, Melchert A: Shark oil pneumonia: An overlooked entity. Chest 103:976, 1993.
3. Ayed AD: Resection of the right middle lobe and lingula in children for middle lobe/lingula syndrome. Chest 125:38, 2004.
4. Barish CF, Wu WC, Castell DO: Respiratory complications of gastroesophageal reflux. Arch Intern Med 145:1882, 1985.
5. Becton DL, Lowe JE, Falletta JM: Lipoid pneumonia in an adolescent girl secondary to use of lip gloss. J Pediatr 105:421, 1984.
6. Bertelsen S, Struve-Christensen E, Aasted A, Sparup J: Isolated middle lobe atelectasis: Aetiology, pathogenesis,

and treatment of the so-called middle lobe syndrome. Thorax 35:449, 1980.
7. Bhaget R, Holmes IH, Kulaga A, et al: Self-injection with olive oil. A cause of lipoid pneumonia. Chest 107:875, 1995.
8. Borrie J, Gwynne JF: Paraffinoma of lung: Lipoid pneumonia. Report of two cases. Thorax 28:214, 1973.
9. Burke M, Fraser R: Obstructive pneumonitis: A pathologic and pathogenetic reappraisal. Radiology 166:699, 1988.
10. Chien H-P, Lin T-P, Chen H-L, Huang TW: Right middle lobe atelectasis associated with endobronchial silicotic lesions. Arch Path Lab Med 124:1619, 2000.
11. Collins KA, Geisinger KR, Wagner PH, et al: The cytologic evaluation of lipid-laden alveolar macrophages as an indicator of aspiration pneumonia in young children. Arch Pathol Lab Med 119:229, 1995.
12. Colombo JL, Hallberg TK: Recurrent aspiration in children: Lipid-laden alveolar macrophage quantitation. Pediatr Pulmonol 4:86, 1987.
13. Corwin RW, Irwin RS: The lipid-laden alveolar macrophage as a marker of aspiration in parenchymal lung disease. Am Rev Respir Dis 132:576, 1985.
14. Dines DE, Titus JL, Sessler AD: Aspiration pneumonitis. Mayo Clin Proc 45:347, 1970.
15. Eisenberg RS, Valdesuso C: Middle lobe syndrome secondary to allergic bronchopulmonary aspergillosis. Ann Allergy 44:217, 1980.
16. Glynn KP, Gale NA: Exogenous lipoid pneumonia due to inhalation of spray lubricant (WD-40 lung). Chest 97:1265, 1990.
17. Greenberger PA, Katzenstein A-LA: Lipid pneumonia with atypical mycobacterial colonization. Association with allergic bronchopulmonary aspergillosis. Arch Intern Med 143:2003, 1983.
18. Heckers H, Melcher FW, Dittmar K, et al: Long-term course of mineral oil pneumonia. Lung 155:101, 1978.
19. Hutchins GM, Boitnott JK: Atypical mycobacterial infection complicating mineral oil pneumonia. JAMA 240:539, 1978.
20. James CE, Modell JH: Pulmonary aspiration. Semin Anesth 2:177, 1983.
21. Kaplan SL, Gnepp DR, Katzenstein A-LA, et al: Miliary pulmonary nodules due to aspirated vegetable particles. J Pediatr 92:449, 1978.
22. Kwon KY, Myers JL, Swensen SJ, Colby TV: Middle lobe syndrome: A clinicopathological study of 21 patients. Hum Pathol 26:302, 1995.
23. Langston C, Pappin A: Lipid-laden alveolar macrophages as an indicator of aspiration pneumonia. Arch Pathol Lab Med 120:326, 1996.
24. Lauque D, Dongay G, Levade T, Caratero C, Carles P: Bronchoalveolar lavage in liquid paraffin pneumonitis. Chest 98:1149, 1990.
25. Lipinski J, Weisbrod G, Sanders D: Exogenous lipoid pneumonitis: Pulmonary patterns. AJR Am J Roentgenol 136:931, 1981.

26. Livingston GL, Holinger LD, Luck SR: Right middle lobe syndrome in children. Int J Pediatr Otorhinolaryngol 13:11, 1987.

27. Miller GJ, Ashcroft MT, Beadnell HM, et al: The lipoid pneumonia of blackflat tobacco smokers in Guyana. Q J Med 40:457, 1971.

27a. Mukhopadhyay S, Katzenstein A-LA: Occult aspiration of gastric contents in biopsy/resection specimens: An often unrecognized cause of lung infiltrates and nodules. Mod Pathol 19 (suppl 1):313A, 2006.

28. Nelson HS: Gastroesophageal reflux and pulmonary disease. J Allergy Clin Immunol 73:547, 1984.

29. Nussbaum E, Maggi JC, Mathis R, Galant SP: Association of lipid-laden alveolar macrophages and gastroesophageal reflux in children. J Pediatr 110:190, 1987.

30. Oldenburger D, Maurer WJ, Beltaos E, et al: Inhalation lipoid pneumonia from burning fats. A newly recognized industrial hazard. JAMA 222:1288, 1972.

31. Orenstein SR, Orenstein DM: Gastroesophageal reflux and respiratory disease in children. J Pediatr 112:847, 1988.

32. Reich JM, Johnson RE: *Mycobacterium avium* complex pulmonary disease presenting as an isolated lingular or middle lobe pattern: The Lady Windermere syndrome. Chest 101:1605, 1992.

33. Rosenbloom SA, Ravin CE, Putman CE, et al: Peripheral middle lobe syndrome. Radiology 14:17, 1983.

34. Saha SP, Mayo P, Long GA, McElvein RB: Middle lobe syndrome: Diagnosis and management. Ann Thorac Surg 33:28, 1982.

35. Verbeken EK, Remedts M, Vanwing J, et al: Pulmonary phospholipid accumulation distal to an obstructed bronchus. A morphologic study. Arch Pathol Lab Med 113:886, 1989.

36. Wagner RB, Johnston MR: Middle lobe syndrome. Ann Thorac Surg 35:679, 1983.

37. Waterfall WE, Craven MA, Allen CJ: Gastroesophageal reflux: Clinical presentation, diagnosis and management. Can Med Assoc J 135:1101, 1986.

Lung Abscess

38. Alexander JC, Wolfe WG: Lung abscess and empyema of the thorax. Surg Clin North Am 60:835, 1980.

39. Asher MI, Spier S, Beland M, et al: Primary lung abscess in childhood. The long-term outcome of conservative management. Am J Dis Child 136:491, 1982.

40. Estrera AS, Platt MR, Mills LJ, et al: Primary lung abscess. J Thorac Cardiovasc Surg 79:275, 1980.

41. Hagan JL, Hardy, JD: Lung abscess revisited. A survey of 184 cases. Ann Surg 197:755, 1983.

42. Shanks GD, Berman JD: Anaerobic pulmonary abscesses. Hematogenous spread from head and neck infections. Clin Pediatr 25:520, 1986.

43. Steyer BJ, Sobonya RE: Pasteurella multocida lung abscess. A case report and review of the literature. Arch Intern Med 144:1081, 1984.

44. Weber TR, Vane DW, Krishna G, et al: Neonatal lung abscess: Resection using one-lung anesthesia. Ann Thorac Surg 36:464, 1983.

Non-neoplastic Masses

45. Chung-Park M, Tomashefski JF Jr, Cohen AM, et al: Shrinking pleuritis with lobar atelectasis, a morphologic variant of "round atelectasis". Hum Pathol 20:382, 1989.

46. Dernevik L, Gatzinsky P: Pathogenesis of shrinking pleuritis with atelectasis-'rounded atelectasis'. Eur J Respir Dis 71:244, 1987.

47. Hershey CO, Panaro V: Round pneumonia in adults. Arch Intern Med 148:1155, 1988.

48. Hillerdal G: Rounded atelectasis. Clinical experience with 74 patients. Chest 95:836, 1989.

49. Matsubara O, Tan-Liu NS, Kenney RM, Mark E: Inflammatory pseudotumors of the lung: Progression from organizing pneumonia to fibrous histiocytoma or to plasma cell granuloma in 32 cases. Hum Pathol 19:807, 1988.

50. Menzies R, Fraser R: Round atelectasis: Pathologic and pathogenetic features. Am J Surg Pathol 11:674, 1987.

51. Smith LS, Schillaci RF: Rounded atelectasis due to acute exudative effusion: Spontaneous resolution. Chest 85:830, 1984.

52. Stark P: Round atelectasis: Another pulmonary pseudotumor. Am Rev Respir Dis 125:248, 1982.

53. Voisin C, Fisekci F, Voisin-Saltiel S, Ameille J, Brochard P, Pairon J-C: Asbestos-related rounded atelectasis: Radiologic and mineralogic data in 23 cases. Chest 107:477, 1995.

54. Yousem SA: Pulmonary apical cap: A distinctive but poorly recognized lesion in pulmonary surgical pathology. Am J Surg Pathol 25:679, 2001.

Disorders of Large Airways

Bronchiectasis

55. Barker AF: Bronchiectasis. N Engl J Med 346:1383, 2002.

56. Bateman ED, Hayashi S, Kuwano K, Wilke TA, Hogg JC: Latent adenoviral infection in follicular bronchiectasis. Am J Respir Crit Care Med 151:170, 1995.

57. Conlan AA, Hurwitz SS, Knige L, et al: Massive hemoptysis. Review of 123 cases. J Thorac Cardiovasc Surg 85:120, 1983.

58. Hoeffler HB, Schweppe HI, Greenberg SP: Bronchiectasis following pulmonary ammonia burn. Arch Pathol Lab Med 106:686, 1982.

59. Kang EY, Miller RR, Müller NL: Bronchiectasis: Comparison of preoperative thin-section CT and pathologic findings in resected specimens. Radiology 195:649, 1995.

60. McGuinness G, Naidich DP, Leitman BS, McCauley DI: Bronchiectasis: CT evaluation. AJR Am J Roentgenol 160:253, 1993.

61. Newman KB, Beam WR: Congenital bronchiectasis in an adult. Am J Med 91:198, 1990.

62. Nicotra MB, Rivera M, Dale AM, et al: Clinical, pathophysiologic, and microbiologic characterization of bronchiectasis in an aging cohort. Chest 108:955, 1995.

63. Pasteur MC, Helliwell SM, Houghton SJ, et al: An investigation into causative factors in patients with bronchiectasis. Am J Respir Crit Care Med 162:1277, 2000.

64. Stockley RA: Bronchiectasis – new therapeutic approaches based on pathogenesis. Clin Chest Med 8:481, 1987.

65. Van der Bruggen-Bogarts BAHA, van der Bruggen HMJG, van Waes PFGM, Lammers J-WJ: Screening for bronchiectasis: A comparative study between chest radiography and high-resolution CT. Chest 109:608, 1996.

Cystic Fibrosis

66. Bedrossian CWM, Greenberg SP, Singer DB, et al: The lung in cystic fibrosis. A quantitative study including prevalence of pathologic findings among different age groups. Hum Pathol 7:195, 1976.

67. Bhargava V, Tomashefski JF Jr, Stern RC, Abramowsky CR: The pathology of fungal infection and colonization in patients with cystic fibrosis. Hum Pathol 20:977, 1989.

68. Carson JL, Collier AM, Gambling TM, et al: Ultrastructure of airway epithelial cell membranes among patients with cystic fibrosis. Hum Pathol 21:640, 1990.

69. Davis PB, Drumm M, Konstan MW: Cystic fibrosis. Am J Respir Crit Care Med 154:1229, 1996.

70. Fernald GW, Boat TF: Cystic fibrosis: Overview. Semin Roentgenol 22:87, 1987.

71. Friedman P, Harwood I, Ellenbogen P: Pulmonary cystic fibrosis in the adult: Early and late radiologic findings with pathologic correlation. AJR Am J Roentgenol 136:1131, 1981.

72. Gilljam H, Motakefi AM, Robertson B, Strandvik B: Ultrastructure of the bronchial epithelium in adult patients with cystic fibrosis. Eur J Respir Dis 71:187, 1987.

73. Griscom NT, Vawter GF, Stigol LC: Radiologic and pathologic abnormalities of the trachea in older patients with cystic fibrosis. AJR Am J Roentgenol 148:691, 1987.

74. Hamutcu R, Rowland JM, Horn MV, et al: Clinical findings and lung pathology in children with cystic fibrosis. Am J Respir Crit Care Med 165:1172, 2002.

75. Oppenheimer EH: Similarity of the tracheobronchial mucous glands and epithelium in infants with and without cystic fibrosis. Hum Pathol 12:36, 1981.

76. Sobonya RE, Taussig LM: Quantitative aspects of lung pathology in cystic fibrosis. Am Rev Respir Dis 134:290, 1986.

77. Sturgess J, Imrie J: Quantitative evaluation of the development of tracheal submucosal glands in infants with cystic fibrosis and control infants. Am J Pathol 106:303, 1982.

78. Tomashefski JF, Christoforidis AJ, Abdullah AK: Cystic fibrosis in young adults. An overlooked diagnosis with emphasis on pulmonary function and radiological patterns. Chest 57:28, 1970.

79. Tomashefski JF Jr, Bruce M, Stern RC, et al: Pulmonary air cysts in cystic fibrosis: Relation of pathologic features to radiologic findings and history of pneumothorax. Hum Pathol 16:253, 1985.

80. Tomashefski JF Jr, Dahms B, Bruce M: Pleura in pneumothorax: Comparison of patients with cystic fibrosis and "idiopathic" spontaneous pneumothorax. Arch Pathol Lab Med 109:910, 1985.

81. Tomashefski JF Jr, Konstan MW, Bruce MC, Abramowsky CR: The pathologic characteristics of interstitial pneumonia in cystic fibrosis. A retrospective autopsy study. Am J Clin Pathol 91:522, 1989.

Intrinsic Obstructive Lesions of Bronchi

82. Arguelles M, Blanco I: Inflammatory bronchial polyps associated with asthma. Arch Intern Med 143:570, 1983.

83. Berman DE, Wright ES, Edstrom HW: Endobronchial inflammatory polyp associated with a foreign body: Successful treatment with corticosteriods. Chest 86:483, 1984.

84. Cahill BC, Harmon KR, Shumway SJ, et al: Tracheobronchial obstruction due to silicosis. Am Rev Respir Dis 145:719, 1992.

85. Conces DJ, Tarver RD, Vix VA: Broncholithiasis: CT features in 15 patients. AJR Am J Roentgenol 157:249, 1991.

86. Conlan AA, Hurwitz SS, Nicolaou N, et al: Broncholithiasis – the endoscopic appearance and review of factors influencing management. A case report. South Med J 63:1016, 1983.

87. Kargi HA, Kuhn C III: Bronchiolitis obliterans: Unilateral fibrous obliteration of the lumen of bronchi with atelectasis. Chest 93:1107, 1988.

88. Nollet AS, Vansteenkiste JF, Demedts MG: Broncholithiasis: Rare but still present. Respir Med 92:963, 1998.

89. Perlman EJ, Lederman HM, Taylor GA, et al: "Bronchitis" obliterans and prolonged transient hypogammaglobulinemia in a child. Pediatr Pulmonol 16:375, 1993.

90. Wedel MK, Hanson AS, Heithoff K: Broncholithiasis. Minn Med 67:139, 1984.

91. Williams DO, Vanecko RM, Glassroth J: Endobronchial polyposis following smoke inhalation. Chest 84:774, 1983.

Primary Ciliary Dyskinesia

92. Afzelius BA: Ultrastructural basis for ciliary motility. Eur J Respir Dis Suppl 128(Pt 1):280, 1983.

93. Afzelius BA, Camner P, Mossberg B: Acquired ciliary defects compared to those seen in the immotile-cilia syndrome. Eur J Respir Dis Suppl 127:5, 1983.

94. Afzelius BA, Gargani G, Romano C: Abnormal length of cilia as a possible cause of defective mucociliary clearance. Eur J Respir Dis 66:173, 1985.

95. Becker B, Morgenroth K, Reinhardt D, Irlich G: The dyskinetic cilia syndrome in childhood. Modifications of ultrastructural patterns. Respiration 46:180, 1984.

96. Buchdahl RM, Reiser J, Ingram D, et al: Ciliary abnormalities in respiratory disease. Arch Dis Child 63:238, 1988.

97. Carson JL, Collier AM, Hu SS: Acquired ciliary defects in nasal epithelium of children with acute viral upper respiratory infections. N Engl J Med 312:463, 1985.

98. Cornillie FJ, Lauweryns JM: Atypical bronchial cilia in children with recurrent respiratory tract infections. Pathol Res Pract 178:595, 1984.

99. de Iongh R, Rutland J: Orientation of respiratory tract cilia in patients with primary ciliary dyskinesia, bronchiectasis, and in normal subjects. J Clin Pathol 42:613, 1989.

100. de Iongh RU, Rutland J: Ciliary defects in healthy subjects, bronchiectasis, and primary ciliary dyskinesia. Am J Respir Crit Care Med 151:1559, 1995.

101. Eavey RD, Nadol JB Jr, Holmes LB, et al: Kartagener's syndrome. A blinded, controlled study of cilia ultrastructure. Arch Otolaryngol 112:646, 1986.

102. Ehouman A, Pinchon MC, Escudier E, Bernandin JF: Ultrastructural abnormalities of respiratory cilia. Descriptive and quantitative study of respiratory mucosa in a series of 33 patients. Virchows Arch B Cell Pathol Incl Mol Pathol 48:87, 1985.

103. Eliasson R, Mossberg B, Camner P, et al: The immotile cilia syndrome. A congenital ciliary abnormality as an etiologic factor in chronic airway infections and male sterility. N Engl J Med 297:1, 1977.

104. Fox B, Bull TB, Arden GB: Variations in the ultrastructure of human nasal cilia including abnormalities found in retinitis pigmentosa. J Clin Pathol 33:327, 1980.

105. Fox B, Bull TB, Oliver TN: The distribution and assessment of electron-microscopic abnormalities of human cilia. Eur J Respir Dis Suppl 127:11, 1983.

106. Gordon RE, Kattan M: Absence of cilia and basal bodies with predominance of brush cells in the respiratory mucosa from a patient with immotile cilia syndrome. Ultrastruct Pathol 6:45, 1984.

107. Handelsman DJ, Conway AJ, Boylan LM, Turtle JR: Young's syndrome. Obstructive azoospermia and chronic sinopulmonary infections. N Eng J Med 310:3, 1984.

108. Heino M: Morphological changes related to ciliogenesis in the bronchial epithelium in experimental conditions and clinical course of disease. Eur J Respir Dis Suppl 151:1, 1987.

109. Howell JT, Schochet SS, Goldman AS: Ultrastructural defects of respiratory tract cilia associated with chronic infections. Arch Pathol Lab Med 104:52, 1980.

110. Katz SM, Holsclaw DS Jr: Ultrastructural features of respiratory cilia in cystic fibrosis. Am J Clin Pathol 73:682, 1980.

111. Kollberg H, Mossberg B, Afzelius BA, et al: Cystic fibrosis compared with the immotile-cilia syndrome. A study of mucociliary clearance, ciliary ultrastructure, clinical picture and ventilatory function. Scand J Respir Dis 59:297, 1978.

112. Kovesi T, Sinclair B, MacCormick J, et al: Primary ciliary dyskinesia associated with a novel microtubule defect in a child with Down's syndrome. Chest 117:1207, 2000.

113. Lee RMK, Rossman CM, O'Brodovich H: Assessment of postmortem respiratory ciliary motility and ultrastructure. Am Rev Respir Dis 136:445, 1987.

114. Lungarella G, De Santi MM, Palatresi R, Tosi P: Ultrastructural observations on basal apparatus of respiratory cilia in immotile cilia syndrome. Eur J Respir Dis 66:165, 1985.

115. Lungarella G, Fonzi L, Burrini AG: Ultrastructural abnormalities in respiratory cilia and sperm tails in a patient with Kartagener's syndrome. Ultrastruct Pathol 3:319, 1982.

116. Neustein HB, Nickerson B, O'Neal M: Kartagener's syndrome with absence of inner dynein arms of respiratory cilia. Am Rev Respir Dis 122:979, 1980.

117. Nielsen MH, Pedersen M, Christensen B, Mygind N: Blind quantitative electron microscopy of cilia from patients with primary ciliary dyskinesia and from normal subjects. Eur J Respir Dis Suppl 127:19, 1983.

118. Noone PG, Leigh MW, Sannuti A, et al: Primary ciliary dyskinesia: Diagnostic and phenotypic features. Am J Respir Crit Care Med 169:459, 2004.

119. Pederson M: Specific types of abnormal ciliary motility in Kartagener's syndrome and analogous respiratory disorders. A quantified microphoto-oscillografic investigation of 27 patients. Eur J Respir Dis Suppl 127:78, 1983.

120. Rayner CFJ, Rutman A, Dewar A, et al: Ciliary disorientation in patients with chronic upper respiratory tract inflammation. Am J Respir Crit Care Med 151:800, 1995.

121. Rayner CFJ, Rutman A, Dewar A, et al: Ciliary disorientation alone as a cause of primary ciliary dyskinesia syndrome. Am J Respir Crit Care Med 153:1123, 1996.

122. Reyes de la Rocha, S, Pysher TJ, Leonard JC: Dyskinetic cilia syndrome: Clinical, radiographic and scintigraphic findings. Pediatr Radiol 17:97, 1987.

123. Rossman CM, Forrest JB, Lee RMKW, et al: The dyskinetic cilia syndrome. Ciliary motility in immotile cilia syndrome. Chest 78:580, 1980.

124. Rossman CM, Newhouse MT: Primary ciliary dyskinesia: Evaluation and management. Pediatr Pulmonol 5:36, 1988.

125. Rutland J, de Iongh RU: Random ciliary orientation: A cause of respiratory tract disease. N Engl J Med 323:1681, 1990.

126. Smallman LA, Gregory J: Ultrastructural abnormalities of cilia in the human respiratory tract. Hum Pathol 17:848, 1986.

127. Stannard W, Rutman A, Wallis C, O'Callaghan C: Central microtubular agenesis causing primary ciliary dyskinesia. Am J Respir Crit Care Med 169:634, 2004.

128. Sturgess JM, Chao J, Turner JAP: Transposition of ciliary microtubules. Another cause of impaired ciliary motility. N Engl J Med 303:318, 1980.

129. Sturgess JM, Chao J, Wong J, et al: Cilia with defective radial spokes: A cause of human respiratory disease. N Engl J Med 300:53, 1979.

130. Torikata C, Kawai T, Nogawa S, et al: Nine Japanese patients with immotile-dyskinetic cilia syndrome: An ultrastructural study using tannic acid-containing fixation. Hum Pathol 22:830, 1991.

131. Tsang KWT, Tipoe G, Sun J, et al: Severe bronchiectasis in patients with "cystlike" structures within the ciliary shafts. Am J Respir Crit Care Med 161:1300, 2000.

132. Van der Baan S, Veerman AJP, Bezemer PD, Feenstra L: Primary ciliary dyskinesia: Quantitative investigation of the ciliary ultrastructure with statistical analysis. Ann Otol Rhinol Laryngol 96:264, 1987.

133. Verra F, Escudier E, Lebargy F, et al: Ciliary abnormalities in bronchial epithelium of smokers, ex-smokers, and nonsmokers. Am J Respir Crit Care Med 151:630, 1995.

134. Verra F, Fleury-Feith J, Boucherat M, et al: Do nasal ciliary changes reflect bronchial changes? An ultrastructural study. Am Rev Respir Dis 147:908, 1993.

135. Wilton LJ, Teichtahl H, Temple-Smith PD, deKretser DM: Kartagener's syndrome with motile cilia and immotile spermatozoa: Axonemal ultrastructure and function. Am Rev Respir Dis 134:1233, 1986.

Small Airways Disease (General)

136. Edwards C, Cayton R, Bryan R: Chronic transmural bronchiolitis: A non-specific lesion of small airways. J Clin Pathol 45:993, 1992.

137. Kindt GG, Weiland JE, Davis WB, et al: Bronchiolitis in adults. A reversible cause of airway obstruction associated with airway neutrophils and neutrophil products. Am Rev Respir Dis 140:483, 1989.

138. Macklem PT, Thurlbeck WM, Fraser RO: Chronic obstructive disease of small airways. Ann Intern Med 74:167, 1971.

139. Ryu JH, Myers JL, Swensen SJ: Bronchiolar disorders. Am J Respir Crit Care Med 168:1277, 2003.

140. Thurlbeck WM: The pathology of small airways in chronic airflow limitation. Eur J Respir Dis Suppl 121:9, 1982.

Respiratory Bronchiolitis

141. Brody A, Craighead J: Cytoplasmic inclusions in pulmonary macrophages of cigarette smokers. Lab Invest 32:125, 1975.

142. Fraig M, Shreesha U, Savici D, Katzenstein A-LA: Respiratory bronchiolitis: A clinicopathologic study in current smokers, ex-smokers, and never-smokers. Am J Surg Pathol 26:647, 2002.

143. Myers JL, Veal CF, Shin MS, Katzenstein A-LA: Respiratory bronchiolitis causing interstitial lung disease. Am Rev Respir Dis 135:880, 1987.

144. Niewoehner DE, Kleinerman J, Rice DB: Pathologic changes in peripheral airways of young cigarette smokers. N Engl J Med 291:755, 1974.

145. Yousem SA, Colby TV, Gaensler E: Respiratory bronchiolitis-associated interstitial lung disease and its relationship to desquamative interstitial pneumonia. Mayo Clin Proc 64:1373, 1989.

Diffuse Panbronchiolitis

146. Akira M, Higashihara T, Sakatani M, Hara H: Diffuse panbronchiolitis: Follow-up CT examination. Radiology 189:559, 1993.

147. Akira M, Kitatani F, Yong-Sik L, et al: Diffuse panbronchiolitis: Evaluation with high-resolution CT. Radiology 168:433, 1988.

148. Baz MA, Kussin PS, Van Trigt P, et al: Recurrence of diffuse panbronchiolitis after lung transplantation. Am J Respir Crit Care Med 151:895, 1995.

149. Fisher MS, Rush WL, Rosado-de-Christenson M, et al: Diffuse panbronchiolitis: Histologic diagnosis in unsuspected cases involving North American residents of Asian descent. Arch Pathol Lab Med 122:156, 1997.

150. Fitzgerald JE, King TEJr, Lynch DA, et al: Diffuse panbronchiolitis in the United States. Am J Respir Crit Care Med 154:497, 1996.

151. Homer RJ, Khoo L, Walker Smith GJ: Diffuse panbronchiolitis in a Hispanic man with travel history to Japan. Chest 107:1176, 1995.

152. Homma H, Yamanaka A, Tanimoto S, et al: Diffuse panbronchiolitis: A disease of the transitional zone of the lung. Chest 83:63, 1983.

153. Iwata M, Colby TV, Kitaichi M: Diffuse panbronchiolitis: Diagnosis and distinction from various pulmonary diseases with centrilobular interstitial foam cell accumulations. Hum Pathol 25:357, 1994.

154. Kadota J, Mukae H, Fujii T, et al: Clinical similarities and differences between human T-cell lymphotropic virus type 1-associated bronchiolitis and diffuse panbronchiolitis. Chest 125:1239, 2004.

155. Maeda M, Saiki S, Yamanaka A: Serial section analysis of the lesions in diffuse panbronchiolitis. Acta Pathol Jpn 37:693, 1987.

156. Nishimura K, Kitaichi M, Izumi T, Itoh H: Diffuse panbronchiolitis: Correlation of high-resolution CT and pathologic findings. Radiology 184:779, 1992.

157. Randhawa P, Hoagland MH, Yousem SA: Diffuse panbronchiolitis in North America: Report of three cases and review of the literature. Am J Surg Pathol 15:43, 1991.

158. Sugiyama Y, Kudoh S, Maeda H, et al: Analysis of HLA antigens in patients with diffuse panbronchiolitis. Am Rev Respir Dis 141:1459, 1990.

159. Todate A, Chida K, Suda T, et al: Increased numbers of dendritic cells in the bronchiolar tissues of diffuse panbronchiolitis. Am J Respir Crit Care Med 162:148, 2000.

Constrictive Bronchiolitis Obliterans

160. Abernathy EC, Hruban RH, Baumgartner WA, Reitz BA, Hutchins GM: The two forms of bronchiolitis obliterans in heart-lung transplant recipients. Hum Pathol 22:1102, 1991.

161. Akpinar-Elci M, Travis WD, Lynch DA, Kreiss K: Bronchiolitis obliterans syndrome in popcorn production plant workers. Eur Respir J 24:298, 2004.

162. Chan C, Hyland R, Hutcheson M, et al: Small-airways disease in recipients of allogeneic bone marrow transplants. An analysis of 11 cases and a review of the literature. Medicine (Baltimore) 66:327, 1987.

163. Chang H, Wang J-S, Tseng H-H, et al: Histopathological study of *Sauropus androgynus*-associated constrictive bronchiolitis obliterans: A new cause of constrictive bronchiolitis obliterans. Am J Surg Pathol 21:35, 1997.

164. Chang Y-L, Yao Y-T, Wang N-S, Lee Y-C: Segmental necrosis of small bronchi after prolonged intakes of *Sauropus androgynus* in Taiwan. Am J Respir Crit Care Med 157:594, 1998.

165. Geddes DM, Corrin B, Brewerton D, et al. Progressive airway obliteration in adults and its association with rheumatoid disease. Q J Med 46:427, 1977.

166. Hawley PC, Whitcomb ME: Bronchiolitis fibrosa obliterans in adults. Arch Intern Med 141:1324, 1981.

167. Holness L, Tenenbaum J, Cooter NBE, Grossman RF: Fatal bronchiolitis obliterans associated with chrysotherapy. Ann Rheum Dis 42:593, 1983.

168. Iannuzzi MC, Farhi DC, Bostrom PD, et al: Fulminant respiratory failure and death in a patient with idiopathic bronchiolitis obliterans. Arch Intern Med 145:733, 1985.

169. Jacobs, P, Bonnyns M, Depierreux M, et al: Rapidly fatal bronchiolitis obliterans with circulating antinuclear and rheumatoid factors. Eur J Respir Dis 65:384, 1984.

170. Kim CK, Kim SW, Kim JS, et al: Bronchiolitis obliterans in the 1990s in Korea and the United States. Chest 120:1101, 2001.

171. Kim MJ, Lee KY: Bronchiolitis obliterans in children with Stevens-Johnson syndrome: Follow-up with high resolution CT. Pediatr Radiol 26:22, 1996.

172. Kraft M, Mortenson RL, Colby TV, et al: Cryptogenic constrictive bronchiolitis: A clinicopathologic study. Am Rev Respir Dis 148:1093, 1993.

173. Kogutt MS, Swishuk LE, Goldblum R: Swyer-James syndrome (unilateral hyperlucent lung) in children. Am J Dis Child 125:614, 1973.

174. Kreiss K, Gomaa A, Kullman G, et al: Clinical bronchiolitis obliterans in workers at a microwave-popcorn plant. N Engl J Med 347:330, 2002.

175. Lebargy F, Wolkenstein P, Gisselbrecht M, et al: Pulmonary complications in toxic epidermal necrolysis: A prospective clinical study. Intensive Care Med 23:1237, 1997.

176. Markopolou KD, Cool CD, Elliot TL, et al: Obliterative bronchiolitis: Varying presentations and clinicopathological correlation. Eur Respir J 19:20, 2002.

177. Murphy KC, Atkins CJ, Offer RC, et al: Obliterative bronchiolitis in two rheumatoid arthritis patients treated with penicillamine. Arthritis Rheum 24:557, 1981.

178. Nousari HC, Deterding R, Wojtczack H, et al: The mechanism of respiratory failure in paraneoplastic pemphigus. N Engl J Med 340:1406, 2004.

179. Stokes D, Sigler A, Khouri N, Talamo R: Unilateral hyperlucent lung (Swyer-James syndrome) after severe *Mycoplasma pneumoniae* infection. Am Rev Respir Dis 117:145, 1978.

180. Turton C, Williams G, Green M: Cryptogenic obliterative bronchiolitis in adults. Thorax 36:805, 1981.

181. Urbanski SJ, Kossakowska AE, Curtis J, et al: Idiopathic small airways pathology in patients with graft-versus-host disease following allogeneic bone marrow transplantation. Am J Surg Pathol 11:965, 1987.

182. Yousem S, Burke C, Billingham M: Pathologic pulmonary alterations in long-term human heart-lung transplantation. Hum Pathol 16:911, 1985.

Emphysema

183. Askin FB, McCann BG, Kuhn C: Reactive eosinophilic pleuritis. A lesion to be distinguished from pulmonary eosinophilic granuloma. Arch Pathol Lab Med 101:187, 1977.

184. Barnes PT: Chronic obstructive pulmonary disease. N Engl J Med 343:269, 2000.

185. Bergin C, Muller N, Nichols DM, et al: The diagnosis of emphysema. A computed tomographic-pathologic correlation. Am Rev Respir Dis 133:541, 1986.

186. Cardoso WV, Sekhon HS, Hyde DM, Thurlbeck WM: Collagen and elastin in human pulmonary emphysema. Am Rev Respir Dis 147:975, 1993.

187. Fidler ME, Koomen M, Sebek B, et al: Placental transmogrification of the lung, a histologic variant of giant bullous emphysema: Clinicopathological study of three further cases. Am J Surg Pathol 19:563, 1995.

188. Foster WL Jr, Pratt PC, Roggli VL, et al: Centrilobular emphysema: CT-pathologic correlation. Radiology 159:27, 1986.

189. Gillooly M, Lamb D, Farrow ASJ: New automated technique for assessing emphysema on histological sections. J Clin Pathol 44:1007, 1991.

190. Goldstein DS, Karpel JP, Appel D, Williams MH Jr: Bullous pulmonary damage in users of intravenous drugs. Chest 89:266, 1986.

191. Hochholzer L, Moran CA, Koss MN: Pulmonary lipomatosis: A variant of placental transmogrification. Mod Pathol 10:846, 1997.

192. Hruban RH, Meziane MA, Zerhouni EA, et al: High resolution computed tomography of inflation-fixed lungs. Pathologic-radiologic correlation of centrilobular emphysema. Am Rev Respir Dis 136:935, 1987.

193. Imai K, Dalal SS, Chen ES, et al: Human collagenase (matrix metalloproteinase-1): Expression in the lungs of patients with emphysema. Am J Respir Crit Care Med 163:786, 2001.

194. Johnson MK, Smith RP, Morrison D, et al: Large lung bullae in marijuana smokers. Thorax 55:340, 2000.

195. Linhartova A: Lesions in resected lung parenchyma with regard to possible initial phase of pulmonary emphysema. Pathol Res Pract 181:71, 1986.

196. Luna E, Tomashefski JE Jr, Brown D, et al: Reactive eosinophilic pulmonary vascular infiltration in patients

with spontaneous pneumothorax. Am J Surg Pathol 18:195, 1994.

197. Mark EJ, Muller K-M, McChesney T, et al: Placentoid bullous lesion of the lung. Hum Pathol 26:74, 1995.

198. McDonnell TJ, Crouch EC, Gonzalez JG: Reactive eosinophilic pleuritis: A sequela of pneumothorax in pulmonary eosinophilic granuloma. Am J Clin Pathol 91:107, 1989.

199. Morgan MDL, Edwards CW, Morris J, Matthews HR: Origin and behaviour of emphysematous bullae. Thorax 44:533, 1989.

200. Nagai A, Yamawaki I, Thurlbeck WM, Takizawa T: Assessment of lung parenchymal destruction by using routine histologic tissue sections. Am Rev Respir Dis 139:313, 1989.

201. Ohata M, Suzuki H: Pathogenesis of spontaneous pneumothorax with special reference to the ultrastructure of emphysematous bullae. Chest 77:771, 1980.

202. Schmidt RA, Glenny RW, Godwin JD, et al: Panlobular emphysema in young intravenous Ritalin abusers. Am Rev Respir Dis 143:649, 1991.

203. Snider GL: Emphysema: The first two centuries and beyond. A historical overview, with suggestions for future research: Part 1. Am Rev Respir Dis 146:1334, 1992.

204. Stern EJ, Webb WR, Weinacker A, Muller NL: Idiopathic giant bullous emphysema (vanishing lung syndrome): Imaging findings in nine patients. AJR Am J Roentgenol 162:279, 1994.

205. Thurlbeck WM: *Chronic Airflow Obstruction in Lung Disease*. Philadelphia, Saunders, 1976.

206. Tomashefski JF Jr, Crystal RG, Wiedemann HP, et al: The bronchopulmonary pathology of alpha-1 antitrypsin (AAT) deficiency: Findings of the Death Review Committee of the national registry for individuals with Severe Deficiency of Alpha-1 Antitrypsin. Hum Pathol 35:1452, 2004.

207. Wright JL: Emphysema: Concepts under change – a pathologist's perspective. Mod Pathol 8:873, 1995.

208. Wright JL, Barry W, Pare PD, Hogg JC: Ranking the severity of emphysema on whole lung slices. Concordance of upper lobe, lower lobe, and entire lung ranks. Am Rev Respir Dis 133:930, 1986.

209. Xu R, Murray M, Jagirdar J, et al: Placental transmogrification of the lung is a histologic pattern frequently associated with pulmonary fibrochondromatous hamartoma. Arch Pathol Lab Med 126:562, 2002.

Pulmonary Calcification and Ossification

210. Bein ME, Lee DBN, Mink JH, Dickmeyer J: Unusual case of metastatic pulmonary calcification. AJR Am J Roentgenol 132:812, 1979.

211. Bestetti-Bosisio M, Cotelli F, Schiaffino E, et al: Lung calcification in long-term dialysed patients: A light and electronmicroscopic study. Histopathology 8:69, 1984.

212. Bloodworth J, Tomashefski JF Jr: Localised pulmonary

metastatic calcification associated with pulmonary artery obstruction. Thorax 47:174, 1992.

213. Breitz HB, Sirotta PS, Nelp WB, et al: Progressive pulmonary calcification complicating successful renal transplantation. Am Rev Respir Dis 136:1480, 1987.

214. Chan ED, Morales DV, Welsh CH, et al: Calcium deposition with or without bone formation in the lung. Am J Respir Crit Care Med 165:1654, 2002.

215. Conger JD, Hammond WS, Alfrey AC, et al: Pulmonary calcification in chronic dialysis patients. Clinical and pathologic studies. Ann Intern Med 83:330, 1975.

216. Felson B, Schwarz J, Lukin RR, Hawkins HH: Idiopathic pulmonary ossification. Radiology 153:303, 1984.

217. Firooznia H, Pudlowski R, Golimbu C, et al: Diffuse interstitial calcification of the lungs in chronic renal failure mimicking pulmonary edema. AJR Am J Roentgenol 129:1103, 1977.

218. Fried ED, Godwin TA: Extensive diffuse pulmonary ossification. Chest 102:1614, 1992.

219. Gilman M, Nissim JA, Terry P, Whelton A: Metastatic pulmonary calcification in the renal transplant recipient. Am Rev Respir Dis 121:415, 1980.

220. Green JD, Harle TS, Greenberg SD, et al: Disseminated pulmonary ossification. A case report with demonstration of electron-microscopic features. Am Rev Respir Dis 101:293, 1970.

221. Heath D, Robertson AJ: Pulmonary calcinosis. Thorax 32:606, 1977.

222. Hodges MK, Israel E: Tracheobronchopathia osteochondroplastica presenting as right middle lobe collapse. Diagnosis by bronchoscopy and computerized tomography. Chest 94:842, 1988.

223. Joines RW, Roggli VL: Dendriform pulmonary ossification: Report of two cases with unique findings. Am J Clin Pathol 91:398, 1989.

224. Justrabo E, Genin R, Rifle G: Pulmonary metastatic calcification with respiratory insufficiency in patients on maintenance haemodialysis. Thorax 34:384, 1979.

225. Kayser K, Stute H, Tuengerthal S: Diffuse pulmonary ossification associated with metastatic melanoma of the lung. Respiration 52:221, 1987.

226. Kim TS, Han J, Chung MP, Choi YS: Disseminated dendriform pulmonary ossification associated with usual interstitial pneumonia: Incidence and thin-section CT-pathologic correlation. Eur Radiol 15:1581, 2005.

227. Lundgren R, Stjernberg NL: Tracheobronchopathia osteochondroplastica. A clinical bronchoscopic and spirometric study. Chest 80:706, 1981.

228. Milliner DS, Lieberman E, Landing BH: Pulmonary calcinosis after renal transplantation in pediatric patients. Am J Kidney Dis 7:495, 1986.

229. Muller K-M, Friemann J, Stichnoth E: Dendriform pulmonary ossification. Pathol Res Pract 168:163, 1980.

230. Ndimbie OK, Williams CR, Lee MW: Dendriform pulmonary ossification. Arch Pathol Lab Med 111:1062, 1987.

231. Popelka CG, Kleinerman J: Diffuse pulmonary ossification. Arch Intern Med 137:523, 1977.

232. Pounder DJ, Pieterse AS: Tracheopathia osteoplastica: A study of the minimal lesion. J Pathol 138:235, 1982.

233. Pounder DJ, Pieterse AS: Tracheopathia osteoplastica: Report of four cases. Pathology 14:429, 1982.

234. Prakash UBS, McCullough AE, Edell ES, Nienhuis DM: Tracheopathia osteoplastica: Familial occurrence. Mayo Clin Proc 64:1091, 1989.

235. Sanders C, Frank MS, Rostand SG, et al: Metastatic calcification of the heart and lungs in end-stage renal disease: Detection and quantification of dual-energy digital chest radiography. AJR Am J Roentgenol 149:881, 1987.

236. van Nierop MA, Wagenaar SS, van den Bosch JM, Westermann CJ: Tracheobronchopathia osteochondroplastica. Report of four cases. Eur J Respir Dis 64:129, 1983.

237. Wright J, Jones E: Diffuse calcification of the airways. Mod Pathol 14:717, 2001.

238. Young RH, Sandstrom RE, Mark GJ: Tracheopathia osteoplastica. J Thorac Cardiovas Surg 79:537, 1980.

17

TRANSBRONCHIAL LUNG BIOPSY

Transbronchial lung biopsy (TBB) is a widely used, relatively noninvasive and safe method of obtaining lung tissue that may obviate the need for thoracotomy.[62,80] In well-selected patients, it has few complications; pneumothorax occurs in less than 5% and clinically significant bleeding in less than 2%.[4,9,17,28,42,46] Deaths from complications are rare, having been reported in 0.1% to 0.2% of cases.[28,80] The tissue that is obtained consists of one or more pieces of lung averaging 1 to 2 mm in greatest dimension. Most large series report a diagnostic accuracy approaching 50% to 70%.[4,5,14,18,21–24,27,33,41,43,46,47,51,52,55,64,70,71,77] The greatest diagnostic yield is obtained in patients with diffuse infiltrates, whereas biopsies of solitary peripheral nodules are least productive. Accuracy can be enhanced when the results of bronchial washings, bronchial brushings, and bronchoalveolar lavage are combined with TBB.[19,31,39,49,55,65]

Although the size of the tissue sampled by TBB is small, a surprisingly large amount of helpful information can be obtained. The role of the pathologist is to provide as much information for the clinician as possible, with the aim of sparing the patient a thoracotomy, while being careful not to overlook treatable diseases that might require open biopsy for diagnosis. To be successful in this endeavor, the pathologist must be meticulous in examining the tissue, and good communication with the patient's physicians is essential. Although knowledge of the clinical and radiographic findings is important in interpreting even large open lung biopsy specimens, *this knowledge is mandatory* for evaluating the small amount of tissue obtained by TBB.

The following discussion attempts to outline for the pathologist a practical approach to evaluating TBB specimens; detailed descriptions of specific disease processes are presented in other chapters. Interpretation of TBB is discussed separately for immunocompromised and nonimmunocompromised patients, since the clinical and radiographic manifestations, the pathologic findings, and the reasons for biopsy may differ depending on the immunologic status of the patients.

HANDLING OF TBB SPECIMENS

Appropriate handling of TBB specimens requires effort from both the bronchoscopist and pathologist, as outlined in Table 17–1. Cultures should be performed in all cases, and unless infection is highly suspected clinically, use of bronchial washings or bronchoalveolar lavage fluid rather than a tissue piece is adequate. It is important that as many tissue fragments as possible be sent to pathology for histologic examination, since the amount of tissue obtained is so limited. The bronchoscopist should be advised to place the specimen for surgical pathology directly from the biopsy forceps into formalin, because exposing the tissue to air for any length of time will cause atelectasis and drying artifact. We discourage sending aliquots for electron microscopy or immunofluorescence, since as much tissue as possible is needed for light microscopic examination. Although the bronchoscopist may perceive that he or she has submitted multiple tissue pieces, often they consist only of clusters of detached bronchial epithelium or clotted blood. Also, even when multiple lung fragments are received, only one or two may contain abnormal areas sufficient for diagnosis.

The pathologist must handle the small tissue fragments gently, being careful not to crush or otherwise distort them. They should be wrapped in moist lens paper before placing in a cassette, and should never

Table 17–1 Handling of Transbronchial Lung Biopsy Specimens

Bronchoscopist
Send lavage fluid or tissue piece to microbiology for culture.
Place remaining pieces *immediately* in formalin (do not allow to be exposed to air).
Do *not* separate aliquots for special studies (electron microscopy or immunofluorescence) unless there are unusually compelling circumstances.

Pathologist
Wrap tissue in moist lens paper. Do not place between sponges.
Examine at least three H and E-stained step sections initially.
Perform special stains (AFB, GMS) for organisms routinely in immunocompromised patients.
Select special stains or additional studies in immunocompetent patients, depending on the tissue reaction.

be placed between sponges. The latter technique not only causes artifactual atelectasis, but it also produces irregular, geometric spaces in the tissue (so-called sponge artifact) that make evaluation difficult.[38]

In evaluating TBB specimens, at least three hematoxylin and eosin (H and E)-stained slides should be prepared initially from step sections of each block; more can be prepared subsequently if the amount of tissue appears to be inadequate or a diagnosis cannot be established.[48,66] In addition, all TBB specimens from immunocompromised patients should be stained routinely for acid-fast bacilli, other bacteria, fungi, and pneumocystis, regardless of the histologic findings. In nonimmunocompromised patients, special stains for organisms can be selected depending on the histologic appearance of the tissue reaction. We prefer the Ziehl–Neelsen (AFB), Brown–Brenn or Brown–Hopps, and Grocott–Gomori methenamine silver (GMS) stains, as outlined in Chapter 10, but a variety of other stains are equally effective. Additional histochemical or immunohistochemical stains can be performed as indicated.

ASSESSING ADEQUACY OF TBB

An important component of examining a TBB specimen is to determine whether or not the tissue is adequate for diagnosis and to communicate this finding to the clinician. We consider a TBB adequate when at least one fragment of alveolated lung parenchyma is present, although others suggest that at least 20 alveoli are needed for an adequate biopsy.[25] A TBB specimen is inadequate for diagnosis when alveolated lung parenchyma is absent and the tissue present shows no features diagnostic of a specific entity. Occasionally, a biopsy specimen may lack alveoli but contain fragments of bronchial wall in which specific lesions, such as granulomas or tumor, for example, can be found, and obviously this would not be considered inadequate. Even when tissue fragments are absent in a TBB, the specimen may be adequate if, for example, organisms can be identified within exudates or debris, or viral inclusions or cytologic features of malignancy can be found in detached clusters of cells. Therefore, the designation 'tissue inadequate for diagnosis' is reserved for those specimens that lack alveoli and, after careful examination, including special stains for organisms, show no features diagnostic of a specific disease.

Although the pathologist may risk offending the bronchoscopist by labeling the tissue inadequate, knowledge of adequacy (or inadequacy) is extremely important in determining whether additional biopsies would be productive and what kind of procedure should be undertaken. This knowledge also helps the clinician interpret results in other situations. For example, occasionally the microbiology laboratory identifies an organism but the surgical pathology laboratory receives an inadequate specimen lacking lung parenchyma. For the clinician to assess whether or not the organism is pathogenic, he or she must be aware that the biopsy does not contain sufficient lung tissue for evaluation. Without this knowledge, the clinician may incorrectly conclude that the organism is only a saprophyte, since evidence of infection was not noted by the pathologist. Communication of tissue adequacy also serves to build the clinician's confidence in the significance of a truly negative but adequate biopsy. Failure to exclude inadequate TBB specimens when assessing overall accuracy of TBB may explain a low reported diagnostic yield for this procedure in some studies.[32,68]

COMMON ARTIFACTS IN TBB SPECIMENS

A number of artifacts are frequently encountered in TBB specimens. They are listed in Table 17–2 along with important histologic features that help distinguish them from disease processes with which they may be confused. *Atelectasis* is probably the most commonly observed artifact (Fig. 17–1). It is present to some degree in almost all specimens, but it can be so severe in some that interstitial and airspace compartments cannot be distinguished. As noted previously, atelectasis can be minimized by the bronchoscopist if the tissue is placed immediately after biopsy into formalin rather than being exposed to air for any length of time.

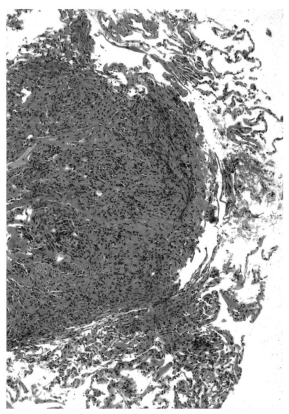

Figure 17–1 Artifactual atelectasis on TBB. The central portion of this tissue fragment is entirely atelectatic. The juxtaposition of normal alveoli next to the atelectatic area without transition helps to distinguish atelectasis from fibrosis, where there is a gradual transition from abnormal to normal.

Difficulty in distinguishing atelectatic lung from bona fide interstitial pneumonia can occur, however, and emphasizes the need for caution in evaluating interstitial lung disease in general (see later on) on tissue obtained by TBB. A helpful histologic feature is the

Table 17–2	Common Artifacts on Transbronchial Biopsy Specimens	
Artifact	**Differential Diagnosis**	**Helpful Histologic Features**
Atelectasis	Interstitial pneumonia/fibrosis	Abrupt transitional to normal alveolar septa at periphery; absent hyperplastic alveolar pneumocytes
Hemorrhage	Alveolar hemorrhage syndromes	No hemosiderin
Bubbles	Exogenous lipid pneumonia	No histiocytes around spaces
Pleura	Carcinoma, lymphoma	Cells form lining on fibrous tissue or fat; mucin stains negative; immunostains (cytokeratin, calretinin, WT-1, CD68, etc.) can help in difficult cases

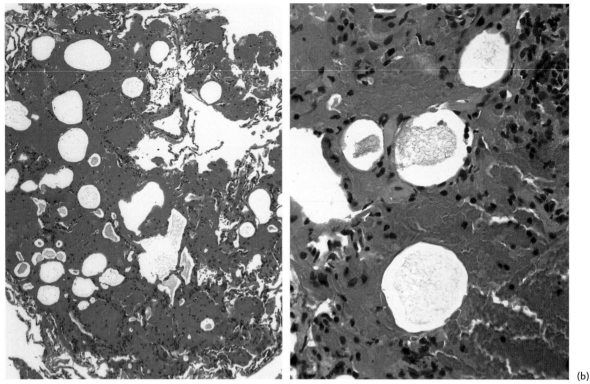

(a)

(b)

Figure 17–2 Intraalveolar hemorrhage on TBB. (a) Fresh blood fills many alveoli in this example. The absence of hemosiderin indicates that the blood is recent and likely secondary to the biopsy procedure. Note also the focal bubble artifact. **(b)** Higher magnification showing the intraalveolar erythrocytes. Round spaces (bubble artifact) without surrounding cellular reaction are also present, and a fibrinous exudate is present in some.

finding of normal alveolar septa directly adjacent to the atelectatic zone, in contrast to a gradual transition from abnormal to normal in cases of interstitial pneumonia. Also, alveolar pneumocyte hyperplasia is usually found in areas of interstitial pneumonia but is absent in atelectasis.

Intraalveolar hemorrhage related to the biopsy procedure itself is another common finding (Fig. 17–2). The presence of hemosiderin in addition to erythrocytes is necessary before the hemorrhage can be considered significant on a TBB. Correlation with the clinical situation should also be helpful, since most patients with intraalveolar hemorrhage have hemoptysis or other signs of pulmonary bleeding.

Occasional TBB specimens will contain a so-called *bubble artifact*, in which the parenchyma is distorted by round spaces of varying sizes (Fig. 17–3).[16] The importance of this artifact is that it can be confused with lipid droplets as occur in exogenous lipid pneumonia (see Chapter 16). It differs from the latter condition, however, in that the spaces are surrounded by lung tissue and not by histiocytes.

Sometimes, bits of *pleura* are included in TBB specimens, and they may cause considerable difficulty in diagnosis. They are most easily recognized when composed of a single layer of low cuboidal, often hobnail-shaped epithelium covering fibrous tissue. Sometimes, portions of pleura are invaginated into the tissue, and they may be lined by hyperplastic mesothelial cells (Fig. 17–4). The bland appearance of the cells as well as the surrounding fibrosis should suggest the correct diagnosis. Occasionally, even parietal pleura (mesothelial-covered fat) is encountered on a TBB specimen (Fig. 17–5). When the mesothelial cells appear hyperplastic and disorganized, they may be difficult to distinguish from atypical alveolar or bronchial epithelial cells. Immunohistochemical stains for calretinin, WT-1, and TTF-1 should clarify the issue. Detached cellular clusters containing a mixture of mesothelial cells and histiocytes (so-called nodular histiocytic/mesothelial hyperplasia) are sometimes encountered (Fig. 17–6).[12,50] When eosinophils are present, the findings resemble the cellular pleural exudates observed in reactive eosinophilic pleuritis (see Chapter 16). These

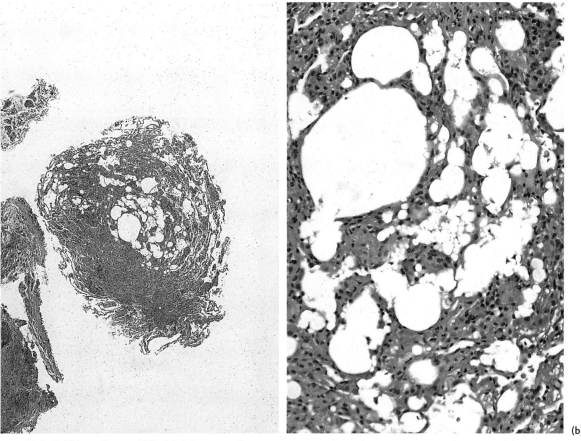

(a)   (b)

Figure 17-3 Bubble artifact on TBB. (a) At low magnification, varying sized round spaces are seen in the center of the tissue. **(b)** Higher magnification shows the numerous round spaces that are distinguished from the lipid droplets of exogenous lipoid pneumonia by the absence of a surrounding histiocytic reaction.

densely cellular aggregates can be prominent and may raise the question of carcinoma. Immunohistochemical stains (especially cytokeratin, calretinin, WT-1, and CD68) can be helpful in such cases. but probably the most important element in diagnosis is to think about the possibility of mesothelium and associated cellular reactions in cases of unusual cellular infiltrates. Also, of course, knowledge of the clinical situation should help in the differential diagnosis.

TBB IN IMMUNOCOMPROMISED PATIENTS

Clinical Features

Immunocompromised patients who undergo TBB usually arc acutely ill with fever, cough, and shortness of breath, and they often develop progressive hypoxemia.

They may present initially with localized infiltrates on chest radiographs, but diffuse pulmonary infiltrates frequently develop by the time of biopsy. The main lesions in the differential diagnosis include infection, drug reactions, radiation effect, and recurrent malignancy.[59] The biopsy specimen is taken in the hope of finding a treatable disease.

Efficacy of TBB

A specific etiologic diagnosis can be established by TBB in 40% to over 80% of immunocompromised patients with diffuse pulmonary infiltrates, and most will represent infections or recurrent malignancy (Table 17-3).[11,18,23,31,34,65,78] A wide variety of infectious agents may be encountered, and the incidence varies among institutions because of differences in both patient populations and endogenous microbiologic

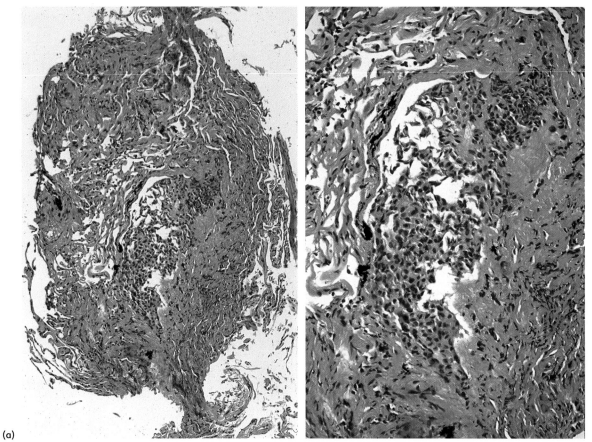

(a)   (b)

Figure 17–4 Entrapped mesothelial cells on TBB. (a) A cluster of mesothelial cells are seen in the middle of this partially atelectatic but otherwise unremarkable tissue fragment. **(b)** At higher magnification, the cells are bland and uniform and are surrounded by a thin fibrous rim that represents invaginated pleura.

Table 17–3	Efficacy of TBB

- Greatest diagnostic yield in *diffuse lung infiltrates*

- In **immunocompromised patients**, greatest accuracy in diagnosing *infection* and *malignancy*

- In **nonimmunocompromised patients**:
    Extremely reliable in confirming diagnosis of *sarcoidosis*
    Reliable in diagnosing *malignancy, infection*
    Often productive in diagnosing lung diseases that have specific pathologic findings (*bronchiolitis obliterans–organizing pneumonia, Langerhans cell histiocytosis (eosinophilic granuloma), lymphangiomyomatosis, pulmonary alveolar proteinosis, amyloidosis, Goodpasture's syndrome,* etc.)
    May confirm clinical diagnosis of *usual interstitial pneumonia, acute interstitial pneumonia* and certain *pneumoconioses*

flora.[59] Although ordinary bacteria constitute important causes of pneumonia, they are usually diagnosed by microbiologic techniques performed on sputum, fluids, or other non-tissue specimens. When tissue samples are needed for diagnosis, other organisms are more frequently identified, such as *Pneumocystis carinii*, aspergillus and other fungi, nocardia, Legionella, various mycobacteria, and herpesvirus and cytomegalovirus (CMV), for example. TBB are also highly accurate in monitoring rejection in lung allograft recipients (see Chapter 6).

Nonspecific histologic changes in which a cause is not identifiable are also commonly encountered in immunocompromised patients. Most cases resemble diffuse alveolar damage (DAD) or a cellular chronic interstitial pneumonia (see further on). The evidence from several studies suggests that when such nonspecific changes are the only abnormalities found, and

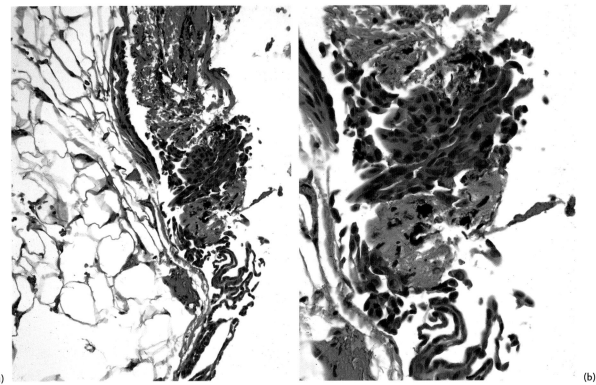

(a)   (b)

Figure 17–5 Parietal pleura on TBB. (a) A fragment of adipose tissue lined by a single layer of mesothelium in some places and clusters of cells as well as a proteinaceous exudate in other places is present in this biopsy specimen. (b) Higher magnification shows the bland appearance of the mesothelial cell clusters.

provided that patients have *diffuse lung infiltrates*, a specific treatable process, especially an infection, is unlikely to be found by additional biopsies. For example, in Katzenstein and Askin's[34] study of immuno-compromised patients with diffuse infiltrates, 40% of 50 TBB specimens showed only nonspecific findings. There was no evidence that an infection or other treatable process was missed in these cases; subsequent open biopsies in two patients and autopsies in three confirmed the initial TBB findings of DAD without organisms. Similarly, no cases of infection were over-looked in TBB specimens from 35 patients with diffuse infiltrates in the study by Williams et al.[76] In a review of 108 biopsies in patients with diffuse infiltrates, Poe et al[54] found that only four infections were missed. In one of these cases, pneumocystis was identified on a simultaneously obtained bronchial brushing specimen.

Not surprisingly, due to sampling difficulties, the efficiency of TBB is less in patients with radiographically localized lung lesions than in patients with diffuse infiltrates.[68] Of course, obtaining adequate biopsy specimens is another factor that influences the yield

of TBB, and the diagnostic accuracy will also depend on the effort expended by the pathologist in searching for infectious agents. Certain specific infections such as aspergillosis may be especially difficult to diagnose on TBB, and there are varied reasons for this difficulty.[3]

These findings emphasize that TBB is a highly reliable technique for diagnosing infection in immuno-compromised patients with diffuse infiltrates. Additional lung biopsy procedures should not be necessary when DAD or other nonspecific inflammatory changes without identifiable infectious agents are found, provided that the TBB specimen is adequate and that special stains for organisms have been carefully examined. It may seem surprising, but open lung biopsy does not appear to be significantly more effective than TBB in establishing a specific diagnosis in similar cases, with reported diagnostic yields ranging from 34% to 75%.[13,15,26,29,40,58,60,63,72] In fact, infections can sometimes be missed even in open lung biopsy specimens.[44,45,60] It should be remembered, however, that TBB is considerably less reliable than open lung biopsy in evaluating localized pulmonary infiltrates because of sampling errors, and, depending

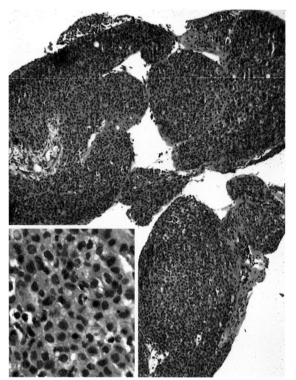

Figure 17–6 Nodular histiocytic/mesothelial hyperplasia on TBB. Large sheet-like masses of epithelioid cells are seen. Inset shows the uniform appearance of bland cells with abundant cytoplasm. Scattered eosinophils are seen in the background.

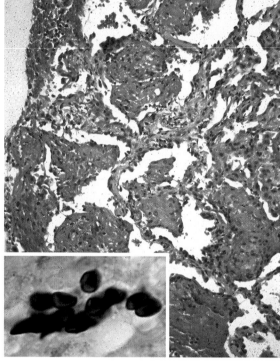

Figure 17–7 Pneumocystis pneumonia on TBB. The alveolar spaces in this example are filled with a proteinaceous exudate. Although the characteristic frothy exudate was absent, a GMS stain demonstrated numerous organisms (inset).

on the clinical situation, additional biopsy techniques may be warranted in such cases when the TBB is nondiagnostic.

Pathologic Findings

Infections

The inflammatory reactions to infectious organisms that are expected in patients possessing intact immune systems are often absent in immunocompromised patients (see Chapter 10). Rather, the most common histologic manifestation of infection is DAD or another nonspecific reaction.[34] *Pneumocystis carinii* pneumonia, especially, can manifest as DAD, in addition to nonspecific fibrosis, chronic inflammation, or a proteinaceous intraalveolar exudate (Fig. 17–7). The classic intraalveolar froth is seen most commonly in AIDS patients. Viral infections such as herpes and, less often, CMV can cause DAD with prominent hyaline membranes. Intraalveolar proteinaceous exudates and DAD may be

the only manifestations of nearby invasive fungal infections (Fig. 17–8). Sometimes, sheets of organisms within a proteinaceous exudate with minimal inflammation constitute the only finding. These observations underscore the need to examine carefully special stains for organisms in all TBB specimens showing nonspecific changes from immunocompromised patients, even though the histologic changes initially may not be suggestive of infection.

A nonspecific type of chronic interstitial pneumonia characterized by a scant lymphocytic and plasma cell infiltrate within alveolar septa associated with alveolar lining cell hyperplasia is typical of CMV pneumonia. The diagnostic enlarged cells with intranuclear and intracytoplasmic inclusions may be sparse and difficult to find, however. Serial sections should be carefully examined for appropriate inclusions in all examples of chronic interstitial pneumonia in immunocompromised patients, especially in individuals who have received bone marrow, heart, or lung transplants. Immunohistochemical stains for CMV antigens as well as in situ

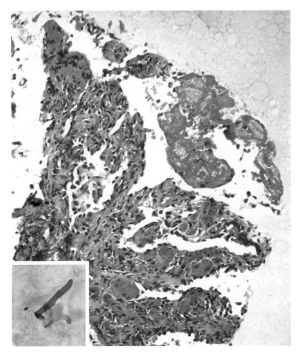

Figure 17–8 Aspergillus pneumonia on TBB. An intraalveolar proteinaceous exudate was the main finding in this example, along with alveolar septal fibrosis and chronic inflammation. Rare fungal hyphae were identified with the GMS stain (inset). This patient had chronic myelogenous leukemia. Bronchial washings grew A. Niger.

hybridization techniques for viral DNA (see Chapter 10) may also facilitate diagnosis. Occasionally, CMV inclusions are seen in TBB specimens unaccompanied by interstitial pneumonia or other tissue reactions, and the significance of this finding will depend on the clinical situation.

Nonspecific Changes

DAD and its variants are the most common findings in cases lacking an identifiable causal agent.[18,24,34,49,54] Because the tissue samples are so small and severe crush artifact is frequently present, the entire spectrum of histopathologic features constituting DAD is not always found. For example, rather than finding well-formed hyaline membranes, there may be intraalveolar fibrinous or proteinaceous exudates, often admixed with erythrocytes, macrophages, and other inflammatory cells (Fig. 17–9). Interstitial inflammation and alveolar lining cell hyperplasia usually accompany the intraalveolar changes.

A number of factors, either alone or in combination, may produce DAD in such individuals, including drug

toxicity and radiation effect as well as sepsis, shock, disseminated intravascular coagulation, and similar complications common in this patient population (see Chapter 2). It should be emphasized that the diagnosis of any of these entities is a diagnosis of exclusion, because there are no specific histologic features. Diagnosis requires careful scrutiny of the tissue for organisms, negative culture results, and a detailed assessment of the clinical history and laboratory findings.

Other nonspecific changes in addition to DAD occur in biopsy specimens from immunocompromised patients.[34] A uniform-appearing chronic interstitial pneumonia unassociated with viral inclusions, interstitial or intra-alveolar fibrosis, acute and chronic inflammation, intraalveolar hemorrhage, and hemosiderin-filled macrophages are some examples that may be encountered. As mentioned previously, special stains for organisms need to be carefully examined in these cases.

Prognosis and TBB Findings

It is interesting that the TBB findings in immuno-compromised patients may not significantly influence survival rates. In the study by Katzenstein and Askin,[34] mortality rates were similar for patients with non-specific changes (35%) and those with specific diagnoses (40%), although DAD unrelated to infection was associated with a somewhat higher mortality (56%). Other investigators have also reported little difference in survival whether specific or nonspecific findings were obtained at TBB,[76] and similar conclusions have been drawn from studies of open lung biopsy results as well.[19,44,45,60,72] A few series of TBB cases or open lung biopsies have shown either improved or worse prognoses in patients with nonspecific findings.[18,26]

Conclusions

TBB is an accurate means of diagnosing infection in immunocompromised patients with diffuse lung infil-trates. Because infection in these cases frequently manifests nonspecific pathologic changes such as DAD or interstitial pneumonia and minimal cellular response, special stains for organisms must be examined routinely in all cases. A repeat biopsy may be indicated if the initial TBB specimen is inadequate or shows normal lung in a patient with diffuse chest infiltrates, or if the TBB is nondiagnostic in a patient with a localized infiltrate and the clinical situation requires a tissue diagnosis. A repeat biopsy may not be necessary when

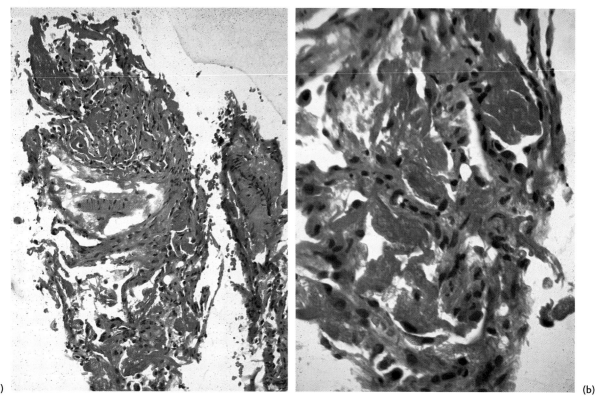

(a)   (b)

Figure 17–9 DAD on TBB. (a) At low magnification a prominent proteinaceous exudate with focal hyaline membrane formation fills many alveoli. **(b)** Higher magnification shows the proteinaceous exudate with focal hyaline membranes. This patient had acute lymphocytic leukemia and developed bilateral lung infiltrates. All stains and cultures were negative. Autopsy showed DAD.

only nonspecific findings are present on an adequate TBB specimen from a patient with diffuse infiltrates.

TBB IN NONIMMUNOCOMPROMISED PATIENTS

Clinical Features

In contrast to immunocompromised patients, most nonimmunocompromised patients who undergo TBB are not critically ill. They may present because of longstanding progressive dyspnea or because of an abnormal chest radiograph associated with relatively few symptoms. In some cases, an acute exacerbation of a preexistent lung disease may be the cause for biopsy, whereas in a few individuals systemic complaints dominate the clinical presentation. The most common role for TBB is to diagnose malignancy in patients with localized masses or infiltrates. In patients with diffuse infiltrates, TBB is usually undertaken to confirm the clinical impression of a chronic infiltrative lung disease

and to exclude other diagnoses such as malignancy or infection.

Efficacy of TBB

As in immunocompromised patients, TBB in nonimmunocompromised patients is most informative when diffuse lung infiltrates are present; 50–80% of such biopsies will either establish a specific diagnosis or produce findings consistent with the clinical impression (see Table 17–3).[4,14,21,23,27,54,64,70,77] Not surprisingly, the diagnostic yield increases in proportion to the number of pieces sampled by the biopsy procedure.[46,52] Accuracy is least in patients who have peripheral masses or localized infiltrates, with specific diagnoses reported in less than 20% of cases.[77] In most patients with peripheral masses and initially nonspecific TBB specimens, subsequent procedures demonstrate neoplasms, whereas most individuals with localized infiltrates have a benign follow-up. Therefore, knowledge of the radiographic manifestations as well as the clinical impression is necessary, not only for interpreting the

TBB findings but also for evaluating the need for more extensive biopsies in patients with nonspecific findings.

Specific Diagnoses

In general, TBB specimens are less productive of a specific diagnosis in nonimmunocompromised patients than they are in immunocompromised patients. In certain selected clinical situations, however, they are especially useful. For example, TBB specimens are highly effective in demonstrating non-necrotizing granulomas in cases of suspected sarcoidosis (Fig. 17–10). In some series, greater than 95% accuracy of TBB is reported when there are radiographically evident parenchymal infiltrates.[36,37,52,56,57,66] Positive biopsy specimens can also be obtained in more than half of cases without radiographic evidence of parenchymal infiltrates.

TBB can be productive in any other disease that has specific histologic features and can be adequately sampled by TBB. For example, TBB is useful in diagnosing carcinoma, especially in patients with diffuse lymphangitic spread, airway obstruction, or evidence of atelectasis.[6,53] It is also accurate in diagnosing infections, and immunohistochemistry and other more sophisticated techniques can add to the diagnostic accuracy.[74] Various other conditions that cause localized infiltrates or involve the lung diffusely may also be diagnosed by TBB, such as Goodpasture's syndrome,[1,7,67] pulmonary alveolar proteinosis,[61] Langerhans cell histiocytosis (eosinophilic granuloma),[30] lymphangiomyomatosis,[10] amyloidosis,[35] eosinophilic pneumonia, alveolar microlithiasis, and metastatic calcification, for example.

Idiopathic BOOP (see Chapter 2) is a common cause of radiographically patchy lung infiltrates in patients with subacute and often mild symptoms, and the diagnosis can frequently be established by TBB (Fig. 17–11).[20,79] BOOP is easily recognized by the characteristic patchy airspace plugs of fibroblasts and chronic inflammation within lightly stained myxoid-appearing stroma. The significance of finding BOOP on a TBB specimen has to be interpreted with caution, however, because BOOP can occur as a nonspecific reactive change on the periphery of a variety of other processes. Careful correlation of

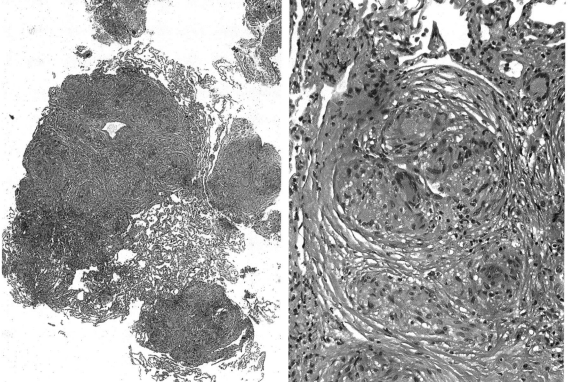

(a)   (b)

Figure 17–10 Sarcoidosis on TBB. (a) Low magnification showing well-circumscribed non-necrotizing granulomas in the interstitium and around blood vessels. Note the adjacent normal alveolar septa without significant inflammation. **(b)** Higher magnification showing the well-circumscribed nature of the granulomas that are surrounded by a thin rim of fibroblasts.

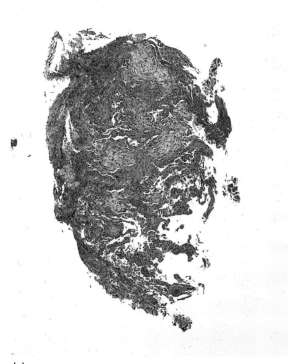

(a)

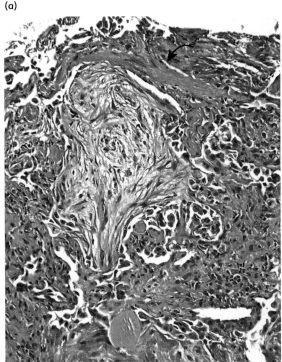

(b)
Figure 17–11 BOOP on TBB. (a) Low magnification view showing the filling of airspaces by lightly staining plugs of fibroblasts. **(b)** Higher magnification of a typical fibroblast plug filling an alveolar duct. Note the surrounding smooth muscle layer of the alveolar duct at top (arrow).

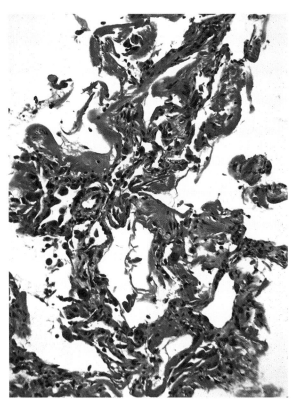

Figure 17–12 DAD in a nonimmunocompromised patient. Hyaline membranes are prominent in this example. This patient became ill several days after being accidentally sprayed by a cropduster.

the clinical and radiographic findings with the pathologic findings, therefore, is needed to determine whether the BOOP is causing the radiographic infiltrates or whether it is a nonspecific reaction.

DAD is also easily recognized on TBB, both in the early stages when hyaline membranes are prominent, and in the organizing stage when interstitial fibroblast proliferation is present (Fig. 17–12).

Interpretation of Nonspecific Findings

Nonspecific findings are common in TBB specimens from nonimmunocompromised individuals and include such changes as fibrosis, inflammation, proteinaceous exudates, macrophages, and hemosiderin. Although none of these findings by themselves would be diagnostic of a specific entity, taken in the context of a particular clinical setting they may be considered consistent with a specific disease. Care must be taken, however, not to overdiagnose a disease based on nonspecific findings alone. For example, it should be remembered that interstitial inflammation and fibrosis

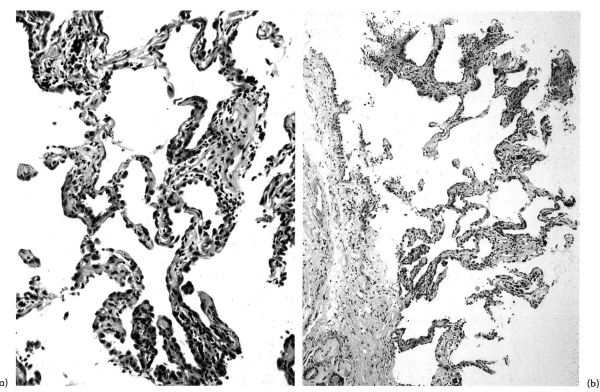

(a)

(b)

Figure 17–13 Nonspecific interstitial inflammation on TBB. (a) There is uniform alveolar septal thickening by chronic inflammation associated with mild alveolar pneumocyte hyperplasia. If these changes were widespread, they would fit with nonspecific interstitial pneumonia. (b) At low magnification, however, the changes are seen to be present adjacent to the bronchial wall (left). The patient had undergone TBB to evaluate a cavitary mass associated with hemoptysis. Interstitial lung disease was not present radiographically.

are common incidental findings in peribronchial interstitium, precisely the location sampled by TBB (Figs 17–13 and 17–14).[2] Therefore, the diagnosis of a chronic interstitial pneumonia should not be suggested based on these findings alone in a patient who lacks clinical and radiographic evidence of a diffuse interstitial process. The accumulation of macrophages within peribronchiolar airspaces is a common finding in cigarette smokers (respiratory bronchiolitis, see Chapter 16) and it should not be overdiagnosed as desquamative interstitial pneumonia (see later on) (Fig. 17–15). Lymphoid aggregates are occasionally encountered and their presence should not conjure up the diagnosis of a lymphoproliferative disorder unless they are extensive or atypical.

Role of TBB in Idiopathic Interstitial Pneumonia and Pneumoconiosis

The use of TBB in excluding infection and malignancy in the evaluation of the idiopathic interstitial pneumonias

is widely appreciated, but its role in diagnosing specific forms of interstitial pneumonia is limited.[73] The problem is that since alveolar septal chronic inflammation and fibrosis are common findings in peribronchial parenchyma, it is difficult to know on a TBB specimen whether interstitial inflammation and/or fibrosis is a localized reaction or part of a diffuse interstitial process. If the findings are striking and uniform in multiple pieces, however, and the patient has radiographic evidence of interstitial lung disease, the generic diagnosis of 'chronic interstitial pneumonia' can be made.[75] Occasionally, specific findings are present that allow a more definitive diagnosis (see further on), but TBB should not be used to quantitate the amount of fibrosis present or estimate the activity of the disease. Moreover, the diagnosis of a chronic interstitial pneumonia should not be considered in the absence of clinical and radiographic evidence of diffuse interstitial lung disease.

Usual interstitial pneumonia (UIP, see Chapter 3) is characterized by specific histologic features, including patchy areas of honeycomb change alternating with

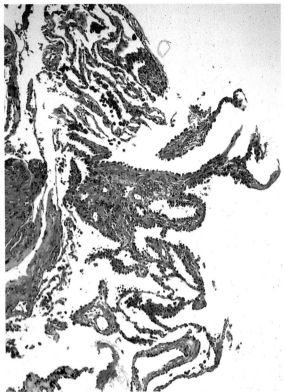

Figure 17–14 Nonspecific interstitial fibrosis in TBB.
Prominent alveolar septal fibrosis and alveolar pneumocyte
hyperplasia are seen in this example. Pigmented intraalveolar
macrophages are also present at the top and reflect cigarette
smoking (respiratory bronchiolitis). This patient was being
evaluated for a mass that proved to be carcinoma. There was
no evidence of interstitial lung disease radiographically.

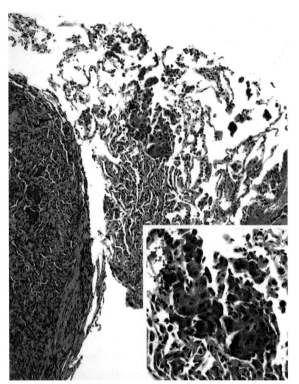

**Figure 17–15 Nonspecific intraalveolar macrophage
accumulation in TBB.** Low magnification view shows clusters
of macrophages within airspaces. A fragment of atelectatic
parenchyma is seen on the left. The inset is a higher
magnification illustrating the lightly pigmented cytoplasm of
the macrophages that is typical of smokers' macrophages.
The findings should not be overinterpreted as DIP.

normal lung, and a mixture of collagen-type fibrosis
and active fibrosis (fibroblast foci). In the right clinical
setting of a patient with a slowly progressive interstitial
lung disease and compatible radiographic findings,
the presence of one or more of these latter features on
TBB can be considered consistent with UIP (Figs 17–16
and 17–17).[8] UIP is an almost uniformly fatal disease
that shows little, if any, response to therapy, and TBB
may obviate the need for a more invasive diagnostic
procedure in these terminally ill patients.

Acute interstitial pneumonia (AIP, see Chapter 3) is
a rapidly progressive and fulminant form of idiopathic
interstitial pneumonia with high mortality rates. It
is characterized pathologically by the presence of DAD,
usually in the organizing stage. TBB is a reliable method
of diagnosis since the findings of alveolar septal
fibroblast proliferation and alveolar pneumocyte
hyperplasia, often with hyaline membranes, are easily

recognizable. Clinical information, however, is necessary
to separate AIP from DAD due to known causes.

Although respiratory bronchiolitis can be readily
diagnosed on TBB by the presence of increased numbers
of pigmented macrophages within airspaces, the related
entities of respiratory bronchiolitis interstitial lung
disease (RBILD) and desquamative interstitial pneumonia
(DIP, see Chapter 3) cannot, since the characteristic
peribronchiolar and diffuse lung distribution, respectively, cannot be distinguished. Likewise, lymphoid
interstitial pneumonia (LIP) cannot be diagnosed by
TBB, because it cannot be differentiated from either
nonspecific peribronchial chronic inflammation or
follicular bronchiolitis.

TBB can contribute to the evaluation of suspected
cases of pneumoconiosis. As with the chronic interstitial pneumonias, the TBB findings must be carefully
correlated with the radiographic and clinical manifestations. Most often, nonspecific findings such as fibrosis,

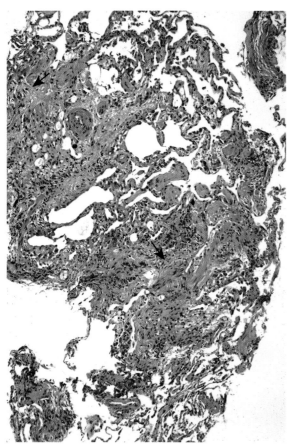

Figure 17–16 UIP on TBB. At low magnification, the typical variegated appearance of UIP can be appreciated with alternating zones of collagen-type fibrosis, active fibrosis (fibroblast foci, arrows), and normal lung.

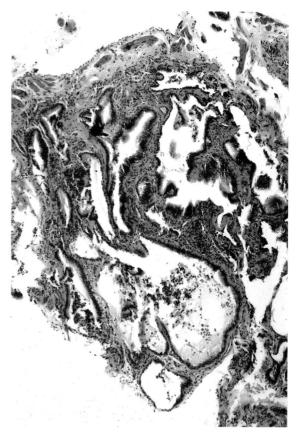

Figure 17–17 Honeycomb change on TBB. Restructured, enlarged airspaces are seen beneath the bronchial wall (top), which is recognized by the presence of the typical bronchial smooth muscle bundles. In the right clinical setting, this finding is highly suggestive of UIP.

asbestos bodies, or pigment deposition are seen, and the changes when interpreted in light of the radiographic and clinical findings may be considered consistent with a particular disease. In a few cases, diagnostic features such as silicotic nodules or giant cell interstitial pneumonia (see Chapter 5) are found. As with the chronic interstitial pneumonias, quantitation of the extent or activity of the disease should not be attempted.

Conclusions

TBB in nonimmunocompromised patients is most productive in individuals with diffuse pulmonary infiltrates. Correlation of the clinical and radiographic manifestations with the pathologic findings is necessary in order to interpret the TBB specimen adequately. Although a specific etiologic diagnosis is established relatively infrequently, the results of a TBB often can be

used to confirm the clinical impression and thus may obviate the need for additional biopsies. TBB should not be used for quantitating the extent of fibrosis or activity of disease in the chronic interstitial pneumonias. An open lung biopsy may be indicated when the pathologic changes found in the TBB specimen do not correlate with the clinical findings.

REFERENCES

1. Abboud R, Chase W, Ballon H, et al: Goodpasture's syndrome: Diagnosis by transbronchial lung biopsy. Ann Intern Med 89:635, 1978.
2. Aisner SC, Albin RJ: Diffuse interstitial pneumonitis and fibrosis in sarcoidosis. Chest 94:193, 1988.
3. Albelda SM, Talbot GH, Gerson SL, et al: Role of fiberoptic bronchoscopy in the diagnosis of invasive pulmonary aspergillosis in patients with acute leukemia. Am J Med 76:1027, 1984.

4. Anders GT, Johnson JE, Bush BA, Matthews JI: Transbronchial biopsy without fluoroscopy. A seven year perspective. Chest 94:557, 1988.

5. Anderson HA: Transbronchial lung biopsy for diffuse pulmonary diseases. Results in 939 patients. Chest 73:734, 1978.

6. Aranda C, Sidhu G, Sasso LA, Adams FV: Transbronchial lung biopsy in the diagnosis of lymphangitic carcinomatosis. Cancer 42:1995, 1978.

7. Beechler C, Enquist R, Hunt K, et al: Immunofluorescence of transbronchial biopsies in Goodpasture's syndrome. Am Rev Respir Dis 121:869, 1980.

8. Berbescu E, Zisman D, Katzenstein A-LA, et al: Utility of transbronchial lung biopsy in usual interstitial pneumonia. Chest, in press, 2006.

9. Blasco LH, Sanchez Hernandez IMS, Garrido VV, et al: Safety of the transbronchial biopsy in outpatients. Chest 99:562, 1991.

10. Bonetti F, Chiodera PL, Pea M, et al: Transbronchial biopsy in lymphangiomyomatosis of the lung. HMB45 for diagnosis. Am J Surg Pathol 17:1092, 1993.

11. Cazzadori A, DiPerri G, Todeschini G, et al: Transbronchial biopsy in the diagnosis of pulmonary infiltrates in immunocompromised patients. Chest 107:101, 1995.

12. Chan JKC, Loo KT, Yau BKC, et al: Nodular histiocytic/mesothelial hyperplasia: A lesion potentially mistaken for a neoplasm in transbronchial biopsy. Am J Surg Pathol 21:658, 1997.

13. Cheson BD, Samlowski WE, Tang TT, Spruance SL: Value of open-lung biopsy in 87 immunocompromised patients with pulmonary infiltrates. Cancer 55:453, 1985.

14. Clark RA, Gray PB, Townshend RH, Howard P: Transbronchial lung biopsy: A review of 85 cases. Thorax 32:546, 1977.

15. Cockerill FR III, Wilson WR, Carpenter HA, et al: Open lung biopsy in immunocompromised patients. Arch Intern Med 145:1398, 1985.

16. Colby T, Yousem S: Pulmonary histology for the surgical pathologist. Am J Surg Pathol 12:223, 1988.

17. Cordasco EM Jr, Mehta AC, Ahmad M: Bronchoscopically induced bleeding: A summary of nine years' Cleveland Clinic experience and review of the literature. Chest 100:1141, 1991.

18. Cunningham JH, Zavala DC, Corry RJ, Keim LW: Trephine air drill, bronchial brush, and fiberoptic transbronchial lung biopsies in immunocompromised patients. Am Rev Respir Dis 115:213, 1977.

19. De Blic J, McKelvie P, Le Bourgeois M, et al: Value of bronchoalveolar lavage in the management of severe acute pneumonia and interstitial pneumonitis in the immunocompromised child. Thorax 42:759, 1987.

20. Dina R, Sheppard M: The histological diagnosis of clinically documented cases of cryptogenic organizing pneumonia: Diagnostic features in transbronchial biopsies. Histopathology 23:541, 1993.

21. Ellis JH: Transbronchial lung biopsy via the fiberoptic bronchoscope. Experience with 107 consecutive cases and comparison with bronchial brushing. Chest 68:524, 1975.

22. Fan LL, Kozinetz CA, Wojtczak HA, et al: Diagnostic value of transbronchial, thoracoscopic, and open lung biopsy in immunocompetent children with chronic interstitial lung disease. J Pediatr 13:565, 1997.

23. Fechner RE, Greenberg SD, Wilson RK, Stevens PM: Evaluation of transbronchial biopsy of the lung. Am J Clin Pathol 68:17, 1977.

24. Feldman NT, Pennington JE, Ehrie MG: Transbronchial lung biopsy in the compromised host. JAMA 238:1377, 1977.

25. Fraire AE, Cooper SP, Greenberg SD, et al: Transbronchial lung biopsy: Histopathologic and morphometric assessment of diagnostic utility. Chest 102:748, 1992.

26. Greenman RL, Goodall PT, King D: Lung biopsy in immunocompromised hosts. Am J Med 59:488, 1975.

27. Hanson RR, Zavala DC, Rhodes ML, Keim LW, Smith JD: Transbronchial biopsy via flexible fiberoptic bronchoscope: Results in 164 patients. Am Rev Respir Dis 114:67, 1976.

28. Herf SM, Suratt PM: Complications of transbronchial lung biopsies. Chest 73:759, 1978.

29. Hiatt JR, Gong H, Mulder DG, Ramming KP: The value of open lung biopsy in the immunosuppressed patient. Surgery 92:285, 1982.

30. Housini I, Tomashefski JF Jr, Cohen A, et al: Transbronchial biopsy in patients with pulmonary eosinophilic granuloma. Comparison with findings on open lung biopsy. Arch Pathol Lab Med 118:523, 1994.

31. Jain P, Sandur S, Meli Y, et al: Role of flexible bronchoscopy in immunocompromised patients with lung infiltrates. Chest 125:712, 2004.

32. Jenkins R, Myerowitz RL, Kavic T, Slasky S: Diagnostic yield of transbronchoscopic biopsies. Am J Clin Pathol 72:926, 1979.

33. Joyner LR, Scheinhorn DJ: Transbronchial forceps lung biopsy through the fiberoptic bronchoscope. Diagnosis of diffuse pulmonary disease. Chest 67:532, 1975.

34. Katzenstein AA, Askin FB: Interpretation and significance of pathologic findings in transbronchial lung biopsy. Am J Surg Pathol 4:223, 1980.

35. Kline LR, Dise CA, Ferro TJ, Hansen-Flaschen JH: Diagnosis of pulmonary amyloidosis by transbronchial biopsy. Am Rev Respir Dis 132:191, 1985.

36. Koerner SK, Sakowitz AJ, Appelman RI, Becker NH, Schoenbaum SW: Transbronchial lung biopsy for the diagnosis of sarcoidosis. N Engl J Med 293:268, 1975.

37. Koontz CH, Joyner LR, Nelson RA: Transbronchial lung biopsy via the fiberoptic bronchoscope in sarcoidosis. Ann Intern Med 85:64, 1976.

38. Landas S, Bromley CM: Sponge artifact in biopsy specimens. Arch Pathol Lab Med 114:1285, 1990.

39. Lauver GL, Hasan FM, Morgan RB, Campbell SC: The usefulness of fiberoptic bronchoscopy in evaluating new pulmonary lesions in the compromised host. Am J Med 66:580, 1979.

40. Leight GS Jr, Michaelis LL: Open lung biopsy for the

diagnosis of acute, diffuse pulmonary infiltrates in the immunocompromised patient. Chest 73:477, 1978.

41. Levin DC, Wides AB, Ellis JH Jr: Transbronchial lung biopsy via the fiberoptic bronchoscope. Am Rev Respir Dis 110:4, 1974.

42. Lukomsky GI, Ovchinnikov AA, Bilal A: Complications of bronchoscopy. Comparison of rigid bronchoscopy under general anesthesia and flexible fiberoptic bronchoscopy under topical anesthesia. Chest 79:316, 1981.

43. Matthay RA, Farmer WC, Odero D: Diagnostic fiberoptic bronchoscopy in the immunocompromised host with pulmonary infiltrates. Thorax 32:539, 1977.

44. McCabe RE, Brooks RG, Mark JBD, Remington JS: Open lung biopsy in patients with acute leukemia. Am J Med 78:609, 1985.

45. McKenna RJ Jr, Mountain CF, McMurtrey MJ: Open lung biopsy in immunocompromised patients. Chest 86:671, 1984.

46. Milman N, Faurschou P, Munch EP, Grode G: Transbronchial lung biopsy through the fibre optic bronchoscope. Results and complications in 452 examinations. Respir Med 88:749, 1994.

47. Mitchell D, Emerson C, Collins J, Stableforth D: Transbronchial lung biopsy with the fiberoptic bronchoscope. Analysis of results in 433 patients. Br J Dis Chest 75:258, 1981.

48. Nagata N, Hirano H, Takayama K, et al: Step section preparation of transbronchial lung biopsy: Significance in the diagnosis of diffuse lung disease. Chest 100:959, 1991.

49. Nishio J, Lynch J III: Fiberoptic bronchoscopy in the immunocompromised host: The significance of a "non-specific" transbronchial biopsy. Am Rev Respir Dis 121:307, 1980.

50. Ordonez NG, Ro JY, Ayala AG: Lesions described as nodular mesothelial hyperplasia are primarily composed of histiocytes. Am J Surg Pathol 22:285, 1998.

51. Pennington JE, Feldman NT: Pulmonary infiltrates and fever in patients with hematologic malignancy. Assessment of transbronchial biopsy. Am J Med 62:581, 1977.

52. Poe RH, Israel RH, Utell MJ, Hall WJ: Probability of a positive transbronchial lung biopsy result in sarcoidosis. Arch Intern Med 139:761, 1979.

53. Poe RH, Ortiz C, Israel RH, et al: Sensitivity, specificity, and predictive values of bronchoscopy in neoplasm metastatic to lung. Chest 88:84, 1985.

54. Poe RH, Utell MJ, Israel RH, Hall WJ, Eshleman JD: Sensitivity and specificity of the nonspecific transbronchial lung biopsy. Am Rev Respir Dis 119:25, 1978.

55. Poletti V, Patelli M, Poggi S, et al: Transbronchial lung biopsy and bronchoalveolar lavage in diagnosis of diffuse infiltrative lung diseases. Respiration 54(Suppl l):66, 1988.

56. Poletti V, Patelli M, Spiga I: Transbronchial lung biopsy in pulmonary sarcoidosis. Is it an evaluable method in detection of disease activity? Chest 89:361, 1986.

57. Puar H, Young R Jr, Armstrong E: Bronchial and transbronchial lung biopsy without fluoroscopy in sarcoidosis. Chest 87:303, 1985.

58. Ray JF III, Lawton BR, Myers WO, et al: Open pulmonary biopsy. Nineteen-year experience with 116 consecutive operations. Chest 69:43, 1976.

59. Rosenow EC, Wilson WR, Cockerill FR: Pulmonary disease in the immunocompromised host (first of two parts). Mayo Clin Proc 60:473, 1985.

60. Rossiter SJ, Miller DC, Churg AM, Carrington CB, Mark JD: Open lung biopsy in the immunocompromised patient. J Thorac Cardiovasc Surg 77:338, 1979.

61. Rubinstein I, Mullen JBM, Hoffstein V: Morphologic diagnosis of idiopathic pulmonary alveolar lipoproteinosis – revisited. Arch Intern Med 148:813, 1988.

62. Shure D: Transbronchial biopsy and needle aspiration. Chest 95:1130, 1989.

63. Singer C, Armstrong D, Rosen PP, Walzer PD, Yu B: Diffuse pulmonary infiltrates in immunocompromised patients. Prospective study of 80 cases. Am J Med 66:110, 1979.

64. Smith CW, Murray GF, Wilcox BR, Starek PJ, Delany DI: The role of transbronchial lung biopsy in diffuse pulmonary disease. Ann Thorac Surg 24:54, 1977.

65. Stover D, Zaman M, Hajdu S, et al: Bronchoalveolar lavage in the diagnosis of diffuse pulmonary infiltrates in the immunosuppressed host. Ann Intern Med 101:1, 1984.

66. Takayama K, Nagata N, Miyagawa Y, et al: The usefulness of step sectioning of transbronchial lung biopsy specimen in diagnosing sarcoidosis. Chest 102:1441, 1992.

67. Teichman S, Briggs W, Knieser M, Enquist R: Goodpasture's syndrome: Two cases with contrasting course and management. Am Rev Respir Dis 113:223, 1976.

68. Toledo-Pereyra L, DeMeester T, Kinealey A, et al: The benefits of open lung biopsy in patients with previous nondiagnostic transbronchial lung biopsy. A guide to appropriate therapy. Chest 77:647, 1980.

69. Trulock EP, Ettinger NA, Brunt EM, et al: The role of transbronchial lung biopsy in the treatment of lung transplant recipients. Chest 102:1441, 1992.

70. Valenti S, Scordamaglia A: Transbronchial lung biopsy with fiberoptic bronchoscope. Scand J Respir Dis 59:243, 1978.

71. Visner GA, Faro A, Zander DS: Role of transbronchial biopsies in pediatric lung diseases. Chest 126:273, 2004.

72. Walker WA, Cole FH Jr, Khandekar A, et al: Does open lung biopsy affect treatment in patients with diffuse pulmonary infiltrates? J Thorac Cardiovasc Surg 97:534, 1989.

73. Wall C, Gaensler E, Carrington C, Hayes J: Comparison of transbronchial and open biopsies in chronic infiltrative lung diseases. Am Rev Respir Dis 123:280, 1981.

74. Wallace J, Deutsch A, Harrell J, Moser K: Bronchoscopy and transbronchial biopsy in evaluation of patients with suspected active tuberculosis. Am J Med 70:1189, 1981.

75. Watanabe K, Higuchi K, Ninomiya K, et al: Steroid treatment based on the findings of transbronchial biopsy

in idiopathic interstitial pneumonia. Eur Respir J 20:1213, 2002.

76. Williams D, Yungbluth M, Adams G, Glassroth J: The role of fiberoptic bronchoscopy in the evaluation of immunocompromised hosts with diffuse pulmonary infiltrates. Am Rev Respir Dis 131:880, 1985.

77. Wilson RK, Fechner RE, Greenberg SD, Estrada R, Stevens PM: Clinical implications of a "nonspecific" transbronchial biopsy. Am J Med 65:252, 1978.

78. Wilson WR, Cockerill FR, Rosenow EC: Pulmonary disease in the immunocompromised host (second of two parts). Mayo Clin Proc 60:610, 1985.

79. Yoshinouchi T, Ohtsuki Y, Kubo K, Shikata Y: Clinicopathological study on two types of cryptogenic organizing pneumonitis. Respir Med 89:271, 1995.

80. Zavala D: Transbronchial biopsy in diffuse lung disease. Chest 73:727, 1978.

Index